Skin Barrier

Skin Barrier

edited by

Peter M. Elias
VA Medical Center
University of California
San Francisco, California, U.S.A.

Kenneth R. Feingold
VA Medical Center
University of California
San Francisco, California, U.S.A.

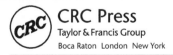 **CRC Press**
Taylor & Francis Group
Boca Raton London New York

CRC Press is an imprint of the
Taylor & Francis Group, an **informa** business

A SPON PRESS BOOK

CRC Press
Taylor & Francis Group
6000 Broken Sound Parkway NW, Suite 300
Boca Raton, FL 33487-2742

First issued in paperback 2019

© 2006 by Taylor & Francis Group, LLC
CRC Press is an imprint of Taylor & Francis Group, an Informa business

No claim to original U.S. Government works

ISBN-13: 978-0-8247-5815-8 (hbk)
ISBN-13: 978-0-367-39210-9 (pbk)

Library of Congress Cataloging-in-Publication Data

Catalog record is available from the Library of Congress

Visit the Taylor & Francis Web site at
http://www.taylorandfrancis.com

and the CRC Press Web site at
http://www.crcpress.com

Preface

The skin is an underappreciated organ playing a crucial role in the survival of animals and humans. The major role of the skin is to provide a barrier between a hostile external environment and the organism. Even modest defects in this barrier can have catastrophic impacts on the organism, threatening its survival. Whereas many of the body's organs have an enormous functional reserve (e.g., one kidney can be removed with minimal impact), the skin barrier must be completely intact and functional for good health. Even relatively minor defects in the stratum corneum can lead to abnormalities in water and electrolyte balance, increase the risk of infection, and result in localized and systemic inflammation. The barrier functions of the skin are primarily mediated by the stratum corneum—the outermost layer of the epidermis.

The stratum corneum is derived from the terminal differentiation of the epidermis. It is a complex structure consisting of corneocytes surrounded by lipid membranes, which allows it to subserve numerous barrier functions, including serving as a barrier to the movement of water and electrolytes, blocking the entry of microorganisms and xenobiotics, as well as providing strength and resistance to external mechanical trauma. Yet, its outermost cells must desquamate invisibly from the skin surface allowing for the continual renewal of the stratum corneum.

The aim of this book is to describe in detail the structure and function of the stratum corneum. In addition, the factors that regulate the formation of the stratum corneum and the abnormalities of the stratum corneum that occur secondary to various disease states will be discussed. In the last several years, innumerable advances in our understanding of the structure, function, and formation of the stratum corneum have occurred and much of this new information has been incorporated into the various chapters with the goal of providing as up-to-date a review as possible. This book will provide, in a single source, comprehensive information on the stratum corneum and its multiple barrier functions. It can be read in its entirety or individual chapters referred to as needed to provide an up-to-date review of specific topics of interest. We are confident that it will be a standard reference for obtaining information on the stratum corneum.

This book will be of interest to dermatologists, skin biologists, individuals developing skin-care products, and scientists concerned with the effect of toxic compounds on the skin. It is expected that readers of this book will emerge with an enhanced understanding and appreciation of the importance of the stratum corneum.

Part I provides definitions and broad concepts regarding stratum corneum function. In addition, chapters by Albert M. Kligman and Peter M. Elias review the history of the development of our current concepts of the stratum corneum from the days when the stratum corneum was considered akin to "Saran® wrap" to our current concepts of the stratum corneum as a dynamic biosensor with multiple integrated functions.

Part II focuses on the structure of the stratum corneum with detailed information on the lipid and protein components. In addition, information on the structural integration of these components will be presented.

Part III discusses the dynamic properties of the stratum corneum. The role of pH and lipid processing by enzymes localized to the stratum corneum will be detailed.

Part IV presents current information on the formation of the stratum corneum during fetal development and in adults. In addition, the factors that regulate the formation of the stratum corneum are discussed.

Part V provides information on the various functions of the stratum corneum including the permeability barrier, microbial defense, antioxidant barrier, hydration, and the formation of vitamin D.

Part VI examines the abnormalities that occur in the stratum corneum including abnormalities in permeability barrier function, diseases of cornification and desquamation, occupational disorders, and atopic dermatitis. In addition, this section also discusses the effect of aging, psychological stress, and various cutaneous disorders on stratum corneum structure and function.

Last, Part VII discusses strategies for improving stratum corneum barrier function.

Thus, this book provides the reader with a single complete source of information on the stratum corneum and should serve as a definitive reference when one seeks information pertaining to stratum corneum structure, function, or disorders.

Kenneth R. Feingold
Peter M. Elias

Contents

Preface . . . . *iii*
Contributors . . . . *xv*

PART I. INTRODUCTION
  **1. Stratum Corneum Barrier Function: Definitions and
  Broad Concepts** *1*
  Peter M. Elias and Kenneth R. Feingold
  Why a Barrier and What Do We Mean
  by "Barrier Function"? 1
  How Are the Various Barrier Functions Mediated? 1
  Evolving Concepts of the SC Barrier 2

  **2. Defensive Functions of the Stratum Corneum:
  Integrative Aspects** *5*
  Peter M. Elias
  Protective Functions Are Linked 5
  Multiple Defensive Functions Can Be Altered by
  a Single Stressor 8
  Perturbations of One Function Can Alter Other
  Defensive Functions 11
  References 12

  **3. A Brief History of How the Dead Stratum Corneum
  Became Alive** *15*
  Albert M. Kligman
  Coda 22
  References 23

  **4. The Epidermal Permeability Barrier: From Saran®
  Wrap to Biosensor** *25*
  Peter M. Elias
  Introduction 25
  References 30

PART II. STRUCTURE OF THE STRATUM CORNEUM

5. Biochemistry of Human Stratum Corneum Lipids *33*
Philip W. Wertz
Composition of Human Stratum Corneum Lipids 33
Biosynthetic Pathways 37
References 40

**6. Stratum Corneum Ceramides: Function, Origins,
and Therapeutic Applications** *43*
Yoshikazu Uchida and Sumiko Hamanaka
Introduction 43
What Is a Ceramide? 44
Why Are Stratum Corneum Ceramides Unique? 45
Generation of Stratum Corneum Ceramides 48
Therapeutic Applications 53
Summary 58
References 58

7. Structure of the Skin Barrier *65*
Joke A. Bouwstra, Gonneke S. K. Pilgram, and Maria Ponec
Introduction 65
Stratum Corneum Lipid Composition and Organization
in Normal Skin 66
Barrier Function in Human Skin Equivalents 78
Relation Between Lipid Composition and Organization 81
A Unique Molecular Arrangement in the Long
Periodicity Phase 85
Extrapolation of In Vitro Findings to the Lipid Composition and
Organization in Diseased and in Xerotic Skin 88
Conclusions 88
References 89

8. Cornified Envelope and Corneocyte-Lipid Envelope *97*
Peter J. Koch, Dennis R. Roop, and Zhijian Zhou
Introduction 97
The Life-Cycle of Keratinocytes and the Histo-Architecture of
the Epidermis 98
Formation of the CE and the CLE 100
Conclusions and Future Directions 105
References 106

**9. Profilaggrin and the Fused S100 Family
of Calcium-Binding Proteins** *111*
Richard B. Presland, Joseph A. Rothnagel, and Owen T. Lawrence
Introduction 111
Profilaggrin / Filaggrin 114

Filaggrin-2: A Filaggrin-Related
   Protein 125
Hornerin 127
Trichohyalin 127
Repetin 128
C1ORF10 (Cornulin) 129
Summary and Concluding Remarks 130
References 132

10. **The Role of Keratins in Epithelial Homeostasis** *141*
   Thomas M. Magin, Julia Reichelt, and Jian Chen
   Introduction 141
   Keratin Complexity, Nomenclature, and
      Genome Organization 141
   Nomenclature of Keratins 142
   The Mammalian Keratin Type I
      Clusters 142
   The Mammalian Keratin Type II
      Clusters 145
   Domain Structure, Assembly, and Protein
      Modifications 146
   Gene Regulation and Expression 148
   Keratinopathies 151
   Keratins and Signaling 152
   Keratin Knockout Mice and Other
      Functional Studies 153
   Conclusions and Perspectives 159
   References 160

11. **Corneodesmosomes: Pivotal Actors in the Stratum Corneum
   Cohesion and Desquamation** *171*
   Marck Haftek, Michel Simon, and Guy Serre
   Structural Aspects 171
   Biochemical Analysis 176
   Functional Correlates 181
   References 185

12. **Epidermal Barrier Function: Role of Tight
   Junctions** *191*
   Johanna M. Brandner and Ehrhardt Proksch
   Introduction 191
   Tight Junctions (TJ) in Simple Epithelia 192
   Tight Junctions in the Skin 196
   Barrier Function of TJ in the Skin 200
   Future Aspects 202
   References 202

13. **What Makes a Good Barrier? Adaptive Features of
    Vertebrate Integument** *211*
    Gopinathan K. Menon
    Introduction 211
    Impact Resistance of the Integument 213
    Permeability Barrier 214
    Facultative Waterproofing 215
    Why Do Lessons from Comparative Biology Matter
      to the Barrier Researchers? 219
    References 220

PART III. DYNAMIC PROPERTIES OF THE STRATUM CORNEUM

14. **SC pH: Measurement, Origins, and Functions** *223*
    Theodora M. Mauro
    Introduction 223
    SC pH: Measurement 223
    SC pH: Origin 224
    SC pH: Functions Impacted 225
    Conclusion 227
    References 227

15. **Stratum Corneum Lipid Processing: The Final Steps
    in Barrier Formation** *231*
    Walter M. Holleran and Yutaka Takagi
    Introduction 231
    Lamellar Membrane Structures in Mammalian
      Stratum Corneum 231
    Glucosylceramides as a Major Source of Stratum
      Corneum Ceramides 233
    Glucosylceramide Processing Is Required for Epidermal
      Barrier Function 236
    Regulation of GlcCer'ase Activity in the
      Epidermis and SC 237
    Lipid Processing of the Corneocyte Lipid Envelope 239
    Sphingomyelinase Activity in the Generation of SC
      Barrier Lipids 240
    Processing of Glycerophospholipids by
      Secretory Phospholipases 242
    Ceramidases in Epidermal Lipid Processing and Function 243
    Processing of Cholesterol Sulfate
      by Steroid Sulfatase 244
    Lipid Processing Alterations in Atopic Dermatitis 245
    Altered Lipid Processing in Psoriasis 247
    Altered Lipid Processing with Aging 248
    Summary 249
    References 249

PART IV. REGULATION OF STRATUM CORNEUM FORMATION

**16. The Epidermal Lamellar Body as a Multifunctional
Secretory Organelle** *261*
Peter M. Elias, Kenneth R. Feingold, and Manigé Fartasch
Lamellar Bodies—Species and Tissue Distribution as an
   Indicator of Permeability Barrier Function 261
Regulation of Lamellar Body Secretion 265
Pathophysiology of Lamellar Body Secretion 269
References 269

17. Skin Structural Development *273*
Mathew J. Hardman and Carolyn Byrne
Introduction 273
Development of Human Skin 273
Periderm—the Embryonic Skin Layer of
   Unknown Function 275
Conclusion 283
References 284

**18. Epidermal Calcium Gradient and the
Permeability Barrier** *289*
Gopinathan K. Menon and Seung Hun Lee
Introduction 289
The Epidermal Calcium Gradient 290
Altered Calcium Gradient in Skin
   Dysfunctions 292
Calcium Gradient and Permeability Barrier:
   Experimental Studies 295
Regulation of the Calcium Gradient 297
Implications of Epidermal Calcium Gradient
   for Skin Biologists 300
References 301

**19. The Role of the Primary Cytokines, TNF, IL-1, and IL-6, in
Permeability Barrier Homeostasis** *305*
Biao Lu, Peter M. Elias, and Kenneth R. Feingold
Introduction 305
Interleukin-1 Family 305
TNF Family 308
Interleukin-6 Family 309
Effect of Barrier Disruption on Cytokine Homeostasis
   in the Epidermis 310
Role in Barrier Repair 312
Pathophysiologic Consequences 313
Summary 313
References 314

20. **Nuclear Hormone Receptors: Epidermal Liposensors** *319*
    Matthias Schmuth and Kenneth R. Feingold
    The Nuclear Hormone Receptor Super Family 319
    Mechanism of Action 319
    Ligands 322
    Peroxisome Proliferator–Activated Receptors (PPAR) 322
    PPAR-Alpha 322
    PPAR-Delta 325
    PPAR-Gamma 327
    Liver X Receptor (LXR) 329
    Crosstalk Between Lipids and Proteins in the Epidermis 332
    References 333

PART V. FUNCTIONS OF THE STRATUM CORNEUM
21. **Permeability Barrier Homeostasis** *337*
    Peter M. Elias and Kenneth R. Feingold
    Structural and Biochemical Basis for the Stratum
        Corneum Barrier 337
    Metabolic Regulation of Permeability Barrier Homeostasis 346
    Extracellular Signals of Barrier Homeostasis 352
    References 354

22. **Cutaneous Barriers in Defense Against Microbial Invasion** *363*
    Anna Di Nardo and Richard L. Gallo
    Introduction 363
    Skin Surface pH 364
    The Skin Lipid Barrier 365
    Antimicrobial Peptides 365
    Other Proteins and Peptides with Antimicrobial
        Peptide Functions 369
    Enzymes 371
    Barrier Implications 372
    Concluding Remarks 373
    References 373

23. **The Epidermal Antioxidant Barrier** *379*
    Jens J. Thiele
    Introduction 379
    Generation of Reactive Oxygen Species and
        Oxidative Stress 379
    Physiological Barrier Antioxidants 380
    Vitamin E 381
    Vitamin C, Glutathione, and Uric Acid 382
    Enzymatic Antioxidants in the Stratum Corneum 383
    Impact of Environmental Factors on Barrier Antioxidants 384
    Physiological Mechanisms of Barrier Antioxidant Repletion 387

Clinical Implications 389
References 393

24. **Sources and Role of Stratum Corneum Hydration** *399*
    A. V. Rawlings
    Introduction 399
    Stratum Corneum Hydration and Water Content 401
    Stratum Corneum Water Retention Capacity 405
    Stratum Corneum Lipid and NMF Gradients 409
    The Effect of the Seasons and Atmospheric Conditions
       on the Stratum Corneum 410
    The Role of Water in the Stratum Corneum 414
    Conclusions 420
    References 422

25. **Vitamin D and the Epidermis** *427*
    Daniel D. Bikle
    Introduction 427
    Vitamin D Production and Metabolism
       in the Epidermis 427
    Role of Vitamin D_3 in Epidermal Differentiation 431
    References 437

PART VI. ABNORMALITIES IN THE STRATUM CORNEUM
26. **Diseases That Affect Barrier Function** *447*
    Hachiro Tagami and Katsuko Kikuchi
    Introduction 447
    In Vivo Functional Assessment of the SC Barrier 448
    Measurements of Skin Surface Hydration State 449
    Assessment of Skin Barrier Function
       in Dermatoses 450
    SC Changes That Occur Later in Life in Those with Normal
       Healthy Skin 460
    Concluding Remarks 462
    References 463

27. **Pathogenesis of the Barrier Abnormalities**
    in Disorders of Cornification *469*
    Matthias Schmuth, Peter M. Elias, and Mary L. Williams
    Introduction 469
    Abnormalities in Extracellular Lipid Lamellar Structures and
       Other Lipid Metabolic Defects 477
    Acquired Ichthyoses Due to Unknown
    Molecular Defects 486
    Abnormalities of Corneocytes 486
    Abnormalities in Intercellular Communication
       (Gap Junctions) 495

Abnormalities in Corneocyte Cohesion Due to Abnormal
Proteolysis of Desmosomes 497
References 498

28. Pathogenesis of Desquamation and Permeability Barrier
Abnormalities in RXLI 511
Peter M. Elias, Debra Crumrine, Ulrich Rassner, Gopinathan K. Menon,
Kenneth R. Feingold, and Mary L. Williams
The Molecular and Biochemical Basis for
Recessive X-Linked Ichthyosis 511
Steroid Sulfatase and Cholesterol Sulfate
in Normal Epidermal Physiology 512
Regulation of Differentiation by Cholesterol Sulfate 513
Mechanisms Proposed to Perturb Permeability
Barrier Homeostasis in RXLI 514
Mechanisms Proposed as Causes of Abnormal Desquamation
in RXLI 514
References 515

29. Prevention and Repair of Barrier Disruption
in Occupational Dermatology 519
Nanna Y. Schürer and Hans J. Schwanitz
Introduction 519
Primary Individual Prevention 521
Secondary Individual Prevention 527
Tertiary Individual Prevention 529
References 530

30. The Aged Epidermal Permeability Barrier: Basis for
Functional Abnormalities 535
Chantal O. Barland, Peter M. Elias, and Ruby Ghadially
Structure, Function, Lipid Composition, and Metabolism
of the Barrier 535
Regulation of the Normal Epidermal Barrier 537
The Aged Epidermal Barrier 538
Barrier Repair Strategies for Aged Epidermis 545
Clinical Implications 546
References 547

31. Psychological Stress and the Barrier:
The Psychosensory Interface 553
Mitsuhiro Denda
Introduction 553
Animal Model 554
Human Experiments 559
Effect of Odorant Inhalation on Barrier Homeostasis 562

Epidermis and Endocrine System   562
Epidermis and Neurotransmitters   563
Conclusion   564
References   565

**32. The Stratum Corneum of the Epidermis
in Atopic Dermatitis** *569*
Jens-Michael Jensen, Ehrhardt Proksch, and Peter M. Elias
Normal Stratum Corneum: Composition and Function   569
Atopic Dermatitis: Genetics   570
Atopic Dermatitis: Function   571
Basis for Barrier Abnormalities   572
Clinical Manifestations Resulting from Impaired
   Barrier Function   578
Therapeutic Implications   580
References   581

PART VII. IMPROVING BARRIER FUNCTION
Epilogue: Fixing the Barrier—Theory and Rational Deployment *591*
Peter M. Elias
Introduction   591
Dynamics of Barrier Recovery   591
Clinical Applications of the Cutaneous Stress Test   592
Individual Lipid Requirements for the Barrier   593
The Three Key SC Lipids Are Required in an
   Equimolar Distribution   593
Non-Physiologic Lipids—Mechanism of Action   593
Potential of Barrier Repair Therapy   595
References   597

Index *601*

Contributors

Chantal O. Barland Department of Dermatology, and Dermatology Service, VA Medical Center, University of California, San Francisco, California, U.S.A.

Daniel D. Bikle Professor of Medicine and Dermatology, Endocrine Research Unit, VA Medical Center, University of California, San Francisco, California, U.S.A.

Joke A. Bouwstra Leiden/Amsterdam Center for Drug Research, Gorlaeus Laboratories, Leiden University, Leiden, The Netherlands

Johanna M. Brandner Department of Dermatology and Venerology, University Hospital Hamburg Eppendorf, Hamburg, Germany

Carolyn Byrne Queen Mary School of Medicine and Dentistry, University of London, London, U.K.

Jian Chen Institut für Physiologische Chemie, Abteilung für Zellbiochemie, Bonner Forum Biomedizin and LIMES, Universitätsklinikum Bonn, Nussallee, Bonn, Germany

Debra Crumrine Department of Dermatology and Dermatology Service, University of California, VAMC, San Francisco, California, U.S.A.

Mitsuhiro Denda Shiseido Life Science Research Center, Yokohama, Japan

Anna Di Nardo Department of Medicine–Dermatology Section, University of California, San Diego, California, U.S.A.

Peter M. Elias Dermatology Service, VA Medical Center, and Department of Dermatology, University of California, San Francisco, California, U.S.A.

Manigé Fartasch Department of Dermatology, University of Erlanger, Federal Republic of Germany

Kenneth R. Feingold Department of Medicine and Dermatology, University of California, San Francisco, California, U.S.A.

Richard L. Gallo   Department of Medicine–Dermatology Section, University of California, San Diego, California, U.S.A.

Ruby Ghadially   Department of Dermatology, and Dermatology Service, VA Medical Center, University of California, San Francisco, California, U.S.A.

Marek Haftek   Department of Dermatology, Hôpital E. Herriot, Université Lyon I, Lyon, France

Sumiko Hamanaka   Department of Life Sciences, Graduate School of Arts and Sciences, University of Tokyo, Tokyo, Japan, and Department of Dermatology, Saitama Medical School, Saitama, Japan

Mathew J. Hardman   School of Biological Sciences, University of Manchester, Manchester, U.K.

Walter M. Holleran   Departments of Dermatology and Pharmaceutical Chemistry, Schools of Medicine and Pharmacy, VAMC, San Francisco, California, U.S.A.

Jens-Michael Jensen   Department of Dermatology, University Hospitals of Schleswig-Holstein, Campus Kiel, Kiel, Germany

Katsuko Kikuchi   Department of Dermatology, Tohoku University School of Medicine, Sendai, Japan

Albert M. Kligman   Department of Dermatology, Hospital of the University of Pennsylvania, Philadelphia, Pennsylvania, U.S.A.

Peter J. Koch   Departments of Dermatology and Molecular and Cellular Biology, Baylor College of Medicine, Houston, Texas, U.S.A.

Owen T. Lawrence   Department of Oral Biology, University of Washington, Seattle, Washington, U.S.A.

Seung Hun Lee   Department of Dermatology, Yonsei University College of Medicine, Seoul, Korea

Biao Lu   Department of Medicine and Dermatology, VA Medical Center, University of California, San Francisco, California, U.S.A.

Thomas M. Magin   Institut für Physiologische Chemie, Abteilung für Zellbiochemie, Bonner Forum Biomedizin and LIMES, Universitätsklinikum Bonn, Nussallee, Bonn, Germany

Theodora M. Mauro   Department of Dermatology, University of California, San Francisco, California, U.S.A.

Gopinathan K. Menon Department of Dermatology and Dermatology Medical Service, University of California, San Francisco, California, U.S.A.

Gonneke S. K. Pilgram Department of Dermatology, Leiden University Medical Center, Leiden, The Netherlands

Maria Ponec Department of Dermatology, Leiden University Medical Center, Leiden, The Netherlands

Richard B. Presland Departments of Oral Biology and Medicine (Dermatology), University of Washington, Seattle, Washington, U.S.A.

Ehrhardt Proksch Department of Dermatology, University of Kiel, Kiel, Germany

Ulrich Rassner Departments of Dermatology and Dermatology and Medical Service, University of California, and VAMC, San Francisco, California, U.S.A.

A. V. Rawlings AVR Consulting Ltd., Northwich, Cheshire, U.K.

Julia Reichelt Institut für Physiologische Chemie, Abteilung für Zellbiochemie, Bonner Forum Biomedizin and LIMES, Universitätsklinikum Bonn, Nussallee, Bonn, Germany

Dennis R. Roop Departments of Dermatology and Molecular and Cellular Biology, Baylor College of Medicine, Houston, Texas, U.S.A.

Joseph A. Rothnagel Department of Biochemistry and Molecular Biology, and the Institute for Molecular Bioscience, University of Queensland, St. Lucia, Queensland, Australia

Matthias Schmuth Department of Dermatology, Medical University Innsbruck, Innsbruck, Austria

Nanna Y. Schürer Department of Dermatology, Environmental Medicine and Health Theory, University of Osnabrück, Osnabrück, Germany

Hans J. Schwanitz Department of Dermatology, Environmental Medicine and Health Theory, University of Osnabrück, Osnabrück, Germany

Guy Serre Différenciation Épidermique et Autoimmunité Rhumatoïde, CNRS-UPS UMR5165, Toulouse, France

Michel Simon Différenciation Épidermique et Autoimmunité Rhumatoïde, CNRS-UPS UMR5165, Toulouse, France

Hachiro Tagami Department of Dermatology, Tohoku University School of Medicine, Sendai, Japan

Yutaka Takagi Biological Science Laboratories, Kao Corporation, Haga-gun, Tochigi, Japan

Jens J. Thiele   Department of Dermatology, Northwestern University, Chicago, Illinois, U.S.A.

Yoshikazu Uchida   Department of Dermatology, School of Medicine, University of California, San Francisco, California, U.S.A.

Philip W. Wertz   Dows Institute, University of Iowa, Iowa City, Iowa, U.S.A.

Mary L. Williams   Department of Dermatology and Pediatrics, University of California, San Francisco, California, U.S.A.

Zhijian Zhou   Department of Molecular and Cellular Biology, Baylor College of Medicine, Houston, Texas, U.S.A.

1

Stratum Corneum Barrier Function: Definitions and Broad Concepts

Peter M. Elias
*Dermatology Service, VA Medical Center, and Department of Dermatology,
University of California, San Francisco, California, U.S.A.*

Kenneth R. Feingold
*Department of Medicine and Dermatology, University of California,
San Francisco, California, U.S.A.*

WHY A BARRIER AND WHAT DO WE MEAN BY "BARRIER FUNCTION"?

Life in a terrestrial environment threatens mammals with desiccation, if transcutaneous water loss is unrestricted. In addition, the external skin layers must defend the organism from mechanical insults and pathogenic microbes, as well as from continuous bombardment by both UV-irradiation and free radicals generated from the ozone and other environmental pollutants. In addition, the barrier layers must also desquamate invisibly; trap appropriate amounts of water (hydration); metabolize exogenous xenobiotics; and even transduce sensory signals, i.e., they serve as a psychosensory interface. This volume devotes one or more chapters to most of these important protective ("barrier") functions. Yet, it is the structural, biochemical, regulatory, and pathophysiologic mechanisms that sustain permeability barrier homeostasis, which are justifiably the major emphasis of this book. Unfortunately, other worthy "barrier" mechanisms, such as epidermal UV filtration by endogenous molecular filters, are not included, in part because of space considerations, and also because of a dearth of current research activity and interest. Perhaps future editions of this volume will do greater justice to this and other topics. In Chapter 2, we discuss how several of these protective functions are linked topographically, structurally, or biochemically, and how many of these functions are co-regulated.

HOW ARE THE VARIOUS BARRIER FUNCTIONS MEDIATED?

It is now generally accepted that most of the defensive (barrier) functions of the epidermis localize to the stratum corneum (SC), a two-compartment system of corneocytes embedded in a lipid-enriched extracellular matrix. These various barrier functions further localize either to the corneocyte or to the extracellular matrix, and it is the latter site that mediates the majority of these functions. Yet, as described in Chapter 2, these functions do not work in isolation—each often influences other functions that exist either within the same, or in the adjacent compartment. For example, as described by Schmuth et al. (Chap. 27), defects in the corneocyte brick that lead to ichthyosis alter the extracellular lamellar membrane structure, and thereby the permeability barrier function. Clearly, the localization and organization of secreted hydrophobic lipids into characteristic lamellar membrane structures is critical for permeability barrier function (Chaps. 7 and 15). Yet, tight junctions (zonulae occuludentes, ZO) appear to be required for permeability barrier development. While their constituent proteins (e.g., occludin and claudin) persist in adult epidermis, complete ZO are not present. Whether these incomplete junctions or their constitutive proteins still regulate barrier function by other mechanisms, e.g., by targeting of lamellar body secretion to the apical plasma membrane of the granular cell, remains unknown (Chap. 12).

EVOLVING CONCEPTS OF THE SC BARRIER

Although the two-component ("bricks and mortar") model still provides a reasonable metaphor for the structure and composition of the SC, it is an inherently static concept (Table 1). A revised model that has emerged in recent years emphasizes the SC both as metabolically active, with multiple types of catalytic (primarily catabolic) activity in the cytosolic and membrane/extracellular compartments (Chaps. 9, 11 and 24), and as adaptive (the SC as a "smart tissue" Chap. 13). Instead, through its persistent metabolic activities, the SC self-regulates several of its key functions, such as permeability barrier formation, desquamation, maintenance of mechanical integrity, and the generation of osmotically active humectants (hydration). Separate chapters in this volume discuss the various types of metabolic activity that localize to the cytosolic, extracellular, or cornified envelope compartments.

　　As noted above, the SC barrier is not only metabolically active, but also adaptive (biosensor concept). In response to external perturbations or even alterations in humidity, signaling molecules, such as cytokines, are activated and elaborated. As described in Chap. 2, alterations in humidity alone not only modulate permeability barrier status, but also regulate epidermal cell kinetics and even the initiation of inflammation. These signals regulate the epidermal metabolic responses that sustain

Table 1 Current Concepts of Stratum Corneum

Two-compartment organization ("bricks and mortar")
Microheterogeneity within extracellular spaces ("there's more to the mortar than lipid")
Persistent metabolic activity (distinct enzymatic mechanisms in the cytosol, corneocyte
 periphery, and SC interstices)
Functional regulation of metabolism in the nucleated cell layers (barrier requirements
 regulate epidermal DNA and lipid synthesis)
Pathophysiologic links to deeper skin layers (barrier abrogation +/− epidermal injury
 initiates epidermal hyperplasia and inflammation)
Stratum corneum as a biosensor (humidity regulates proteolysis of filaggrin and epidermal
 DNA synthesis)

---

permeability barrier function, and perhaps other barriers as well (e.g., human β-defensin activation after cytokine signaling) (Chaps. 2, 22). Finally, while we have emphasized here the metabolic responses that maintain barrier homeostasis, these signaling molecules are also classic two-edged swords, capable of initiating inflammation (Chap. 19).

2

Defensive Functions of the Stratum Corneum: Integrative Aspects

Peter M. Elias

Dermatology Service, VA Medical Center, and Department of Dermatology, University of California, San Francisco, California, U.S.A.

PROTECTIVE FUNCTIONS ARE LINKED

Co-Localization of Defensive Functions

Virtually all epidermal functions (with the exception of vitamin D production) can be considered protective, and perhaps more specifically, defensive. Most of these critical protective functions reside in the stratum corneum (SC) (Table 1) (1,2). Yet, as will be discussed below, many individual functions are linked structurally, biochemically, or by common regulatory mechanisms to one or more of the other defensive functions of the SC (Table 2). The structural organization of the SC into a two-compartment system of corneocytes embedded in a lipid matrix further underlies the localization of defensive functions to either the extracellular or cytosolic compartments (Table 1). It is the lamellar body (LB) secretory system that dictates several functions that reside in the SC interstices (Fig. 1), because in addition to secreting lipids, LB delivers hydrolytic enzymes which both process lipid precursors into their respective products, and at least one serine protease and a variety of glycosidases with uncertain substrates (Chap. 16) (3,4), and orchestrates desquamation (Chap. 11) (5). LB secrete not only lipids and enzymes, but also certain structural proteins, enzyme inhibitors, and antimicrobial peptides to extracellular domains. These include: (i) corneodesmosin (6), a novel protein of the outer epidermis that coats the external face of corneodesmosomes, rendering these junctions resistant to premature proteolysis (Chap. 11); (ii) at least two antimicrobial peptide, human β-defensin 2 (hBD2) and the cathelicidin product LL-37 (Chaps. 2,22); (iii) and at least three protease inhibitors, elafin (SKALP), cystatin C/K, and the lymphoepithelial kazal-type inhibitor (LEKTI) (Chap. 16).

Relationship of Permeability and Antimicrobial Barriers

In addition to encountering an imposing physical barrier at the environmental interface, pathogenic microbes must pass a gauntlet of SC antimicrobial lipids, peptides, and enzyme inhibitors which, together with epidermal toll-like receptors and chemokines, comprise cutaneous innate immunity. The ability to restrict water loss out of

Table 1 Protective Functions of Mammalian Stratum Corneum

Function	Localization
Permeability barrier[a]	Extracellular
Initiation of inflammation (cytokine activation)[a]	Corneocyte
Cohesion (integrity) → desquamation[a]	Extracellular
Antimicrobial barrier (innate immunity)[a]	Extracellular
Mechanical (impact and shear resistance)	Corneocyte
Toxic chemical/antigen exclusion	Extracellular
Selective absorption	Extracellular
Hydration	Corneocyte
UV barrier	Corneocyte
Psychosensory interface	Unknown
Thermal barrier	Unknown

[a]Regulated by SC pH.

the body, while simultaneously blocking the ingress of microbial pathogens, is a further attribute of the SC's organization into a two-component system of lipid-depleted corneocytes embedded in a lipid-enriched extracellular matrix (7). While it is the (i) absolute quantities, (ii) hydrophobic character, (iii) lipid distribution, and (iv) supramolecular organization of its constituent lipids into a series of lamellar bilayers (8), which together account for the permeability barrier, at least three of these same SC lipids exhibit robust antibacterial activity [i.e., free fatty acids (FFA), glucosylceramides, the Cer hydrolytic product, sphingosine (9,10)]. The potential importance of this mechanism is shown in atopic dermatitis (AD), where increased colonization of *Staphylococcus aureus* is linked to depletion of sphingosine (11), the most potent of the three endogenous antimicrobial lipids.

Mammalian epidermis expresses three major families of antimicrobial peptides, the α- and β-defensins, hNP 1 and 2, and hBD 1–4, and a cathelicidin, hCAP-18 (12,13). Defensins comprise small, cationic, and cysteine-enriched members of a highly conserved gene family, consisting of α- and β subtypes, which differ slightly in their disulfide-bond pairing, genomic organization, and tissue distribution (12). They exhibit potent overlapping antimicrobial activity against a variety of gram-negative and gram-positive bacteria, yeast, and viruses. While α-defensins are present in low levels in the epidermis, β-defensins are more strongly expressed, and of the four mammalian hBDs, hBD1, and -2 predominate (12). hBD2 further localizes to the outer epidermis (14), where it translocates from the endoplasmic reticulum to LB following IL-α stimulation (15). Finally, hBD2 further immunolocalizes to SC membrane domains in inflammatory dermatoses (16).

Table 2 Integrative Defensive Functions of the Stratum Corneum

Defensive functions	How linked
Permeability and antimicrobial	Biochemical overlap; co-localize to extracellular domains
Hydration; UV-L; Immunosuppression; acidification	Down-stream products of filaggrin proteolysis and histidase pathway; co-localize to corneoctye cytosol

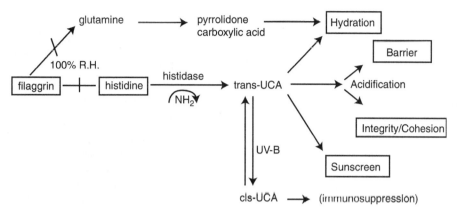

Figure 1 Filaggrin products influence multiple defensive function of stratum corneum.

Human epidermis also expresses the cathelicidin, hCAP-18 (13). Cathelicidins are a class of small cationic peptides with a highly-conserved NH-terminal cathelin segment, and a C-terminal segment, LL-37, which possesses antiviral, anti-gram-negative, and anti-streptococcal, but not anti-staphylococcal activity (13,17). The importance of this mechanism for antimicrobial defense is shown by the increased incidence of skin infections in cathelicidin knock out mice. Like hBD2, LL-37 immu-nolocalizes to the outer epidermis (13), where it also localizes to LB (Chap. 4). These findings clearly demonstrate that the permeability and antimicrobial barriers both co-localize and overlap biochemically (Table 2). As additional antimicrobial activities sequester to the SC interstices, it is clear that these activities are perfectly positioned to intercept pathogenic microbes before they can penetrate between corneocytes.

The Histidase Pathway Links Multiple Functions in the Corneocyte Cytosol

Other defensive functions co-localize to the corneocyte ("brick") cytosol (Table 1). In addition to providing resistance of the skin to mechanical or blunt injury, corneocytes generate amino acids and their deiminated products from filaggrin, which along with sebaceous gland–derived glycerol (18), regulate SC hydration (Chap. 24). Early in cornification, filaggrin—the predominant, histidine-enriched, basic protein in F-type keratohyalin granules disperses around keratin filaments within the stratum compac-tum (19). At ambient humidities; i.e., above the stratum compactum, filaggrin is largely hydrolyzed into free fatty acids, including histidine, glutamine (glutamic acid), and argi-nine (20,21) (Fig. 1). Whereas the still-uncharacterized cytosolic (aspartate) protease that generates these hygroscopically active molecules is inhibited at the high humidities present in the stratum compactum (21), activation occurs only after hydration levels begin to decline in the outer SC (i.e., <80% relative humidity). These amino acids, along with their more distal products (urocanic acid, pyrrolidone carboxylic acid, and ornithine/citrulline/aspartic acid), comprise much of the osmotically active mate-rial that regulates SC hydration (22). Proteolysis of filaggrin to histidine is followed by nonoxidative deimination of histidine to its acidic polar metabolite, trans-urocanic acid (tUCA) by the enzyme, histidine ammonia lyase (histidase). tUCA, in turn, can be photoisomerized by UV-B to cisUCA, acting in the process as an endogenous sunsc-reen, while simultaneously generating a potent immunosuppressive molecule (23) (Fig. 1). Finally, tUCA could be a major contributor to SC acidification with several pH-dependent functions impacted by this mechanism (24) (Chap. 2). Thus, products of the histidase pathway regulate several critical defensive functions of the SC.

Table 3 Stressor Effects on Multiple Defensive Functions

Stressor	Co-regulated functions
Barrier perturbation/external injury	Permeability barrier Inflammation
Psychologic stress	Permeability barrier SC integrity/cohesion
Increased pH	Permeability barrier SC integrity/cohesion Cytokine activation (inflammation) Antimicrobial barrier

MULTIPLE DEFENSIVE FUNCTIONS CAN BE ALTERED BY A SINGLE STRESSOR

Although it is both appropriate and convenient to classify each of the defensive functions of the SC as a discrete process, several of these functions are co-regulated in response to common stressors (Table 3).

External Injury Regulates Permeability Barrier Homeostasis and Initiates Inflammation

Current fashion views the skin as a pro-inflammatory tissue, e.g., distinctive T-cell abnormalities occur in common dermatoses, such as psoriasis, contact dermatitis, and atopic dermatoses. Yet, these diseases are often initiated and sustained by external perturbations (e.g., Koebner phenomenon in psoriasis). Indeed, most cutaneous immune phenomena are triggered by the release of a preformed pool of the primary cytokines, IL-1α, IL-1β, and TNFα, from the corneocyte and granular cell cytosol, along with other signaling molecules, in response to minimal external (barrier) perturbations (25) (Chap. 19). Following their release, these cytokines signal divergent, downstream pathways that initiate both homeostatic (repair-related) and pro-inflammatory processes.

According to this view, inflammation is merely a byproduct of permeability barrier perturbations, because this often-pathogenic sequence is linked to the cutaneous defensive function of greatest importance, i.e., maintenance of a competent permeability barrier. While external perturbations initiate a signal cascade that stimulates homeostatic processes that repair the barrier, the same signals also stimulate cutaneous inflammation through downstream recruitment/entrapment of inflammatory cells (Fig. 2). Accordingly, many cutaneous inflammatory phenomena, including disease-specific T-cell responses, are recruited merely as incidental participants in a defensive sequence aimed at normalizing SC function (2,25). Thus, the cutaneous permeability barrier and inflammatory signaling can be considered two distinct defensive functions of the epidermis that are linked to a common stressor, i.e., barrier perturbation.

Psychological Stress Alters Both Barrier Function and SC Integrity/Cohesion

Another pertinent example of linked functions that are altered in response to a common stressor is psychological stress, which is now well known to exert negative effects on permeability barrier function (26,27) (Chap. 2). However, by stimulating an increase in endogenous glucocorticoids (28), as will be discussed below, stress

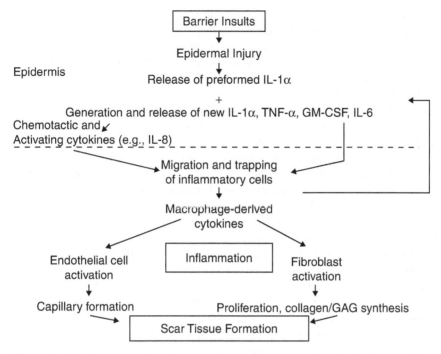

Figure 2 Barrier insults stimulate not only repair responses, but also initiate cytokine cascade.

impacts not only barrier functions, but also SC integrity/cohesion. The negative effects of glucocorticoids, in turn, can be attributed to suppression of epidermal lipid synthesis and LB production (Fig. 3). The stress-induced abnormalities can all be recapitulated by short-term administration of either systemic or topical steroids (29), and blocked by glucocorticoid-receptor antagonists (28). Interestingly, not only the stress-induced barrier abnormality, but also the abnormality in SC integrity can be reversed (overridden) by a mixture of physiologic lipids, containing all three key SC species (i.e., ceramides, free fatty acids, and cholesterol) (29). Thus, psychological stress represents a second example of a single stressor with multiple downstream functional consequences.

Elevations of SC pH Can Alter Multiple Defensive Functions

A third stressor that can impact multiple defensive functions comprises the set of alterations induced by an elevated SC pH. Indeed, the "acid mantle" of the SC orchestrates at least three, and probably four, key SC functions (Chap. 14). The most widely accepted hypothesis about the role of the SC acid mantle is in antimicrobial defense (30). Pathogenic bacteria, such as *S. aureus*, grow best at a neutral pH, while conversely, normal flora (coagulase-negative staphylococci, propionibacteriae) grow

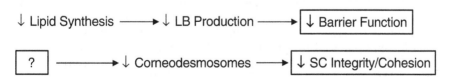

Figure 3 Psychologic stress and glucocorticoids rapidly compromise epidermal function.

best at a more acidic pH (30). The potential importance of pH for antimicrobial function is underscored in neonatal skin, which displays a neutral pH coupled with an enhanced risk of infection, as well as inflammation, impaired SC integrity/cohesion, and a subtle barrier abnormality (31). Although the density and composition of the cutaneous normal flora are dependent on a variety of factors, including hydration and occlusion, pH appears to be pre-eminent (32). Pertinently, both intertriginous and inflamed skin display an increased pH (33,34), as does newborn SC, which only gradually develops an acidic pH over the first one-to-three months of life (35). Hence, the reduced resistance to pathogens that characterizes these settings. The developmental delay in acidification in neonates is complicated further by a vicious circle of increased hydration, a defective barrier, and urea/fecal contamination, all of which can further increase pH, with enhanced risk of infections and/or diaper dermatitis.

The importance of SC pH for a second function, permeability barrier homeostasis, is suggested both by the worsening of barrier function when intact skin is exposed to an alkaline pH (36) and by the delay in barrier recovery that occurs when perturbed skin is exposed to a neutral pH (37). pH could influence barrier function directly through its effects on membrane bilayer organization (38) and/or secondarily through its regulation of extracellular lipid processing (37). Lipid processing refers to the post-secretory conversion of secreted, LB-derived, polar lipid precursors into their non-polar lipid products, a sequence that, generates the extracellular lamellar bilayers that mediate barrier function (Chap. 15). Two of the hydrolytic enzymes critical for bilayer generation exhibit acidic pH optima [β-glucocerabrosidase (-GlcCer'-ase) and acidic sphingomyelinase (aSMase)], while two others [group 1 secretory phospholipase A2 (sPLA$_2$) and steroid sulfatase (SSase)] display neutral-to-alkaline pH optima, suggesting that the SC pH gradient could orchestrate lipid processing.

SC integrity/cohesion, which is inversely related to rates of corneocyte shedding (desquamation) (Chap. 11), represents a third SC function that is pH-dependent. Integrity/cohesion is thought to be regulated predominantly by two proteolytic enzymes: the epidermis-specific kallikrains (KIK) SC chymotryptic (SCCE) and tryptic (SCTE) serine proteases. Since SCCE (KIK) and SCTE (KIKS) exhibit neutral-to-alkaline pH optima, they are likely to be active at an elevated pH, as occurs in inflammatory dermatoses. But proteolysis, sufficient to sustain low rates of normal desquamation, almost certainly occurs in normal SC, particularly in the lower layers. In fact, these enzymes exhibit residual activity at an acidic pH, but other proteases with acidic pH optima could become operative (e.g., aspartate and cysteine proteases); and hence, even more important in the outer SC (39,40). However, it is likely that SCCE/SCTE activities would dominate at all SC levels in pathological skin, which is characterized by optimal conditions for serine protease activation at all levels (i.e., increased pH, hydration, and presence of Ca^{++} in SC).

An acidic SC pH could also restrict the initiation of cutaneous inflammation. The corneocyte cytosol contains substantial reservoirs of precursors of both IL-1α and IL-1β, and these cytokines are activated, along with another primary cytokine of the outer epidermis, TNFα, in response to external perturbations (41). Release of these cytokines is mediated by pH-dependent activation of SC serine proteases. The serine protease, SCCE, is capable of activating IL-1β in vitro at several sites N-terminal to ASP 116, generating fragments with variable activity (42). Although the cleavage sites for pro–IL-1α lie between either Phe (43) and Leu (44), or Tyr (45) and Glu (46), whether SCCE or SCTE can also activate this cytokine is not known. However, though an elevated pH alone suffices to initiate cytokine activation, inflammation does not result from this mechanism alone (47). Additional triggers must co-exist, e.g., barrier abnormality. Pertinently, the pH of dermatitic (inflamed) skin is generally about one unit higher than that of normal SC (33).

In summary, the impact of an elevated SC pH on SC integrity/cohesion and cytokine activation involves a common mechanism, i.e., activation of serine, and perhaps other proteases, but the responsible mechanisms diverge following enzyme activation. pH also can alter barrier function in a serine protease–dependent fashion, because sustained serine protease (SP) further alters barrier function through degradation of the lipid processing enzymes, β-glucocerebrosidase and acidic sphin-gomyelinase (aSMase) (48). The negative consequences of an elevated pH on SC integrity/cohesion and cytokine activation can be explained by other SP-catalyzed reactions, which result in degradation of corneodesmosomes and activations of cytokines, respectively.

PERTURBATIONS OF ONE FUNCTION CAN ALTER OTHER DEFENSIVE FUNCTIONS

Alterations in Hydration Influence Permeability Barrier

The interactivity of certain defensive functions is further demonstrated by instances in which perturbations in one function impact other functions (Table 4). Important examples are variations in external humidity, and their effects first on SC hydration (Chap. 24), which then can provoke alterations in permeability barrier function (Fig. 3). Whereas prolonged exposure to a humid environment (>80%) results in a gradual deterioration in barrier function, exposure to low relative humidities (<20%) enhances barrier homeostasis (49). Thus, changes in hydration stimulate alterations in permeability barrier function that are appropriate for environmental conditions. Yet, sudden switches in hydration extremes, i.e., from skin previously exposed to a humid milieu to a dry environment paradoxically produce a profound, though temporary, deficit in barrier function (50) (Fig. 4). The mechanism that is responsible for the barrier abnormality in this instance appears to be the inability of humid-adapted cells of the granular layer (SG) to respond, i.e., they fail to upregulate the metabolic and secretory machinery necessary to maintain barrier homeostasis. Though humans often travel between such extremes in humidity, the barrier defect fortunately is transient, as defective cells are quickly replaced by a new generation of functionally competent arrivals to the outer epidermis

Alterations in Mechanical Barrier Influence Permeability Barrier

Another pertinent example of one function impacting a second is shown by the role of the cornified envelope (CE) to act not only as a mechanical barrier, but also as a scaffold necessary for the organization of secreted lipids into continuous lamellar membrane structures, which mediate permeability barrier function. Defective lamel-lar structures and increased transcutaneous water loss occur in both transglutami-nase 1 (TG1)–deficient lamellar ichthyosis and loricrin keratoderma (Vohwinkel's

Table 4 Perturbations in One Function Can Alter Other Defensive Functions

1° Perturbed function	2° Affected function(s)
Hydration	Permeability barrier
Mechanical	Permeability barrier

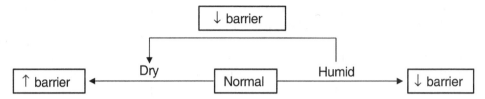

Figure 4 Changes in external humidity regulate permeability barrier status.

disease). Both of these inherited diseases display attenuated or fragile CE that provoke abnormalities in adjacent membranes, which result in altered barrier function (51,52) (Chap. 28).

In summary, we have shown how many defensive functions of the SC are co-localized or co-regulated, and how alterations in one defensive function can, in turn, impact other key defensive functions.

REFERENCES

1. Elias PM, Feingold KR. Skin as an organ of protection. In: Freedberg I et al. eds. Fitzpatrick's Dermatology in General Medicine. Philadelphia: McGraw-Hill, 1999:164–174.
2. Chuong CM, Nickoloff BJ, Elias PM, Goldsmith LA, Macher E, Maderson PA, Sundberg JP, Tagami H, Plonka PM, Thestrup-Pederson K, Bernard BA, Schroder JM, Dotto P, Chang CM, Williams ML, Feingold KR, King LE, Kligman AM, Rees JL, Christophers E. What is the "true" function of skin? Exp Dermatol 2002; 11:159–187.
3. Abraham W, Wertz PW, Landmann L, Downing DT. Stratum corneum lipid liposomes: calcium-induced transformation into lamellar sheets. J Invest Dermatol 1987; 88:212–214.
4. Aioi A, Tonogaito H, Suto H, Hamada K, Ra CR, Ogawa H, Maibach H, Matsuda H. Impairment of skin barrier function in NC/Nga Tnd mice as a possible model for atopic dermatitis. Br J Dermatol 2001; 144:12–18.
5. Alaiti S, Kang S, Fiedler VC, Ellis CN, Spurlin DV, Fader D, Ulyanov G, Gadgil SD, Tanase A, Lawrence I, Scotellaro P, Raye K, Bekersky I. Tacrolimus (FK506) ointment for atopic dermatitis: a phase I study in adults and children. J Am Acad Dermatol 1998; 38:69–76.
6. Alibek K. Biohazard: The Chilling True Story of the Largest Covert Biological Weapons Program in the World, Told from the Inside by the Man who Ran It. New York: Random House, 1999.
7. Elias PM. Epidermal lipids, barrier function, and desquamation. J Invest Dermatol 1983; 80(suppl):44s–49s.
8. Elias PM, Menon GK. Structural and lipid biochemical correlates of the epidermal permeability barrier. Adv Lipid Res 1991; 24:1–26.
9. Miller SJ, Aly R, Shinefeld HR, Elias PM. In vitro and in vivo antistaphylococcal activity of human stratum corneum lipids. Arch Dermatol 1988; 124:209–215.
10. Bibel DJ, Miller SJ, Brown BE, Pandey BB, Elias PM, Shinefield HR, Aly R. Antimicrobial activity of stratum corneum lipids from normal and essential fatty acid-deficient mice. J Invest Dermatol 1989; 92:632–638.
11. Arikawa J, Ishibashi M, Kawashima M, Takagi Y, Ichikawa Y, Imokawa G. Decreased levels of sphingosine, a natural antimicrobial agent, may be associated with vulnerability of the stratum corneum from patients with atopic dermatitis to colonization by *Staphylococcus aureus*. J Invest Dermatol 2002; 119:433–439.
12. Ganz T. Defensins: antimicrobial peptides of innate immunity. Nat Rev Immunol 2003; 3:710–720.

13. Gallo RL, Nizet V. Endogenous production of antimicrobial peptides in innate immunity and human disease. Curr Allergy Asthma Rep 2003; 3:402–409.
14. Ong PY, Ohtake T, Brandt C, Strickland I, Boguniewicz M, Ganz T, Gallo RL, Leung DY. Endogenous antimicrobial peptides and skin infections in atopic dermatitis. N Engl J Med 2002; 347:1151–1160.
15. Oren A, Ganz T, Liu L, Meerloo T. In human epidermis, beta-defensin 2 is packaged in lamellar bodies. Exp Mol Pathol 2003; 74:180–182.
16. Huh WK, Oono T, Shirafuji Y, Akiyama H, Arata J, Sakaguchi M, Huh NH, Iwatsuki K. Dynamic alteration of human beta-defensin 2 localization from cytoplasm to intercellular space in psoriatic skin. J Mol Med 2002; 80:678–684.
17. Zaiou M, Gallo RL. Cathelicidins, essential gene-encoded mammalian antibiotics. J Mol Med 2002; 80:549–561.
18. Fluhr JW, Mao-Qiang M, Brown BE, Wertz PW, Crumrine D, Sundberg JP, Feingold KR, Elias PM. Glycerol regulates stratum corneum hydration in sebaceous gland deficient (asebia) mice. J Invest Dermatol 2003; 120:728–737.
19. Dale BA, Presland RB, Lewis SP, Underwood RA, Fleckman P. Transient expression of epidermal filaggrin in cultured cells causes collapse of intermediate filament networks with alteration of cell shape and nuclear integrity. J Invest Dermatol 1997; 108:179–187.
20. Scott IR. Factors controlling the expressed activity of histidine ammonia-lyase in the epidermis and the resulting accumulation of urocanic acid. Biochem J 1981; 194:829–838.
21. Scott IR, Harding CR. Filaggrin breakdown to water binding compounds during development of the rat stratum corneum is controlled by the water activity of the environment. Dev Biol 1986; 115:84–92.
22. Harding CR, Watkinson A, Rawlings AV, Scott IR. Dry skin, moisturization, and corneodesmolysis. Int J Cosm Sci 2000; 22:21–52.
23. Noonan FP, De Fabo EC. Immunosuppression by ultraviolet B radiation: initiation by urocanic acid. Immunol Today 1992; 13:250–254.
24. Krien P, Kermici M. Evidence for the existence of a self-regulated enzymatic process within human stratum corneum-an unexpected role for urocanic acid. J Invest Dermatol 2000; 115:414–420.
25. Elias PM, Wood LC, Feingold KR. Epidermal pathogenesis of inflammatory dermatoses. Am J Contact Dermat 1999; 10:119–126.
26. Garg A, Chren MM, Sands LP, Matsui MS, Marenus KD, Feingold KR, Elias PM. Psychological stress perturbs epidermal permeability barrier homeostasis: implications for the pathogenesis of stress-associated skin disorders. Arch Dermatol 2001; 137:53–59.
27. Altemus M, Rao B, Dhabhar FS, Ding W, Granstein RD. Stress-induced changes in skin barrier function in healthy women. J Invest Dermatol 2001; 117:309–317.
28. Denda M, Tsuchiya T, Elias PM, Feingold KR. Stress alters cutaneous permeability barrier homeostasis. Am J Physiol Regul Integr Comp Physiol 2000; 278:R367–R372.
29. Kao JS, Fluhr JW, Man MQ, Fowler AJ, Hachem JP, Crumrine D, Ahn SK, Brown BE, Elias PM, Feingold KR. Short-term glucocorticoid treatment compromises both permeability barrier homeostasis and stratum corneum integrity: inhibition of epidermal lipid synthesis accounts for functional abnormalities. J Invest Dermatol 2003; 120:456–464.
30. Korting HC, Hubner K, Greiner K, Hamm G, Braun-Falco O. Differences in the skin surface pH and bacterial microflora due to the long-term application of synthetic detergent preparations of pH 5.5 and pH 7.0. Results of a crossover trial in healthy volunteers. Acta Derm Venereol 1990; 70:429–431.
31. Fluhr J, Behne M, Brown BE, Moskowitz DG, Selden C, Mauro T, Elias PM, Feingold K. Stratum corneum acidification in neonatal skin: I. Secretory phospholipase A2 and the NHE1 antiporter acidify neonatal rat stratum corneum. J Invest Dermatol 2004; 122:320–329.
32. Aly R, Shirley C, Cunico B, Maibach HI. Effect of prolonged occlusion on the microbial flora, pH, carbon dioxide and transepidermal water loss on human skin. J Invest Dermatol 1978; 71:378–381.

33. Beare JM, Cheeseman EA, Gailey AA, Neill DW. The pH of the skin surface of children with seborrhoeic dermatitis compared with unaffected children. Br J Dermatol 1958; 70:233–241.

34. Yosipovitch G, Tur E, Cohen O, Rusecki Y. Skin surface pH in intertriginous areas in NIDDM patients. Possible correlation to candidal intertrigo. Diab Care 1993; 16:560–563.

35. Visscher MO, Chatterjee R, Munson KA, Pickens WL, Hoath SB. Changes in diapered and nondiapered infant skin over the first month of life. Pediatr Dermatol 2000; 17:45–51.

36. Thune P, Nilsen T, Hanstad IK, Gustavsen T, Lovig Dahl H. The water barrier function of the skin in relation to the water content of stratum corneum, pH and skin lipids. The effect of alkaline soap and syndet on dry skin in elderly, non-atopic patients. Acta Derm Venereol 1988; 68:277–283.

37. Mauro T, Holleran WM, Grayson S, Gao WN, Man MQ, Kriehuber E, Behne M, Feingold KR, Elias PM. Barrier recovery is impeded at neutral pH, independent of ionic effects: implications for extracellular lipid processing. Arch Dermatol Res 1998; 290:215–222.

38. Bouwsta JA, Gooris GS, Dubbelaar FE, Ponec M. Phase behaviour of skin barrier model membranes at pH 7.4. Cell Mol Biol (Noisy-le-grand) 2000; 46:979–992.

39. Horikoshi T, Arany I, Rajaraman S, Chen SH, Brysk H, Lei G, Tyring SK, Brysk MM. Isoforms of cathepsin D and human epidermal differentiation. Biochimie 1998; 80:605–612.

40. Suzuki Y, Nomura J, Hori J, Koyama J, Takahashi M, Horii I. Detection and characterization of endogenous protease associated with desquamation of stratum corneum. Arch Dermatol Res 1993; 285:372–377.

41. Wood LC, Jackson SM, Elias PM, Grunfeld C, Feingold KR. Cutaneous barrier perturbation stimulates cytokine production in the epidermis of mice. J Clin Invest 1992; 90:482–487.

42. Nylander-Lundqvist E, Egelrud T. Formation of active IL-1 beta from pro-IL-1 beta catalyzed by stratum corneum chymotryptic enzyme in vitro. Acta Derm Venereol 1997; 77:203–206.

43. Sondell B, Thornell LE, Stigbrand T, Egelrud T. Immunolocalization of stratum corneum chymotryptic enzyme in human skin and oral epithelium with monoclonal antibodies: evidence of a proteinase specifically expressed in keratinizing squamous epithelia. J Histochem Cytochem 1994; 42:459–465.

44. Grubauer G, Elias PM, Feingold KR. Transepidermal water loss: the signal for recovery of barrier structure and function. J Lipid Res 1989; 30:323–333.

45. Ghadially R, Brown BE, Sequeira-Martin SM, Feingold KR, Elias PM. The aged epidermal permeability barrier. Structural, functional, and lipid biochemical abnormalities in humans and a senescent murine model. J Clin Invest 1995; 95:2281–2290.

46. Scheuplein RJ, Blank IH. Permeability of the skin. Physiol Rev 1971; 51:702–747.

47. Hachem JP, Crumrine D, Fluhr J, Brown BE, Feingold KR, Elias PM. pH directly regulates epidermal permeability barrier homeostasis, and stratum corneum integrity/cohesion. J Invest Dermatol 2003; 121:345–353.

48. Hachem JP, Man MQ, Crumrine D, Uchida Y, Brown BE, Feingold KR, Elias PM. Consequences of a sustained increase in pH for stratum corneum permeability barrier homeostasis and integrity. J Invest Dermatol. In press.

49. Denda M, Sato J, Masuda Y, Tsuchiya T, Koyama J, Kuramoto M, Elias PM, Feingold KR. Exposure to a dry environment enhances epidermal permeability barrier function. J Invest Dermatol 1998; 111:858–863.

50. Sato J, Denda M, Chang S, Elias PM, Feingold KR. Abrupt decreases in environmental humidity induce abnormalities in permeability barrier homeostasis. J Invest Dermatol 2002; 119:900–904.

51. Elias PM, Schmuth M, Uchida Y, Rice RH, Behne M, Crumrine D, Feingold KR, Holleran WM, Pharm D. Basis for the permeability barrier abnormality in lamellar ichthyosis. Exp Dermatol 2002; 11:248–256.

52. Schmuth M, Fluhr J, Crumrine D, Uchida Y, Hachem JP, Behne M, Feingold K, Elias PM. Structural and functional consequences of loricrin mutations in human loricrin keratoderma (Vohwinkel syndrome with ichthyosis). J Invest Dermatol 2004; 122:909–922.

3

A Brief History of How the Dead Stratum Corneum Became Alive

Albert M. Kligman
Department of Dermatology, Hospital of the University of Pennsylvania, Philadelphia, Pennsylvania, U.S.A.

Judging by the more than 500 articles that have been published about the stratum corneum over the last 10 years in seven different languages the world over, this structure is surely one of the most fascinating and interesting tissues in mammalian biology.

The stratum corneum has intrigued a remarkable confederation of scientists from many unrelated disciplines, including geneticists, biochemists, physicists, anatomists, physiologists, engineers, material scientists, immunologists, and even psychologists! One might argue that this diverse and dedicated interest simply reflects the fact that without the stratum corneum, occupation of dry land would have been impossible. A seal against diffusional water loss is an absolute prerequisite. Further, extremely premature infants with a defective horny layer cannot survive, and those with hereditary malformations of the horny layer cannot thrive. Toxic chemicals are impeded from penetration. It was this knowledge that led early investigators to use the term "barrier" as short-hand for the stratum corneum. This usage stresses the traditional concept that the role of the stratum corneum was to prevent diffusional loss of vital substances from the inside to the outside, and to prevent diffusion of exogenous substances into the inside.

Thus, the "barrier" has been traditionally viewed as a two-way seal, serving as an inert wrapping to separate the internal and external environments.

More recent studies have made it clear that this view is a vast oversimplification. Far from being a dead, inert wrapping, the stratum corneum has turned out to be a remarkably dynamic tissue with a multiplicity of functions which continue to surprise and excite us.

The daunting question before us is how can a structure as dead as a door nail serve so many disparate functions? One might ask whether this intense interest is purely an academic pursuit to satisfy intellectual curiosity. The answer is much more complex upon analysis.

Firstly, even a moderately defective horny layer is a very disagreeable feature which adversely affects the quality of life. An abnormal horny layer is dry, rough, scaly, brittle, cracked, and often itchy, provoking scratching, initiating an itch-scratch vicious cycle for which topical remedies provide little relief. This itchy xerotic skin has

15

many different unrelated causes, and is the basis of a huge skin care industry aimed at overcoming dry, scaly, roughness by making the surface smooth, supple, and comfortable, agreeable to both sight and touch. More than 90% of adult women use "moisturizers" every day for decades, stretching into old age, when xerosis is both universal and severe.

A great deal of what we now know about the consequences of defective horny layers derives from the far-reaching investigations of scientists working for large, international cosmetic and skin care companies (who incidentally receive too little praise and recognition from medical academicians). These industries have produced a remarkable array of useful products that bring relief from rough xerotic skin, regardless of cause.

Secondly, there is a distressing variety of hereditary and congenital skin disorders in which derangements of the horny layer are far more severe. These unfortunates are encased in thick, fissured, extremely rough and scaly, unsightly integuments which severely limit daily activities, requiring enormous efforts to provide something resembling a normal life. It is understandable then that pharmaceutical companies and academic scholars have invested heavily in trying to understand the pathogenesis of these devastating disorders. The payoff has been the development of some systemic drugs which can moderate and partially normalize this grossly abnormal stratum corneum, greatly improving the quality of life.

Thirdly, the concept has slowly developed that the "barrier" may not be so completely impenetrable as to resist all the repeated efforts to breach it. In truth, the barrier may be 100 times more permeable to some agents than others. What determines permeability? On the face of it, topical drugs are an extremely inefficient way to treat diseases of the skin. For most agents, especially that old war horse corticosteroids, only 3% to 4% of the applied drug is absorbed. The rest is wasted! These are sound reasons for seeking ways to enhance the penetration of topical drugs. Oral drugs not only face problems of absorption through the gut, but are subject to the first-pass phenomenon of being metabolized by the liver, reducing the concentration that reaches diseased skin. Moreover, oral drugs exhibit the well-known rollercoaster highs and lows of serum levels, when the highs may be toxic and the lows may lack efficacy. By contrast, steady-state serum levels can be obtained when the drug is applied in a reservoir device applied to normal skin. This is a wonderfully innovative idea, since the famous impenetrable barrier is no longer a barrier to thinking about ways of targeting skin as a potential portal of entry, a concept that was unimaginable 50 years ago. We are no longer shocked when physicists announce—as they did in 2000—that the "epidermal permeability barrier is a porous medium consisting of permeable and impermeable regions" (1).

This approach is already something of a therapeutic triumph, in that there are currently on the market transdermal patch test systems for the delivery of at least six different drugs, including hormones, anti-hypertensives, nicotine, nitroglycerin, and others. Furthermore, it is becoming increasingly possible by physical means (photomechanical waves and ultrasound) as well as with liposomal small-particle systems (transfersomes) to achieve therapeutic benefits without irreversibly damaging the stratum corneum. The possibilities for breaching the barrier for therapeutic purposes seem endless.

In sum, scientific interest in the stratum corneum has produced a solid body of knowledge of how the stratum corneum is built and how it functions.

My intent in this essay is to tell the story of how the dead stratum corneum became so alive. The state of knowledge of the horny layer, a half century ago, was summarized by Rothman in his landmark text, *Physiology and Biochemistry of Skin* (2). He depicted the horny layer as an amorphous, loose mass of keratin fibrils, the product of living keratinocytes, which disintegrated as they moved upward in the process of differentiation, dumping their horny contents onto the surface. He viewed this as a holocrine process similar to the production of sebum by the sebaceous gland. The stratum corneum was viewed as a kind of graveyard of insoluble keratin fibrils, an amorphous mass lacking a cellular structure.

No description could be more fallacious. How could one of the giants of dermatologic research go so anatomically astray? Enlightenment began 10 years later in 1964 when I wrote what many regard as a seminal article entitled the "Biology of the Stratum Corneum"(3). Some of the current major players in this field have told me that their interest in the stratum corneum was inspired by this account. Accordingly, I have the conceit to say that I am the father of corneobiology, the study of the structure and function of the stratum corneum. In brief, I showed that the stratum corneum was a genuine tissue made up of well-defined sturdy cells which I named corneocytes, also called horny cells. It turned out that the image that histopathologists had been looking at in formalin-fixed specimens for more than a hundred years was false.

In such preparations, no cells are visible. Instead one sees fine laminae or fibrils, separated by wide spaces, a loose airy mass which histologists to this very day describe as having a "basket-weave" appearance, descriptively accurate but misleading (Fig. 1). I showed that this appearance was an artifact of formalin fixation which literally tears the stratum corneum apart, ruining it beyond recognition. The basket-weave appearance posed a paradox for physiologists since there was already evidence in the mid-century that the horny layer actually did provide a barrier to the

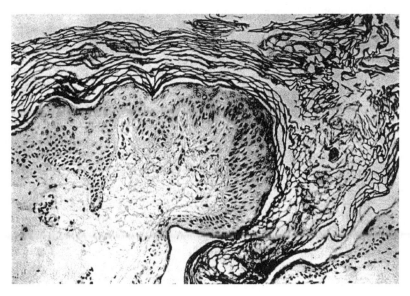

Figure 1 This is the famous "basket-weave" appearance of the stratum corneum. It apparently consists of amorphous laminae or filaments, separated by wide spaces. How such a loose, airy structure could serve as a "barrier" was incomprehensible. This image is entirely false, an artifact of formalin fixation and paraffin processing, which violates the tissue beyond recognition (H&E, × 40).

diffusion of substances into and out of the skin. The intriguing question was: How could such a loose, airy structure impede penetration when it looked completely permeable? Szakall tried to solve the paradox by proposing that the real barrier was a very thin, histologically invisible impermeable membrane at the bottom of the basket-weave stratum corneum which he could isolate after repeated strippings (4). No one could confirm this.

In 1944, Winsor and Burch had found that the skin became freely permeable to water and dissolved substances after the horny layer had been removed by sandpapering, a convincing proof of its barrier function (5). Further evidence was provided by Monash, an imaginative clinician in private practice, who observed in 1957 that high concentrations of topical anesthetic agents applied to human skin did not provide anesthesia to painful stimuli. After stripping away the horny layer with tape, anesthesia was rapidly induced, such that even very low concentrations of anesthetic agents blocked sensory perception of pain (6). There could no longer be any doubt that the stratum corneum was "the barrier." In 1958, Malkinson, too, found that only 1% to 2% of radiolabeled hydrocortisone could penetrate native human skin whereas more than 90% was absorbed through stripped skin (7).

In my 1954 paper, I described a series of studies that finally resolved the basket-weave paradox. Using surgically excised or cadaver skin, we found that heating full-thickness samples of human skin at 60°C for one minute yielded a thin, tough, transparent membrane, which was rather stiff when dry, becoming very pliable when moistened with water (Fig. 2). When wet, this membrane could be stretched considerably without tearing or cracking, enabling it to conform to physical deformations, a highly desirable property for a body wrapping. I likened it to a tough plastic sheet which encased the body as a kind of dead shroud. Christophers, in my laboratory, then showed that sheets of stratum corneum could be obtained in vivo by raising up a blister with cantharidin, which produces mid-epidermal cleavage (8). Matoltsy et al. later noted in passing that sheets of stratum corneum in vivo floated free when whole skin was immersed in strong concentrations of urea (9).

I then went on to show that the stratum corneum was made up of polygonal corneocytes, mostly pentagons and hexagons, about 30 microns in diameter and less than 0.5 microns in width. The next objective was to determine how many layers of corneocytes comprised the stratum corneum of the general body surface. Christophers and I did this by immersing the sheets in sodium hydroxide which caused the corneocytes to swell greatly owing to dissolution of keratin filaments, making the cells transparent for easy counting (10). This simple technique yielded an incidental finding, later shown to be of great importance to the stability of the stratum corneum, that the swollen cells were bounded by well-defined, sturdy envelopes. The composition, function, and nature of the corneocyte envelope have since received an enormous amount of investigative attention (Fig. 3), properly so in proportion to its biologic importance.

We went on to show that the number of corneocytes making up the thickness of the stratum corneum on most body sites was in the range of 14 to 16, sometimes stacked one above the other in neat columns.

Mackenzie et al. later provided many examples of this columnar architecture, which makes sound structural sense as a protection against physical forces (11). We found, however, that the neat columns, so routinely evident in mice, were often disturbed, evident in some segments, but more random in others. I suspected that the lack of columns in human skin was due to the constant friction imposed upon the

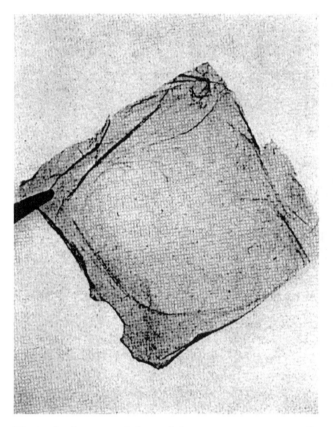

Figure 2 A separated sheet of the stratum corneum was formalin-fixed, stained with H&E, and mounted for horizontal viewing. This was the first demonstration that the stratum corneum was made up of well-defined polygonal, horny cells (corneocytes) that are tightly bound to each other. The dark dots covering the surface are probably corneodesmosomes, which rivet the cells together.

horny layer by clothing, washing, and daily physical activities. This was confirmed when I raised up cantharadin blisters on two patients with fractures who had worn plaster casts for one month. Immediately after removing the casts, the corneocytes were organized into beautiful columnar arrays. One month later, the columns were in random arrangement. How corneocytes, which are passively pushed to the surface, can become oriented into columns, notably in protected sites, is still a mystery.

Stimulated by these findings, I made a bold statement which has since been often quoted that "the raison d'etre of the viable epidermis was to make a horny layer, its specific biologic mission." This view has turned out to be both naïve and inaccurate, revealing how little we knew about epidermal biology four decades ago. We know now that keratinocytes possess a variety of capabilities, subserving hormonal, immunologic, semiotic neurosensory, antibacterial, antiviral, and biochemical functions that make the epidermis one of the most complex tissues in the body.

The advent of transmission electron microscopy established beyond doubt that the corneocytes were tightly bound together, separated by narrow intercellular

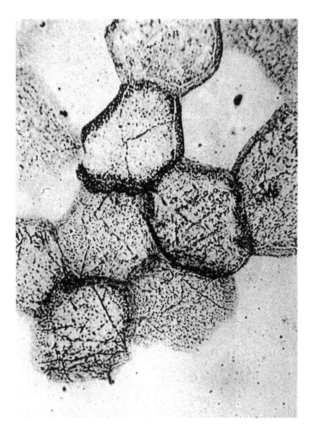

Figure 3 The stratum corneum, after separation from the viable epidermis by a brief immersion in water at 60°C, is a transparent, tough sheet made up of coherent corneocytes, brittle when dry and pliable when wet.

spaces, forming a coherent membrane except near the surface where they become progressively detached for shedding. At first, the intercellular spaces seemed curiously empty and structureless. This turned out to be another fixation and processing artifact. The development of post-fixation staining with ruthenium tetroxide showed that the spaces were filled with stacks of alternating electron-dense and electron-lucent membranes, the so-called Landman units. The physico-chemical nature of these membranes came under intense scrutiny, culminating in the surprising concept that these spaces comprised the actual pathways through which xenobiotics, whether water or lipid soluble, had to pass to reach the viable tissues below (12). It is now appreciated that it is these long tortuous pathways between the corneocytes that actually constitute the barrier to inward or outward diffusion of substances. Thus, it became necessary to revise the notion of direct transmembrane diffusion across the stratum corneum, proposed in the pioneering work on permeability by Scheuplein and Blank, using in vitro diffusion chambers (13). A number of proposals made regarding the possible routes of penetration of exogenous substances, viz., appendageal shunts, direct transcorneal, or via extracellular spaces between corneocytes, directed attention to the physico-chemical properties of the stratum corneum giving rise to a vast literature of its own.

These observations culminated in the concept of the "brick and mortar" model of the structural organization of the stratum corneum, created by the foremost master of corneobiology, Peter Elias, and his collaborators. No one can have a good grasp of the structure and function of the stratum corneum without reading the many illuminating papers published by this fertile group (14–16).

According to this model, now enshrined in all text book accounts, the bricks are the corneocytes containing densely packed hydrophilic keratin filaments, while the mortar comprises the intercellular spaces made up of hydrophobic, lipid-soluble bilaminar membranes. Instead of being a homogeneous plastic wrapping, as I had suggested, the stratum corneum was organized into a two-compartment system, each with quite different physical, mechanical, and physiological functions.

The brick and mortar two-compartment model has been of enormous heuristic value by emphasizing the complex organization of the stratum corneum. Nonetheless, the brick and mortar model is an oversimplification, and may actually be misleading. Marks and Leveque, corneobiologists with substantial bona fides, share this view, stating somewhat more bluntly that "the brick and mortar model is misleading and false."

The fact is that a steady stream of advances using sophisticated, powerful methodologies by a small army of investigators has made it necessary to revise the brick and mortar model to make it more compatible with anatomical and physiological realities. To start with, the term "mortar" suggests that it is a fairly homogeneous substance, a kind of cement that holds the "bricks" together. In fact, the mortar does not play a cementing role. The corneocytes are physically bound to each other by corneodermosomes, the end product of epidermal dermosomes. These act as rivets spaced along the surface of corneocytes. It is only after the corneosomes are digested by proteolytic enzymes in the intercellular spaces that the corneocytes are set free near the surface to be shed individually in the process of desquamation. It becomes evident that the hydrophobic, lipoidal intercellular spaces also contain water-soluble proteases and glycosidases that regulate gradients across the stratum corneum. The complexity of the stratum corneum seems all the more remarkable when it is realized that the pH gradient across the stratum corneum ranges from about 7 at the bottom to about 5 at the top, a one-hundred–fold difference, closely regulated to permit activation of different enzymes concerned with different biochemical activities at various levels within the stratum corneum (17).

The "bricks" too are not a complete description. The corneocytes are actually bounded and encased by well-defined thick, tough, cornified envelopes. The chemical complexity of these rigid cornified envelopes is simply astounding. These include such unfamiliar names as involucrin, loricin, cornatin, cystatin A, elastin, fillagrin, endoplakin, sciellin, annexin, plasminogen activator, and so on. The list of unpronounceable proteins is still growing! How these interact to provide stability and strength to individual corneocytes is under intense investigation. In any event, budding corneobiologists are hereby cautioned that this is not a field for dilettantes.

The brick and mortar model, as useful as it has been, should be regarded only as a graphic that does not do justice to the extraordinarily complex architecture and heterogeneity of the stratum corneum. The reports by Swartzendruber et al. on the lipid biochemistry of the stratum corneum further emphasizes this point. They found that extensive extraction of the intercellular lipids leaves behind a thin lucent band made up of tightly packed hydroxy-acylsphingosine molecules linked to proteins on the corneocyte surface (18). Thus, each corneocyte envelope is bounded by its own lipid envelope that not only reinforces the cohesion between corneocytes, but also provides a barrier to passage of water into and/or out of the corneocyte.

These and other ingenious studies reveal that the stratum corneum is anything but a static structure. Instead, it is now seen as a plastic, dynamic tissue that can adaptively respond in a variety of ways to the external environment. The work of Menon and Elias vividly portrays this. They applied hydrophilic and hydrophobic substances under basal conditions as well as after various physical and chemical penetration enhancers. They observed that dilatations of the intercellular spaces occurred at regular intervals in normal stratum corneum forming what they called "lacunae." After the imposition of various penetration enhancers, these interspersed lacunae fused to form a continuous network of widened spaces (19). Dermatologists had earlier observed that water itself was a penetration enhancer. Topical medicaments, such as corticosteroids, penetrate more readily through hydrated tissue, markedly enhancing therapeutic efficacy. Menon and Elias' ingenious studies explained why occlusive dressings were a practical means of opening up the horny layer barrier. Warner et al. too showed that exposure to water alone in vitro could disrupt the intercellular bilaminar membranes, creating widened lacunae through which hydrophilic and hydrophobic substances could diffuse more readily (20). To top it all off, physical chemists in the Netherlands showed that hydration created water pools in the intercellular domains of the stratum corneum, especially in the outermost desquamating region (21).

Concepts of the ultrastructural organization of the stratum corneum are constantly changing. For example, high-pressure cryofixation, which avoids artifacts induced by the customary method of embedding tissue in plastic for electron microscopy, shows that the peripheral apical surfaces of corneocytes have vellus-like projections into the undersurface of the corneocyte above, forming hooks or clumps that further add to the great mechanical strength of the horny layer; moreover, cyrofixation followed by low-temperature embedding yields surprising new ultrastructural findings, which again have obliged us to take another look at the images that conventional methods have presented to us. They found that the distribution of organelles within keratinocytes was not uniform as we had thought, but existed in "microdomains" or clusters (22). Once again, fixation artifacts have fooled us. Perhaps, we should no longer be surprised by the continuous revelations made possible by newer more powerful techniques.

CODA

In my 1954 paper, which established that the horny layer was a tissue made up of corneocytes, I could not have dreamed of the spectacular advances that have been brought to light by an international school of corneobiologists. I did not go any further than asserting that the stratum was a cellular barrier, the end product of a viable epidermis whose raison d'etre was to produce the dead stratum corneum. I did not have the vision to foresee that the stratum corneum would become very much alive, subserving a variety of important functions that include being: a biosensor of environmental changes; a reservoir of drugs and chemicals, and innate molecules such as pro-inflammatory cytokines; a primary immunologic defense system against bacterial, viral, and fungal infections; a regulator of homeostatic restoration after disruption by disease or exogenous insults; the producer of the natural moisturizing factor, which keeps the stratum corneum soft, smooth, supple, and hydrated against a dry environment in cold, northern climates; and still others (21).

I cite this multiplicity of functions as a preface to a treatise I am now writing on corneotherapy, a novel approach to the treatment of chronic dermatoses, focusing on repair and reinforcement of these dysfunctional stratum corneums as a primary therapeutic target. This concept has already been presaged by Elias in what he calls "outside-in" therapy, in contrast to traditional inside-out interventions based on anti-inflammatory topical drugs (14).

This volume, edited by Maestro Elias, is a magnum opus, the first of its kind, which brings us completely up to date on every aspect of the structure and function of the stratum corneum in health and disease. For medical professionals, this text portrays a unique version of the pathophysiology of skin disease, and is a required reading for those charged with preventing, moderating, and curing the many hundreds of skin disorders that undermine good health and degrade the quality of life.

REFERENCES

1. Kitron N, Thewalt JL. Hypothesis: the epidermal permeability barrier is a porous medium. Acta Derm Venereol 2000; 208:12.
2. Rothman S. Physiology and Biochemistry of Skin. Chicago, IL: University of Chicago Press, 1954:64.
3. Kligman AM. The biology of the stratum corneum. In: Montagna W, ed. The Epidermis. New York: Academic Press Inc., 1964.
4. Szakall A. Experimentelle daten zus klärung der funktion der wasser barrier in epidermis des lebinden. Menschen-Berufsdermatosen 1958; 6:171.
5. Winsor T, Burch GE. Rate of invisible perspiration through living and dead stratum corneum. Arch Int Med 1944; 74:437.
6. Monash H. Location of the superficial barrier to skin penetration. J Invest Derm 1957; 29:367.
7. Malkinson FD. Studies of the percutaneous absorption of C14 labeled steroid by use of the gas flow cell. J Invest Derm 1958; 31:19.
8. Kligman AM, Christophers E. Preparation of isolated sheets of human stratum corneum. Arch Dermatol 1964; 88:702.
9. Matoltsy AG, Schuagei II, Matolsty MN. Observations on regeneration of the skin barrier. J Invest Derm 1962; 38:251.
10. Christophers E, Kligman AM. Visualization of the cell layers of the stratum corneum. J Invest Derm 1964; 42:407.
11. Mackenzie IC, Zimmerman K, Peterson L. The pattern of cellular organization of human epidermis. J Invest Derm 1981; 76:459.
12. Elias PM, Menon GK. Structural and lipid biochemical correlates of the epidermal permeability barrier. Adv Lipid Res 1991; 24:1.
13. Schueplein RJ, Blank IH. Permeability of the skin. Physiol Rev 1971; 51:702.
14. Williams ML, Elias PM. From basket-weave to barrier. Arch Dermatol 1993; 129:626.
15. Elias PM, Menon GK. Structural and lipid biochemical correlates of the epidermal permeability barrier. Adv Lipid Res 1991; 1:24.
16. Menon GK, Williams ML, Ghadially R, Elias PM. Lamellar bodies as delivery systems of hydrolytic enzymes: implications for normal cohesion and abnormal desquamation. Br J Dermatol 1992; 126:337.
17. Uhman H, Vahlquest A. In vivo studies concerning a pH gradient in human stratum corneum. Acta Derm Venereol 1994; 74:375.

18. Swartzendruber DC, Wertz DW, Madison MD, Downing DT. Evidence that the corneocyte envelope has a chemically bound lipid envelope. J Invest Derm 1987; 88:709.
19. Menon GK, Elias PM. Morphologic basis for a pore-pathway in mammalian stratum corneum. Skin Pharmacol 1997; 10:235.
20. Warner RR, Boissy YL, Spears MJ, Marshall JL, Stone RJ. Water disrupts the stratum corneum lipid lamellae: damage is similar to surfactants. J Invest Derm 1999; 113:966.
21. Egelrud T. Desquamation. In: Loden M, Maibach HI, eds. Dry Skin and Moisturizers. New York: CRC Press, Chapter 9, 2000.
22. Pfeiffer S, Vielhaber G, Vieteke J, Wittern KP, Hentz V, Wepf R. High pressure freezing provides new information on human epidermis. Simultaneous protein antigen and lamellar lipid structure preservation. J Invest Derm 2000; 114:1030.

4

The Epidermal Permeability Barrier: From Saran® Wrap to Biosensor

Peter M. Elias

Dermatology Service, VA Medical Center, and Department of Dermatology, University of California, San Francisco, California, U.S.A.

INTRODUCTION

Perhaps no tissue is so *physically* maligned by processing for light/electron microscopy as is the stratum corneum (SC). To further complicate matters, no tissue of such critical importance for survival has been so *intellectually* maligned as well. Because routine microscopic images of normal SC depict loosely attached corneocytes ("basket-weave pattern"), until the 1960s the barrier was thought to reside not in the SC but rather in the outer stratum granulosum (SG) (Table 1). The key breakthroughs came from Albert M. Kligman's group (Chap. 3), who found isolated SC to be not friable, but rather extremely durable (1), and from the work of Irvin Blank and Robert Scheuplein in Thomas Fitzpatrick's department at Harvard, who further demonstrated the highly impermeable nature of the SC (2,3). Because Blank and Scheuplein found the water-transport characteristics of human SC to be similar to those of a plastic wrap, the SC soon was analogized to a sheet of plastic or "Saran®" wrap (Table 1). According to this model, which still dominates the world view of many skin biophysicists and physical chemists, hydrophilic and lipophilic molecules traverse a uniform SC "membrane" via a transcellular route without regard to tissue architecture or metabolic activity (2). Accordingly, percutaneous penetration is determined by the chemical characteristics of the penetrating molecule, as well as by the diffusion path-length across the SC (thickness of the membrane), as embodied in Fick's law (3). Although common sense alone (e.g., the hyperpermeability of the thickened SC of the palms and soles to water) immediately invalidates the "plastic wrap" model, the seminal work of Blank and Scheuplein nevertheless established the importance of the SC as the critical tissue determinant of the cutaneous permeability barrier. Perhaps of greater importance is that it spawned an entirely new industry devoted to transdermal drug delivery.

Developments after 1970 showed that the plastic wrap model did justice neither to the structural heterogeneity nor to the metabolic activity of the SC. Frozen sections of the SC revealed the compression of corneocytes into exquisite geometric stacks of interlocking tetracaidodecahedra (24-sided cells) (1,4). Frozen sections and

25

Table 1 Evolving Concepts of Stratum Corneum

Outdated
Disorganized; no functional significance ("basket-weave")
Homogenous film ("Saran® wrap")
Current
Two-compartment organization ("bricks and mortar")
Microheterogeneity within extracellular spaces ("there's more to the mortar than lipid")
Persistent metabolic activity (dynamic changes in cytosol, cornified envelope, and interstices
 from inner to outer SC)
Homeostatic links to the nucleated cell layers (barrier function regulates epidermal DNA and
 lipid synthesis)
Pathophysiologic links to deeper skin layers (barrier abrogation initiates epidermal
 hyperplasia and inflammation)
Stratum corneum as a biosensor (changes in external humidity alone regulate proteolysis of
 filaggrin, epidermal DNA/lipid synthesis, and initiation of inflammation)

freeze-fracture images revealed lipid stacks, localized to the intercellular spaces (5),
which were shown to derive from the secreted contents of epidermal lamellar or
Odland bodies (George Odland first realized the novelty and potential importance
of this organelle, previously thought to be an effete mitochondrion) (6). Lipid biochemistry, coupled with lipid histochemistry, revealed a unique, extracellular, extremely hydrophobic, membrane system devoid of phospholipids, relying instead
on an equimolar mixture of ceramides, cholesterol, and non-essential free fatty acids
to form extracellular membranes (7,8), which are riveted into parallel structures by
ω-hydroxy ceramides bearing the esterified essential fatty acid, linoleic acid (acylceramides) (9). Hence, the still-current, two-compartment "bricks and mortar" model
of the SC (Table 1).

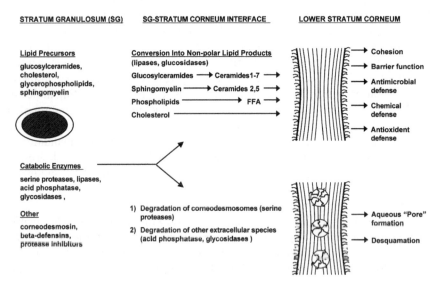

Figure 1 Lamellar body secretion dictates localization of multiple functions to the extracellular compartment.

Table 2 Enzymatic Contents of Epidermal Lamellar Bodies

Enzymes	Function
Lipid hydrolases[a]	
β-Glucocerebrosidase[b]	Converts glycosylceramides to ceramides
Acidic asphingomyelinase	Converts sphingomyelin to ceramides
Secretory phospholipase A2 (Group I)[b]	Converts phospholipids to free fatty acids
Acidic lipase	? Deacylates ω-esterified ceramides
Proteases	
SC chymotryptic enzyme (SCCE)	Degrades corneodesmosomes; activates IL-1β
Aspartate proteases (e.g., Cathepsin L)	Desquamation
Glycosidases	? Desquamation
Acid phosphatase	Unknown
Protease inhibitors[c]	
Serine protease inhibitors (SKALP)	Desquamation, ? Cytokine activation
Cysteine protease inhibitors	Desquamation

[a]Recent studies suggest that an additional lipid hydrolase, steroid sulfatase, is also present.
[b]Mucosal epithelia and perhaps cetacean epidermis, display reduced β-glycocerebrosidase and secretory phospholipase.
[c]Recent studies have shown that additional serine protease inhibitor, LEKTI, is present.

Awareness that the lamellar body is rich in hydrolytic enzymes initially led to speculation that this organelle could be a modified lysosome, whose primary function lay in desquamation (Fig. 1 and Table 2) (9,10). Indeed, that suspicion has been borne out by recent studies, which have demonstrated a role for lamellar body–derived enzymes (and structural proteins) in desquamation (Chap. 11). Yet, while the lamellar body may be in the lysosomal lineage, it is also clearly a secretory organelle (11). Even more important than its role in desquamation is its role in the delivery to the SC interstices of a family of lipid hydrolases, which metabolize polar lipid precursors (cholesterol sulfate, phospholipids, sphingomyelin, and glucosylceramides) into their more non-polar products, which together form the extracellular lamellar membrane system (12). This critical sequence, together called "lipid processing" (Chap. 15), also provides powerful evidence that the SC is not metabolically inert, but possesses several types of metabolic activity (Table 3). In fact, each SC subcellular compartment, i.e., corneocyte

Table 3 Examples of Metabolic Activity in Stratum Corneum

Corneocyte cytosol
  Filaggrin catabolism to amino acids and their deiminated products
Cornified envelope
  Complete degradation of plasma membrane
  Progressive transglutaminase-mediated cross-linking of cornified envelope
  Covalent attachment of hydroxyceramide enriched-external envelope (the corneocyte lipid envelope)
Extracellular processing
  Proteolysis of desmosomes (formation of "pore pathway")
  Catabolism of lamellar body–derived polar lipids:
      Secretory phospholipase(s)
      β-Glucocerebrosidase
      Steroid sulfatase
      Acidic sphingomyelinase

cytosol, cornified envelope, and extracellular domains, contains its own array of metabolic activities. Finally, recent studies have shown that changes in extracellular acidity regulate the extracellular, enzymatic processes that lead to both barrier formation (13,14) and desquamation (Chap. 14).

Not only lipids, but also specialized junctional structures called corneodesmosomes (CDs) localize to SC intercellular domains. While these simplified junctions lack many of the proteins of their counterparts in lower epidermal layers, they are rich in desmoglein 1 (DSGl), desmocollin 1 (DSCl), and a novel protein, corneodesmosin, which appears to coat their external surfaces by making CDs initially resistant to proteolysis (15). However, CDs and their constituent proteins eventually succumb to the relentless attack of secreted proteases (primarily serine, but also aspartate and thiol proteases), which degrade not only corneodesmosin, but also DSG1 and DSC1 (16,17). Many of the key participants in SC cohesion/desquamation, including corneodesmosin, the serine protease, SC chymotryptic (SCCE) and other serine, aspartate, and cysteine proteases, and their respective inhibitors, as well as glycosidases, whose specific roles are less well-understood, also are lamellar body products (Fig. 1, Table 2). Interestingly, like every known structure in the SC, even the lacunae that result from CD degradation mediate a key function; i.e., they form an aqueous, expansile "pore" penetration pathway that becomes interconnected, bypassing both corneocytes and adjacent lamellar bilayers (18).

Recent studies suggest that both the initial cohesion and the ultimate desquamation of corneocytes from the SC surface may be orchestrated by localized changes in pH, which selectively activate different classes of extracellular proteases in a pH-dependent fashion (Chap. 14). The most rigorously studied participants are the epidermis-specific serine proteases, the SCCE and SC tryptic (SCTE) enzymes, kallikreins 7 and 5, respectively (17), which both exhibit neutral-to-alkaline pH optima. Because an acidic pH dominates in normal SC, we suspect that two other protease family members, thiol (cysteine) proteases (cathepsin L2) and an aspartate protease, cathepsin D (Cath D) (16,19), mediate desquamation in the outer layers of the normal SC, while SCCE/SCTE could initiate CD degradation in the inner layers of the normal SC, as well as in dermatitic skin, where a neutral pH predominates at all SC levels. Thus, permeability barrier homeostasis and cohesion/desquamation are both exquisitely programmed processes that localize to the SC interstices and are pH-dependent.

The SC cytosol is also far from inert. A cascade of hydrolytic and deiminating enzymes that localize to the corneocyte cytosol have been linked to several key SC functions, including SC hydration, UV filtration, and UV-induced immunosuppression, favoring skin cancer development, as well as possibly both antimicrobial activity and cytokine activation. The filaggrin–histidine–urocanic acid (UCA) pathway generates not only critical humectants, but also the H^+ donor, UCA, which could mediate one or more of the pH-dependent functions (Chap. 9, 24) (20,21). Importantly, the putative aspartate protease (cathepsin E) that initiates this cascade is inversely regulated by changes in external humidity (20). Thus, the capacity of the corneocyte to hydrate above the stratum compactum is largely dependent upon the activation of this pathway in response to a reduction in external humidity. Yet, several other mechanisms, e.g., glycine deimination to pyrrolidone carboxylic acid, arginine deimination to citrulline by arginase, and glycerol generation from sebaceous gland–derived glycerol (22), also contribute to the hydration of the corneocyte cytosol.

The most dynamic view of the SC depicts this tissue as an exquisite biosensor (Table 1). In response to barrier abrogation, external injury, altered pH, or even

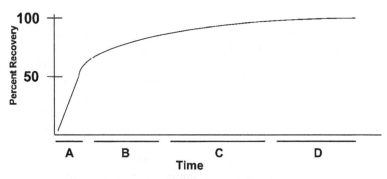

A: Secretion of pre-formed pool of lamellar bodies
B: Increased cholesterol/fatty acid synthesis
   Accelerated lamellar body formation/secretion
C: Increased ceramide synthesis
   Increased glucosylceramide processing
D: Increased DNA synthesis

Figure 2 The cutaneous stress test: multiple applications in dermatologic settings.

extremes of humidity alone, the SC initiates a set of homeostatic responses that rapidly adjust permeability barrier status (23). The rate of barrier recovery after acute abrogations constitutes a type of cutaneous stress test ("Cutaneous Treadmill Exam"), which was deployed initially to discern a sequence of metabolic processes such as increased lipid synthesis, lamellar body production/secretion, DNA synthesis, and lipid processing, linked specifically to the maintenance of barrier function (Fig. 2) (23). Subsequently, the cutaneous stress test has also been deployed (i) to identify the underlying pathology in situations, such as for aged skin (24), where the basal function was normal; (ii) in the development and comparison of various "barrier repair" preparations (25); and (iii) to identify metabolic approaches that enhance transdermal drug delivery (26) (Fig. 2).

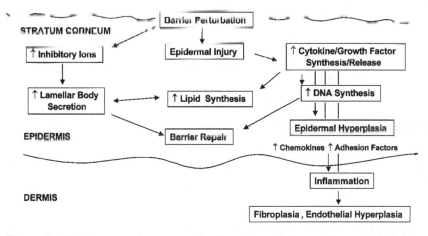

Figure 3 Cytokine cascade can provoke downstream inflammation, endothelial hyperplasia, and fibrosis.

The "biosensor" concept implies the existence of signaling mechanisms between the SC and the nucleated cell layers, and recent studies have identified both extra- and intracellular processes that are stimulated by barrier abrogation. One of the best-characterized classes of extracellular signaling molecules are primary cytokines, principally IL-1α and -β, released in a non–energy-dependent fashion from their pre-formed pools in corneocytes subsequent to barrier abrogation (27), which then appear to regulate downstream processes such as keratinocyte proliferation and lipid synthesis (23). A second, unrelated class of extracellular signals comprises alterations in ion concentrations, particularly that of calcium, in the outer epidermis. Fluctuations in calcium regulate both lamellar body secretion (28) and epidermal differentiation (29).

It is worth emphasizing again that the primary purpose of all these signaling events is to upregulate metabolic processes that normalize permeability barrier status, the principal function of the skin, allowing life in a terrestrial environment. But permeability barrier function is not the sole function of the SC, and as described extensively and eloquently elsewhere in this volume, the SC mediates a host of critical defensive functions, which are often linked and/or co-regulated. Finally, the biosensor concept, with its signal cascade, can be a cruel, two-edged sword. If sustained, the signals that stimulate homeostatic responses ultimately can initiate a "cytokine cascade" that leads to inflammation and epidermal hyperplasia (23) (Fig. 3).

REFERENCES

1. Christophers E, Kligman AM. Visualization of the cell layers of the stratum corneum. J Invest Dermatol 1964; 42:407–409.
2. Blank IH. Transport across the stratum corneum. Toxicol Appl Pharmacol 1969; 3(suppl):23–29.
3. Scheuplein RJ, Blank IH. Permeability of the skin. Physiol Rev 1971; 51:702–747.
4. Menton DN, Eisen AZ. Structure and organization of mammalian stratum corneum. J Ultrastruct Res 1971; 35:247–264.
5. Elias PM, Friend DS. The permeability barrier in mammalian epidermis. J Cell Biol 1975; 65:180–191.
6. Odland G, Reed T. Epidermis. In: Zelickson A, ed. Ultrastructure of Normal and Abnormal Skin. Philadelphia: Lea & Febiger, 1967:54–75.
7. Elias PM, Brown BE, Fritsch P, Goerke J, Gray GM, White RJ. Localization and composition of lipids in neonatal mouse stratum granulosum and stratum corneum. J Invest Dermatol 1979; 73:339–348.
8. Gray GM, Yardley HJ. Different populations of pig epidermal cells: isolation and lipid composition. J Lipid Res 1975; 16:441–447.
9. Wertz PW, Downing DT. Covalently bound omega-hydroxyacylsphingosine in the stratum corneum. Biochem Biophys Acta 1987; 917:108–111.
10. Wolff K, Holubar K. Keratinosomes as epidermal lysosomes. Arch Klin Exp Dermatol 1967; 231:1–19.
11. Elias PM, Cullander C, Mauro T, Rassner U, Komuves L, Brown BE, Menon GK. The secretory granular cell: the outermost granular cell as a specialized secretory cell. J Invest Dermatol Symp Proc 1998; 3:87–100.
12. Elias PM, Menon GK. Structural and lipid biochemical correlates of the epidermal permeability barrier. Adv Lipid Res 1991; 24:1–26.
13. Fluhr JW, Kao J, Jain M, Ahn SK, Feingold KR, Elias PM. Generation of free fatty acids from phospholipids regulates stratum corneum acidification and integrity. J Invest Dermatol 2001; 117:44–51.

14. Behne MJ, Meyer JW, Hanson KM, Barry NP, Murata S, Crumrine D, Clegg RW, Gratton E, Holleran WM, Elias PM, Mauro TM. NHE1 regulates the stratum corneum permeability barrier homeostasis. Microenvironment acidification assessed with fluorescence lifetime imaging. J Biol Chem 2002; 277:47399–47406.
15. Lundstrom A, Serre G, Haftek M, Egelrud T. Evidence for a role of corneodesmosin, a protein which may serve to modify desmosomes during cornification, in stratum corneum cell cohesion and desquamation. Arch Dermatol Res 1994; 286:369–375.
16. Horikoshi T, Igarashi S, Uchiwa H, Brysk H, Brysk MM. Role of endogenous cathepsin D-like and chymotrypsin-like proteolysis in human epidermal desquamation. Br J Dermatol, 1999; 141:453–459.
17. Eckholm IE, Brattsand M, Egelrud T. Stratum corneum tyrptic enzyme in normal epidermis: a missing link in the desquamation process. J Invest Dermatol 2000; 114:56–63.
18. Menon GK, Elias PM. Morphologic basis for a pore-pathway in mammalian stratum corneum. Skin Pharmacol 1997; 10:235–246.
19. Bernard D, Mehul B, Thomas-Collignon A, Simonetti L, Remy V, Bernard MA, Schmidt R. Analysis of proteins with caseinolytic activity in a human stratum corneum extract revealed a yet unidentified cysteine protease and identified the so-called "stratum corneum thiol protease" as cathepsin l2. J Invest Dermatol 2003; 120:592–600.
20. Scott IR, Harding CR. Filaggrin breakdown to water binding compounds during development of the rat stratum corneum is controlled by the water activity of the environment. Dev Biol 1986; 115:84–92.
21. Krien P, Kermici M. Evidence for the existence of a self-regulated enzymatic process within human stratum corneum—an unexpected role for urocanic acid. J Invest Dermatol 2000; 115:414–420.
22. Fluhr JW, Mao-Qiang M, Brown BE, Wertz PW, Crumrine D, Sundberg JP, Feingold KR, Elias PM. Glycerol regulates stratum corneum hydration in sebaceous gland deficient (asebia) mice. J Invest Dermatol 2003; 120:728–737.
23. Elias PM, Wood LC, Feingold KR. Epidermal pathogenesis of inflammatory dermatoses. Am J Contact Dermatol 1999; 10:119–126.
24. Ghadially R, Brown BE, Sequeira-Martin SM, Feingold KR, Elias PM. The aged epidermal permeability barrier. Structural, functional, and lipid biochemical abnormalities in humans and a senescent murine model. J Clin Invest 1995; 95:2281–2290.
25. Mao-Qiang M, Brown BE, Wu-Pong S, Feingold KR, Elias PM. Exogenous nonphysiologic vs. physiologic lipids. Divergent mechanisms for correction of permeability barrier dysfunction. Arch Dermatol, 1995; 131:809–816.
26. Elias PM, Tsai J, Menon GK, Holleran WM, Feingold KR. The potential of metabolic interventions to enhance transdermal drug delivery. J Investig Dermatol Symp Proc 2002; 7:79–85.
27. Wood LC, Elias PM, Calhoun C, Tsai JC, Grunfeld C, Feingold KR. Barrier disruption stimulates interleukin-1 alpha expression and release from a pre-formed pool in murine epidermis. J Invest Dermatol 1996; 106:397–403.
28. Menon GK, Price LF, Bommannan B, Elias PM, Feingold KR. Selective obliteration of the epidermal calcium gradient leads to enhanced lamellar body secretion. J Invest Dermatol 1994; 102:789–795.
29. Elias PM, Ahn SK, Denda M, Brown BE, Crumrine D, Kimutai LK, Komuves L, Lee SH, Feingold KR. Modulations in epidermal calcium regulate the expression of differentiation-specific markers. J Invest Dermatol 2002; 119:1128–1136.

5

Biochemistry of Human Stratum Corneum Lipids

Philip W. Wertz

Dows Institute, University of Iowa, Iowa City, Iowa, U.S.A.

COMPOSITION OF HUMAN STRATUM CORNEUM LIPIDS

The intercellular lipids of the human stratum corneum (SC) are unique in composition and quite different from the lipids found in most biological membranes (1).

History

Early evidence indicating a significant role for lipids in the barrier function of the skin came from experiments in which removal of lipids from the skin in vitro by extraction with organic solvents resulted in increased permeability (2). A more detailed understanding of the roles of membrane lipids in the formation and function of the epidermal barrier was based on electron microscopic observations made in the early 1970s (3,4). In transmission electron micrographs, lamellar granules were shown to extrude their membranous contents into the intercellular space at the boundary between the granular layer and the SC, and the freeze–fracture technique revealed, for the first time, that the intercellular spaces of the SC contain broad, multiple membranous structures (5). In addition, the use of water-soluble tracers to monitor the movement of water in the skin by electron microscopy demonstrated that the entire SC was essentially water impermeable (3,4). A major finding that emerged from this body of work was that molecules traversing the SC do so by passive diffusion through the intercellular spaces. This was most clearly indicated by an experiment in which *n*-butanol was allowed to diffuse across the tissue prior to exposure to osmium vapor, which reacts with the butanol and precipitates in situ (6).

Major Components

The major lipids of the human SC are ceramides, cholesterol, and fatty acids, comprising approximately 50%, 25%, and 10% of the total lipid mass, respectively (7). From early work of Long (8) on cow snout epidermis and of Kooyman (9) on human palmar and plantar epidermis, it was recognized that the nature of the polar lipid components of the SC lipids differs markedly from that of the phospholipids in the viable portion of the epidermis. The inner epidermis contained high levels of phospholipids, but the phospholipids were replaced by cholesterol, fatty acids, and other neutral lipids as the SC was approached. Unfortunately, due to the specialized nature of the epidermis used in these early studies it was not certain that the results would generally apply to other regions of the skin. In 1965, Nicolaides identified ceramide as a quantitatively significant polar SC lipid (10). Work with a porcine model (1,11), human epidermis from different anatomic sites (1,12), and epidermal cysts (13) established that cholesterol, fatty acids, and ceramides are the major human SC lipids.

The early findings of Nicolaides went largely unappreciated until the mid-1970s and the efforts of Gray and Yardley (1,11) (reviewed in Ref. 14). These workers published a complete lipid class composition of human SC (1,14) and demonstrated that the ceramides are structurally heterogenous (15). They identified normal and α-hydroxyacids, sphingosine and phytosphingosine among the ceramide components. They also showed that there was a great deal of similarity between human and porcine SC lipids.

Subsequently, the detailed structures of the porcine ceramides were determined (16), and all of the same structural types were found among the human SC lipids (13,17). However, new ceramides continue to be discovered (18–20). Representative chemical structures of the known human SC ceramides are summarized in Figure 1. In addition to the fatty acid and long-chain base components originally identified by Gray and White (21), the human ceramides include ω-hydroxyacids and 6-hydroxysphingosine as building blocks. All combinations of sphingosine,

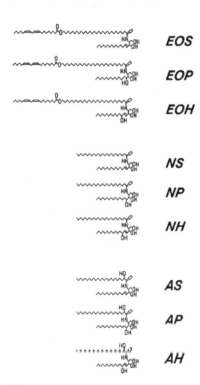

EOS

EOP

EOH

NS

NP

NH

AS

AP

AH

Figure 1 Representative chemical structures of the free ceramides from human stratum corneum.

phytosphingosine, and 6-hydroxysphingosine bearing amide-linked normal fatty acid, α-hydroxyacid, and ω-O-linoleoylfatty acid have been identified (20). This would seem to be all inclusive; however, the possibility of a future identification of yet another to date unresolved fatty acid or long-chain base cannot be ruled out.

Figure 1 also includes abbreviations for ceramide structures as proposed by Motta et al. (22). This system is much more useful than the earlier identification of ceramides by fraction number (16). The Motta system overcomes several potentially confusing problems: 1. Two of the human ceramides are not generally resolved on thin-layer chromatograms (20). 2. Different development regimens used in different laboratories can result in different numbers of chromatographic fractions. 3. Common animal models contain different numbers of ceramide fractions compared to human. Within this system, the presence of normal fatty acid, α-hydroxyacid, or ω-hydroxyacids is designated by N, A, or O, respectively. Sphingosine, phytosphingosine, and 6-hydroxysphingosine are indicated by S, P, and H, respectively, and the presence of ester-linked fatty acid is indicated by the prefix E.

The linoleate- and ω-hydroxyacid–containing acylceramides (CER EOS, CER EOH, and CER EOP) are the most unusual of the SC ceramides (16,18,20). In each case the ω-hydroxyacids are 30–34 carbons in length, and the most abundant ester-linked fatty acid is linoleic acid (20). It has been shown that extracted SC lipids can reconstitute lamellae with the same pattern of organization seen in native SC; however, if CER EOS is removed from the lipid mixture, only simple bilayers are generated (23). In essential fatty acid deficiency, oleate replaces linoleate in CER EOS, and this is accompanied by a decreased barrier function (24). While it seems likely that the same fatty acid substitution occurs with CER EOH and CER EOP, there are presently no data on this point. There is essentially no information on the possible functional roles or relative significance of CER EOH and CER EOP.

Cholesterol is the only major sterol in human SC (1). This is also true of the porcine model system (1) but not of rodent models, where cholest-7-ene-3-β-ol is also present in significant amounts (1). As phospholipids are being degraded in the final stages of the keratinization process, the remaining unsaturated fatty acids, mostly oleic acid, become transferred to cholestrol to produce cholesteryl esters (13). It has been suggested that these unsaturated cholesteryl esters separate into liquid phase pockets within the intercellular space of the SC and that this provides a mechanism for keeping unsaturated fatty acids out of the lamellar phase domains (25).

The free fatty acids in human SC are predominantly straight-chain saturated species ranging from 14 to 28 carbons in length (7). They are mainly 20 carbons and longer, with the 22- and 24-carbon entities being the most abundant. The fatty acids are the only ionizable major lipids in human SC. As such, they may be necessary for the formation of lamellae.

Minor Components

Cholesterol sulfate is a minor SC lipid that has been implicated in the regulation of the desquamation process (26–29). It has been demonstrated both with mouse ear skin organ cultures (26) and with human skin in vivo (27) that hydrolysis of cholesterol sulfate accompanies cell shedding. Moreover, in the genetic disease recessive X-linked ichthyosis, where sterol sulfatase is defective, desquamation does not proceed normally (28,29). The skin can become very scaly. More recently, it has been shown that cholesterol sulfate can inhibit the serine proteases that normally degrade desmosomal proteins as part of the desquamation process (30). Recessive X-linked ichthyosis is discussed in greater detail in Chapter 27.

Another important but minor type of lipids in the SC are the free long-chain bases (31). These are thought to be released through the action of ceramidases on ceramides (32). Both an acid ceramidase and an alkaline ceramidase have been detected, and there appears to be a sphingosine gradient across the epidermis. This gradient could be important for providing a potent antimicrobial to the skin surface (33) and, through the ability of sphingosine to inhibit protein kinase C, for regulating of the keratinization process (34).

Contaminants

When working with human skin, other than that from the palmar and plantar regions, sebaceous lipids are always present (35). The major uniquely sebaceous lipids present at the human skin surface are squalene, wax esters, and triglycerides. Due to partial hydrolysis of sebaceous triglycerides by lipases of both bacterial and epidermal origin, sebaceous fatty acids will contribute to the fatty acid fraction. The sebaceous fatty acids are mainly shorter than 20 carbons in length, while the SC fatty acids are mainly 20 carbons long and longer. This difference can be used to distinguish sebaceous from SC fatty acids by gas chromatographic analysis of the methyl esters. The cholesterol and cholesterol ester fractions are also of mixed epidermal and sebaceous origin. In addition, subcutaneous fat is very fluid, and the SC surface of excised human skin is invariably contaminated with large amounts of subcutaneous triglycerides. Like the sebaceous triglycerides, the subcutaneous triglycerides can undergo time-dependent hydrolysis to release fatty acids. Finally, various contaminants including hydrocarbons can be present on the skin surface as a result of the use of emollients and cosmetic products.

Covalently Bound Lipids

Covalently bound lipids were first detected in porcine epidermal SC (36,37), and were subsequently found in human tissue (38). The principal covalently bound lipids are ω-hydroxyceramides that appear to be derived from the analogous acylceramides. They are attached to the outer surface of the cornified envelope through ester linkages that may be generated through the action of transglutaminase 1 (39). The first covalently bound hydroxyceramide to be identified in human SC was ω-hydroxyacylsphingosine, which is also the principal covalently bound lipid in porcine SC (37,38). However, in the human there was a second hydroxyceramide that subsequently proved to be ω-hydroxyacyl-6-hydroxysphingosine (18). By analogy with the acylceramides, it can be anticipated that one of the minor unidentified components among the human covalently bound lipids is probably ω-hydroxyacylphytosphingosine. In addition to the ω-hydroxyceramides, there are small proportions of covalently bound fatty acids and ω-hydroxyacids among the bound lipids in human SC (38). The covalently attached ω-hydroxyacids are likely generated through the action of a ceramidase on covalently bound ω-hydroxyceramides. This action would also release free sphingosine, which is both a potent inhibitor of protein kinase C and a broad acting antimicrobial. This system for the generation of a free long-chain base could be significant in the regulation of the keratinization process through the inhibition of protein kinase C. It could also, through the antimicrobial properties of sphingosine, be part of the innate immune system of the skin.

BIOSYNTHETIC PATHWAYS

Cholesterol

Basal keratinocytes derive some of their cholesterol from the circulation by means of plasma membrane–associated LDL receptors (40); however, the cholesterol that accumulates with increasing differentiation is synthesized from acetate de novo (41). The main intermediates in the cholesterol biosynthetic pathway are summarized in Figure 2 (42). The first part of the pathway involves the conversion of three molecules of acetyl-CoA into one β-hydroxymethylglutaryl CoA (HMG-CoA). The next step requires two molecules of NADPH to reduce one HMG-CoA to mevalonate-CoA. This is the rate-limiting step in cholesterol biosynthesis and is catalyzed by HMG-CoA reductase. The CoA thioester is then hydrolyzed to release free mevalonic acid, which is then phosphorylated at the expense of two ATPs to produce 5-pyrophospomevalonic acid. An additional phosphorylation produces an unstable intermediate which spontaneously releases one phosphate group and CO_2 yielding 3-isopentenylpyrophosphate. This metabolite equilibrates with its isomer, 3,3'-dimethylallyl pyrophosphate. These two isomers undergo condensation with the release of pyrophosphate to form *trans, trans*-geranyl pyrophosphate. Another isoprenyl pyrophosphate is condensed with this metabolite, again with the loss of pyrophosphate, to produce *trans,trans*-farnesyl pyrophosphate, which equilibrates with

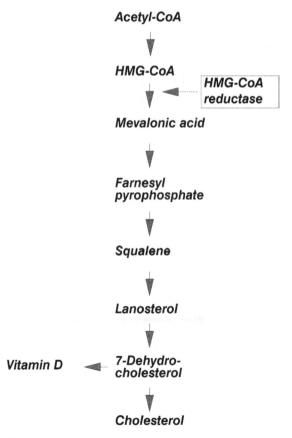

Figure 2 A summary of main steps in the biosynthetic pathway leading to cholesterol.

its isomer, nerolidol pyrophosphate. These two intermediates are reductively condensed in a step requiring NADPH and yielding squalene. Squalene is oxidized to squalene 2,3-epoxide, which is then converted into lanosterol, a tetracyclic triterpene. Conversion of lanosterol into cholesterol involves 19 discrete enzymatic steps. All of the enzymes involved in this conversion are membrane associated. One of the intermediates in this conversion, 7-dehydrocholesterol, is the precursor of vitamin D in the skin (43). The production of vitamin D from 7-dehydrocholesterol requires exposure to ultraviolet light and is non-enzymatic.

As is often the case with rate-limiting enzymes, HMG-CoA reductase is regulated by the state of phosphorylation (44). Phosphorylation inactivates the enzyme, while removal of phosphate activates it. Evidence in support of the concept that the messenger RNA level and phosphorylation status of HMG-CoA reductase are regulated by permeability barrier requirements, has been reviewed (45).

Fatty Acids

The main source of carbon for lipid synthesis appears to be acetate from the circulation (41). Acetate thiokinase converts acetate into acetyl-CoA at the expense of one ATP. Acetyl-CoA carboxylase, a biotin-dependent enzyme, converts acetyl-CoA into malonyl-CoA at the cost of one ATP (46). This conversion is the rate-limiting step in fatty acid synthesis. Acetate and malonate are transferred from the CoA thioesters to acyl carrier protein (ACP) in the cytosolic fatty acid synthetase complex. Basically, this complex condenses seven malonates and one acetate to produce palmitate, as indicated in Figure 3. One CO_2 is liberated and two NADPHs are consumed in each condensation step.

The palmitoyl group is either hydrolyzed from ACP, yielding free palmitic acid, or transferred to CoA to produce palmitoyl-CoA. Palmitoyl-CoA can be extended in length through the action of a fatty acid elongase system located within the endoplasmic reticulum (47). The ω-hydroxyacids found in the acylceramides are thought to be produced by a cytochrome p450–mediated hydroxylation of the methyl terminus of a fatty acid when it has been extended just enough to span the endoplasmic

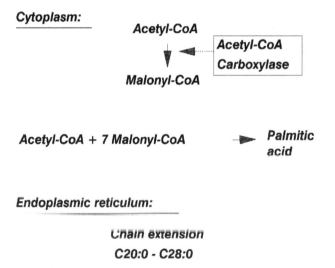

Figure 3 A summary of key features of fatty acid biosynthesis.

reticular membrane. Double bonds can also be introduced through the action of fatty acid desaturases, which are also located in the endoplasmic reticulum (48).

As was the case with HMG-CoA reductase, acetyl-CoA carboxylase is regulated by phosphorylation (49). The phosphorylated enzyme is inactive, while the dephosphorylated form is active. There is also allosteric activation by citrate.

Ceramides and Glucosylceramides

Serine palmitoyl transferase is the rate-determining enzyme in sphingolipid biosynthesis (50). It condenses serine with palmitoyl-CoA in an NADPH-dependent reaction to produce 3-ketodihydrosphingosine as shown in Figure 4. The ketone group in this intermediate is reduced to dihydrosphingosine by an NADPH-requiring reductase, and N-acylation then produces a ceramide. The dihydrosphingosine moiety of the simple ceramide can then be hydroxylated to produce a phytosphingosine-containing ceramide, or a trans double bond can be introduced between carbons 4 and 5 to yield a sphingosine-containing ceramide. A sphingosine-containing ceramide can in turn be hydroxylated to convert the base moiety into 6-hydroxysphingosine. Hydroxylation of the fatty acid moieties results in the production of α- and ω-hydroxyacids. The hydroxylation reactions that produce the more polar ceramides are vitamin C–dependent (51).

Ceramides are glycosylated in the Golgi apparatus. This is mediated by the enzyme ceramide glucosyltransferase, which utilizes UDP-glucose and is located on the cytosolic surface of this organelle. The Golgi apparatus is the likely site of lamellar granule origin.

After lipids and enzymes are extruded from the lamellar granules into the intercellular space, the phospholipids and the glycosylceramides are acted upon by the hydrolytic enzymes to produce the mature ceramide, cholesterol, and fatty acid mixture that constitutes the barrier. This enzymatic lipid processing is discussed in detail in Chapter 15.

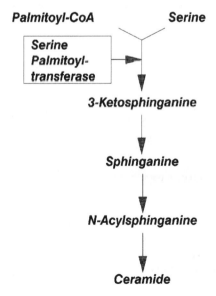

Figure 4 A summary of key steps in the biosynthesis of sphingolipids.

REFERENCES

1. Gray GM, Yardley HJ. Lipid compositions of cells isolated from pig, human, and rat epidermis. J Lipid Res 1975; 16:434–440.
2. Sweeney TM, Downing DT. The role of lipids in the epidermal barrier to water diffusion. J Invest Dermatol 1970; 55:135–140.
3. Squier CA. The permeability of keratinized and nonkeratinized oral epithelium to horse-radish peroxidase. J Ultrastruct Res 1973; 43:160–177.
4. Elias PM, Friend DS. The permeability barrier in mammalian epidermis. J Cell Biol 1975; 65:180–191.
5. Breatnach AS, Goodman T, Stolinski C, Gross M. Freeze–fracture replication of cells of stratum corneum of human epidermis. J Anat 1973; 114:65–81.
6. Namanic MK, Elias PM. In situ precipitation: a novel cytochemical technique for visualization of permeability pathways in mammalian stratum corneum. J Histochem Cytochem 1980; 28:573–578.
7. Wertz P, Norlen L. "Confidence intervals" for the "true" lipid composition of the human skin barrier? In: Forslind B, Lindberg M, eds. Skin, Hair, and Nails. Structure and Function. New York: Marcel Dekker Inc., 2003:85–106.
8. Long VJW. Variations in lipid composition at different depths in the cow snout epidermis. J Invest Dermatol 1970; 55:269–273.
9. Kooyman DJ. Lipids in the skin. Some changes in the lipids of the epidermis during the process of keratinization. Arch Dermatol Syph 1932; 25:444–450.
10. Nicolaides N. Skin lipids. II. Lipid class composition of samples from various species and anatomical sites. J Am Oil Chem Soc 1965; 42:691–702.
11. Gray GM, Yardley HJ. Different populations of pig epidermal cells: isolation and lipid composition. J Lipid Res 1975; 16:441–447.
12. Lampe MA, Burlingame AL, Whitney J, Williams ML, Brown BE, Roitman E, Elias PM. Human stratum corneum lipids: characterization and regional variation. J Lipid Res 1983; 24:120–130.
13. Wertz PW, Swartzendruber DC, Madison KC, Downing DT. The composition and morphology of epidermal cyst lipids. J Invest Dermatol 1987; 89:419–425.
14. Yardley HJ, Summerly R. Lipid composition and metabolism in normal and diseased epidermis. Pharmacol Ther 1981; 13:357–383.
15. Gray GM, White RJ. Glycosphingolipids and ceramides in human and pig epidermis. J Invest Dermatol 1978; 70:336–341.
16. Wertz PW, Downing DT. Ceramides of pig epidermis: structure determination. J Lipid Res 1983; 24:759–765.
17. Wertz PW, Miethke MC, Long SA, Strauss JS, Downing DT. The composition of the ceramides from human stratum corneum and from comedones. J Invest Dermatol 1985; 84:410–412.
18. Robson KJ, Stewart ME, Michelsen S, Lazo ND, Downing DT. 6-Hydroxy-4-sphengenine in human epidermal ceramides. J Lipid Res 1994; 35:2060–2068.
19. Stewart ME, Downing DT. A new 6-hydroxysph-4,5-sphingenine-containing ceramide in human skin. J Lipid Res 1999; 40:1434–1439.
20. Ponec M, Weerheim A, Lankhorst P, Wertz P. New acylceramide in native and reconstructed epidermis. J Invest Dermatol 2003; 120.581–588.
21. Gray GM, White RJ. Glycosphingolipids and ceramides in human and pig epidermis. J Invest Dermatol 1978; 70:336–341.
22. Motta SM, Monti M, Sesana S, Caputo R, Carelli S, Ghidoni R. Ceramide composition of the psoriatic scale. Biochim Biophys Acta 1993; 1182:147–151.
23. Kuempel D, Swartzendruber DC, Squier CA, Wertz PW. In vitro reconstitution of stratum corneum lipid lamellae. Biochim Biophys Acta 1998; 1372:135–140.

24. Melton JL, Wertz PW, Swartzendruber DC, Downing DT. Effects of essential fatty acid deficiency on O-acylsphingolipids and transepidermal water loss in young pigs. Biochim Biophys Acta 1987; 921:191–197.
25. Wertz PW. Lipids and barrier function of the skin. Acta Derm Venereol 2000; 208:1–5.
26. Ranasinghe AW, Wertz PW, Downing DT, Mackenzie IC. Lipid composition of cohesive and desquamated corneocytes from mouse ear skin. J Invest Dermatol 1986; 86:187–190.
27. Long SA, Wertz PW, Strauss JS, Downing DT. Human stratum corneum polar lipids and desquamation. Arch Dermatol Res 1985; 277:284–287.
28. Elias PM, Williams ML, Maloney ME, Bomifas JA, Brown BE, Grayson S, Epstein EH Jr. Stratum corneum lipids in disorders of cornification. Steroid sulfatase and cholesterol sulfate in normal desquamation and the pathogenesis of recessive X-linked ichthyosis. J Clin Invest 1984; 74:1414–1421.
29. Elias PM. Epidermal lipids, barrier function, and desquamation. J Invest Dermatol 1983; 80(suppl):44s–49s.
30. Sato J, Denda M, Nakanishi J, Nomura J, Koyama J. Cholesterol sulfate inhibits proteases that are involved in desquamation of stratum corneum. J Invest Dermatol 1998; 111:189–193.
31. Wertz PW, Downing DT. Free sphingosine in human epidermis. J Invest Dermatol 1990; 94:159–161.
32. Wertz PW, Downing DT. Ceramidase activity in porcine epidermis. FEBS Lett 1990; 268:110–112.
33. Bibel DJ, Aly R, Shinefield HR. Antimicrobial activity of sphingosines. J Invest Dermatol 1992; 98:269–273.
34. Hannun YA, Loomis CR, Merrill AH Jr, Bell RM. Sphingosine inhibition of protein kinase C activity and of phorbol dibutyrate binding in vitro and in human platelets. J Biol Chem 1986; 261:12604–12609.
35. Strauss JS, Pochi PE, Downing DT. The sebaceous glands: twenty-five years of progress. J Invest Dermatol 1976; 67:90–97.
36. Wertz PW, Downing DT. Covalent attachment of ω-hydroxyacid derivatives to epidermal macromolecules: a preliminary characterization. Biochem Biophys Res Commun 1986; 137:992–997.
37. Wertz PW, Downing DT. Covalently bound ω-hydroxyacylsphingosine in the stratum corneum. Biochim Biophys Acta 1987; 917:108–111.
38. Wertz PW, Madison KC, Downing DT. Covalently bound lipids of human stratum corneum. J Invest Dermatol 1989; 91:109–111.
39. Nemes Z, Marekov LN, Fesus L, Steinert PM. A novel function for transglutaminase 1: attachment of long-chain omega-hydroxyceramides to involucrin by ester bond formation. Proc Natl Acad Sci USA 1999; 96:8402–8407.
40. Ponec M, te Pas MF, Havekes L, Boonstra J, Mommaas AM, Vermeer BJ. LDL receptors in keratinocytes. J Invest Dermatol 1992; 98(suppl):50s–56s.
41. Hedberg CL, Wertz PW, Downing DT. The time course of lipid biosynthesis in pig epidermis. J Invest Dermatol 1988; 91:169–174.
42. Russell DW. Cholesterol biosynthesis and metabolism. Cardiovasc Drugs Ther 1992; 6:103–110.
43. Webb AR, DeCosta BR, Holick MF. Sunlight regulates the cutaneous production of vitamin D3 by causing its photodegradation. J Clin Endocrin Metabol 1989; 68:882–887.
44. Beg ZH, Shonik JA, Brewer HB Jr. 3-Hydroxy-3-methylglutaryl coenzyme A reductase: regulation of enzymatic activity by phosphorylation and dephosphorylation. Proc Natl Acad Sci USA 1978; 75:3678–3682.
45. Feingold KR. The regulation and role of lipid synthesis. Adv Lipid Res 1991; 24:57–82.
46. Slabas AR, Brown A, Sinden BS, Swinhoe R, Simon JW, Ashton AR, Whitfield PR, Elborough KM. Pivotal reactions in fatty acid synthesis. Prog Lipid Res 1994; 33:39–46.

47. Inagaki K, Aki T, Fukuda Y, Kawamoto S, Shigeta S, Ono K, Suzuki O. Identification and expression of a rat fatty acid elongase involved in biosynthesis of C18 fatty acids. Biosci Biotech Biochem 2002; 66:613–621.
48. Periera SL, Leonard AE, Mukerji P. Recent advances in the study of fatty acid desaturases from animals and lower eukaryotes. Prostaglandins Leukot Essential Fatty Acids 2003; 68:97–106.
49. Munday MR. Regulation of mammalian acetyl-CoA carboxylase. Biochem Soc Trans 2002; 30:1059–1064.
50. Radin NS. Biosynthesis of the sphingoid bases: a provocation. J Lipid Res 1984; 25:1536–1540.
51. Ponec M, Weerheim A, Kempenaar J, Mulder A, Gooris GS, Bouwstra JA, Mommaas AM. The formation of competent barrier lipids in reconstructed human epidermis requires the presence of vitamin C. J Invest Dermatol 1997; 109:348–355.

6

Stratum Corneum Ceramides: Function, Origins, and Therapeutic Applications

Yoshikazu Uchida
Department of Dermatology, School of Medicine, University of California,
San Francisco, California, U.S.A.

Sumiko Hamanaka
Department of Life Sciences, Graduate School of Arts and Sciences,
University of Tokyo, Tokyo and Department of Dermatology,
Saitama Medical School, Saitama, Japan

INTRODUCTION

Over the past 10+ years, the number of research reports related to ceramides (Cer) has dramatically increased in biological and biomedical fields. Most of these reports focus on the regulation of cellular proliferation, apoptosis, and cell senescence in a variety of cell types. The attention to Cer in the cutaneous research field began in the late 1970s. Pioneering analytical studies by Gray and co-workers (1–4) elucidated the Cer concept of epidermal lipids, which stimulated a host of other researchers. Later, Downing and Wertz, and others including ourselves (5–17), further explored the structural analysis of epidermal sphingolipids. A summary of these studies showed that the epidermis displays a unique Cer molecular profile, i.e., bulk amount, molecular heterogeneity, chemical structures, etc. Concurrently, the physiological relevance of epidermal sphingolipids for epidermal permeability barrier function was elucidated by Elias and co-workers (18–20), and those suffering from skin diseases with barrier defects, e.g., atopic dermatitis (21–24), psoriasis (25,26), and ichthyosis (27), were shown to have alterations in the stratum corneum (SC) Cer profile. These studies stimulated further epidermal sphingolipid research. The importance of sphingolipids in cellular function has led to the use of sphingolipids and their metabolic inhibitors for therapeutic purposes, e.g., in sphingolipidosis (28), cancer (29), and cardiovascular disease (30,31), with the development of approved drugs that have not yet been launched. Cer and its metabolic activators have already been utilized for improving epidermal permeability barrier function and/or to treat dry skin symptoms. The purpose of the following review is to summarize what is currently known about the unique Cer content of the SC, its origins, function, and therapeutic applications.

WHAT IS A CERAMIDE?

Cer is an amide-linked fatty acid (FA) containing a long-chain amino alcohol. This amino alcohol is named as sphingoid base or sphingol (Fig. 1). The carbon chain lengths of amide-linked FA and sphingol in most mammalian tissues are 16–26 and 18–20, respectively, although there is a molecular heterogeneity, particularly in the epidermis, as described below. Cer is the backbone structure of all sphingolipids. The 1-position of Cer is glycosylated to glycosphingolipid, choline phosphorylated to sphingomyelin (SM) or to Cer-1-phosphate. Although sphingolipids, including glycosphingolipids and phosphosphingolipids, are ubiquitously distributed in mammalian tissues, a tissue-specific molecular distribution has been described; e.g., glucosylceramide (GlcCer) is enriched in epidermis and spleen, while galactosylceramide (GalCer) is enriched in brain, but not detected in keratinocytes (KC). The molecular heterogeneity of sphingolipids is due to the molecular variation of (i) carbohydrate in glycosphingo-lipids, (ii) carbon chain length of amide-linked FA, and (iii) hydroxylation of both amide-linked FA and sphingol.

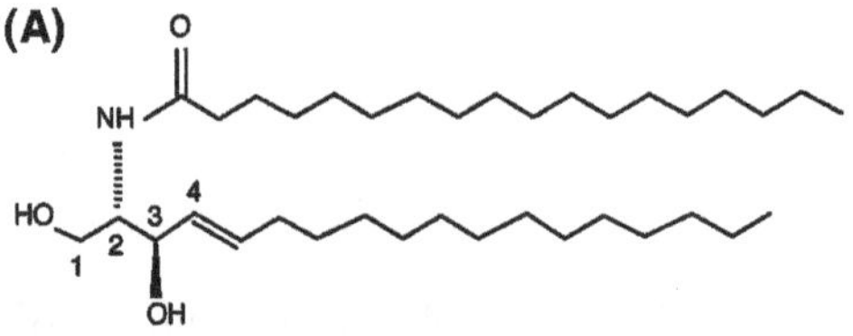

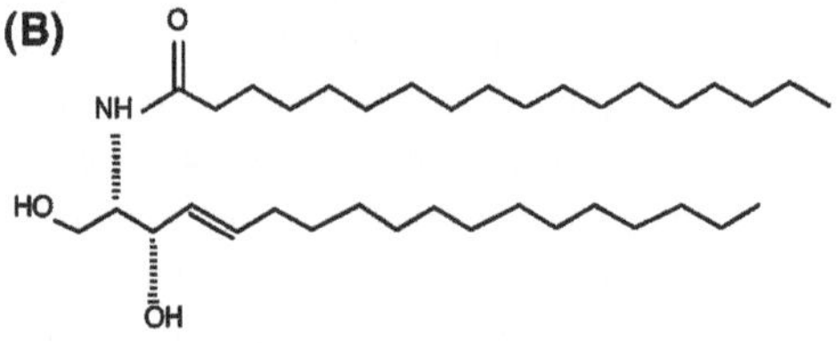

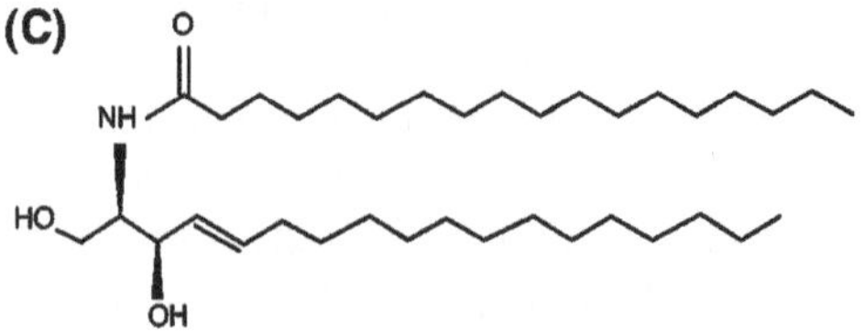

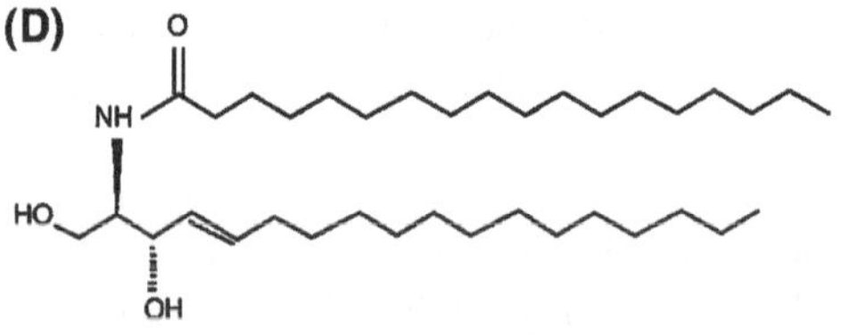

Figure 1 Structures of ceramides. (A) (2S,3R,4E)-2-(octadecanoylamino)-4-octadecene-1,3 diol or N-acyl-D-*erythro*-sphingosine (natural form). (B) (2S,3S,4E)-2-(octadecanoylamino)-4-octadecene-1,3 diol or N-acyl-D-*threo*-sphingosine. (C) (2R,3R,4E)-2-(octadecanoylamino)-4-octadecene-1,3 diol or N-acyl-D-threo-sphingosine. (D) (2R,3S,4E)-2-(octadecanoylamino)-4-octadecene-1,3 diol or N-acyl-L-*erythro*-sphingosine.

Since Cer or the Cer moiety of sphingolipids has both a proton donor, the amide NH group, and a proton acceptor, the OH group on C3 carbon, sphingolipids can form intermolecular hydrogen bonds with other molecules. An interaction between SM and cholesterol has been well characterized (32), i.e., the amide group of SM and 3-OH group of cholesterol forms an intermolecular hydrogen bond (33). Indeed, in vivo, SM and cholesterol are co-localized in the same membrane domains (32).

Sphingol has two asymmetric carbon atoms (C2 and C3 carbon), suggesting that, in theory, there are four isomers (Fig. 1). However, the structure of sphingol moiety of natural sphingolipids is restricted to 2S,3R- (or D-*erythro*) configuration, e.g., (2S,3R,4E)-2-(octadecanoylamino)-4-octadecene-1,3 diol or N-acyl-D-*erythro*-sphingosine (Fig. 1A). A stereoisomer (2S,3S- or L-*threo* configuration) of natural SM (2S,3R- or D-*erythro*) has less capability to interact with cholesterol (34). In another example, D-MAPP (D-*erythro*-2-(N-myristoylamino)-1-phenyl-1-propanol), which is a synthetic compound based on a part of the Cer structure, inhibits ceramidase which cleaves the amide-linkage of Cer and results in generating sphingol and FA, while a stereo isomer of D-MAPP, the L-MAPP, does not inhibit ceramidase but is a substrate of ceramidase (35). These suggest that isomer(s) of Cer behave as different compounds in cells. In addition, *trans*(4E)—double bond also affects the strength of intramolecular hydrogen bonding (36). Although further studies are required to elucidate the relationship between Cer structures, including configurations, presence of double bond or hydroxy group, its biochemical and/or physical properties, the stereo structures of Cer as well as the chemical structure should be important for lamellar bilayer formation with cholesterol and FA in the SC. Thus, if synthetic Cer or sphingolipids are utilized for therapeutic applications, the appropriate stereo structures will be required. However, it is noted that the configurations of most of the SC Cer, i.e., Cer 3, Cer 4, Cer 6, Cer 7, Cer 8, and Cer 9 (see below, also c.f. Fig. 3) have not yet been identified.

WHY ARE STRATUM CORNEUM CERAMIDES UNIQUE?

Cer is ubiquitously distributed in almost all mammalian tissues, while epidermal Cer is different in (i) content, (ii) molecular heterogeneity, (iii) localization, and (iv) function compared with Cer in other tissues.

Content

Whereas Cer is a minor lipid component, which comprises less than 10% of cholesterol or phospholipids in other mammalian tissues, Cer in the SC is the major lipid component, accounting for 30–40% of SC lipids by weight (1,37), e.g., 50-fold vs. liver, kidney, 35-fold vs. brain (38), and 9-fold vs. dermis (14). Moreover, such a high content of Cer in the SC is not observed in the epidermal stratum granulosum (SG), stratum spinosum (SP), or stratum basale (SB) (39). This also suggests that terminal differentiation is a key factor in generating and/or accumulating Cer.

Molecular Heterogeneity

Cer containing non-OH FA as amide-linked FA and sphingenine as sphingol is a major Cer molecule in most mammalian tissues. Phytosphingosine is the sphingol in sphingolipids of plants and yeast, while sphingolipid species containing α-hydroxy

(α-OH) FA are also commonly present in yeast. Although Cer containing α-OH FA
or phytosphingosine are present in mammalian extracutaneous tissues [liver, kidney,
and brain (40)], they are minor components. Likewise, Cer containing non-OH FA
and sphingenine is a predominant major Cer molecule in the undifferentiated KC
(Fig. 2). In contrast, at least twelve molecular groups of Cer (ten as unbound forms
and two as protein bound forms) have been identified in the human SC (Fig. 3)
(9,15,17). KC differentiation induces the syntheses of a variety of Cer molecules,
including Cer containing α-OH FA, ω-hydroxy (ω-OH) FA, phytosphingosine, and
trihydroxysphingenine. Molecules containing hydroxylated FA are >62% of total
Cer in the SC (13). Finally, the synthesis and content of Cer containing ω-OH FA in
murine epidermis are decreased by the topical application of aminobenzotriazole, a
suicide inhibitor of CYP4 ω-hydroxylase, indicating that the type 4 subfamily of
cytochrome P450 (CYP4) appears to be responsible for ω-OH Cer formation (41).
On the other hand, ω-OH FA are generated as catabolites of FA, e.g., arachidonic acid,
by the CYP4 series of enzymes in mammalian tissues, e.g., liver, kidney (42). Conjugated lipids, i.e., sphingolipids or phospholipids containing ω-OH FA, have not been
found. In addition, although differentiated KC synthesize very long chain ω-OH FA,
this FA is only utilized for Cer and GlcCer but not other lipid synthesis. Moreover,
whereas very long chain ω-OH FA (C-26–32) are found in wool wax (43) and giant-ring
lactones in the skin surface lipids (44,45), the involvement of these very long chain
ω-OH FA in epidermal Cer synthesis has not yet been elucidated.

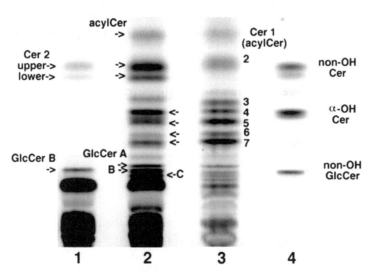

Figure 2 Thin layer chromatography of GlcCer and ceramide of both undifferentiated and
differentiated cultured human KC and SC. Lane 1, undifferentiated KC; lane 2, differentiated
KC; lane 3, human SC; lane 4, contains standard non-OH Cer, α-OH Cer, and GlcCer. Human
KC derived from newborn foreskins were cultured in serum-free KC growth medium, containing 0.07 mM calcium, and grown to 90–100% confluence (undifferentiated KC). The medium
then was switched to Dulbecco's medium and Ham F-12 (2:1, v/v) containing 1.2 mM calcium,
supplemented with 10% FBS, 10 µg/mL insulin, 0.4 µg/mL hydrocortisone and ascorbic acids
(final concentration of 50 µg/mL) (119) for 12 days (differentiated KC). SC was obtained from
normal subject. Total lipids were extracted from cell and from SC and separation of individual
lipid species was achieved by high-performance thin layer chromatography (119).

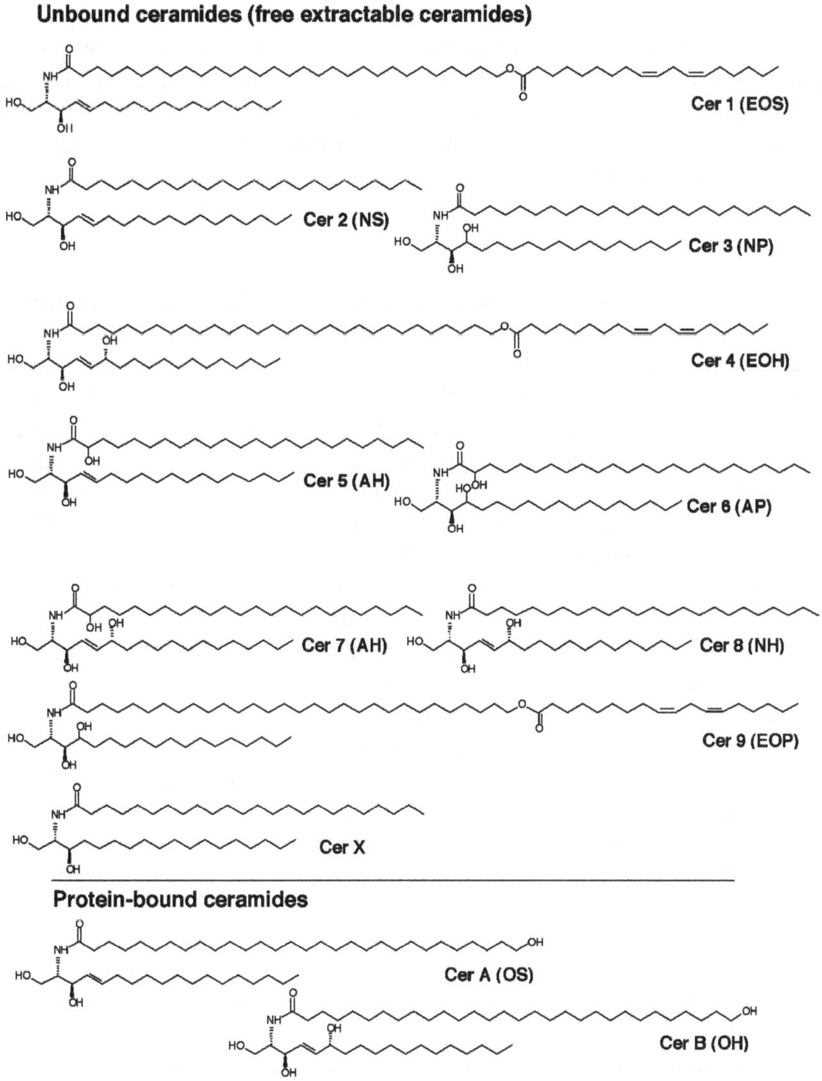

Unbound ceramides (free extractable ceramides)

Protein-bound ceramides

Figure 3 Structures of human SC ceramides (6,8,15,17). Abbreviation for Cer structures are according to Wertz and Downing (8) and Robson et al. (6). A stereo structure of Cer B was determined by Mori and Masuda as (2S,3R,4E,6R)-N-(30-hydroxytriacontanoyl)-6-hydroxy-4-sphingenine (120).

Localization

While Cer is one of the cellular membrane components, albeit quantitatively a minor component, it is more prominently represented in three sites within the epidermis and in two forms in the SC. (i) As the epidermis undergoes a differentiation of SG to SC, the plasma membrane is replaced by a protein-dominant cornified envelope. The ω-position of amide-linked FA of ω-hydroxylated Cer is covalently bound to the carboxy terminal of cornified envelope proteins at the extracellular surface of the corneocyte forming the corneocyte lipid envelope (CLE) (bound form); (ii) Lamellar bodies (LB) (known organelles of lipid storage and secretion in lung, intestinal tract, and epidermis) in the SG, which have been shown to contain the essential lipid components and their precursors for permeability barrier formation in the SC (46,47), included Cer (46); (iii) As lipids are extruded into the extracellular domains of the SC, they undergo a transition to lipid bilayer structures, and Cer are key components of these lamellae. Cer are also found in the SC in unbound form, as are other major SC lipids i.e., cholesterol, FA.

Function

Alteration of cellular Cer levels in response to cellular stimulus, e.g., cytokine, radiation, oxidative stress via activation of SM hydrolysis, and/or de novo synthesis leads to cell cycle arrest, cellular differentiation, apoptosis, and cell senescence in a variety of cells (48), including KC (49,50). In an effort to mimic these Cer-metabolic changes, cellular Cer levels are experimentally modified by exogenously adding more cell-permeable Cer containing shorter carbon chain lengths of amide-linked FA (N-acetyl, N-caproyl or N-octanoylsphingosine), natural Cer, bacterial SM'ase treatment, or Cer metabolic inhibitors. Previous studies suggest that Cer containing non-OH FA is more potent in inducing apoptosis on U939 human promonocytic cells than Cer containing α-OH FA (51). In addition, sphingol, including sphingosine and phytosphingosine, a metabolite of Cer by ceramidase, induces apoptosis (52,53). While a further distal metabolite of Cer, sphingosine-1-phosphate, which is generated from sphingosine by sphingosine kinase, stimulates cellular proliferation and protects cells from apoptosis in a variety of cell types including skin fibroblasts (54,55), sphingosine-1-phosphate inhibits proliferation and induces differentiation in KC (55). Thus, Cer and its distal metabolites have potential role(s) in regulating KC function in nucleated layers of the epidermis. However, it has not yet been examined whether acylCer or ω-OH Cer alters cellular function. Moreover, little is known on whether SC Cer or their metabolite(s) are taken into the nucleated layers of epidermis and then influence differentiation and/or apoptosis.

In addition to these bioregulatory roles that it plays, Cer is critical for epidermal barrier function (19). Both unbound and bound Cer are essential lipid components in forming lamellar bilayer structures, which serve in the barrier function (41). The competent lamellar bilayer formation is dependent not only on bulk amounts of Cer but also heterogeneous molecules of Cer (56,57). In particular, two of the SC Cer, Cer 1 and Cer 3, are important for forming the long periodicity phase in the lamellar bilayer structures in the SC (57) (Chap. 7). All types of SC Cer levels decreased in the SC of atopic dermatitis patients (22–24). In particular, Cer 1 (acylCer) is significantly reduced in both lesional and non-lesional SC (21,23,24). Levels of Cer 1 are also reportedly decreased in the SC of lamellar icthyosis and Sjogren–Larssen syndrome (27). Total Cer levels are not altered in psoriatic scale, while acylCer species and Cer containing phytosphingosine decrease (25). These changes in Cer profiles in the SC are likely to account for the barrier abnormality in these diseases.

GENERATION OF STRATUM CORNEUM CERAMIDES

Generation of Epidermal Sphingolipids

Major epidermal sphingolipids are limited to five classes: Cer, acylCer, GlcCer, acylGlcCer, and SM. De novo syntheses of Cer and acylCer, and the conjugated sphingolipids, which are GlcCer, acylGlcCer, and SM, occur in the nucleated KC,

SB, SP, and SG. The initial rate-limiting step in sphingolipid synthesis initiates the enzymatic condensation of L-serine and palmitoyl-CoA by serine palmitoyltransferase, generating the precursor of all sphingols, 3-kctosphinganinc, followcd by a rcduction to sphinganine by 3-ketosphinganine reductase (58). Two subsequent steps lead to Cer formation: first, the amino group of sphinganine is acylated to form dihydro-Cer by Cer synthase, and finally, dihydroCer is desaturated (C4–5 *trans*) to Cer by dihydroCer desaturase (58). This desaturase can also occur with hydroxylation at the 4 position of carbon in the sphingol of Cer, thereby forming Cer containing phytosphingosine (59). Yet, GlcCer and SM levels are higher than Cer levels in suprabasal epidermis, suggesting that the newly synthesized Cer are quickly converted to GlcCer or SM. GlcCer and SM are synthesized in differcnt subcellular sitcs: Ccr glucosylation occurs on the cytosolic aspect of the endoplasmic reticulum (ER) and proximal Golgi, while SM synthesis is localized to the luminal side (60). Recent studies demonstrated that translocation of Cer from ER to Golgi for SM synthesis is an ATP-dependent pathway mediated by a cytoplasmic protein, ceramide transfer protein (CERT), while the translocation of Cer for GlcCer synthesis is not ATP/CERT-dependent (61,62). Specific molecular species of Cer are utilized for GlcCer or SM synthesis in the epidermis (as described below), while the selective mechanism of specific Cer molecules for either GlcCer or SM synthesis is not known. Synthesized GlcCer, SM and Cer are subsequently transferred to the cellular membrane fractions and thereafter become membrane components. GlcCer and SM are also transferred to LB in the differentiated KC.

Origins of Stratum Corneum Ceramides

Generation of Cer, which alters cellular function as described above, is due to either increasing de novo synthesis or a hydrolysis of SM by various stimuli. However, these metabolic pathways cannot fully explain the generation of unique Cer in the SC.

Gaucher type 2 patients who lack a β-GlcCer'ase activity display significant epidermal barrier abnormalities (63). The mouse model of Gaucher disease demonstrates the accumulation of GlcCer and a decrease in SC Cer, as well as altering the SC Cer composition (63,64). In another sphingolipidosis, Niemann–Pick disease, which has decreased sphingomyelinase (SM'ase) activity, abnormal barrier recovery is observed following an acute barrier disruption, indicating that SM'ase–mediated hydrolysis of SM is also involved in the epidermal permeability barrier (65,66). Furthermore, in both cases, blockade of β-GlcCer'ase or SM'ase activity using specific enzyme inhibitors delayed the recovery of epidermal permeability barrier following an acute barrier perturbation (65). These studies indicate that (i) the conversion of GlcCer and SM to SC Cer is required for the barrier function (Chap. 15) and (ii) GlcCer and SM are immediate precursors for SC Cer generation.

Origin of Each Unbound Ceramide Molecular Species

Stratum Corneum Ceramides from Glucosylceramide and Acylglucosylceramide. GlcCer is a glycosphingolipid composed of one mole each of glucose, FA and sphingol (Fig. 4), and distributed widely in mammalian tissues. In the epidermis, GlcCer was the first reported glycosphingolipid (67), and then, a unique acylated GlcCer (acylGlcCer) was found in pig and human epidermis (4). Subsequent mammalian epidermal glycosphingolipid analyses (5,7,10,11,14,16,46,68,69) suggest that the GlcCer is a predominant glycosphingolipid and other complex glycosphingolipid families

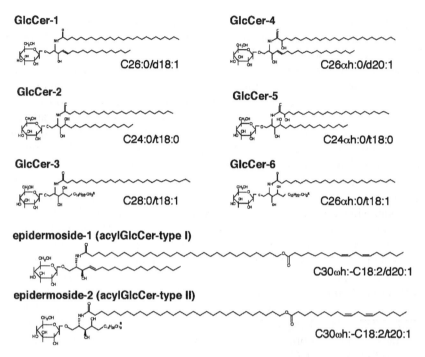

Figure 4 Structures of human epidermal GlcCer (1) and acylGlcCer (2) (11,13). The number before and after colon delineates carbon chain length and the number of double bonds, respectively. **h**, **d**, and **t** indicate hydroxy, dihydroxy, and trihydroxy, respectively. **a** indicates the position of double bond which is not determined.

(e.g., lactosylceramide, globoside, Forssman active glycolipid or gangliosides) are either absent or present in trace amounts in the epidermis. These results also suggest that the de novo synthesized GlcCer but not the catabolites of other glycosphingolipids by deglyco-sylation are potential precursors of Cer in the SC.

The Cer moieties of GlcCer in the human epidermis are composed of combinations of at least six different sphingols (d18:1, d20:1, t18:0, t20:0, t18:1, and t20:1) and 13 amide-linked FA (C16:0, C17:0, C18:0, C24:0, C25:0, C26:0, C27:0, C28:0, C29:0, C30:0, C24αOH:0, C25αOH:0, and C26αOH:0) (13). In addition to these molecules, acylGlcCer contain more than 10 species (11). The epidermal GlcCer family in the SC displays a remarkable heterogeneity that is not seen in other tissues/organs, which could be the source of the similarly diverse Cer population in the SC. The comparison of generated Cer from human GlcCer by recombinant β-GlcCer'ase with SC Cer demonstrated that epidermal GlcCer contain Cer backbone structures that are equivalent to SC Cer, indicating that GlcCer, including acylGlcCer are major precursors of SC Cer (13) (Table 1). Moreover, we detected a small amount of Glc-C24:0αh/d18:0 (molecular weight 829) by Fast atom bombardment–mass spectrometry (unpublished data). This molecular species is equivalent to SC Cer X (N-acylsphinganine, C24–33:0/C18:0) (15).

Acylgalactosylceramides, which are 2-O- or 3-O-acyl galactosylceramides, have been found in mammalian brain, i.e., whale, bovine, and human (70,71), while acyl glucosylceramide (acylGlcCer) (Fig. 4) have been shown to be present only in differentiated KC (72,73). This unique epidermal acylated GlcCer, acylGlcCer, has been investigated in the process of research on essential FA and their deficient conditions,

Table 1 Deduced Precursors, Conjugated Sphingolipids, of SC Cer

	Conjugated sphingolipids	
	Cer moieties of most abundant molecule (M.W.)[a]	Generated SC Cer (6,15,17)
Glycosphingolipids		
AcylGlcCer		
Epidermoside-1	C30ωh:0-C18:2/d20:1 (1201)	Cer 1 (EOS) & Cer A
	C32ωh:1-C18:2/d20:1 (1227)	
Epidermoside-2	C30ωh:0-C18:2/t20:1 (1217)	Cer 4 (EOH) & Cer B
Unidentified minor epidermoside		Cer 9
GlcCer-1	C26:0/d18:1 (839)	Cer 2 (NS)
GlcCer-2	C24:0/t18:0 (829)	Cer 3 (NP)
GlcCer-3	C28:0/t20:1 (911)	Cer 8 (NH)
GlcCer-4	C26αh:0/d20:1 (883)	Cer 5 (AS)
GlcCer-5	C24αh:0/t18:0 (845)	Cer 6 (AP)
GlcCer-6	C26αh:0/t18:1 (871)	Cer 7 (AH)
Phosphosphingolipids		
SM-1	C24:0/d18:1 (814)	Cer 2 (NS)
SM-2	C16:0/d18:1 (702)	—
SM-3	C16αh:0/d18:1 (718)	Cer 5 (AS)

[a]Molecular weight determined by fast atom bombardment-mass spectrometry (5, 11–13).

In 1930, Burr and Burr demonstrated that certain polyunsaturated FA are essential in the diet of growing rats (74). One of the outstanding symptoms of essential FA deficiency was an increase in water loss from the skin (75). Extracellular lamellar bilayer structures in the SC were disorganized in essential FA–deficient murine skin (76). This abnormality was fully restored by the addition of linoleic acid to the diet or even by topical application of linoleic acid to the skin (74,75,77,78). These patho-physiological findings led to the study of linoleate-enriched lipid molecular species. Structural analyses of several mammalian epidermal lipids revealed that acylGlcCer, which is GlcCer with a very long chain ω-OH FA esterified with linoleic acid through the ω-OH group (4,10,11,14,16,46,69), has been identified as an epidermis-specific linoleate-enriched molecule. In humans, epidermal acylGlcCer contain more than 95% linoleic acid, but this figure is 75–77% in pigs (3,69), 32% in rats (46), 45% in mice (79), and 84% in guinea pigs (14). More than 50% of glucosylsphingolipids are acylGlcCer in human epidermis (68). Since acylGlcCer carrying linoleic acid are involved in the physiologic maintenance of the epidermal permeability barrier (80), they were named epidermosides (11,81). Moreover, human acylGlcCer are subdivided into type 1 and type 2, which are present at a 1.5:1.0 mol ratio (11), while type 2 acylGlcCer has not been reported in other mammalian epidermis. The structure of type 1 is glucosyl β1-*N*-(ω-*O*-linoleyl)-acylsphingosines, whereas type 2 is characterized by a novel sphingosine, trihydroxysphingosine, having a double bond. In epidermoside 1 and 2, at least 10 different ω-OH FA (C26ωh:0, C28ωh:0, C30ωh:0, C32ωh:0, C34ωh:0, C26ωh:1, C28ωh:1, C30ωh:1, C32ωh:1, and C34ωh:1) represent the amide-linked FA component (11). Enzymatic hydrolysis by β-GlcCer'ase showed that epidermoside 1 and 2 generate Cer 1 and Cer 4, respectively (Fig. 5). The structure of the Cer moiety of epidermoside 1 is the same as Cer 1. On the other hand, the sphingosine of Cer 4 is reported to be 6-hydroxy-4-sphingenine, which is different from that of epidermoside 2 (4-hydroxy-

Ceramides
non-OH Cer
α-OH Cer
GlcCer
1
2
3
4
5
6
7
1
2
3
4
5
6
7
8

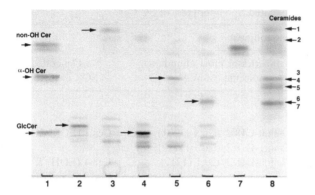

Figure 5 Generation of acylceramides (Cer 1 and Cer 4) from acylGlcCer (epidermoside 1 and 2) by β-glucocerebrosidase treatment (13). Lane 1 contains standard non-OH Cer, α-OH Cer, and GlcCer. Lanes 2 and 4 contain epidermosides I and II, respectively, indicated by arrows. Lanes 3 and 5 contain Cer obtained by β-GlcCer'ase treatment of either epidermoside I or II, respectively. Lane 6 contains Cer with ω-OH FA obtained from acylceramides in lane 5 by saponification. Lane 7 contains non-OH Cer as a standard. Lane 9 shows Cer species obtained from human SC.

sphingosine; the position of the double bond has not yet been determined). It is still an open question whether epidermoside 2 is a precursor of Cer 4. Although an acylGlcCer fraction containing a Cer 9 backbone has not yet been identified, minor components detected (other than those in epidermoside 1 and 2) in our previous studies might be a precursor of Cer 9 (11).

Stratum Corneum Ceramides from Sphingomyelin. SM is a sphingophospholipid, which contains phosphorylcholine attached to a Cer backbone (Fig. 6). SM is a common membrane component of all mammalian cells that is concentrated primarily in the outer leaflet of the plasma membrane (82,83). In general, the amide-linked

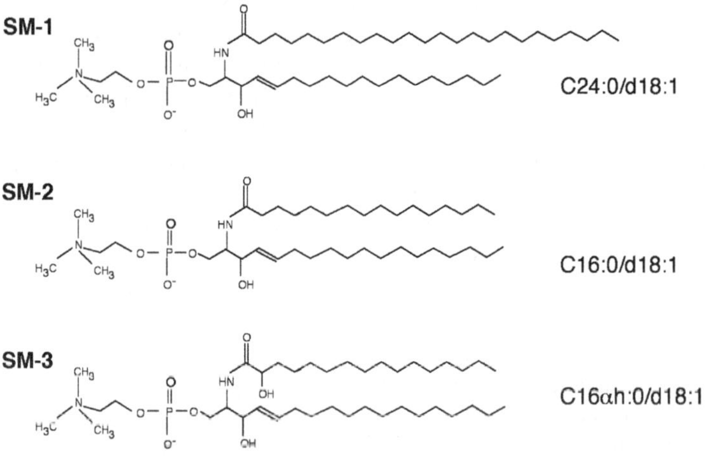

SM-1
C24:0/d18:1
SM-2
C16:0/d18:1
SM-3
C16αh:0/d18:1

Figure 6 Structures of human and murine sphingomyelins. Most-abundant SM species from both murine and human epidermis are shown. The number before and after colon delineates carbon chain length and the number of double bonds, respectively. d indicates dihydroxy. *Source*: From Ref. 12.

FA of SM is non–OH acid with a carbon chain length of C16–24 (2,84,85) with palmitic acid (C16 FA) as the predominant FA. A recent study revealed that epidermal SM contained α-OH palmitic acid as well as non-OH C16 and C24 FA as the N-acyl FA components (12). The relatively hydrophilic SM with α-OH palmitic acid is not widely distributed in mammalian tissues although it is detected in other tissues/ organs (84,86–88). Based on the FA composition, epidermal SM were subdivided into three molecular species: long-chain FA (SM-1; C22–26), short-chain FA (SM-2; primarily C16), and short-chain α-OH FA (SM-3; C16–18) (12). In contrast, only trace quantities of ω-OH FA were present (12). Comparison of these SM with corresponding SM'ase–generated epidermal Cer and SC Cer revealed that the Cer moieties of SM-1 and SM-3 are equivalent to Cer 2 and Cer 5, respectively (Fig. 6 and Table 1) (12). Moreover, both Cer 2 and Cer 5 were found in Gaucher SC, which does not generate Cer from GlcCer (see above), whereas other Cer subfractions did not occur. This suggests that all Cer species, including Cer 1 and Cer 3, which are important in the formation of the lamellar bilayer structures in the SC (57), are derived from the GlcCer precursor, but not from SM, while Cer 2 and Cer 5 are derived from SM. This is likely to be one of the reasons why the barrier impairment is severe in patients with Gaucher's disease compared to the patients with Niemann–Pick disease.

Origins of Bound Ceramide Molecular Species

AcylGlcCer, especially epidermosides, appear to be precursors of Cer A and B (Fig. 3) of CLE. Studies on Gaucher transgenic mice and transgenic mice deficient in prosaposin (sphingolipid-activating proteins that stimulate enzymatic hydrolysis of sphingolipids) demonstrated that the glucosylated ω-OH Cer are first covalently bound to the envelope proteins and then are hydrolyzed by β-GlcCer'ase (89–91). In addition, immunohistochemical staining with anti-GlcCer antibody revealed that GlcCer is present in the cornified envelopes of the cells only in the first layer of the SC and absent in the upper SC (92). Moreover, free ω-OH GlcCer are not detected in human epidermis (13), suggesting that acylGlcCer but not free ω-OH GlcCer is a precursor of CLE-Cer. These results support the hypothesis of Doering et al. that acylGlcCer are the precursors of ω-OH Cer, by releasing linoleic acid and binding to the proteins, followed by deglucosylation to ω-OH Cer, Cer A, and Cer B (89,90). Steinert and co-workers discovered a novel function of transglutaminase 1, which generates isopeptide bonds, and forms the ester linkage between involucrin and a synthetic pseudo-ω-OH Cer[16-(16-hydroxyhexadecyl) oxypalmitoyl sphingenine] (93). They hypothesized that the thioester bond between transglutaminase 1 and a Gln residue of involucrin is replaced by the ω-OH group of ω-OH Cer, forming a Glu-O-Cer linkage. Thus, acylGlcCer may be hydrolyzed to ω-OH GlcCer, followed by a nucleophilic ω-OH attack on the thioester bond. As Doering et al. (90) suggested, it is also possible that transesterification occurs between acylGlcCer and the carboxy group of CE proteins, resulting in the formation of CE-ω-O-Cer and the subsequent release of linoleic acid, mediated by an as yet unknown enzyme(s) or by a non-enzymatic reaction.

THERAPEUTIC APPLICATIONS

The epidermal barrier function is easily disrupted by mechanical stress and dehydration due to soap, detergents, and/or organic solvents. The injured barrier increases a transepidermal water loss (TEWL) and causes pro-inflammatory cytokine production in the skin. Furthermore, antigens and/or irritants can easily penetrate the impaired barrier. Subsequently, eczematous lesions with scales develop. These phenomena are seen in several skin diseases including contact dermatitis, atopic dermatitis, xerotic dermatitis, and ichthyosis, as well as skin problems observed in sensitive and irritable conditions. Topically applied agents have been utilized in attempts to restore the impaired epidermal barrier function. Prior to identifying the functional roles of specific sphingolipids in the epidermis, sphingolipid-enriched fractions from central nervous system tissues were patented for dermatological uses by Hoffmann–La Rosch (#399655, Switzerland). Later, based on the importance of Cer for epidermal barrier function, several experimental and clinical trials of the topical application of sphingolipids, i.e., Cer, pseudoceramides, and GalCer, have been performed and the results have led to the development of new skin care products. (Table 2).

Ceramide Agents

Independent research groups have studied the effects of topical application of Cer on the epidermal barrier function and dry skin symptoms. First, topical application of the

Table 2   Clinical Trials of Sphingolipids and Pseudosphingolipids

Agents	Subjects	References
Cer enriched SC agent	Damaged skin on the healthy volunteers	94
Cer 2, Cer 5	Damaged skin on the healthy volunteers	95
	Chronologically aged skin	96 etc.
Cer 3, Cer 3B	Damaged skin on the healthy volunteers	97
	Irritable contact dermatitis, allergic contact dermatitis	99
Cer 3, Cer 3B, Cer 6	Damaged skin on the healthy volunteers	98
Pseudoceramide[a]	Atopic dermatitis	103 and 104
Pseudoceramide[b]	Childhood atopic dermatitis	106–108
Pseudoceramide[c]	Xerotic dermatitis	109
GalCer	Xerotic dermatitis, atopic dermatitis, psoriasis vulgaris, ichthyosis vulgaris, RXLI, cutaneous amyloidosis	112
GalCer enriched agent	Atopic dermatitis, irritable hand eczema, xerotic dermatitis	115
Pseudogalactosylceramide	Not tested in human subjects	

The structures of compounds are shown in Figure 2 (Cer), Figure 7 (pseudoceramides), and Figure 8 (GalCer and pesudogalactosylceramdide).
[a]Kao Co.
[b]NeoPharm Co. Ltd.
[c]Pacific R&D Center.

Cer-rich SC lipid fraction was demonstrated to significantly enhance the recovery of the water-holding capacity of human skin in which barrier function was abrogated by a mixture of acetone and diethylether treatment (94). Second, the effect of authentic Cer samples (Sigma Chem. Co., St Louis, Missouri, U.S.A.) corresponding to Cer 2 and Cer 5 in the SC on barrier recovery was investigated using a murine experimental model (95). Whereas Cer alone delayed the barrier recovery following an acute barrier disruption by tape-stripping, the combination of Cer with cholesterol and FA, at the mol ratio of 1:1:1, accelerated barrier recovery (95). In addition, the barrier recovery in aged human skin was accelerated by the application of a mixture of cholesterol, Cer, essential FA (linoleic acid), and non-essential FA (palmitic acid) at the mol ratio of 3:1:1:1 (96). These studies also demonstrated that externally applied Cer traversed the SC and entered the nucleated epidermis where they were subsequently incorporated into LB and secreted to form extracellular lamellar bilayers in the SC (95). Moreover, ultrastructural studies showed that the SC was largely replete with lamellar unit structures in the sites treated with the optimal lipid mixture (95). In addition to these studies using natural Cer, a new method for the semichemical synthesis of Cer allows us to commercially synthesize Cer 3 (N-stearoyl-phytosphingosine) and Cer 3B (N-oleoyl-phytosphingosine) (Fig. 3), which correspond to Cer 3 in the SC (Cosmoferm, Delft, Netherlands). These Cer 3 and Cer 3B are chemically prepared from biosynthesized phytosphingosine using yeast and FA. Although four isomers are present in sphingol (Fig. 1), yeast selectively produces a natural form of sphingol isomers, $2S,3S,4R$ configurations. These semichemical synthetic Cer were applied to the skin whose epidermal barrier was abrogated by treatment with organic solvent (acetone), detergent (sodium lauryl sulfate), or sequential tape-stripping (97,98). An emollient containing Cer 3 and Cer 3B did not show significant effects on barrier recovery compared with vehicle control (97), while the combination of Cer 3, Cer 3B, and Cer 6 (containing non-OH FA and phytosphingosine) with phytosphingosine, cholesterol, and linoleic acid accelerated the barrier recovery (98). Moreover, a large-scale clinical study of the effects of a topically applied cream comprising a physiological lipid mixture containing Cer 3, cholesterol, palmitic acid, and oleic acid at the 3:2:2:2 mol ratio (Yamanouchi Co., Tokyo, Japan) in patients with irritant contact dermatitis, allergic contact dermatitis, and atopic dermatitis demonstrated that the barrier repair cream significantly improved the barrier function besides ameliorating the clinical symptoms, including dryness, scaling, erythema, pruritus, fissuring, and overall disease severity (99). These studies clearly define Cer as an essential component of lipids required for barrier integrity.

Pseudoceramides

Synthetic compounds have been developed for dermatological uses; these are based on the structure of Cer but whose molecules do not have a sphingol structure. These are defined as "pseudoceramidies." One of these pseudoceramides [N-(3-hexadecy-loxy-2-hydroxypropyl)-N-2-hydroxyethylhexadecanamide] (Fig. 7A) (Kao Co., Tokyo, Japan), which is based on Cer-containing non-OH FA and sphingosine (Cer 2, which is one of the major SC Cer species) is capable of forming lamellar structures with cholesterol and FA (100–102). The cream containing this pseudoceramide (8%) improved the cutaneous symptoms of atopic dermatitis, but did not alter TEWL levels in patients receiving this cream (103,104). Another pseudoceramide, N-(2-hydro-xyethyl)-2-pentadecanolylhexadecanamide (NeoPharm Co. Ltd., Taejeon, Korea) (Fig. 7B), can form multilamellar structures with cholesterol and stearic acid (105). A Cer-dominant formulation containing this pseudoceramide, cholesterol, and FA

(A)

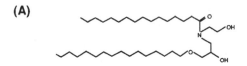

(B)

(C)

Figure 7 Structures of pseudoceramides. (A) *N*-(3-Hexadecyloxy-2-hydroxypropyl)-*N*-2-hydroxyethylhexadecanamide (100). (B) *N*-(2-Hydroxyethyl)-2-pentadecanolylhexadecanamide (105). (C) *N,N'-bis*bis(2-hydroxyethyl)-*N,N'*-bisoctadecanoyl-1,3-diamino-2-propanol (109).

(3:1:1 mol ratio) (TriCeram, Osmotics Corp., Denver, Colorado, U.S.A.) was applied to children with stubborn-to-recalcitrant atopic dermatitis and resulted in improvement of clinical symptoms, TEWL, and SC integrity (cohesion) (106,107). Moreover, this new barrier repair complex accelerated the formation of extracellular lamellar membranes in the SC (106). Another formula, which is a multilamellar emulsion containing *N*-(2-hydroxyethyl)-2-pentadecanolylhexadecanamide, also improves the symptoms of childhood atopic dermatitis (108). In addition to these two pesudoceramides, *N,N'-bis*(2-hydroxyethyl)-*N,N'-bis*octadecanoyl-1,3-diamino-2-propanol (Pacific R&D Center, Yongin, Korea) (Fig. 7C) was demonstrated to decrease scaliness and increase water content in the SC in patients with xerosis (109).

Drug–design technology based on Cer structure and Cer derivatives could lead to the development of numerous new barrier repair agents. However, the metabolic pathways that these pseudo-compounds enter could be different from those of natural Cer. Thus, therapeutic applications accompanied by extensive studies, e.g., absorption, fates, must be carried out to minimize and avoid adverse effects and toxicities.

Stimulation of Endogenous Ceramide Production

Topical mixtures containing both acylCer (Cer 1 or Cer 4) and Cer 3, which are important molecules for the formation of lamellar bilayer structures (57), have not yet been developed. Because the cost of formulations containing these Cer is currently very high, whether they will be developed is uncertain.

Another approach to enhancing barrier function would be to find ways to stimulate SC Cer production.

Galactosylceramide

Whereas GalCer (Fig. 8) is commonly present on mammalian cellular membranes, especially nervous issues, GalCer is not detected in the KC. GalCer reported in the epidermis might be derived from melanocytes or other non-KC cells (5,110). Interestingly,

GalCer

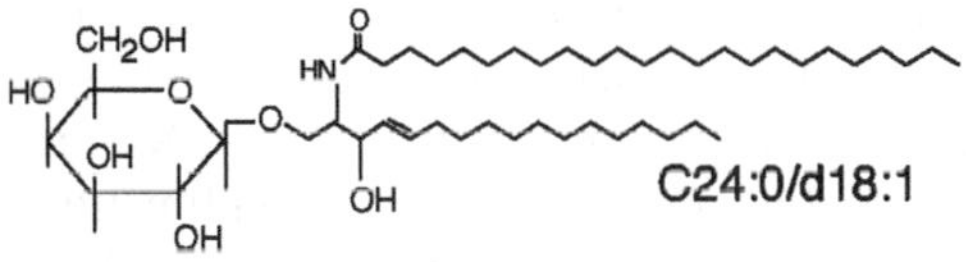

pseudogalactosylceramide

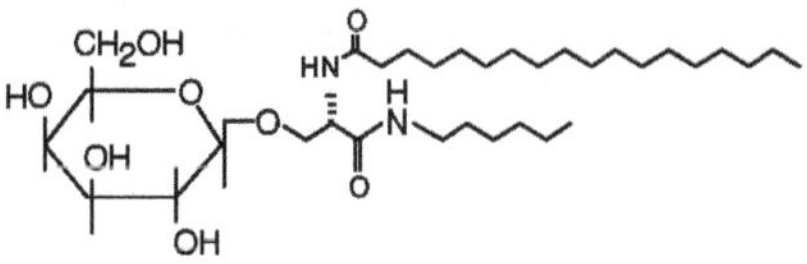

Figure 8 Structures of galactosylceramide and pseudogalactosylceramide (116).

however, GalCer significantly increased the β-GlcCer'ase activity, which is a key enzyme in the production of SC Cer from GlcCer, in both cultured human KC and in vivo murine epidermis (111). In contrast to Cer or pseudoceramide agents that are directly utilized for lamellar bilayer components, GalCer increased the endogenous production of all SC Cer molecular species (111). Not only does it increase the conversion of GlcCer to Cer by activating β-GlcCer'ase but it also accelerates the de novo sphingolipid synthesis. The mechanisms for these effects have not yet been elucidated.

A cream containing GalCer (1%) (Kanebo Ltd., Tokyo, Japan) was applied to the dry and scaly skin of patients with atopic dermatitis, xerosis, psoriasis vulgaris, ichthyosis vulgaris, recessive X-linked ichthyosis (RXLI), and cutaneous amyloidosis (112). The dry skin improved, showing the disappearance of scales and pruritus, and the inflammatory reaction reduced. The ear lesions that occur in patients with RXLI showed marked amelioration. The levels of prosapocin, which is an endogenous activator of β-GlcCer'ase, are reportedly decreased in, at least, atopic dermatitis (113) and psoriasis (114). GalCer may compensate for the decrease in an activator of β-GlcCer'ase in the skins of these patients. Thus, although there is no direct evidence linking the improvement in skin symptoms and normalization of Cer profiles in these patients, GalCer increasing β-GlcCer'ase may be responsible for the improvement of barrier function in these diseases.

In addition, a cream containing a GalCer-rich lipid mixture, GalCer 70%, phospholipids (PM, phosphatidylethanolamine, and phosphatidylcholine) 20%, and cholesterol 1% (Rozett Co., Tokyo, Japan) was shown to improve the overall symptoms of atopic dermatitis (115).

Pseudogalactosylceramide

As with pseudoceramides, pseudgalactosylceramides are synthesized based on natural GalCer structure. As seen with natural GalCer, one of the chemically synthesized pseudogalactosylceramides (Fig. 8) increased β-GlcCer'ase and also improved the barrier recovery in a murine experimental dry skin model (116). A clinical trial of this pseudogalactosylceramide has not yet been reported.

Niacin

Nicotinic acid (or niacin) and nicotin amide (niacin amide), which are defined as vitamin B3, are incorporated into nicotinamide adenine dinucleotide (NAD) or nicotinamide adenine phosphate (NADP). These pyridine nucleotides serve as cofactors in more than two hundred enzymatic reactions. A deficiency of niacin or niacin amide causes pellagra, which is characterized by symmetric photosensitive skin eruption, gastrointestinal manifestations, and neurological disturbances (117). Niacin has been utilized in skin care products. A recent study demonstrated a novel function for niacin: the stimulation of sphingolipid synthesis in cultured human KC (118). The increases in sphingolipid production, including all molecular species of Cer, are accounted for by an increase in the serine palmitoyl transferase gene expression (118). The cream containing niacin amide improved the barrier recovery in human subjects with xerosis compared with vehicle control (118).

SUMMARY

Sphingolipids are recognized as critical components of the SC and are required for epidermal homeostasis. Cer has a dual role in the epidermis: (i) It is an essential component for epidermal barrier function and (ii) it can modulate proliferation and differentiation, and induce apoptosis in KC. The findings from the studies of epidermal barrier function and the role of sphingolipids have already been translated into therapeutic applications. Topical application of Cer or pseudoceramide is a direct approach to supplying Cer for improving the barrier function, while a stimulation of all SC Cer molecules by GalCer or niacin is an alternative strategy. Moreover, the development of pseudoceramide and pseudogalactosylceramide allows for a more cost effective approach as well as perhaps for more potent effects. In addition to its utilization for epidermal barrier function, Cer can be applied to regulate KC function by inhibiting proliferation and inducing differentiation in the treatment of cutaneous diseases characterized by hyperplasia. Finally, inducing apoptosis in epidermal cells by Cer could be applicable to the therapy of skin tumors.

REFERENCES

1. Gray GM, Yardley HJ. Different populations of pig epidermal cells: isolation and lipid composition. J Lipid Res 1975; 16:441–447.
2. Gray GM, King IA, Yardley HJ. The plasma membrane of granular cells from pig epidermis: isolation and lipid and protein composition. J Invest Dermatol 1978; 71:131–135.
3. Gray GM, White RJ. Glycosphingolipids and ceramides in human and pig epidermis. J Invest Dermatol 1978; 70:336–341.
4. Gray GM, White RJ, Majer JR. 1-(3′-O-acyl)-beta-glucosyl-N-dihydroxypentatriacontadienoylsphingosine, a major component of the glucosylceramides of pig and human epidermis. Biochim Biophys Acta 1978; 528:127–137.
5. Hamanaka S, Takemoto T, Hamanaka Y, Asagami C, Suzuki M, Suzuki A, Otsuka F. Structure determination of glycosphingolipids of cultured human keratinocytes. Biochim Biophys Acta 1993; 1167:1–8.
6. Robson KJ, Stewart ME, Michelsen S, Lazo ND, Downing DT. 6-Hydroxy-4-sphingenine in human epidermal ceramides. J Lipid Res 1994; 35:2060–2068.
7. Wertz PW, Downing DT. Glucosylceramides of pig epidermis: structure determination. J Lipid Res 1983; 24:1135–1139.
8. Wertz PW, Downing DT. Ceramides of pig epidermis: structure determination. J Lipid Res 1983; 24:759–765.

9. Stewart ME, Downing DT. A new 6-hydroxy-4-sphingenine-containing ceramide in human skin. J Lipid Res 1999; 40:1434–1439.
10. Abraham W, Wertz PW, Downing DT. Linoleate-rich acylglucosylceramides of pig epidermis: structure determination by proton magnetic resonance. J Lipid Res 1985; 26:761–766.
11. Hamanaka S, Asagami C, Suzuki M, Inagaki F, Suzuki A. Structure determination of glucosyl beta 1-N-(omega-O-linoleoyl)-acylsphingosines of human epidermis. J Biochem (Tokyo) 1989; 105:684–690.
12. Uchida Y, Hara M, Nishio H, Sidransky E, Inoue S, Otsuka F, Suzuki A, Elias PM, Holleran WM, Hamanaka S. Epidermal sphingomyelins are precursors for selected stratum corneum ceramides. J Lipid Res 2000; 41:2071–2082.
13. Hamanaka S, Hara M, Nishio H, Otsuka F, Suzuki A, Uchida Y. Human epidermal glucosylceramides are major precursors of stratum corneum ceramides. J Invest Dermatol 2002; 119:416–423.
14. Uchida Y, Iwamori M, Nagai Y. Distinct differences in lipid composition between epidermis and dermis from footpad and dorsal skin of guinea pigs. Jpn J Exp Med 1988; 58:153–161.
15. Vietzke JP, Strassner M, Hintze U. Separation and identification of ceramides in the human stratum corneum by high-performance liquid chromatography coupled with electrospray ionization mass spectrometry and electrospray multiple-stage spectrometry prolifing. Chromatographica 1999; 50:15–20.
16. Bowser PA, Nugteren DH, White RJ, Houtsmuller UM, Prottey C. Identification, isolation and characterization of epidermal lipids containing linoleic acid. Biochim Biophys Acta 1985; 834:419–428.
17. Ponec M, Weerheim A, Lankhorst P, Wertz P. New acylceramide in native and reconstructed epidermis. J Invest Dermatol 2003; 120:581–588.
18. Elias PM, Tsai J, Menon GK, Holleran WM, Feingold KR. The potential of metabolic interventions to enhance transdermal drug delivery. J Invest Dermatol Symp Proc 2002; 7:79–85.
19. Elias PM, Menon GK. Structural and lipid biochemical correlates of the epidermal permeability barrier. Adv Lipid Res 1991; 24:1–26.
20. Elias PM, Feingold KR. Coordinate regulation of epidermal differentiation and barrier homeostasis. Skin Pharmacol Appl Skin Physiol 2001; 1(suppl 14):28–34.
21. Imokawa G, Abe A, Jin K, Higaki Y, Kawashima M, Hidano A. Decreased level of ceramides in stratum corneum of atopic dermatitis: an etiologic factor in atopic dry skin? J Invest Dermatol 1991; 96:523–526.
22. Melnik B, Hollmann J, Plewig G. Decreased stratum corneum ceramides in atopic individuals—a pathobiochemical factor in xerosis? [letter]. Br J Dermatol 1988; 119: 547–549.
23. Yamamoto A, Serizawa S, Ito M, Sato Y. Stratum corneum lipid abnormalities in atopic dermatitis. Arch Dermatol Res 1991; 283:219–223.
24. Di Nardo A, Wertz P, Giannetti A, Seidenari S. Ceramide and cholesterol composition of the skin of patients with atopic dermatitis. Acta Derm Venereol 1998; 78:27–30.
25. Motta S, Monti M, Sesana S, Caputo R, Carelli S, Ghidoni R. Ceramide composition of the psoriatic scale. Biochim Biophys Acta 1993; 1182:147–151.
26. Motta S, Monti M, Sesana S, Mellesi L, Ghidoni R, Caputo R. Abnormality of water barrier function in psoriasis. Role of ceramide fractions. Arch Dermatol 1994; 130: 452–456.
27. Paige DG, Morse-Fisher N, Harper JI. Quantification of stratum corneum ceramides and lipid envelope ceramides in the hereditary ichthyoses. Br J Dermatol 1994; 131:23–27.
28. Abe A, Wild SR, Lee WL, Shayman JA. Agents for the treatment of glycosphingolipid storage disorders. Curr Drug Metab 2001; 2:331–338.
29. Kolesnick R. The therapeutic potential of modulating the ceramide/sphingomyelin pathway. J Clin Invest 2002; 110:3–8.

30. Charles R, Sandirasegarane L, Yun J, Bourbon N, Wilson R, Rothstein RP, Levison SW, Kester M. Ceramide-coated balloon catheters limit neointimal hyperplasia after stretch injury in carotid arteries. Circ Res 2000; 87:282–288.

31. Bourbon NA, Sandirasegarane L, Kester M. Ceramide-induced inhibition of Akt is mediated through protein kinase Czeta: implications for growth arrest. J Biol Chem 2002; 277:3286–3292.

32. Ohvo-Rekila H, Ramstedt B, Leppimaki P, Slotte JP. Cholesterol interactions with phospholipids in membranes. Prog Lipid Res 2002; 41:66–97.

33. Veiga MP, Arrondo JL, Goni FM, Alonso A, Marsh D. Interaction of cholesterol with sphingomyelin in mixed membranes containing phosphatidylcholine, studied by spin-label ESR and IR spectroscopies. A possible stabilization of gel-phase sphingolipid domains by cholesterol. Biochemistry 2001; 40:2614–2622.

34. Ramstedt B, Slotte JP. Interaction of cholesterol with sphingomyelins and acyl-chain-matched phosphatidylcholines: a comparative study of the effect of the chain length. Biophys J 1999; 76:908–915.

35. Bielawska A, Greenberg MS, Perry D, Jayadev S, Shayman JA, McKay C, Hannun YA. (1S,2R)-D-erythro-2-(N-myristoylamino)-1-phenyl-1-propanol as an inhibitor of cera-midase. J Biol Chem 1996; 271:12646–12654.

36. Talbott CM, Vorobyov I, Borchman D, Taylor KG, DuPre DB, Yappert MC. Confor-mational studies of sphingolipids by NMR spectroscopy. II. Sphingomyelin. Biochim Biophys Acta 2000; 1467:326–337.

37. Weerheim A, Ponec M. Determination of stratum corneum lipid profile by tape strip-ping in combination with high-performance thin-layer chromatography. Arch Dermatol Res 2001; 293:191–199.

38. Schoephoerster RT, Wertz PW, Madison KC, Downing DT. A survey of polar and non-polar lipids of mouse organs. Comp Biochem Physiol [B] 1985; 82:229–232.

39. Lampe MA, Williams ML, Elias PM. Human epidermal lipids: characterization and modulations during differentiation. J Lipid Res 1983; 24:131–140.

40. Iwamori M, Costello C, Moser HW. Analysis and quantitation of free ceramide containing nonhydroxy and 2-hydroxy fatty acids, and phytosphingosine by high-performance liquid chromatography. J Lipid Res 1979; 20:86–96.

41. Behne M, Uchida Y, Seki T, de Montellano PO, Elias PM, Holleran WM. Omega-hydroxyceramides are required for corneocyte lipid envelope (CLE) formation and nor-mal epidermal permeability barrier function. J Invest Dermatol 2000; 114:185–192.

42. Powell PK, Wolf I, Jin R, Lasker JM. Metabolism of arachidonic acid to 20-hydroxy-5,8,11,14-eicosatetraenoic acid by P450 enzymes in human liver: involvement of CYP4F2 and CYP4A11. J Pharmacol Exp Ther 1998; 285:1327–1336.

43. Downing DT, Kranz ZH, Murray KE. Studies in waxes. XIV. An investigation of the aliphatic constituents of hydrolyzed wool wax by gas chromatography. Aust J Chem 1960; 13:80–94.

44. Downing DT, Colton SWT. Skin surface lipids of the horse. Lipids 1980; 15:323–327.

45. Wertz PW, Colton SWT, Downing DT. Comparison of the hydroxyacids from the epi-dermis and from the sebaceous glands of the horse. Comp Biochem Physiol [B] 1983; 75:217–220.

46. Wertz PW, Downing DT, Freinkel RK, Traczyk TN. Sphingolipids of the stratum cor-neum and lamellar granules of fetal rat epidermis. J Invest Dermatol 1984; 83:193–195.

47. Grayson S, Johnson-Winegar AG, Wintroub BU, Isseroff RR, Epstein EH Jr, Elias PM. Lamellar body-enriched fractions from neonatal mice: preparative techniques and partial characterization. J Invest Dermatol 1985; 85:289–294.

48. Hannun YA, Obeid LM. The Ceramide-centric universe of lipid-mediated cell regula-tion: stress encounters of the lipid kind. J Biol Chem 2002; 277:25847–25850.

49. Uchida Y, Nardo AD, Collins V, Elias PM, Holleran WM. De novo ceramide synthesis participates in the ultraviolet B irradiation-induced apoptosis in undifferentiated cultured human keratinocytes. J Invest Dermatol 2003; 120:662–669.

50. Geilen CC, Bektas M, Wieder T, Kodelja V, Goerdt S, Orfanos CE. 1 alpha, 25-dihydroxyvitamin D3 induces sphingomyelin hydrolysis in HaCaT cells via tumor necrosis factor alpha. J Biol Chem 1997; 272:8997–9001.
51. Ji L, Zhang G, Uematsu S, Akahori Y, Hirabayashi Y. Induction of apoptotic DNA fragmentation and cell death by natural ceramide. FEBS Lett 1995; 358:211–214.
52. Cuvillier O. Sphingosine in apoptosis signaling. Biochim Biophys Acta 2002; 1585: 153–162.
53. Park MT, Kang JA, Choi JA, Kang CM, Kim TH, Bae S, Kang S, Kim S, Choi WI, Cho CK, Chung HY, Lee YS, Lee SJ. Phytosphingosine induces apoptotic cell death via caspase 8 activation and bax translocation in human cancer cells. Clin Cancer Res 2003; 9:878–885.
54. Spiegel S, Milstien S. Sphingosine 1-phosphate, a key cell signaling molecule. J Biol Chem 2002; 277:25851–25854.
55. Vogler R, Sauer B, Kim DS, Schafer-Korting M, Kleuser B. Sphingosine-1-phosphate and its potentially paradoxical effects on critical parameters of cutaneous wound healing. J Invest Dermatol 2003; 120:693–700.
56. Bouwstra J, Pilgram G, Gooris G, Koerten H, Ponec M. New aspects of the skin barrier organization. Skin Pharmacol Appl Skin Physiol 2001; 14:52–62.
57. de Jager MW, Gooris GS, Dolbnya IP, Bras W, Ponec M, Bouwstra JA. The phase behaviour of skin lipid mixtures based on synthetic ceramides. Chem Phys Lipids 2003; 124:123–134.
58. Merrill AH Jr. De novo sphingolipid biosynthesis: a necessary, but dangerous, pathway. J Biol Chem 2002; 277:25843–25846.
59. Ternes P, Franke S, Zahringer U, Sperling P, Heinz E. Identification and characterization of a sphingolipid delta 4-desaturase family. J Biol Chem 2002; 277:25512–25518.
60. Ichikawa S, Hirabayashi Y. Glucosylceramide synthase and glycosphingolipid synthesis. Trends Cell Biol 1998; 8:198–202.
61. Fukasawa M, Nishijima M, Hanada K. Genetic evidence for ATP-dependent endoplasmic reticulum-to-Golgi apparatus trafficking of ceramide for sphingomyelin synthesis in Chinese hamster ovary cells. J Cell Biol 1999; 144:673–685.
62. Hanada K, Kumagai K, Yasuda S, Miura Y, Kawano M, Fukasawa M, Nishijima M. Molecular machinery for non-vesicular trafficking of ceramide. Nature 2003; 426:803–809.
63. Holleran WM, Ginns EI, Menon GK, Grundmann JU, Fartasch M, McKinney CE, Elias PM, Sidransky E. Consequences of beta-glucocerebrosidase deficiency in epidermis. Ultrastructure and permeability barrier alterations in Gaucher disease. J Clin Invest 1994; 93:1756–1764.
64. Holleran WM, Takagi Y, Menon GK, Legler G, Feingold KR, Elias PM. Processing of epidermal glucosylceramides is required for optimal mammalian cutaneous permeability barrier function. J Clin Invest 1993; 91:1656–1664.
65. Schmuth M, Man MQ, Weber F, Gao W, Feingold KR, Fritsch P, Elias PM, Holleran WM. Permeability barrier disorder in Niemann–Pick disease: sphingomyelin-ceramide processing required for normal barrier homeostasis. J Invest Dermatol 2000; 115:459–466.
66. Jensen JM, Schütze S, Förl M, Krönke M, Proksch E. Roles for tumor necrosis factor receptor p55 and sphingomyelinase in repairing the cutaneous permeability barrier. J Clin Invest 1999; 104:1761–1770.
67. Gray GM, Yardley HJ. Lipid compositions of cells isolated from pig, human, and rat epidermis. J Lipid Res 1975; 16:434–440.
68. Hamanaka S, Asagami C, Kobayashi K, Ishibashi Y, Otsuka F. Sphingoglycolipids in human cultured keratinocytes. Arch Dermatol Res 1990; 282:345–347.
69. Wertz PW, Downing DT. Acylglucosylceramides of pig epidermis: structure determination. J Lipid Res 1983; 24:753–758.
70. Yasugi E, Saito E, Kasama T, Kojima H, Yamakawa T. Occurrence of 2-O-acyl galactosyl ceramide in whale brain. J Biochem (Tokyo) 1982; 91:1121–1127.

71. Yasugi E, Kasama T, Kojima H, Yamakawa T. Occurrence of 2-O-acyl galactosyl ceramide in human and bovine brains. J Biochem (Tokyo) 1983; 93:1595–1599.

72. Ponec M, Weerheim A, Kempenaar J, Mommaas AM, Nugteren DH. Lipid composition of cultured human keratinocytes in relation to their differentiation. J Lipid Res 1988; 29:949–961.

73. Madison KC, Swartzendruber DC, Wertz PW, Downing DT. Murine keratinocyte cultures grown at the air/medium interface synthesize stratum corneum lipids and "recycle" linoleate during differentiation. J Invest Dermatol 1989; 93:10–17.

74. Burr GO, Burr MM. On the nature and role of fatty acids essential in nutrition. J Biol Chem 1930; 86:587–621.

75. Basnayake HM, Sinclair V. The effect of deficiency of essential fatty acids upon the skin. In: Popjak G, LeBreton E, eds. Biochemical Problems of Lipids. London: Butterworth Scientific Publications, 1957:476–484.

76. Hou SY, Mitra AK, White SH, Menon GK, Ghadially R, Elias PM. Membrane structures in normal and essential fatty acid-deficient stratum corneum: characterization by ruthenium tetroxide staining and X-ray diffraction. J Invest Dermatol 1991; 96:215–223.

77. Prottey C, Hartop PJ, Press M. Correction of the cutaneous manifestations of essential fatty acid deficiency in man by application of sunflower-seed oil to the skin. J Invest Dermatol 1975; 64:228–234.

78. Houtsmuller UM, van der Beek A. Effects of topical application of fatty acids. Prog Lipid Res 1981; 20:219–224.

79. Wertz PW, Downing DT. Linoleate content of epidermal acylglucosylceramide in newborn, growing and mature mice. Biochim Biophys Acta 1986; 876:469–473.

80. Hansen HS, Jensen B, von Wettstein-Knowles P. Apparent in vivo retroconversion of dietary arachidonic to linoleic acid in essential fatty acid-deficient rats. Biochim Biophys Acta 1986; 878:284–287.

81. Hamanaka S, Suzuki M, Suzuki A, Yamakawa T. Epidermosides: structure and function of skin-specific glycolipids. Proc Japan Acad 2001; 77:51–56.

82. Allan D, Quinn P. Resynthesis of sphingomyelin from plasma-membrane phosphatidylcholine in BHK cells treated with Staphylococcus aureus sphingomyelinase. Biochem J 1988; 254:765–771.

83. Slotte JP, Bierman EL. Depletion of plasma-membrane sphingomyelin rapidly alters the distribution of cholesterol between plasma membranes and intracellular cholesterol pools in cultured fibroblasts. Biochem J 1988; 250:653–658.

84. Kitano Y, Iwamori Y, Kiguchi K, DiGiovanni J, Takahashi T, Kasama K, Niwa T, Harii K, Iwamori M. Selective reduction in alpha-hydroxypalmitic acid-containing sphingomyelin and concurrent increase in hydroxylated ceramides in murine skin tumors induced by an initiation-promotion regimen. Jpn J Cancer Res 1996; 87:437–441.

85. Barenholz Y, Thompson TE. Sphingomyelins in bilayers and biological membranes. Biochim Biophys Acta 1980; 604:129–158.

86. Breimer ME, Karlsson KA, Samuelsson BE. The distribution of molecular species of monoglycosylceramides (cerebrosides) in different parts of bovine digestive tract. Biochim Biophys Acta 1974; 348:232–240.

87. Yasugi E, Kasama T, Shibahara M, Seyama Y. Composition of long-chain bases in sphingomyelin of the guinea pig Harderian gland. Biochem Cell Biol 1990; 68:154–160.

88. Robinson BS, Johnson DW, Poulos A. Novel molecular species of sphingomyelin containing 2-hydroxylated polyenoic very-long-chain fatty acids in mammalian testes and spermatozoa. J Biol Chem 1992; 267:1746–1751.

89. Doering T, Holleran WM, Potratz A, Vielhaber G, Elias PM, Suzuki K, Sandhoff K. Sphingolipid activator proteins are required for epidermal permeability barrier formation. J Biol Chem 1999; 274:11038–11045.

90. Doering T, Proia RL, Sandhoff K. Accumulation of protein-bound epidermal glucosylceramides in beta-glucocerebrosidase deficient type 2 Gaucher mice. FEBS Lett 1999; 447:167–170.

91. Uchida Y, Sidransky E, Ginns EI, Elias PM, Holleran WM. Formation of the lipid-bound envelope (LBE): insights from glucocerebrosidase-deficient Gaucher mouse epidermis. J Invest Dermatol 1999; 112:543a.

92. Vielhaber G, Pfeiffer S, Brade L, Lindner B, Goldmann T, Vollmer E, Hintze U, Wittern KP, Wepf R. Localization of ceramide and glucosylceramide in human epidermis by immunogold electron microscopy. J Invest Dermatol 2001; 117:1126–1136.

93. Nemes Z, Marekov LN, Fésüs L, Steinert PM. A novel function for transglutaminase 1: attachment of long-chain omega-hydroxyceramides to involucrin by ester bond formation. Proc Natl Acad Sci USA 1999; 96:8402–8407.

94. Imokawa G, Akasaki S, Hattori M, Yoshizuka N. Selective recovery of deranged water-holding properties by stratum corneum lipids. J Invest Dermatol 1986; 87:758–761.

95. Mao-Qiang M, Brown BE, Wu-Pong S, Feingold KR, Elias PM. Exogenous nonphysiologic vs. physiologic lipids. Divergent mechanisms for correction of permeability barrier dysfunction. Arch Dermatol 1995; 131:809–816.

96. Zettersten EM, Ghadially R, Feingold KR, Crumrine D, Elias PM. Optimal ratios of topical stratum corneum lipids improve barrier recovery in chronologically aged skin. J Am Acad Dermatol 1997; 37:403–408.

97. De Paepe K, Derde MP, Roseeuw D, Rogiers V. Incorporation of ceramide 3B in dermatocosmetic emulsions: effect on the transepidermal water loss of sodium lauryl sulphate-damaged skin. J Eur Acad Dermatol Venereol 2000; 14:272–279.

98. De Paepe K, Roseeuw D, Rogiers V. Repair of acetone- and sodium lauryl sulphate-damaged human skin barrier function using topically applied emulsions containing barrier lipids. J Eur Acad Dermatol Venereol 2002; 16:587–594.

99. Berardesca E, Barbareschi M, Veraldi S, Pimpinelli N. Evaluation of efficacy of a skin lipid mixture in patients with irritant contact dermatitis, allergic contact dermatitis or atopic dermatitis: a multicenter study. Contact Dermat 2001; 45:280–285.

100. Imokawa G, Akasaki S, Kawamata A, Yano S, Takaishi N. Water-retaining function in the stratum corneum and its recovery properties by synthetic pseudoceramides. J Soc Cosmet Chem 1989; 40:273–285.

101. Mizushima H, Fukasawa J, Suzuki T. Phase behavior of artificial stratum corneum lipids containing a synthetic pseudo-ceramide: a study of the function of cholesterol. J Lipid Res 1996; 37:361–367.

102. Mizushima H, Fukasawa J, Suzuki T. Intermolecular interaction between a synthetic pseudoceramide and a sterol-combined fatty acid. J Colloid Interface Sci 1997; 195: 156–163.

103. Mizutani H, Takahashi M, Shimizu M, Kariya K, Sato H. The Nishinihon Journal of Dermatology 2001; 63:457–461.

104. Nakamura T, Honma D, Kasiwagi T, Sakai H, Hashimoto Y, Iizuka H. The Nishinihon J Dermatol 1999; 61:671–681.

105. Park BD, Youm JK, Jeong SK, Choi EH, Ahn SH, Lee SH. The characterization of molecular organization of multilamellar emulsions containing pseudoceramide and type III synthetic ceramide. J Invest Dermatol 2003; 121:794–801.

106. Chamlin SL, Kao J, Frieden IJ, Sheu MY, Fowler AJ, Fluhr JW, Williams ML, Elias PM. Ceramide-dominant barrier repair lipids alleviate childhood atopic dermatitis: changes in barrier function provide a sensitive indicator of disease activity. J Am Acad Dermatol 2002; 47:198–208.

107. Chamlin SL, Frieden IJ, Fowler A, Williams M, Kao J, Sheu M, Elias PM. Ceramide-dominant, barrier-repair lipids improve childhood atopic dermatitis. Arch Dermatol 2001; 137:1110–1112.

108. Lee EJ, Suhr KB, Lee JHK, Park JK, Jin CY, Youm JK, Park BD. The clinical efficacy of a multi-lamellar emulsion containing pseudoceramide in childhood atopic dermatitis: an open crossover study. Ann Dermatol 2003; 15:133–138.

109. Park WS, Son ED, Nam GW, Choi EH, Lee SH, Chang IS. Improvement of skin barrier function using lipid mixture. SOFW J 2001; 127:10–18.

110. Hamanaka S, Yamaguchi Y, Yamamoto T, Asagami C. Occurrence of galactosylcera-mide in pig epidermal cells. Biochim Biophys Acta 1988; 961:374–377.
111. Hara M, Uchida Y, Haratake A, Mimura K, Hamanaka S. Galactocerebroside and not glucocerebroside or ceramide stimulate epidermal beta-glucocerebrosidase activity. J Dermatol Sci 1998; 16:111–119.
112. Hamanaka S, Ujihara M, Uchida Y, Mimura K. A trial of galactosylceramide contain-ing cream to the patients with atopic skin and xerosis. Skin Res 1995; 37:619–625.
113. Chang-Yi C, Kusuda S, Seguchi T, Takahashi M, Aisu K, Tezuka T. Decreased level of prosaposin in atopic skin. J Invest Dermatol 1997; 109:319–323.
114. Alessandrini F, Stachowitz S, Ring J, Behrendt H. The level of prosaposin is decreased in the skin of patients with psoriasis vulgaris. J Invest Dermatol 2001; 116:394–400.
115. Horikawa T, Takashima T, Haradaa S, Chihara T, Ichihaashi M. An open clinical trial glycoceramide-containing cream and lotion on dry skin of atopic dermatitis. Hifu 1998; 40:415–419.
116. Fukunaga K, Yoshida M, Nakajima F, Uematsu R, Hara M, Inoue S, Kondo H, Nishimura S. Design, synthesis, and evaluation of beta-galactosylceramide mimics promoting beta-glucocerebrosidase activity in keratinocytes. Bioorg Med Chem Lett 2003; 13:813–815.
117. Karthikeyan K, Thappa DM. Pellagra and skin. Int J Dermatol 2002; 41:476–481.
118. Tanno O, Ota Y, Kitamura N, Katsube T, Inoue S. Nicotinamide increases biosynthesis of ceramides as well as other stratum corneum lipids to improve the epidermal perme-ability barrier. Br J Dermatol 2000; 143:524–531.
119. Uchida Y, Behne M, Quiec D, Elias PM, Holleran WM. Vitamin C stimulates sphingo-lipid production and markers of barrier formation in submerged human keratinocyte cultures. J Invest Dermatol 2001; 117:1307–1313.
120. Mori K, Masuda Y. Synthesis and stereochemistry of ceramide B, (2S,3R,4E,6R)-N-(30-hydroxytriacontanoyl)-6-hydroxy-4-sphingenine, a new ceramide in human epidermis. Tetrahedron Lett 2003; 44:9197–9200.

7

Structure of the Skin Barrier

Joke A. Bouwstra
Leiden/Amsterdam Center for Drug Research, Gorlaeus Laboratories,
Leiden University, Leiden, The Netherlands

Gonneke S. K. Pilgram
Department of Molecular Cell Biology,
Leiden University Medical Center, Leiden, The Netherlands

Maria Ponec
Department of Dermatology, Leiden University Medical Center,
Leiden, The Netherlands

INTRODUCTION

The skin is composed of several morphologically distinct layers. The skin is protected primarily by the stratum corneum (SC). The superficial region, which is only 10–20 μm thick, is the primary barrier to the percutaneous absorption of compounds, as well as to water loss. Underlying the SC is the viable epidermis (50–100 μm thick), which is responsible for generation of the SC. The dermis (1–2 mm thick) is directly adjacent to the epidermis and provides the mechanical support for the skin. The viable epidermis is a stratified squamous epithelium consisting of basal, spinous, and granular cell layers. Each layer is defined by position, shape, morphology, and state of differentiation of keratinocytes. The epidermis is a dynamic, constantly self-renewing tissue, in which the loss of the cells from the surface of the SC (desquamation) is balanced by cell growth in the lower epidermis. Upon leaving the basal layer, keratinocytes begin to differentiate and during their apical migration through the stratum spinosum and stratum granulosum (SG), they undergo a number of changes in both structure and composition. The keratinocytes synthesize and express numerous different structural proteins and lipids during their maturation. The final steps in keratinocyte differentiation are associated with profound changes in their structure resulting in their transformation into corneocytes. The corneocytes are relatively flat, anucleated squamous cells packed mainly with keratin filaments, and surrounded by a cell envelope composed of cross-linked proteins, as well as a covalently bound lipid (CLE) envelope. This corneocyte lipid envelope most probably plays an important role in keeping the osmotically active material inside the corneocytes. Extracellular non-polar lipids surround the corneocytes, forming a hydrophobic matrix. Furthermore, corneodesmosomes interconnect adjacent corneocytes and are important for the SC cohesion.

Late in the process of differentiation, characteristic organelles (lamellar bodies) appear in the granular cells. The lamellar bodies, which play an essential role in SC formation, are ovoid organelles enriched mainly in polar lipids and catabolic enzymes, which deliver the lipids required for the generation of the SC. In response to a certain signal (possibly an increase in calcium concentration), the lamellar bodies move to the apex and periphery of the uppermost granular cells, fuse with the plasma membrane, and secrete their content into the intercellular spaces by exocytosis. The lipids derived from the lamellar bodies are subsequently modified and rearranged into intercellular lamellae orientated approximately parallel to the surface of the cell (1–7). In this orientation process, the corneocyte-bound lipid envelope (8–10) acts most probably as a template.

Lamellar bodies serve as the carriers of precursors of SC barrier lipids, which consist mainly of glycosphingolipids, free sterols, and phospholipids. After the extrusion of lamellar bodies at the SG/SC interface, the polar lipid precursors are enzymatically converted into non-polar products and assembled into lamellar structures surrounding the corneocytes. Hydrolysis of glycolipids generates ceramides (CER), while phospholipids are converted into free fatty acids (FFA). This change in lipid composition and cell structure results in the formation of a very densely packed structure within the SC interstices. Owing to the impermeable character of the cornified envelope (CE), the major route of penetration resides in the tortuous pathway between the corneocytes as revealed by confocal laser scanning microscopy and X-ray microanalysis studies (11,12). It is for this reason that the lipids play an irreplaceable role in the skin barrier. This makes their mutual arrangement into lamellar domains a key process in the formation of the skin barrier.

In the first part of this chapter the lipid organization of the SC of normal, diseased and in vitro–reconstructed skin will be reviewed, and in the second part of the paper we discuss the role of various lipid classes in SC lipid organization, as assessed with lipid mixtures prepared from isolated CER.

STRATUM CORNEUM LIPID COMPOSITION AND ORGANIZATION IN NORMAL SKIN

Lipid Composition in Stratum Corneum

The major lipid classes (13,14) in the SC are CER, cholesterol (CHOL), and FFA. The CER head groups are very small and contain several functional groups that can form lateral hydrogen bonds with adjacent CER molecules. The acyl chain length distribution in the CER is bimodal with the most abundant chain lengths being C24–C26. Only a small fraction of CER has an acyl chain length of C16–C18. The chain lengths of C24 and C26 are much longer than those in phospholipids in plasma membranes. In human SC (15–17) nine subclasses of CER (HCER) have been identified (Fig. 1). These HCER, referred to as HCER 1 to 9, differ from each other by the head group architecture [sphingosine (S), phytosphingosine (P) or 6-hydroxysphingosine (H) base] linked to a fatty acid (N) or an α-hydroxy fatty acid (A) of varying hydrocarbon chain length. Based on the different bases linked to the fatty acids, recently another nomenclature has been introduced for the CER in the skin. The two nomenclatures along with the CER structures are shown in Figure 1. In the human SC, three CER, CER1 (EOS), CER4 (EOH), and CER9 (EOP), have very exceptional molecular

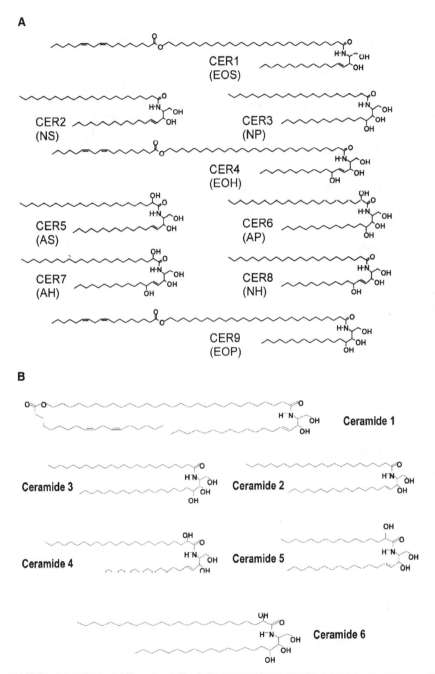

Figure 1 Molecular structure of ceramides: (A) Ceramides in human SC (HCER) and (B) pig SC (pigCER). It is noted that in the HCER mixture both CER1 and CER4 have an ω-hydroxy acyl chain to which a linoleic acid is chemically linked. In pigCER mixture only CER1 has this exceptional molecular structure.

structures. They contain a linoleic acid ester linked to an ω-hydroxy fatty acid (EO) with a chain length of approximately 30–32 C-atoms. In this respect the human CER are different from CER isolated from *pig* SC (pigCER), in which only pigCER1 has this exceptional molecular structure (18) and pigCER5 has an unusual short chain length (acyl chain length of C16–C18). In both species the FFA fraction consists mainly of saturated acids. The major portion of FFA has a chain length of C22 and C24. Another important lipid in SC is cholesterol sulfate. Although cholesterol sulfate is present in a relatively small amount (typically 2–5% w/w), this lipid plays an important role in the desquamation process of SC (19).

Lipid Organization in Stratum Corneum

At the end of the 1950s and in the early 1960s, the lipid organization in human SC (20,21) was measured using X-ray diffraction. The excellent measurements obtained using a conventional camera revealed a similar pattern as observed nowadays with the synchrotron facilities. As no information was available about the lipid organization at an ultrastructural level at that time, the X-ray diffraction patterns were interpreted as being from lipids organized in tubes surrounding keratin filaments. These conclusions were drawn from the similarity between the measured and the calculated diffraction curves, in which the calculated diffraction curves were obtained from Fourier transformations of lipid associates in the geometry of hollow tubes. At least ten years passed before important additional information became available, which provided completely new insights into the lipid organization. Using freeze fracture electron microscopic technique, Breathnach et al. (22,23) reported the presence of lipid lamellae, while the group of Elias proposed the two-compartment model, in which the lamellae are located in the intercellular space (24). This was a big step forward in understanding the structure of the SC.

In transmission electron microscopic studies, the key problem in visualizing lipid lamellae was the saturated nature of the SC lipids, which made their visualization with osmium tetroxide impossible. In 1987, Madison et al. (4,25) used ruthenium tetroxide, a more reactive and electron-dense agent, as a post-fixation agent to preserve the saturated lipids in the SC during the embedding procedure. The subsequent electron microscopic studies revealed a unique lamellar arrangement of a repeating pattern with electron translucent bands in a broad–narrow–broad sequence (26–29). More detailed insights into the SC lipid organization were achieved in the mid-1980s using Fourier transformed infrared (FTIR) spectroscopy and X-ray diffraction techniques. FTIR spectroscopy provides information about the mobility and the lateral packing of the lipids in the SC (30–32), making it possible to distinguish between a hexagonal (gel-phase) and an orthorhombic sub-lattice. The presence of the latter introduces a splitting of the rocking and scissoring frequencies located at approximately 720 and 1460 cm^{-1}, respectively, due to the short-range coupling in the densely packed structure. In addition to the formation of an orthorhombic sub-lattice in the human SC, a small sub-population of lipids also forms a liquid phase. The latter conclusion was based on the presence of CH_2 anti-symmetric and symmetric stretching frequencies at around 2850 and 2920 cm^{-1}, respectively. X-ray diffraction analysis of membrane couplets was also carried out, which revealed that the lateral packing of these couplets was very similar to that of the intact SC (33).

At the end of the 1980s, White et al. (34) performed X-ray diffraction studies with the mouse SC. Using small-angle X-ray diffraction (SAXD) they observed a diffraction pattern of a series of sharp peaks, indicating the presence of a lamellar phase with a periodicity of approximately 13 nm, further referred to as the long periodicity phase (LPP). Furthermore, wide-angle X-ray diffraction (WAXD) studies revealed the presence of an orthorhombic sub-lattice (34) with a transition from an orthorhombic to a hexagonal sub-phase occurring between 30 and 40°C (36). However, in these studies the presence of the hexagonal sub-lattice at room temperature could not be excluded as the reflections based on the hexagonal lateral packing (strong reflection at 0.41-nm spacing) could be obscured by reflections attributed to an orthorhombic phase (strong reflections at 0.41 and 0.37-nm spacings). Besides the orthorhombic phase, liquid lateral packing was also evident. This conclusion was drawn from the detection of a very broad reflection at a spacing of approximately 0.46 nm. However, more recently it became evident that a thick layer of sebum lipids covers the surface of hairless mouse skin (35). Therefore, it cannot be deduced from these X-ray studies whether the detected liquid sub-lattice localizes in the intercellular lipid regions of the SC or in sebum lipids located on the skin surface. Besides the reflections that could be attributed to the presence of crystalline phases, other reflections have also been detected. These reflections could be attributed to the presence of hydrated crystalline CHOL in separate domains. In a more recent publication (36), it became clear that in mouse SC not only is the 13-nm phase present, but also that a small fraction of lipids forms a second phase with a periodicity of approximately 6 nm, further referred to as the short periodicity phase (SPP). The presence of LPP and SPP can be fully ascribed to the extracellular SC lipids, as, after lipid extraction, only reflections attributed to proteins could be detected in the diffraction patterns.

In a more recent series of studies, synchrotron facilities have been used to obtain information about the lipid organization of human and pig SC (37,38). The use of a synchrotron makes it possible to use a very intense and focused X-ray beam, which makes it possible to obtain detailed structural information from the samples. As the SAXD curves of pig and human SC revealed the presence of very broad and partly overlapping peaks, additional information was required to properly interpret the obtained data. These data were obtained in X-ray experiments with the SC in which the lipids were re-crystallized from 120°C to room temperature (Fig. 2). The diffraction curves revealed the presence of a series of sharp peaks, similar to those noted in the mouse SC, indicating that after recrystallization the lipids in human and pig SC were organized in a LPP with a periodicity of approximately 13 nm. Comparing the peak positions in the diffraction patterns obtained before and after recrystallization revealed the presence of at least two lamellar phases: one lamellar phase with a periodicity of approximately 6 nm (SPP), and another phase with a periodicity of approximately 13 nm (LPP) (37,38). As the LPP has been found to be present in all species examined, and because it has a very characteristic molecular organization (see below), it has been suggested that the presence of this phase plays an important role in skin barrier function.

To get more detailed information on the SC lipid organization, changes in diffraction patterns as a function of temperature have also been investigated. These experiments revealed that lipid lamellae persist up to a temperature of around 60°C, after which the lipid lamellae disappear over a temperature range of approximately 10°C (Fig. 2B).

In addition to the lamellar organization, the lateral lipid packing of human and pig SC has also been investigated. In human SC, an orthorhombic lateral packing was observed (39,40), in agreement with the previous FTIR results. It could not be concluded, however, whether a liquid phase co-existed with the orthorhombic lateral packing, as the broad reflection of the liquid phase in the diffraction pattern was obscured by the reflections from soft keratin present with the corneocytes

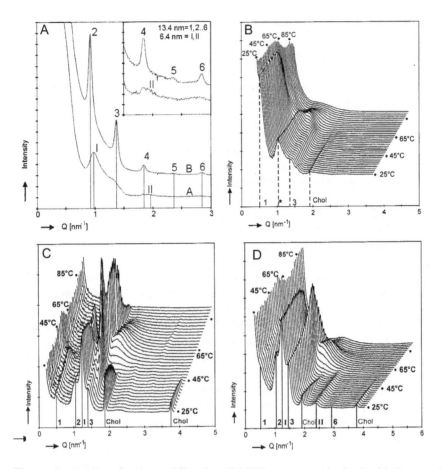

Figure 2 Small-angle X-ray diffraction (SAXD) patterns obtained with human SC and mixtures prepared with isolated lipids from pig SC. In the SAXD curves, the intensity is plotted as a function of Q, the scattering vector. Q is defined as $4\pi \sin \theta / \lambda$, in which θ is the scattering angle and λ is the wavelength of the X-rays. The position of the peaks (Q_1, Q_2, $Q_3 \ldots Q_n$, n being the order of the peak) is related to the periodicity (d) of a lamellar phase by $d = 2n\pi / Q_n$. (A) The SAXD curve of human SC at room temperature and after recrystallization from 120°C. After recrystallization the peaks are located at equal distances, strongly indicating a lamellar phase with a periodicity of 13.4 nm. This phase is referred to as the long periodicity phase (LPP). Comparing this curve with the curve at room temperature revealed the presence of the second lamellar phase in human SC with a periodicity of 6.4 nm, referred to as the short periodicity phase (SPP). In A–D 1, 2, 3, 4, and 6 denote the first, second, third, fourth, and sixth order peak of the pattern based on the LPP. I and II refer to the first and second order of the SPP. (B) The temperature-induced changes in SAXD profiles of human SC. The heating rate was 2°C/min. Each sequential curve has been monitored for 1 min. The lamellar phases disappear between 60 and 75°C. The first order diffraction peak is clearly depicted in this figure. (*) The peak attributed to the first order of the SPP and the second order peak of the LPP. CHOL indicates the peaks attributed to the phase-separated crystalline CHOL. (C) The temperature-induced changes in the SAXD pattern of the equimolar CHOL:pigCER:FFA mixture. The formation of a new peak at 4.3 nm (close to the third order of the LPP) at around 35°C is noted. The lamellar phases disappear between 60 and 80°C, except for the 4.3-nm phase, which is still present at 90°C. CHOL indicates the peaks attributed to phase-separated crystalline CHOL. (D) The temperature-induced changes in the SAXD pattern of the CHOL:pigCER:FFA:cholesterol sulfate (molar ratio: 1:1:1:0.06) mixture. It is noted that the formation of a new peak takes place at much higher temperatures and the intensity of this peak decreased strongly compared with that in C. The phase behavior of this mixture resembles that shown in B. *Source*: From Refs. 37, 87.

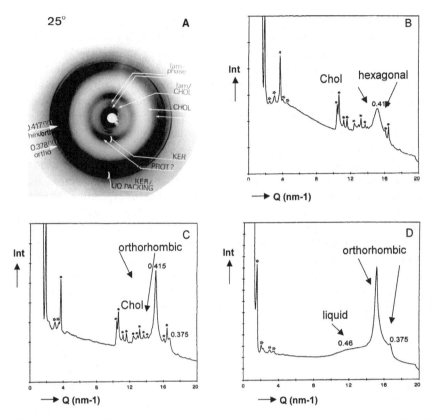

Figure 3 Lateral lipid packing in human SC and in mixtures based on lipids isolated from pig SC. (A) WAXD pattern of human SC orientated parallel to the primary X-ray beam. The diffraction pattern is characterized by two rings, indicating that the lipids are organized in an orthorhombic lateral packing. The rings are stronger in equatorial position, indicating that the lipids are orientated mainly perpendicular to the SC surface. Furthermore, a number of reflections can be attributed to the phase-separated CHOL. The position of the reflection in the pattern indicates that CHOL crystals have a preferred orientation in a similar direction as the lipid lamellae. The strong broad reflections at 0.46 and 0.92 nm can be attributed to soft keratin. (B) One-dimensional WAXD pattern of the equimolar CHOL:pigCER mixture plotted as function of Q (Fig. 4). A broad reflection at 0.415-nm spacing is attributed to the presence of the hexagonal lattice. A large number of sharp reflections are based on the phase-separated CHOL. (C) One-dimensional WAXD pattern of the equimolar CHOL: pigCER:FFA mixture. Two strong sharp reflections indicate the presence of an orthorhombic lateral packing. (D) One-dimensional WAXD pattern of the 1:1:1:0.06 CHOL:pigCER:FFA: cholesterol sulfate mixture. Two strong reflections are attributed to the orthorhombic lateral packing. The broad reflection at 0.46 nm indicates the presence of a liquid phase. It is noted that the reflections attributed to CHOL disappeared due to the presence of cholesterol sulfate. *Source*: From Ref. 86.

(Fig. 3A). In addition, it could not be determined whether a hexagonal phase is present, because the reflections of the orthorhombic phase obscure the reflections from hexagonal lateral packing (40), as in previous observations on the mouse SC. Furthermore, often a crystalline CHOL phase separates from the lamellar phases (38,40). From the orientation of the reflections in the diffraction pattern it could be deduced that the long axis of the CHOL lattice orients perpendicularly to the basal plane of the lamellae. Most probably, the preferred orientation of CHOL crystals is dictated by the orientation of the lipid lamellae, indicating that CHOL is intercalated within the lamellae between the corneocytes. In contrast to the mouse and human SC, no orthorhombic lateral packing was present in pig SC, although a hexagonal lateral packing prevailed. Whether a liquid phase co-exists with the hexagonal sub-lattice is difficult to determine for the same reason as in the case of the human SC. However, after the extraction of the lipids from the pig SC, a reduction in the intensity of the broad reflection at around 0.46 nm was noticed. This reduction in intensity is suggestive of the presence of a liquid phase in the pig SC.

Recently, using the electron diffraction (ED) technique (41), more detailed information has been obtained on the lateral organization of lipids in the human SC. Because a small area with a diameter as small as 1 μm^2 can be selected for exposure to the electron beam, it is possible to obtain reflections only from one or a few crystals. Owing to this small area of exposure, ED provides information on the lateral packing of SC lipids that is supplementary to WAXD. Another advantage of ED is the possibility of obtaining diffraction patterns from SC strips as a function of depth. This allows an in-depth examination of not only an SC lateral packing in vitro, but also in vivo samples.

The diffraction pattern of an orthorhombic single crystal is characterized by two-paired strong reflections at a spacing of approximately 0.406 nm and one pair of strong reflections at a spacing of 0.367 nm. In addition to these strong reflections, higher order reflections can also be detected. The strong reflections are separated by angles that are close but not equal to 60°. A single crystal of a hexagonal sub-lattice is characterized by three-paired diffraction spots separated by angles of 60° at a spacing of 0.41 nm. As spots are detected in these patterns instead of rings, it is possible to distinguish the hexagonal sub-lattice from the orthorhombic one.

In order to determine whether a hexagonal sub-lattice is present in addition to an orthorhombic one, in vivo and ex vivo human skin were studied relative to the depth in the SC. Some characteristic ED patterns are shown in Figure 4. No differences are observed between ED patterns from in vivo and ex vivo SC. The diffraction patterns consist of concentric rings as in WAXD or of opposite arcs/spots at both 0.41 and 0.37 nm, particularly when smaller areas were selected for ED. These latter ED patterns are important to distinguish whether only the orthorhombic packing is present or the hexagonal packing as well. Furthermore, faint reflections at 0.22 and 0.25 nm were recorded occasionally. These reflections can be attributed to other sets of lattice planes within the same crystal. The spacings are in agreement with calculated values, and with the spacings obtained from WAXD.

In order to estimate the frequency of the various detected lattices, the ED patterns were classified into four categories: orthorhombic (ort), orthorhombic in which hexagonal cannot be excluded (ort*), hexagonal (hex), and patterns that are probably hexagonal (hex*). The relative distribution of the ED patterns in these categories was similar for ex vivo and in vivo skin (not shown). The data in Figure 5 are plotted as a function of temperature and show that the percentage of ED patterns attributed to the hexagonal lattice increased at 32°C compared with room temperature. From our studies it was clear that the orthorhombic packing prevails throughout the SC; however, in the upper part of the SC, the hexagonal lattice can occasionally be detected as well. These observations do not confirm the single-phase model recently proposed by Norlen et al. (42), who suggested the formation of a single phase with gel-phase packing.

From the ED studies it was concluded that ED patterns attributed to the hexagonal packing were recorded mainly in the superficial layers of the SC at room temperature and at 32°C. However, in vivo, one would expect to observe the hexagonal

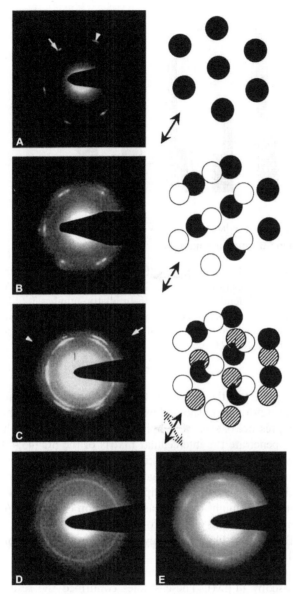

Figure 4 Characteristic electron diffraction (ED) patterns of both in vivo and ex vivo human SC. (A) An orthorhombic sub-lattice that can be found throughout the SC. The *arrow* indicates the 0.41-nm reflections and the *arrowheads* mark the 0.37-nm reflections. (B–C) The second and third orientations of orthorhombic crystals, respectively, rotated approximately 60° with respect to each other. As a consequence, the 0.41-nm reflections are obtained from two differently oriented crystals (41). In (C) higher order reflections are indicated by the *arrowhead* (0.24 nm) at an interplanar angle of 90° with respect to the 0.37-nm reflection, and the *arrow* (0.22 nm). A schematic representation of the corresponding orientations of first, second, and third orientations of the orthorhombic lattice is also shown (A–C), respectively. The double-sided arrows indicate the direction of the 0.37-nm reflection. (D) Two rings at 0.37 and 0.41 nm in which the hexagonal lattice cannot be excluded, as in WAXD patterns. (E) A hexagonal lattice that is mainly found in the outer layers of the SC.

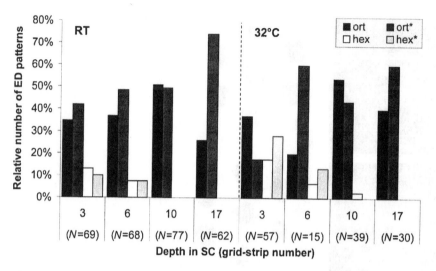

Figure 5 Distribution of the hexagonal and orthorhombic lattices in relation to depth in the ex vivo human SC equilibrated to room temperature or 32°C. The number of recordings (N) shown at the x-axis is set at 100% for each depth indicated by the grid-strip number 3, 6, 10, and 17. The percentage of ED patterns per category is shown along the y-axis (ort, orthorhombic; ort*, orthorhombic; however, the hexagonal lattice cannot be excluded; hex, hexagonal; hex*, probably hexagonal). *Source*: From Ref. 41.

lattice more frequently in the lower part of the SC where the temperature approaches 37°C, but this was not the case. Therefore, there should be another explanation for this phenomenon, which might be the presence of sebaceous lipids that are secreted onto the surface of the skin, and partially penetrate the intercellular matrix of the SC (43,44). These sebaceous lipids could either form a hexagonal packing or alter the phase transition of the endogenous lipids from orthorhombic to hexagonal. FTIR studies by Bommannan et al. (43) showed a fluidization of the upper SC lipids, while Golden et al. (45) have shown that unsaturated fatty acids might function as penetration enhancers. As sebum mainly consists of glycerides, squalene, wax/sterol esters, diesters, as well as (short chain) FFA (unsaturated), it is very likely that they alter the endogenous lipid structure by increasing the alkyl chain mobility.

The orthorhombic to hexagonal phase transition could also be studied on line in the transmission electron microscopy (TEM). These studies confirmed the results observed by X-rays, i.e., an orthorhombic–hexagonal phase transition occurs between 35 and 40°C. It was noticed that the 0.37-nm reflection moves gradually towards the 0.41-nm reflection, indicating that the packing density of the structure is gradually increased. Above 40°C, only the hexagonal packing was detected, and above 80°C the lipids formed a liquid phase (46).

Another striking observation is that the ED patterns frequently display reflections forming three pairs of double arcs at 0.41 and 0.37 nm. These reflections can be assigned to the orthorhombic lattice only by rotating three successive orthorhombic crystals over an angle of 60° relative to each other (Fig. 4). These three orientations may be present within the same lamellae or superimposed on top of each other. The latter possibility could be in good agreement with a recently proposed molecular model for the long-lamellar periodicity (47) and with the broad–narrow–broad (Landmann-unit) sequence visible in RuO$_4$-stained SC sections (25), which suggest that these lamellae consist of three lipid layers. The alignment of the lipid layers is probably of importance for a proper barrier function, because mismatches between crystallites, occurring when the lateral or lamellar organization is not maintained, are sites where permeability of compounds could increase.

X-ray and ED patterns obtained with SC revealed spacings corresponding to 0.406 and 0.367-nm reflections, which are slightly shorter than the orthorhombic and hexagonal lattices observed in phospholipid-based systems. Possibly, due to a strong attractive van der Waals interaction between hydrocarbon chains of the very long hydrocarbon chains of the CER and FFA, a slightly denser packing of the hydrocarbon chains is formed compared with those formed in phospholipid-based systems (48). Furthermore, two decades back, it was shown by Pascher (49,50) that an extensive network of hydrogen bondings exists between the head groups of CER, which promotes the formation of a very dense lattice. The surface area per acyl chain in the structure corresponding to hexagonal and orthorhombic sub-lattice in human skin appears to be approximately 0.190 and 0.179 nm^2, respectively. These surface areas are indeed very small, demonstrating a dense packing of acyl chains in the lipid organization in the SC. This dense packing is most probably crucial for a proper skin barrier.

Lipid Organization in Stratum Corneum with Abnormal Lipid Composition

To determine whether an altered lipid composition results in an altered lipid phase behavior, studies have been carried out with SC derived from xerotic and diseased skin. In the 1980s, the lipid organization in essential fatty acid deficient (EFAD) SC (26,51) was elucidated. Elimination of linoleic acid from the diet resulted in a progressive substitution of oleate with linoleate in the pig epidermal CER1. This increase in CER1-oleate content is accompanied by major abnormalities in the skin sensibility barrier. However, both electron microscopy and X-ray diffraction studies revealed no drastic changes in the SC lipid lamellar organization despite clear evidence found in EFAD skin wherein the lamellar bodies contain amorphous rather than lamellar material (51). In EFAD animals, only a great variability in the number of intercellular lipid lamellae has been reported (26). It seems that other factors, such as a change in lateral packing, may also play a role in the formation of competent skin barrier (see below). The effect of the CER1 oleate/linoleate ratio on barrier properties and lipid organization is of interest, as in normal skin this ratio decreases dramatically during winter months (52). However, at that time the presence of two other ω-hydroxy acyl chain ceramides (Fig. 1) was not yet known.

X-ray diffraction studies performed on xerotic skin and lamellar ichthyosis skin have also been reported. Xerotic skin was selected because of its low content of CER1 (53) and lamellar ichthyosis skin, because of its low content of FFA (54). The only feature in the SAXD pattern, which is uniquely related to the 13-nm phase, is its third order diffraction peak (Fig. 2A). It appeared that when taking all of the volunteers into account in this study, in SC samples in which the third order peak was absent, the contents of CER1 and CER4 (both the ω-hydroxy acyl chain ceramides) were also reduced (55) (Table 1). This relation between CER1/CER4 and the presence of the third order diffraction peak suggests that at a low level of CER1 and CER4, the formation of the 13-nm lamellar phase is reduced in vivo. However, it cannot be excluded whether the decrease in intensity of the third order diffraction peak is caused by a dramatically altered lipid organization within this

Table 1 A Relationship Exists Between the Mean $HCER1/CER_{tot}$ and $HCER4/CER_{tot}$ Ratios and the Presence of the Third Order Reflection of the X-ray Pattern of the LPP

$HCER1/CER_{tot}$	$HCER4/CER_{tot}$	Third order reflection of LPP
0.11 ± 0.02	0.08 ± 0.01	Present
0.05 ± 0.01	0.05 ± 0.03	Absent

The X-ray diffraction profiles of the SC are classified in two populations. In one population the third order reflection of the 13.4-nm phase in the diffraction pattern of SC is absent, while in the other population this reflection is present. The mean HCER1 and HCER4 contents of these populations are also provided. *Abbreviations*: HCER1, human ceramide 1; HCER4, human ceramide 4; CER_{tot}, total ceramides present in human SC.

13-nm phase. It should be noted that in the absence of the third order peak, the reduction in CER1 content is more pronounced than that in CER4 content. In contrast to the studies of Imokawa et al. (53), in this study, no relation was observed between dry skin and a reduced amount of CER1. But this difference might be due to the limited number of volunteers (only 3 or 4) available for each group.

In lamellar ichthyosis (LI) skin, in addition to small changes in CER composition, the content of FFA is strongly reduced compared with that found in the normal SC (Table 2). SAXD studies on the SC of lamellar ichthyosis skin revealed an altered lamellar organization, as it was obvious that the peaks were located at smaller spacings than in the SC of normal skin (56). Recently freeze fracture electron microscopy (FFEM) and ED techniques have been used to study the lipid organization in lamellar ichthyosis patients (56). The lamellae in lamellar ichthyosis skin showed strong undulations compared with that of normal skin, confirming the altered lamellar organization (Fig. 6). A change in lamellar organization was also found by Ghadially et al. (57,62) in the SC of autosomal recessive ichthyosis patients. Whether these changes in lipid organization in diseased and dry skin can be explained by an altered lipid composition or whether other features also play a role can be obtained by systematic studies on the phase behavior of mixtures containing major SC lipids.

The lateral lipid organization in the SC of the flexor forearm of three normal volunteers was compared with that of LI patients (56). The lipids formed a hexagonal lamellar phase co-existing with a small number of crystals, forming an orthorhombic sub-lattice. In Figure 6, some characteristic ED patterns that have been recorded in the SC of normal and LI skin are shown. The recorded ED patterns were classified into the four categories described above (ort, ort*, hex, and hex*) and an additional category pattern, *ort + hex*, i.e., both orthorhombic and hexagonal, is present in the same area selected for ED. The latter category was added because it was observed regularly in the diseased SC. In this category, more crystals of different

Table 2 The Positions of the Peaks in the Diffraction Curves and the FFA/HCER, FFA/CHOL, and HCER/CHOL w/w Ratios of SC from Normal and Lamellar Ichthyosis Skin

	Lamellar ichthyosis	Normal
Peak positions	5.3–5.9 nm	6.4 nm
CHOL/HCER	0.59	0.45
FFA/CHOL	0.18	0.69
FFA/HCER	0.12	0.31

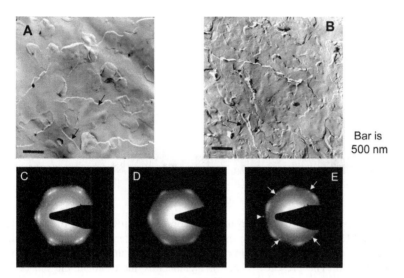

Figure 6 Comparison of lipid structure and lateral organization in the SC derived from healthy subjects and from lamellar ichthyosis patients. (A) Freeze fracture micrograph of the SC of normal skin. The smooth areas indicate the lamellae located between the corneocytes. The sharp edges result from fractures across the lamellae (*arrow*). DD, desmosome; bar = 500 nm. (B) Freeze fracture micrograph of the SC of lamellar ichthyosis skin. The lamellae show undulations, which are absent in normal skin. Furthermore, the fractures across the lamellae result in less sharp edges (*arrow*); bar = 500 nm. (C) Electron diffraction patterns of SC of normal skin. The diffraction pattern shows reflections as two spacings based on various crystals in an orthorhombic packing. (D) Electron diffraction pattern of the SC of lamellar ichthyosis skin. The diffraction pattern shows six reflections separated by angles of 60° at the same distance from the position of the electron beam. This pattern is characteristic of a hexagonal lateral packing. (E) Electron diffraction pattern of SC derived from lamellar ichthyosis skin. A pattern indicative of a hexagonal lateral pattern is observed. However, next to this pattern sharp reflections are present (*arrows*), indicating that a small portion of lipids forms an orthorhombic lateral packing. *Source*: From Ref. 56.

types are present in a relatively small area, which indicates that crystal mismatch occurs more frequently than in normal skin. The distribution profiles of the ED patterns that have been collected from the SC of the normal volunteers and LI patients are depicted in Figure 7.

The changes in the distribution profile of the ED patterns collected from the skin of LI patients were very pronounced. In these patients, the hexagonal lattice in SC was clearly predominant. The appearance of orthorhombic ED patterns differed from control samples as it mainly appeared as small, faint spots next to the hexagonal lattice, and a fluid phase had been clearly observed already at a physiological temperature. The reduced FFA levels in LI patients (Table 2) form the most likely explanation for the predominantly hexagonal packing in the SC of LI patients. However, as a reduction in the chain length of either CER or FFA might also occur, it cannot be excluded that this may play a role as well.

The changes in the lateral lipid organization observed in the SC of LI patients may account for the known aberrations in the SC barrier function (54). Several studies on lipid phase behavior both in phospholipid membranes (58) and in SC (59) have shown that co-existing phases (e.g., during phase transitions) lead to an increased

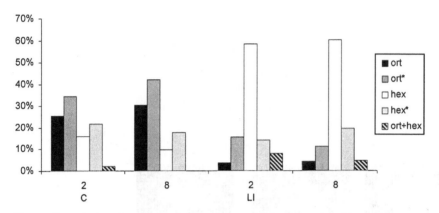

Figure 7 Relative distribution of the electron diffraction (ED) patterns into the five categories from controls, AD, and LI patients. In the graph the ED patterns recorded in samples from healthy volunteers (C) and LI patients in relation to treatment and depth (strip number 2 and 8) are summarized. The presence of *hex* is significantly increased in the SC of LI patients. N is the number of recordings. *Source*: From Ref. 56.

permeability of certain compounds. The reason for this may be an increase of alkyl chain mobility as a result of which compounds can cross lipid layers more readily. Furthermore, lipid layers may show leakage between grain boundaries, which arises at sites where two or more crystals of a different nature fail to form a continuous layer (60). As a result of this, penetration of compounds may be enhanced. Such an effect is likely to occur in the SC of LI patients, as the number of crystal orientations in a certain area selected for diffraction was increased. Furthermore, hexagonal and orthorhombic lattices could be observed in the same ED patterns.

Additionally, other explanations for a defective barrier remain possible as well. Using FFEM, it was shown that aberrations are present with respect to the lamellar organization. Moreover, the morphology of corneodesmosomes was altered (56). The lamellar body extrusion process appears normal in the LI skin, although the reorganization of the lipid stacks into lamellar sheets seems to be incomplete (61,62). Other studies on the LI skin reported changes in the corneocyte envelope (63–65), presumably arising from defects in the gene coding for the enzyme transglutaminase. The latter is involved in the CE formation by catalyzing the cross-linking of precursor proteins such as involucrin (66). These findings may also contribute towards explaining the impaired SC barrier function. Thus, it seems feasible that the SC barrier function depends on both lipid organization and protein structures.

BARRIER FUNCTION IN HUMAN SKIN EQUIVALENTS

Human skin equivalents can be generated by seeding human keratinocytes on an appropriate substrate, with a subsequent culture that follows at the air–liquid interface. Morphological studies have shown that such reconstructed epidermis forms a multilayered epithelium composed of an organized stratum basale, stratum spinosum, SG, and an SC. Furthermore, it displays a characteristic epidermal ultrastructure (67–69), and markers of epidermal differentiation are expressed (70–73).

Ultrastructurally, keratohyalin granules and lamellar bodies are present in the SG. The lamellar bodies are extruded at the SG/SC interface and the SC extracellular spaces are filled with lipid lamellar structures (68). To ensure that the penetration pathway is confined to the intercorneocyte spaces, the presence of a CE with CLE is required. Detailed analysis of the composition of CE proteins of native and reconstructed epidermis revealed great similarities between the two (74). Analysis of CLE revealed also great similarities in composition between reconstructed and native epidermis. In both tissues, comparable amounts of ω-hydroxyceramides were detected. The ω-hydroxyceramide fractions were composed of three major components, which consist of a long chain ω-hydroxyacid amide linked to sphingosine (OS), phytosphingosine (OP), or 6-hydroxy-4-sphingosine (OH), respectively (75). These findings clearly indicate that human keratinocytes in vitro can generate a complete spectrum of CLE. Using confocal laser scanning microscopy, it was established that in reconstructed epidermis the intercorneocyte penetration pathway is the predominating one, as in native skin (76). Furthermore, the CLE could act as a scaffold for the extracellular lipid lamellae as it is assumed to play an important role in the orientation of intercorneocyte lipid lamellae in parallel to the corneocyte surface.

Moreover, the profiles of extractable SC lipids showed a high degree of similarity between native and reconstructed epidermis (68,71,17). All major SC lipid classes, including all CER fractions are synthesized under in vitro conditions (Fig. 8). However, some differences have been noticed, such as lower content of FFA, reduced linoleic acid in acylceramides, and more abundant shorter chain fatty acids in some CER fractions (17). The observed deviations in the lipid composition may contribute to the differences in SC lipid organization between native and reconstructed epidermis (68). Using SAXD technique, two lamellar phases with repeat distances of 13.4 and 6.4 nm have been detected (37) in native human SC, while in reconstructed SC only an LPP of about 12 nm was formed (78). The content of linoleic acid in all three acylceramides [Cer(EOS), Cer(EOH), and Cer(EOP)] is much lower in the reconstructed epidermis than in native tissue (the molecular architecture is provided in Fig. 1). At present it is unclear why the incorporation of linoleic acid into CER in vitro is less efficient than in vivo, in spite of supplementation of culture media with this essential fatty acid (78). The differences in linoleic acid content and enrichment of the Cer(NS) fraction with short chain fatty acids [fraction Cer(NS**)], lower content of free fatty acids (FFA), and the presence of significant amounts of long chain Cer(NS**) may also contribute to the differences in SC lipid organization between native and reconstructed epidermis. Furthermore, using wide-angle and ED techniques (Fig. 9), it has been established that the lateral packing in native SC lipids is predominantly orthorhombic, while the hexagonal packing prevails in reconstructed SC (78,79).

The presence of hexagonal lattice can explain the reduced barrier function in the skin equivalent. The quality of the barrier is strongly dependent on culture conditions used for the establishment of the human skin equivalent. For instance, in reconstructed epidermis generated in the presence of vitamin C, the amount of caffeine that penetrated through the SC was only about two times higher than the penetration through native skin. In the absence of vitamin C, the penetration of caffeine was markedly increased, reaching values 10–15 times higher than in native tissue. These differences in the SC barrier function after different skin culture conditions are probably due to the differences in the CER profile (17), lipid organization (see above), and the permeability of the corneocyte envelope (80,81).

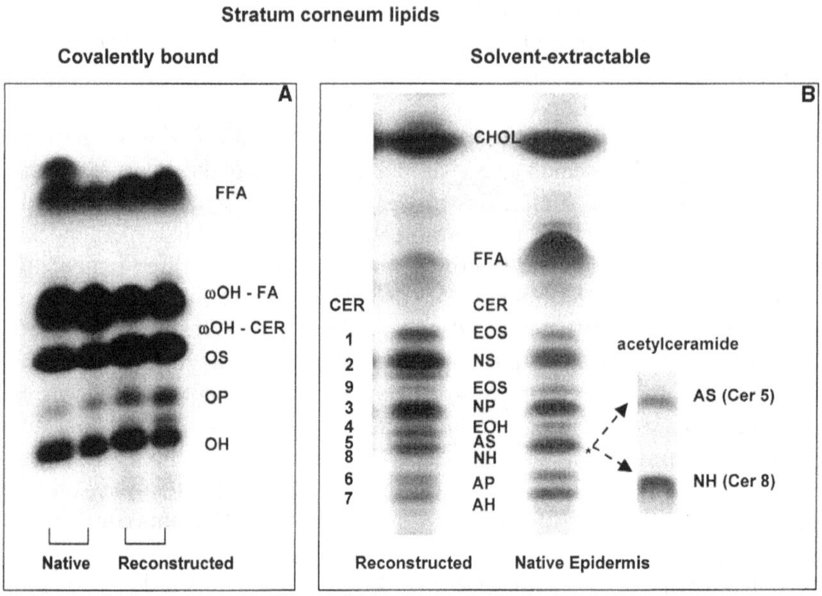

Stratum corneum lipids

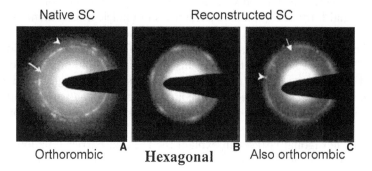

Figure 8 Profile of SC lipids: (A) covalently bound lipids and (B) solvent-extractable lipids. The SC was isolated by enzymatic digestion of viable epidermal cells. The solvent-extractable lipids were extracted from the SC isolated from the native and reconstructed epidermis, and subsequently the residues were subjected to a mild saponification treatment. The solvent-extractable and the released lipids were analyzed by HPTLC using the development system, as described in Ponec et al. (68,17). *Abbreviations*: FFA, free fatty acids; ω-OH–FA, ω-hydroxyacid; CER, ceramides (for ceramide nomenclature, see Fig. 1); CHOL, cholesterol. *Source*: From Ref. 17.

Figure 9 Lateral lipid packing in native and reconstructed SC. Representative electron diffraction (ED) patterns obtained from normal (A) and reconstructed (B, C) SC. The ED of orthorombic sub-lattice is characterized by the presence of two reflections at 0.41 and 0.37 nm and the hexagonal lattice by a 0.41-nm reflection (A). In reconstructed epidermis the 0.41-nm reflections form a ring pattern, indicating that many orientations of the hexagonal packing are present (B). Next to a hexagonal sub-lattice also small amounts of lipids form an orthorhombic sub-lattice, as indicated by the spots at spacings of 0.37 nm (*arrowhead*) and 0.41 nm (*arrows*).

RELATION BETWEEN LIPID COMPOSITION AND ORGANIZATION

The Role of CER, CHOL, and FFA in Lipid Phase Behavior

Owing to the complexity of the native tissue, the role that individual lipids play in the SC lipid organization was studied with mixtures prepared from isolated CER. In our initial studies we used pigCER, as pig SC is readily available and the lipid organization of pig SC is very similar to that of human SC. However, the molecular architecture of pigCER is slightly different from that in human SC (Fig. 1). Over the past 10 years, several studies of lipid phase behavior have examined hydrated lipid mixtures. In such CHOL:pigCER mixtures, two lamellar phases with periodicities of 5.2 and 12.2 nm were formed, mimicking lipid phase behavior in intact SC (82). This phase behavior was observed over a wide range of CHOL:pigCER molar ratios (between 0.4 and 2), indicating that the formation of the lamellar phases is insensitive towards changes in CHOL:pigCER molar ratio. Lowering a CHOL:pigCER molar ratio below 0.4 induces phase separation between lamellar phases and the formation of hydrated crystalline CHOL domains. The high insensitivity of lipid organization to changes in the CHOL:pigCER molar ratio suggests that variations in the CHOL: CER molar ratio do not lead to substantial changes in lipid phase behavior in vivo, because CHOL can form separate crystalline domains when exceeding the amount necessary to saturate the lamellae. The presence of phase-separated CHOL is also observed in the SC (40). In the range of CHOL:pigCER molar ratio between 0.1 and 2, the lipids form a hexagonal lateral packing (Fig. 3B). The phase behavior in CHOL:pigCER mixtures is different from that observed in CHOL:DPPC (dipalmitoylphosphatidylcholine) mixtures, in which a hexagonal lateral packing is observed at a low CHOL content, but at increased CHOL content a phase transition from a hexagonal to an ordered fluid phase has been observed (83–85), demonstrating the important role that CER play in skin barrier function.

In addition to CHOL and CER, FFA belong to the three major SC lipid classes. To mimic the FFA composition in intact SC, an FFA mixture containing predominantly C22:0 and C24:0 fatty acids has been used. Addition of FFA to achieve equimolar CHOL:pigCER:FFA mixtures revealed the presence of two lamellar phases with periodicities of 12.8 and 5.4 nm, which mimics the lipid organization of intact SC even more closely. Addition of long chain FFA induced a phase transition from a hexagonal to an orthorhombic lattice, and therefore they increase the lipid density in the lamellar structures [Fig. 4C and D (86)]. This phase transition was not observed with mixtures containing predominantly short chain (C16 and C18) fatty acids (84). In this study, it was not clear whether, in addition to an orthorhombic and/or hexagonal phase, the liquid phase was also formed as the broad reflection at 0.46 nm (indicative for a liquid phase) might have been obscured by a large series of reflections based on phase-separated crystalline CHOL. The latter is more profoundly present in lipid mixtures than in SC.

Furthermore, although the CHOL:pigCER:FFA mixtures closely mimic the lipid organization of intact SC at room temperature, important differences have been observed at elevated temperatures. As depicted in Figure 2C, at approximately 37°C a strong increase in the intensity of the 4.3-nm peak is observed, indicating the formation of a new phase. In intact pig SC this phase has been detected only at much higher temperatures, while this phase is absent in human SC.

In addition to FFA, CHOL, and pigCER, small amounts of cholesterol sulfate (typically 2–5% w/w of the lipids) are also present in SC. Cholesterol sulfate plays an important role in the inhibition of proteases in SC, enzymes that are important for the degradation of the corneodesmosomes (19). In the superficial SC layers, cholesterol sulfate is metabolized to cholesterol by cholesterol sulfatase, which allows an increased activity of the proteases. These processes promote the degradation of corneodesmosomes (19). Addition of only 2% m/m cholesterol sulfate to an equimolar CHOL:pigCER:FFA mixture resulted in the reduction of the fraction of phase-separated CHOL without affecting the lamellar phase behavior. Moreover, a fluid phase was clearly present in the CHOL:pigCER:FFA:cholesterol sulfate mixture (Fig. 3D). In addition, in the presence of cholesterol sulfate, the formation of the 4.3-nm phase is shifted to higher temperatures, mimicking the lipid phase behavior of intact SC at elevated temperatures, as shown in Figure 2D (87). Thus, cholesterol sulfate appears to stabilize the lipid lamellar phases formed at room temperature. This might be due to the electrostatic interactions induced by the presence of the negatively charged sulfate group. A stabilization of the lamellar phases after introduction of cholesterol sulfate in the mixture has also been observed for both sphingomyelin- and phosphatidylcholin-containing mixtures as well (88,89). When these findings are extrapolated to the in vivo situation, it seems that cholesterol sulfate is required to dissolve CHOL in the lamellar phases and to stabilize SC lipid structure. Therefore, a drop in cholesterol sulfate content in the superficial layers of the SC would be expected to destabilize the lipid lamellar phases and to increase the activity of the proteases (19), events that should facilitate the desquamation process.

Another parameter that may affect the SC lipid behavior is pH. All the phase studies summarized above are carried out with mixtures prepared at pH 5. This pH is chosen, as the pH on the skin surface is slightly acidic (pH 5–6). The pH in the viable epidermis is 7.4 (90,91). For this reason the phase behavior at pH 7.4 is examined as well. At pH 7.4, the formation of the LPP in CHOL:pigCER:FFA mixtures was promoted, indicating that the lipid organization in these mixtures is slightly sensitive to the pH. This suggests that the formation of the LPP in the lowest parts of the SC is promoted by a pH of 7.4. However, the intensity ratios of the diffraction peaks attributed to the LPP are slightly different from those of the LPP prepared at pH 5, indicating a slightly different molecular organization of the LPP at pH 7.4. Furthermore, at elevated temperatures the pH had a dramatic effect on lipid phase behavior: at pH 7.4 it was impossible to select mixtures that mimic SC lipid phase behavior over a wide temperature range. This indicates that the pH in the SC is slightly acidic, confirming the results of Mauro et al. (92). Recently, the slightly acidic environment of human domains at all levels of the SC has been elegantly demonstrated by studies of Behne et al. (93,94) with fluorescence spectroscopy.

The Role of the Various Ceramide Subclasses in Phase Behavior of SC Lipids

Because deviations in CER composition and in lipid organization often occur in diseased skin (55,56,95,96), individual CER subclasses could play an important role in the SC barrier function. To examine whether CER subclasses influence lipid phase behavior, mixtures of varying CER composition were prepared: a mixture lacking ceramide 6 [pigCER (1–5)], a mixture lacking ceramide 1 [pigCER (2–6)], or a mixture containing only ceramides 1 and 2 [pigCER (1,2)] (97–99). These studies revealed that in equimolar CHOL:CER mixtures prepared with pigCER (1–5) or pigCER (1,2), the lipids were organized in the LPP and the SPP with periodicities of approximately 12–13 and 5–6 nm, respectively, similar to that observed in intact

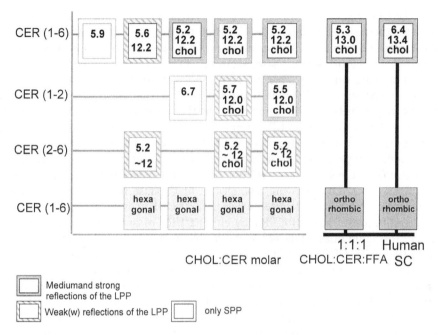

Figure 10 Schematic presentation of the phase behavior of various CHOL:pigCER mixtures as a function of CER composition and of CHOL:CER molar ratio. Mixtures were prepared with full spectrum of CER [CER(1–6)], with CER 1 and 2 [CER(1,2)], or with a CER mixture in which CER1 is absent [CER(2–6)]. In addition, the phase behavior of the equimolar CHOL:CER:FFA mixture and human SC is depicted. The equimolar CHOL:CER (1–6):FFA mixture mimics the phase behavior in human SC most closely. *Source*: From Ref. 99.

SC (Fig. 10). The exception was found with an equimolar CHOL:pigCER (2–6) mixture, in which the LPP was only weakly present (102), indicating that the CER 1 plays a crucial role in the formation of the LPP. In contrast, when the long chain FFA were incorporated into CHOL:pigCER mixtures, they hardly affected the lamellar lipid organization. Again, only pigCER1 has been found to play a crucial role in the formation of the LPP. While in mixtures containing the full spectrum of CER, changes in the CHOL:CER molar ratio over a wide range had no effect on the formation of LPP, the situation changed in mixtures containing only some CER subclasses. This was most clearly observed in mixtures prepared from CHOL and pigCER (1,2): the LPP was only weakly present at a CHOL:pigCER (1,2) molar ratio of 0.6 and absent at lower molar ratios (101). This finding contrasts with the CHOL:pigCER (1–6) mixtures in which this phase was formed even at a molar ratio of 0.2.

Phase Behavior in Mixtures Prepared from Human CER 1–9: The Role of Human CER1

As the access to human skin is limited, only a limited number of phase lipid behavior studies have been carried out with CER isolated from human SC. The lipid phase behavior of mixtures prepared from human CER (100,101) differed slightly from that observed with mixtures prepared from pigCER. For instance, in CHOL:CER mixtures the LPP was dominantly present and only a small fraction of lipids formed the SPP. Furthermore, addition of FFA promoted the presence of the SPP. As in pigCER-containing mixtures, the addition of FFA resulted in a transition from a hexagonal to an orthorhombic phase. However, in mixtures prepared from human CER a liquid phase was clearly present next to the orthorhombic phase. This phase was only noticed in pigCER-containing mixtures in the presence of cholesterol sulfate. As in pigCER-containing mixtures, in the absence of CER1 only a small population of lipids formed the LPP, despite the presence of CER4 and CER9 with a similar molecular structure (Fig. 1A) as CER1. To elucidate the role of fatty acid linked to ω-hydroxyacid in SC lipid organization, natural CER1 was replaced by either *synthetic* CER1-linoleate (CER1-lin), CER1-oleate (CER1-ol) or CER1-stearate (CER1-ste). The following changes in lipid phase behavior were noticed. (i) No liquid phase could be detected when natural CER was substituted by CER1-ste. (ii) Substitution of natural CER1 by either CER1-ol or CER1-lin revealed the presence of the liquid phase. This phase was less prominent in mixtures prepared with CER1-lin than with CER1-ol. (iii) As far as the lamellar phases are concerned, the LPP was not present in CER:CHOL mixtures in which natural CER1 was substituted for CER1-ste. (iv) The 12–13-nm lamellar phase dominated in mixtures in which CER1 was substituted by either CER1-lin or CER1-ol. (v) The addition of FFA to the CER:CHOL mixtures, in which natural CER1 was replaced by CER1-ol, promoted the formation of the SPP. The results of these studies indicate that for the formation of the LPP, a certain (optimal) fraction of lipids is required to form a liquid phase.

Lipid Mixtures Based on Commercially Available and Synthetic Ceramides

In the past, various studies have been performed with mixtures based on commercially available, CER-like bovine-brain CER, not only to mimic lipid phase behavior but also with an aim to use them in topical products. Several studies used model membranes prepared with palmitic acid, CHOL, and bovine-brain CER. The choice of palmitic acid was based on a study by Lampe et al. (102), in which it was stated that most of the free fatty acids in SC have a chain of C16 and C18:1. However, in more recent studies it became clear that this was not a correct choice, and that mainly FFA with chain lengths of C22 and C24 are present in the human SC (102). NMR studies carried out with equimolar mixtures of CHOL and bovine-brain CERIII in the presence or absence of palmitic acid revealed that the main population of lipids (80%) forms a crystalline phase, but also that a small proportion of lipids forms a more mobile phase (104,105). Formation of a crystalline phase in the presence of a substantial amount of CHOL is an exceptional observation for lipid membranes. For example, in phospholipid-containing mixtures, an increasing amount of CHOL, up to a mole ratio of 0.3, results in a transition from a crystalline to a liquid-ordered phase (83–85). The difference in phase behavior might be ascribed to differences in either the head group size or the chain length between phospholipids and CER. The lateral packing was found to depend strongly on the size of the head group. For example, equimolar cholesterol:sphingomyelin mixtures form a liquid phase, while equimolar cholesterol:bovine-brain ceramide III mixtures having the same chain length distribution form a crystalline phase (106). As far as the lateral packing is concerned, mixtures prepared with synthetic CER mimic the SC lipid organization quite closely. However, as shown more recently using the X-ray diffraction technique, the CHOL:bovine-brain CERIII:palmitic acid mixture does not form the characteristic LPP (107,108). However, when synthetic CER1 is present, the LPP can be formed (109) (unpublished results). There is one report on the formation of a 10.5-nm lamellar phase in CHOL:bovine-brain CER mixtures interpreted as a double layer structure. This structure, however, differs from the LPP phase present in the SC (110). In several studies, FTIR spectroscopy measurements were carried out using mixtures prepared from either bovine-brain CERIII, synthetic CER2 or synthetic CER5 (111,112), CHOL and palmitic acid. At a physiological temperature, the CD_2 scissoring mode of palmitic acid and the CH_2 scissoring mode of CER are each split into two components, indicating that these molecules are located in different lattices. Measurements at elevated temperature confirmed that the components were not properly mixed in one orthorhombic lattice, but phase-separated in different lattices. A similar behavior was found when mixing fatty acids with either synthetic CER2 or synthetic CER5 (111). Similarly, FT-Raman spectroscopy was also used to observe the phase separation between CER and saturated fatty acid (113). It should be noted that the components had a uniform chain length. Recently, we have observed that the C22 fatty acid did not mix properly with isolated pigCER and CHOL (Bouwstra et al., unpublished results). However, in earlier publications (82,114) it was reported that the addition of FFA with a chain length distribution between 16 and 24 to the CHOL:pigCER did not show any phase separation. The latter was observed by X-ray diffraction and ED. Therefore, to achieve a proper mixing of FFA and CER the use of mixtures of the FFA containing varying instead of uniform chain length is essential.

In several studies, liposomes were also used as model systems (115–117). Although these systems are excellent models for studying the bilayer permeability, some fundamental problems are encountered when using liposomes as an SC lipid model. For instance, when vesicles were prepared at a pH value ranging between 5 and 7, which approximates the pH in the SC (96,97,118,119) the vesicles show a tendency to fuse. This is probably due to the fact that at pH 5, FFA, CER, and CHOL are not charged, and at pH 7.4, FFA are most probably only partially charged. Furthermore, while lamellar phases are thermodynamically stable phases, liposome formulations are not, which makes liposomes more complicated and more sensitive to small changes in the environment.

A UNIQUE MOLECULAR ARRANGEMENT IN THE LONG PERIODICITY PHASE

In 1989, a model that describes the molecular arrangement in the LPP was proposed for the first time (121). Based on the broad–narrow–broad pattern obtained after fixation with ruthenium tetroxide, a trilayer model was proposed. In this model, the CER are arranged in a planar arrangement and the linoleic moiety of CER1 is not located in the narrow layer, but is randomly distributed in the two broad layers adjacent on both sides of the narrow layer. Furthermore, the CHOL interfacial area is assumed to be similar to that of the CER in planar alignment. Based on more recent knowledge about the lipid phase behavior of CHOL:pigCER and CHOL:HCER mixtures, another trilayer model has been proposed for the molecular arrangement of the LPP (98,101) (Fig. 11). In this model, the CER are either partly

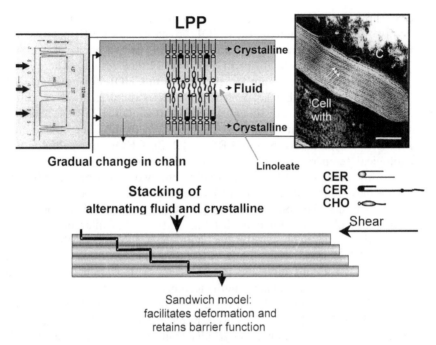

Figure 11 Model of molecular arrangement of the long periodicity phase (LPP). The electron density profile calculated from the ED profile of the LPP indicates the presence of a broad–narrow–broad sequence in the repeating unit of the LPP (arrows) (*left panel*). This is in agreement with the broad–narrow–broad pattern found in RuO₄-fixed SC (*right panel*). Based on these and other (see text) observations, a molecular model is presented (*middle panel*), in which CER1 plays an important role in dictating the broad–narrow–broad sequence. Furthermore, the fluid phase is located in the central narrow band. In adjacent regions the crystalline nature gradually increases from the central layer. Even in the presence of the central fluid layer the barrier function is retained while deformation as a consequence of shear stresses is facilitated. The latter might be of importance for the elastic properties of the skin. *Source*: From Ref. 101.

interdigitated (the broad low-electron density layers) or fully interdigitated (the narrow low-electron density layer in the center of the lamellae), and are arranged tail-to-tail in doublets within the lipid layers. The two broad low-electron density regions are formed by CER with the long chain fatty acids (predominantly C24–C26) linked to the (phyto) sphingosine backbone and by CHOL, while the narrow low–electron density region is formed by CHOL and the unsaturated C18 acyl chain linked to the ω-hydroxy fatty acid. The proposed molecular model is based on the following findings: (i) the electron density profile of the repeating unit calculated from the intensities of the first to the tenth order of the lamellar pattern attributed to the LPP in CHOL:pigCER mixtures (98) resulted in a sequence of broad–narrow–broad low-electron density regions with the in-between higher electron density regions corresponding to the head groups; (ii) the crucial role of CER1 in the formation of the LLP; (iii) the bimodal fatty acid chain-length distribution of the CER (106,17); (iv) the observed phase separation in a mixture containing CER with long acyl chains and short acyl chains (106). The LPP consists of three different regions in which the liquid sub-lattice is located in the central lipid layer. Here, mainly unsaturated linoleic acid and CHOL are present. Adjacent to this central layer, two regions are located in which a gradual change in lipid mobility occurs in the direction perpendicular to the central plane. The decreased mobility in these adjacent layers can be attributed to the presence of less mobile, very long, fully saturated hydrocarbon chains (Fig. 1). As only a small fraction of lipids forms a fluid phase in the SC, it is assumed that this central lipid layer is not a continuous one. Because the lipid lamellae are mainly oriented in a parallel manner to the surface of the corneocytes, substances always have to pass the crystalline lipid lamellar region and partly diffuse through the less densely packed lipid regions parallel to these regions. In this way an excellent barrier is maintained, even when a fluid phase is present. When comparing our model with the model of Swarzendruber et al. (121), our model suggests an approximately equal interfacial area of CHOL and CER with a tail-to-tail arrangement, while Swarzendruber's model suggests an equal interfacial area of CHOL and CER in a planar alignment. Dahler and Pascher reported an interfacial area of CER in a planar arrangement of approximately $0.25 \, nm^2$ (122). This is different from that of CHOL $0.37 \, nm^2$. The interfacial area of CER having a tail-to-tail double arrangement is predicted to be approximately $0.40 \, nm^2$ (122), which is indeed a value close to that of CHOL. Furthermore, in the molecular model proposed by Swarzendruber et al. (121), the presence of a liquid layer is not possible, owing to the random distribution of the linoleate of CER1. It will be a task for future studies to validate whether the proposed "sandwich model" correctly represents the lipid organization of the LPP in the SC. In 1993, another model was proposed by Forslind (123). This model postulated the presence of a continuous liquid phase from the superficial layers of the SC down to the viable epidermis, the so-called domain mosaic model. Although this was the first model that accounted for the presence of a liquid phase in the SC lipid structures, no experimental data have been provided to support this model. In a recent paper, another model has been proposed for the SC lipid organization, called the "Single Gel Phase Model." According to this model, the intercellular lipids within the SC exist as "a single and coherent gel phase" and "this structure has virtually no boundaries" (42). This gel phase is defined as a "crystalline lamellar lipid structure that usually has a hexagonal hydrocarbon chain packing." Although this model is similar to our sandwich model with respect to the absence of grain boundaries, the single phase model proposes either the hexagonal phase or a co-existence of the hexagonal and orthorhombic phases within the deeper layers of the SC such that the orthorhombic phase is located adjacent to the head group region and changes gradually into a hexagonal phase in the central region of the lamellae. If this is the case, the orthorhombic and hexagonal phases should always be present simultaneously. However, as already explained in Section 3, no evidence has been found for the presence of the hexagonal phase in the lower SC regions. In addition, the orthorhombic phase is frequently observed without the presence of the hexagonal phase. Therefore, the "Single Gel Phase Model" is not confirmed by experimental data. Finally, in the "Single Gel Phase Model," no attention has been paid to the role that individual lipids play in the lipid organization; this includes (i) the crucial role of ceramide 1 in the formation of the 13-nm lamellar phase and its influence on the phase behavior and (ii) the presence (or absence) of long chain free fatty acids, which cause the formation of the orthorhombic packing in vitro as well as in vivo, as shown in diseased skin.

EXTRAPOLATION OF IN VITRO FINDINGS TO THE LIPID
COMPOSITION AND ORGANIZATION IN DISEASED
AND IN XEROTIC SKIN

The skin of the patients of atopic dermatitis and xerosis (56,124) shows a reduced CER1 content which alters the organization of lamellar phases (55), reflecting the observations made with lipid mixtures. Here, in the absence of CER1, the formation of the 12–13-nm lamellar phase was reduced, while the formation of the 5–6-nm lamellar phase was strongly promoted (101). In addition, in xerotic skin during the winter season, and in EFAD skin, the CER1-ol content is increased at the expense of CER1-lin (52). One would also expect that changes in lipid phase behavior might occur (54), as the presence of the liquid phase is more prominent in CER1-ol–containing lipid mixtures when compared with CER1-lin–containing mixtures (101). In fact, in EFAD and xerotic skin a reduced skin barrier has been observed (51), while the ultrastructural appearance of the lipid lamellae was still similar to that seen in normal skin (26,51). It can be speculated that the fraction of lipids forming a fluid phase increases due to the presence of a higher fraction of CER1-ol. Although the presence of a sub-population of lipids forming the fluid phase might be required for a proper functioning of the SC, an excessive presence of a fluid phase may lead to the reduction of the barrier function. Furthermore, we have also noticed that a hexagonal lateral packing is formed in CHOL:CER and CHOL:pigCER mixtures and that the presence of FFA facilitates the transformation of the hexagonal into an orthorhombic lateral packing. The prominent presence of the hexagonal lateral packing in lamellar ichthyosis skin (56) might be caused by the observed reduced content of FFA in this skin disease (54). Finally, as cholesterol sulfate promotes the formation of a fluid phase (87), an increase in cholesterol sulfate content, similar to that occurring in recessive x-linked ichthyosis skin (125), could further reduce lattice density, and consequently increase SC permeability, accounting for the observed reduction of barrier function in this skin disease.

CONCLUSIONS

Although in the last 20 years, enormous progress has been made in elucidating the lipid organization in the SC, it is not fully understood. One of the problems in studying SC lipid organization is the complexity of the tissue with its unusual lipid composition. As it appeared to be impossible to selectively extract lipids from the SC, the role that the various lipid classes play in lipid phase behavior could only be studied with isolated lipid mixtures. These studies revealed that mixtures prepared with isolated CER, CHOL, FFA, and cholesterol sulfate mimic the SC lipid organization very closely. Furthermore, until now, deviation in lipid organization in diseased and dry skin could often be explained by the results obtained with the isolated lipid mixtures, illustrating an excellent in vitro–in vivo correlation. Despite the substantial progress made in the last 20 years, further research is required to unravel in detail the organization of the LPP and SPP, focusing on, among others, the distribution of various subclasses between these lamellar phases, and providing additional extensive information on the abnormal phase behavior and lipid composition in diseased skin.

REFERENCES

1. Bowser PA, White RJ, Nugteren DH. Int J Cosmet Sci 1968; 8:125–134.
2. Elias PM, Menon GP. Structural and lipid biochemical corrlates of the epidermal permeability barrier. Adv Lipid Res 1991; 24:1–26.
3. Schurer NY, Elias PM. The biochemistry and function of stratum corneum. Adv Lipid Res 1991; 24:27–54.
4. Madison KC, Swarzendruber DC, Wertz PW, Downing DT. Presence of intact intercellular lipid lamellae in the upper layers of the stratum corneum. J Invest Dermatol 1988; 90:110–116.
5. Downing DT. Lipid and protein structures in the permeability barrier of mammalian epidermis. J Lipid Res 1992; 33:301–314.
6. Swarzendruber DC, Wertz PW, Madison KC, Downing DT. Evidence that the corneocyte has a chemical bound lipid envelope. J Invest Dermatol 1987; 88:709–713.
7. Wertz PW, Madison KC, Downing DT. Covalently bound lipids of human stratum corneum. J Invest Dermatol 1989; 92:109–111.
8. Menon GK, Ghadially RR, Williams ML, Elias PM. Lamellar bodies as delivery systems of hydrolytic enzymes: implications for normal and abnormal desquamation. Br J Dermatol 1992; 126:337–345.
9. Lazo ND, Meine JG, Downing DT. Lipids are covalently attached to rigid corneocyte protein envelopes existing predominantly as beta-sheets: a solid-state nuclear magnetic resonance study. J Invest Dermatol 1995; 105:296–300.
10. Marekov LN, Steinert PM. Ceramides are bound to structural proteins of the human foreskin epidermal cornified cell envelope. J Biol Chem 1998; 273:17763–17770.
11. Simonetti O, Hoogstraate AJ, Bialik W, Kempenaar JA, Schrijvers AHGJ, Bodde HE, Ponec M. Visualization of diffusion pathway across the stratum corneum of native and in-vitro-reconstructed epidermis by confocal laser scanning microscopy. Arch Dermatol Res 1995; 287:465–473.
12. Meuwissen MEMJ, Janssen J, Cullander C, Junginger HE, Bouwstra JA. A cross-section device to improve visualization of fluorescent probe penetration into skin by confocal laser scanning microscopy. Pharm Res 1998; 5:352–356.
13. Ponec M, Weerheim A, Kempenaar J, Mommaas AM, Nugteren DH. Lipid composition of cultured human keratinocytes in relation to their differentiation. J Lipid Res 1988; 29:949–996.
14. Wertz PW, Downing DT. Epidermal lipids. In: Goldsmith LA, ed. Physiology, Biochemistry, and Molecular Biology of the Skin. 2nd ed. Oxford: Oxford University Press, 1991: 205–236.
15. Robson KJ, Stewart ME, Michelsen S, Lazo ND, Downing DT. 6-Hydroxy-4-sphingenine in human epidermal ceramides. J Lipid Res 1994; 35:2060–2068.
16. Stuart ME, Downing DT. 6 Hydroxy-4-sphingenine in human epidermal ceramides J Lipid Res 1999; 40:1434–1439.
17. Ponec M, Lankhorst P, Weerheim A, Wertz P. New acylceramide in native and reconstructed epidermis. J Invest Dermatol 2003; 120:581–588.
18. Wertz PW, Downing DT. Acylglucosylceramides of pig epidermis: structure determination. J Lipid Res 1983; 24:753–758.
19. Sato J, Denda M, Nakanishi J, Nomura J, Koyama J. Cholesterol sulfate inhibits proteases that are involved in desquamation of stratum corneum. J Invest Dermatol 1998; 111:189–193.
20. Swanbeck G, Thyresson N. An X-ray diffraction study of scales from different dermatosis. Acta Derm Venereol 1961; 41:289–296.
21. Swanbeck G, Thyresson N. A study of the state of aggregation of the lipids I normal and psoriatic horny layer. Acta Derm Venereol 1962; 42:445–557.
22. Breathnach AS, Goodman T, Stolinsky C, Gross MJ. Freeze–fracture replication of cells of stratum corneum of human cells. J Anat 1973; 114:65–81.

23. Breathnach AS. Aspects of epidermal structure. J Invest Dermatol 1975; 65:2–12.

24. Elias PM, Friend DS. The permeability barrier in mammalian epidermis. J Cell Biol 1975; 65:180–191.

25. Madison KC, Swarzendruber DC, Wertz PC, Downing DT. Presence of intact intercellular lipid lamellae in the upper layers of the stratum corneum. J Invest Dermatol 1987; 88:714–718.

26. Hou SY, Mitra AK, White SH, Menon GK, Ghadially R, Elias P. Membrane structures in normal and essential fatty acid-deficient stratum corneum: characterization by ruthenium tetroxide staining and X-ray diffraction. J Invest Dermatol 1991; 6:215–223.

27. Fartasch M, Bassakas ID, Diepgen TL. Disturbed extruding mechanism of lamellar bodies in dry noneczematous skin of atopics. Br J Dermatol 1992; 127:221–227.

28. Swartzendruber DC. Studies of epidermal lipids using electron microscopy. Sem Dermatol 1992; 11:157–161.

29. van den Bergh BAI, Swartzendruber DC, Bos-van Geest A, Hoogstraate JJ, Schrijvers AHGL, Boddé HE, Junginger HE, Bouwstra JA. Development of an optimal protocol for the ultrastructural examination of skin by transmission electron microscopy. J Microsc 1997; 87:125–133.

30. Ongpipattanakul B, Francoeur ML, Potts RO. Polymorphism in stratum corneum lipids. Biochim Biophys Acta 1994; 1190:115–122.

31. Naik A, Guy RH. Infrared spectroscopic and differential scanning calorimetric investigations of the stratum corneum barrier function. In: Potts RO, Guy RH, eds. Mechanism of Transdermal Drug Delivery. New York: Marcel Dekkers Inc., 1997:87–163.

32. Gay CL, Guy RH, Golden GM, Mak VM, Francoeur ML. Characterization of low-temperature (i.e., $< 65°C$) lipid transitions in human stratum corneum. J Invest Dermatol 1994; 103:233–229.

33. Elias PM, Bonar L, Grayson S, Baden HP. X-ray diffraction analysis of stratum corneum membrane couplets. J Invest Dermatol 1983; 80:213–214.

34. White SH, Mirejovsky D, King GI. Structure of lamellar lipid domains and corneocyte envelopes of murine stratum corneum. An X-ray diffraction study. Biochemistry 1988; 27:3725–3732.

35. Bouwstra JA, Gooris GS, van der Spek JA, Lavrijsen S, Bras W. The lipid and protein structure of mouse stratum corneum: a wide angle and small angle diffraction study. Biochim Biophys Acta 1994; 1212:183–192.

36. van den Bergh BAI, Bouwstra JA, Junginger HE, Wertz PW. Elasticity of vesicles effects hairless mouse skin structure and permeability. J Control Release 1999; 62:367–379.

37. Bouwstra JA, Gooris GS, van der Spek JA, Bras W. Structural inestigation of human stratum corneum by small angle X-ray scattering. J Invest Dermatol 1991; 97:1005–1012.

38. Bouwstra JA, Gooris GS, Bras W, Downing DT. The lipid organisation of pig stratum corneum. J Lipid Res 1995; 36:685–695.

39. Garson J-C, Doucet J, Lévêque J-L, Tsoucaris GJ. Oriented structure in human stratum corneum revealed by X-ray diffraction. J Invest Dermatol 1991; 96:43–49.

40. Bouwstra JA, Gooris GS, Salomons-de Vries MA, van der Spek JA, Bras W. The influence of alkyl-azones on the ordering of the lamellae in human stratum corneum. Int J Pharm 1992; 84:205–216.

41. Pilgram GSK, Engelsma-van Pelt AM, Bouwstra JA, Koerten HK. Electron diffraction provides new information on human stratum corneum lipid organization studied in relation to depth and temperature. J Invest Dermatol 1999; 133:403–409.

42. Norlen L. Skin barrier structure and function: the single gel phase model. J Invest Dermatol 2001; 117:830–836.

43. Bomommannan D, Potts RO, Guy RH. Examination of stratum corneum barrier function in vivo by infrared spectroscopy. J Invest Dermatol 1990; 95:403–408.

44. Bonte F, Saunois A, Pinguet P, Meybeck A. Existence of lipid gradient in the upper stratum corneum and it's possible biological significance. Arch Dermatol Res 1997; 289:78–82.

45. Golden GM, McKie JE, Potts RO. Role of stratum corneum lipid fluidity in transdermal drug flux. J Pharm Sci 1987; 76:25–28.

46. Pilgram GSK, Engelsma-van Pelt AM, Bouwstra JA, Koerten HK. Electron diffraction provides new information on human stratum corneum lipid organization studied in relation to depth and temperature. J Invest Dermatol 1999; 113:403–409.

47. Bouwstra JA, Dubbelaar FER, Gooris GS, Ponec M. The lipid organisation in the skin barrier. Acta Derm Venereol 2000; 208:23–30.

48. Abrahamsson S, Dahlen B, Löfgren H, Pascher I. Lateral packing of hydrocarbon chains. Prog Chem Fats Lipids 1978; 16:125–143.

49. Löfgren H, Pascher I. Molecular arrangement of sphingolipids. The monolayer approach. Chem Phys Lipids 1977; 20:273–284.

50. Pascher I, Sundell S. Molecular arrangements in sphingolipids—crystal structure of the ceramide N-(2D,3D dihydroxyoctadecanoyl)-phytosphingosine. Chem Phys Lipids 1992; 1:79–86.

51. Melton JL, Wertz PW, Swarzendruber DC, Downing DT. Effects of essential fatty acid defiency epidermal 0-acylsphingolipids and transepidermal water loss in young pigs. Biochim Biophys Acta 1987; 921:191–197.

52. Conti A, Rogers J, Verdejo P, Harding CR, Rawlings AV. Sesonal influences on stratum corneum ceramide 1 fatty acids and the influence of topical essential fatty acids. Int J Cosmet Sci 1996; 15:1–12.

53. Imokawa G, Abe A, Kawashima M, Hidano A. Decreased levels of ceramides in stratum corneum of atopic dermatitis: an etiologic factor in atotic dry skin. J Invest Dermatol 1991; 96:523–526.

54. Lavrijsen APM, Bouwstra JA, Gooris GS, Boddé HE, Ponec M. Reduces skin barrier function parallels. Abnormal stratum corneum lipid organisation in patients with lamellar ichtyosis. J Invest Dermatol 1995; 105:619–624.

55. Schreiner V, Gooris GS, Lanzendörfer G, Pfeiffer S, Wenck H, Diembeck W, Proksch E, Bouwstra JA. Barrier characteristics of different human skin types investigated with X-ray diffraction, lipid analysis and electron microscopy imaging. J Invest Dermatol 2000; 114:654–660.

56. Pilgram GSK, Vissers DCJ, van der Meulen H, Parel S, Lavrijsen SPM, Bouwstra JA, Koerten HK. Abberant lipid organization in stratum corneum of patients with atopic dermatitis and lamellar ichtyosis. J Invest Dermatol 2001; 117:710–717.

57. Ghadially R, Williams ML, Hou SYE, Elias P. Membrane structural abnormalities in the stratum corneum of the autosomal recessive ichthyosis. J Invest Dermatol 1992; 99:755–763.

58. Xiang TX, Anderson BD. Permeability of acetic acid across gel and liquid crystalline lipid bilayers conforms to free-surface-area theory. Biophys J 1997; 72:223–237.

59 Ogiso T, Hirota T, Iwaki M, Hino T, Tanino T. Effect of temperature on percultaneous absorption of terodiline, and relationship between penetration and fluidity of stratum corneum lipids. Int J Pharm 1998; 176:63–72.

60. Langner M, Hui SW. Dthionite penetration through phospholipid bilayers as a measure od defects in lipid molecular packing. Chem Phys Lipids 1993; 65:23–30.

61. Fartash M. Epidermal barrier in disorders of the skin. Microsc Res Tech 1997; 38: 361–372.

62. Ghadially R, Williams ML, Hou SYE, Elias PM. Membrane structural abnormalities in the stratum corneum of autosomal recessive ichthyoses. J Invest Dermatol 1992; 99:755–763.

63. Niemi KM, Kanerva L, Kuokkanen K. Recessive ichtyosis congenita type II. Arch Dermatol Res 1991; 283:211–218.

64. Hoil D, Huber M, Frenk E. Analysis of the cornified cell envelope in lamellar ichthyosis. Arch Dermatol 1993; 129:618–624.

65. Paige DG, Morsefisher N, Harper JL. Quantification of stratum corneum ceramides and lipid envelope ceramides in the hereditary ichtyosis. Br J Dermatol 1992; 131: 23–27.

66. Huber M, Rettler I, Bernasconi K, Frenk E, Lavrijsen APM, Ponec M, Bon A, Lautenslager S, Schorderet DF, Hohl D. Mutations of keratinocyte transglutaminase in lamellar ichtyosis. Science 1995; 267:525–528.

67. Ponec M, Weerheim A, Kempenaar J, Mommaas AM, Nugteren DH. Lipid composition of cultured human keratinocytes in relation to their differentiation. J Lipid Res 1988; 29:949–962.

68. Ponec M, Weerheim A, Kempenaar J, Mulder A, Gooris GS, Bouwstra JA, Mommaas AM. The formation of competent barrier lipids in reconstructed human epidermis requires the presence of vitamin C. J Invest Dermatol 1997; 109:348–355.

69. Ponec M, Gibbs S, Pilgram G, Boelsma E, Koerten H, Bouwstra JA, Mommaas M. Barrier function in reconstructed epidermis and its resemblance to native human skin. Skin Pharmacol Appl Skin Physiol 2001; 14(suppl 1):63–71.

70. Gibbs S, Vicanova Y, Bouwstra JA, Valstar I, Kempenaar J, Ponec M. Culture of reconstructed epidermis in serum free medium at 33°C shows a delayed epidermal maturation, prolonged lifespan and improved stratum corneum. Arch Dermatol Res 1997; 289:585–595.

71. Gibbs S, Boelsma E, Kempenaar J, Ponec M. Temperature-sensitive regulation of epidermal morphogenesis and the expression of cornified envelope precursors by EGF and TGFα. Cell Tissue Res 1998; 292:107–114.

72. El Ghalbzouri A, Gibbs S, Lamme E, van Blitterswijk CA, Ponec M. Effect of fibroblasts on epidermal regeneration in a human skin equivalent. Br J Dermatol 2002; 147:230–243.

73. El Ghalbzouril A, Lamme E, Ponec M. Crucial role of fibroblasts in regulation of epidermal morphogenesis. Cell Tissue Res 2002; 310:189–199.

74. Ponec M. Skin constructs for replacement of skin tissues for in vitro testing. Adv Drug Deliv Rev 2002; 54(suppl 1):S19–S30.

75. Chopart M, Castiel-Higounenc I, Arbey E, Schmidt R. A new type of covalently bound ceramide in human epithelium. Poster, Stratum corneum III meeting, Basel, 2001.

76. Vicanova J, Boelsma E, Mommaas AM, Kempenaar JA, Forslind B, Pallon J, Egelrud T, Koerten HK, Ponec M. Normalization of epidermal calcium distribution profile in reconstructed epidermis is related to improvement of terminal differentiation and stratum corneum barrier formation. J Invest Dermatol 1998; 111:97–106.

77. Bouwstra JA, Gooris GS, Weerheim A, Kempenaar J, Ponec M. Characterization of stratum corneum structure in reconstructed epidermis by X-ray diffraction. J Lipid Res 1995; 36:496–504.

78. Vicanova J, Weerheim A, Kempenaar J, Ponec M. Incorporation of linoleic acid by cultured human keratinocytes. Arch Dermatol Res 1999; 291:405–412.

79. Pilgram GSK, Gibbs S, Ponec M, Koerten HK, Bouwstra JA. The lateral lipid organization in stratum corneum of a human skin equivalent is predominantly hexagonal. In: A Close Look at the Stratum Corneum Organization by Cryo-Electron Diffraction. Ph.D. Thesis, Leiden, 2000.

80. Simonetti O, Hoogstrate JA, Bialik W, Kempenaar JA, Schrijvers AHGJ, Boddé HE, Ponec M. Visualisation of diffusion pathways across the stratum corneum of native and in vitro reconstructed epidermis by confocal laser scanning microscopy. Arch Dermatol Res 1995; 287:465–473.

81. Vicanova J, Boelsma E, Mommaas AM, Kempenaar JA, Forslind B, Pallon J, Egelrud T, Koerten HK, Ponec M. Normalization of epidermal calcium distribution profile in reconstructed epidermis is related to improvement of terminal differentiation and stratum corneum barrier formation. J Invest Dermatol 1998; 111:97–106.

82. Bouwstra JA, Gooris GS, Cheng K, Weerheim A, Bras W, Ponec M. Phase behaviour of isolated skin lipids. J Lipid Res 1996; 37:999–1011.
83. Engelman DM, Rothman J. The planar organization of lecithin-cholesterol bilayers. J Nature 1992; 247:3694–3697.
84. Demel RA, de Kruyff B. Studies of epidermal lipids using electron microscopy. Biochim Biophys Acta 1976; 457:109–132.
85. Liu F, Sugar IP, Chong L-G. Cholesterol and ergosterol superlattices in three-component liquid crystalline lipid bilayers as revealed by dehydroergosterol fluorescence. Biophys J 1997; 72:2243–2254.
86. Bouwstra JA, Gooris GS, Dubbelaar FER, Weerheim A, Ponec M. pH and cholesterol sulfate and fatty acids affect the stratum corneum lipid organization. J Invest Dermatol Symp Proc 1998; 3:69–74.
87. Bouwstra JA, Gooris GS, Dubbelaar FER, Weerheim A, Ponec M. Cholesterol sulfate and calcium affect stratum corneum lipid organization over a wide temperature range. J Lipid Res 1999; 40:2303–2312.
88. Kitson N, Monck M, Wong K, Thewalt J, Cullis P. The influence of cholesterol-3-sulphate on phase behaviour and hydrocarbon order in model membrane systems. Biochim Biophys Acta 1992; 1111:127–133.
89. Cheetham JJ, Chen RJ, Epand RM. Interaction of calcium and cholesterol sulphate induces membrane destabilization and fusion: implications for the acrosome reaction. Biochim Biophys Acta 1990; 1024:367–372.
90. Aly R, Shirley C, Cumico B, Maibach HI. Effect of prolonged occlusion on the mirobial flora, pH, carbon dioxide and transepidermal water loss of human skin. J Invest Dermatol 1978; 70:378–381.
91. Sage BH, Huke RH, McFarland AC, Kowalczyk K. The importance of skin pH in iontophoresis of peptides. In: Brain K, James V, Walters KA, eds. Prediction Percutaneous Penetration. Cardiff: STS Publishing, 1993:410–418.
92. Mauro T, Grayson S, Gao WN, Man MQ, Kriehuber E, Behne M, Feingold KR, Elias PM. Barrier recovery is impeded at neutral pH, independent of ionic effects: implications for extracellular lipid processsing. Arch Derm Res 1998; 290:215–222.
93. Hanson KM, Behne MJ, Barry NP, Mauro TM, Gratton E, Clegg RM. Two-photon fluorescence lifetime imaging of the skin stratum corneum pH gradient. Biophys J 2002; 83:1682–1690.
94. Behne MJ, Barry NP, Hanson KM, Aronchik I, Clegg RW, Gratton E, Feingold K, Holleran WM, Elias PM, Mauro TM. Neonatal development of the stratum corneum pH gradient: localization and mechanisms leading to emergence of optimal barrier function. J Invest Dermatol 2003; 120:998–1006.
95. Motta S, Monti M, Sesana S, Mellesi L, Caputo R, Carelli S, Ghidoni R. Ceramide composition of the psoriatic scale. Biochim Biophys Acta 1993; 1182:147–151.
96. Hara J, Higuchi K, Okamoto R, Kawashima M, Imokawa G. High-expression of sphingomyelin deacylase is an important determinant of ceramide deficiency leading to barrier disruption in atopic dermatitis. J Invest Dermatol 2000; 115:406–413.
97. Bouwstra JA, Cheng K, Gooris GS, Weerheim A, Ponec M. The role of ceramides 1 and 2 in the stratum corneum lipid organisation. Biophys Acta 1996; 1300:177–186.
98. Bouwstra JA, Gooris GS, Dubbelaar FER, Weerheim AM, IJzerman AP, Ponec M. The role of ceramide 1 in the molecular organisation of the stratum corneum. J Lipid Res 1998; 39:186.
99. Bouwstra JA, Dubbelaar FER, Gooris GS, Weerheim AM, Ponec M. The role of ceramide composition in the lipid organisation of the skin barrier. Biochim Biophys Acta 1999; 1419:127–136.
100. Lampe MA, Williams ML, Elias P. Human stratum corneum lipids: characterization and modulations during differentiation. J Lipid Res 1983; 24:131–140.

101. Bouwstra JA, Gooris GS, Dubbelaar FER, Ponec M. Phase behaviour of lipid mixtures based on human ceramides: the role of natural and synthetic ceramide 1. J Invest Dermatol 2002; 118:606–616.

102. Bouwstra JA, Gooris GS, Dubbelaar FER, Ponec M. Phase behaviour of stratum corneum lipid mixtures based on human ceramides: coexistence of crystalline and liquid phases. J Lipid Res 2001; 42:1759–1770.

103. ten Grotenhuis E, Demel RA, Ponec M, de Boer DR, van Miltenburg JC, Bouwstra JA. Phase behaviour of stratum corneum lipids in mixed Langmuir blodgett monolayers. Biophys J 1996; 71:1389–1399.

104. Fenske DB, Thewalt JL, Bloom M, Kitson N. Models of stratum corneum intercellular membranes: 2HnmR of macroscopically oriented multilayers. Biophys J 1994; 67: 1562–1573.

105. Kitson N, Thewalt J, Lafleur M, Bloom M. A model membrane approach to the epidermal permeability barrier. Biochemistry 1994; 33:6707–6715.

106. Thewalt J, Kitson N, Araujo C, MacKay A, Bloom M. Models of stratum corneum intercellular membranes: the sphingolipid headgroup is a determinant of phase behavior in mixed lipid dispersions. Biochem Biophys Comm 1992; 188:1247–1252.

107. Bouwstra JA, Thewalt J, Gooris GS, Kitson N. A model membrane approach to the epidermal barrier, an X-ray diffraction study. Biochemistry 1997; 36:7717–7725.

108. Schückler F, Bouwstra JA, Gooris GS, Lee GJ. An X-ray diffraction study of some model stratum corneum lipids containine azone and dodecyl-l-pyroglutamate. J Control Release 1993; 23:27–36.

109. de Jager MW, Gooris GS, Dolbnya IP, Bras W, Ponec M, Bouwstra JA. The phase behaviour of skin lipid mixtures based on synthetic ceramides. Chem Phys Lipids 2003; 124:123–134.

110. Parrott DT, Turner JE. Mesophase formation by ceramides and cholesterol: a model for stratum corneum lipid packing? Biochim Biophys Acta 1993; 1147:273–276.

111. Moore DJ, Rerek ME. Insights into the molecular organization of lipids in the skin barrier from infrared spectroscopy studies of stratum corneum lipid models. Acta Derm Venereol Suppl 2000; 208:16–22.

112. Moore DJ, Rerek ME, Mendelsohn R. Lipid domains and FTIR spectroscopy studies of the conformational order and phase behavior of ceramides. J Phys Chem 1997; 101:8933–8940.

113. Neubert R, Rettig W, Warterig S, Wegener M, Wienholdt A. Structure of stratum corneum lipids characterized by FT-Raman spectroscopy and DSC. II. Mixtures of ceramides and saturated fatty acids. Chem Phys Lipids 1997; 89:3–14.

114. Pilgram GSK, van Engelsma-Pelt AM, Koerten HK, Bouwstra JA. Study on the lipid organisation of stratum corneum lipid models by cryo-electron diffraction. J Lipid Res 1998; 39:1669–1676.

115. Hatfield RM, Fung LW-M. A new model system for lipid interactions in stratum corneum vesicles: effects of lipid composition, calcium, and pH. Biochemistry 1999; 38:784–791.

116. Hatfield RM, Fung LW-M. Molecular properties of a stratum corneum model lipid system: large unilamellar vesicles. Biophys J 1995; 68:196–207.

117. de la Maza A, Lopez O, Coderch L, Parra JL. Int J Pharm 1998; 171:63–74.

118. Aly R, Shirley C, Cumico B, Maibach HI. Effect of prolongedocculusion on the microbial flora, pH, carbon dioxide and trasepidermal water loss on human skin. J Invest Dermatol 1978; 71:378–381.

119. Turner N, Cullander C, Guy RH. Determination of the pH gradient across the stratum corneum. J Invest Dermatol Symp Proc 1998; 3:110–113.

120. Ohman H, Vahlquist A. The pH gradient over the stratum corneum differs in X-linked recessive and autosomal dominant ichthyosis: a clue to the molecular origin of the "acid skin mantle"? J Invest Dermatol 1998; 111:674–677.

121. Swarzendruber DC, Wertz PW, Kitko DJ, Madison KC, Downing DT. Molecular models of the intercellular lipid lamellae in mammalian stratum corneum. J Invest Dermatol 1989; 92:251–257.
122. Dahlen B, Pascher I. Molecular arrangements in sphingolipids—thermotropic phase-behavior of tetracosanoylphytosphingosine. Chem Phys Lipids 1979; 24:119–133.
123. Forslind B. A domain mosaic model of the skin barrier. Acta Derm Venereol 1994; 74:1–6.
124. Di Nardo A, Wertz P, Giannetti A, Seidenari S. Ceramide and cholesterol composition of the skin of patients with atopic dermatitis. Acta Derm Venereol 1998; 78:27–30.
125. Elias PM, Williams ML, Maloney ME, Bonifas JA, Brown BE, Grayson S, Epstein EH. Stratum corneum lipids in disorders of cornification. Steroid sulfatase and cholesterol sulfate in normal desquamation and the pathogenesis of recessive X-linked ichthyosis. J Clin Invest 1984; 74:1414–1421.

8

Cornified Envelope and Corneocyte-Lipid Envelope

Peter J. Koch and Dennis R. Roop
Departments of Dermatology and Molecular and Cellular Biology,
Baylor College of Medicine, Houston, Texas, U.S.A.

Zhijian Zhou
Department of Molecular and Cellular Biology, Baylor College of Medicine, Houston,
Texas, U.S.A.

INTRODUCTION

The skin of terrestrial animals is the primary interface between their body and the environment. As such, it affects social and sexual behaviors, regulates body temperature, triggers immunological responses to pathogenic microorganisms, and serves as a shield against environmental hazards. Most importantly, the skin provides a barrier that prevents the uncontrolled loss of water and ions. The detrimental effects of a loss of skin barrier function have been demonstrated by the phenotypes observed in animals with mutations in genes that encode either barrier components or enzymes required for barrier assembly. These genetically engineered mouse mutants often die shortly after birth due to uncontrolled transepithelial water loss (TEWL) and hypothermia (see below).

A complete loss of skin barrier function is rare in humans, and modern medicine has dramatically reduced the lethality of infants born with barrier defects. Nevertheless, lack of a functional skin barrier is a major concern, for example, in prematurely born infants. The skin barrier develops late during embryonic development. Based on histological data, it is assumed that a barrier is established by 34 weeks of gestation (1). Premature infants show increased TEWL and are highly susceptible to infections. This clearly demonstrates that understanding the biochemical processes that establish barrier function will help us to develop better treatments for these patients.

Several hereditary skin diseases are caused by mutations in genes that encode structural proteins or enzymes required for barrier formation. We will discuss some of these diseases below. A more complete discussion of hereditary barrier defects can be found in Chaps. 26 to 28.

In this chapter we will summarize our current view of the cell biological basis of skin barrier formation. We will focus mainly on the barrier established in the interfollicular epidermis. We will also discuss various animal models that have highlighted the role of individual genes in this process. Finally, we will discuss open questions and outline new research strategies that will provide insight into the molecular and cellular mechanisms of skin barrier formation.

THE LIFE-CYCLE OF KERATINOCYTES AND THE HISTO-ARCHITECTURE OF THE EPIDERMIS

Although the final goal of cutaneous research is to understand the basic biology of human skin and diseases that affect its structure and function, much of our current knowledge is derived from studying mouse skin. This is largely due to the fact that genetic manipulations of mice are now easily accomplished and allow us to test the function of individual genes in barrier formation. Although human and mouse skin show some obvious differences, it is becoming increasingly clear that the integuments of both species are controlled by very similar genetic and biochemical processes. The following paragraphs are therefore based on knowledge derived from both human and mouse skin.

Figure 1 outlines the histo-architecture of the interfollicular epidermis, a stratified squamous epithelium that is connected to the underlying mesenchymal tissue via a specialized extracellular matrix (ECM), the so-called basement membrane zone (BMZ).

The epithelial component of the skin, the epidermis, is maintained by pluripotent stem cells that reside in the basal cell layer as well as in the bulge region of hair follicles. These stem cells persist for the entire life span of the organism. They divide infrequently, yielding two types of progeny: cells that maintain the stem cell compartments and transient amplifying (TA) cells that undergo a highly regulated differentiation program which establishes and maintains the various strata of the interfollicular epidermis (Fig. 1). TA cells have limited proliferation potential. After a few cell divisions, they loose their contact with the BMZ and begin to migrate toward the skin surface. Concomitantly, these cells undergo morphological and biochemical changes. Changes in the synthesis of cytoskeletal proteins, such as keratins and desmosomal proteins (2,3), have been used as markers to describe this process. TA cells and stem cells, for example, synthesize keratins 5 and 14 (K5, K14). Once these cells leave the BMZ, they begin to express K1 and K10. In the upper spinous and the granular layers, keratinocytes begin to express components of the cornified cell envelope (CE), a structure that eventually replaces the plasma membrane (see below). During the transition from the granular layer to the stratum corneum (SC), keratinocytes loose their nuclei and organelles. Mature corneocytes are dead cells encased by a chemically resistant protein and lipid shell (corneocyte lipid envelope, CLE), and are filled with a matrix that consists mainly of keratin fibrillae. The corneocytes are embedded in a lipid matrix (intercellular lamellar lipids). Both the protein and the lipid components of the SC are essential for establishing normal barrier function.

Eventually, corneocytes loose their contacts, maintained for example by corneodesmosomes, and are sloughed into the environment. It is noteworthy that desmosomes and corneodesmosomes are more than just cell-adhesion junctions that hold epidermal cells (including corneocytes in the lower layers of the stratum corneum) together. Recently, it has been shown that changes in the molecular composition of suprabasal desmosomes and presumably corneodesmosomes affect the structure and function of the stratum corneum. Transgenic mice that over-express the desmosomal transmembrane component, desmoglein 3, in the suprabasal layers of the epidermis show abnormal SCs with a loss of skin barrier function and neonatal death (4).

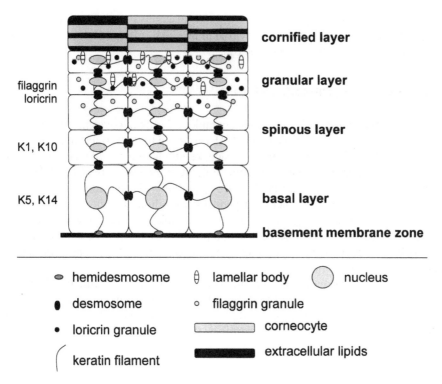

filaggrin
loricrin

K1, K10

K5, K14

cornified layer

granular layer

spinous layer

basal layer

basement membrane zone

⊜ hemidesmosome   θ lamellar body   ◯ nucleus

● desmosome   ○ filaggrin granule

• loricrin granule   ▭ corneocyte

⌠ keratin filament   ▬ extracellular lipids

Figure 1 Histo-architecture of the interfollicular epidermis (newborn mouse). The epidermis is a stratified squamous epithelium that is connected to the underlying mesenchymal tissue via the basement membrane zone (BMZ), a specialized extracellular matrix (ECM). Based on morphological and biochemical criteria, four layers (strata) can be distinguished: basal layer, spinous layer, granular layer, and cornified layer. Marker proteins that assemble into the epidermal cytoskeleton (e.g., hemidesmosomes, desmosomes, and keratin intermediate filaments) are commonly used to identify individual layers (e.g., keratins 5, 14, 1, 10; K5, K14, K1, K10). Note that CE components (e.g., filaggrin, loricrin) are synthesized in the spinous and granular layers. Lamellar bodies are extruded from the granular layer and contribute to the formation of the lipid matrix in which the corneocytes are embedded.

Another type of cell junction, the tight junction (TJ), has recently been shown to play a role in skin barrier formation as well. TJs have long been known to occur in polarized simple epithelia, such as the colon epithelium, where they demarcate the border between apical and basolateral membrane areas of epithelial cells. TJs in these tissues seal the intercellular space and consequently prevent the free paracellular diffusion of water and ions. Whether the TJs are present in stratified epithelia has been controversial in the past. Recent studies, however, have clearly provided evidence for the existence of TJs in the granular layer of the interfollicular epidermis and in the Henle layer of hair follicles (5–7). Although it is not known whether TJ proteins contribute to CE formation, there is emerging evidence that TJs establish an essential water barrier in the suprabasal layers of the epidermis. Recently, claudin 1–deficient mice were generated (8). Claudins are transmembrane components of TJ. These mice die within one day after birth, most likely due to increased TEWL. Furthermore, transgenic mice over-expressing claudin 6 in the suprabasal layers of the epidermis develop a severe barrier defect shortly after birth with a deregulation of certain barrier components (e.g., filaggrin, loricrin, TGase 3, involucrin, and SPRRPs) and abnormal CE morphology (9). These animals also show deregulation of Klf4, a transcription factor that might play a key role in terminal differentiation of keratino-cytes and skin barrier formation (see below).

FORMATION OF THE CE AND THE CLE

The cornified cell envelope (CE) consists of a complex mixture of covalently cross-linked proteins and a layer of characteristic lipids (CLE) attached to the extracellular surface of the protein layer (10–21). On the cytoplasmic side, keratin filaments and their attachment sites at the plasma membrane, the desmosomes (3), are embedded in the CE (22,23). The CE components are cross-linked mainly via ε-(γ-glutamyl) lysine isopeptide bonds, a reaction which is catalyzed by calcium-dependent transglutaminases (TGases, Fig. 2) (17,21,24–26). This cross-linking leads to a protein complex that is highly insoluble and resistant to conventional biochemical extraction procedures. In fact, the standard proce-dure to isolate CEs is boiling skin samples in buffers containing high concentrations of ionic detergents (example in Fig. 3).

The significance of the TGase-mediated cross-linking for skin function has been demonstrated by the discovery that mutations in one of these enzymes (TGase 1) can lead to lamellar ichthyosis, an autosomal recessive skin disease (25,27–30). Patients with this severe disorder develop hyperkeratosis (thickening of the stratum corneum)

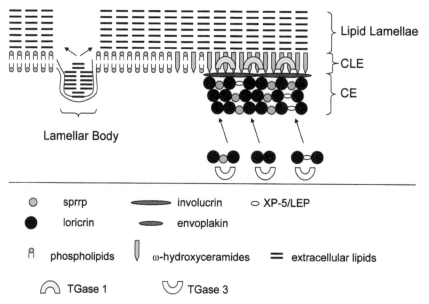

Figure 2   Simplified model of cornified envelope (CE) and corneocyte lipid envelope (CLE) assembly at the interface of granular and cornified cell layers. Initially, TGase 3 is thought to generate soluble complexes of CE components (SPRRPs, loricrin) in the cytoplasm which are then covalently linked to a scaffold consisting of involucrin, periplakin, and envoplakin at the cell periphery by TGase 1. At the same time, lamellar bodies fuse with the apical region of granular cells and extrude their lipid and enzyme contents into the intercellular space (for details see text). Eventually, these lipids will form the lipid lamellae in which corneocytes are embedded. The phospholipid bilayer cell membrane of granular cells is replaced with the CE/CLE.

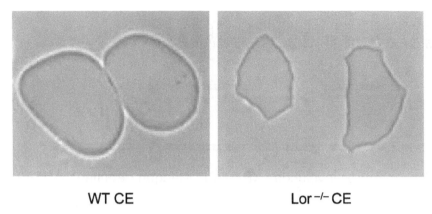

WT CE   Lor⁻/⁻ CE

Figure 3 Microscopic picture of cornified cell envelopes (CE) from newborn wild-type and Lor null mice. CEs are isolated by boiling newborn skin in buffers containing high concentrations of ionic detergents and reducing agents. Note that the wild-type CE appears smooth, whereas the Lor$^{-/-}$ CE displays an irregular shape.

and acanthosis (thickening of the epidermis) due to a failure to form the CE. Furthermore, mice deficient in TGase 1 exhibit a severe defect in epidermal barrier function resulting in neonatal lethality (31).

Several protein components of the CE have been identified; among them are involucrin, members of a family of small proline-rich proteins (SPRRPs), XP-5/late epidermal protein genes (XP-5/LEP), loricrin, cystatin α, desmoplakin, envoplakin, periplakin, elafin, filaggrin, S100 proteins, repetin, and several keratins (11,13,17,32–35). Some of these proteins (involucrin, SPRRPs, XP-5/LEP, loricrin, filaggrin, repetin) are encoded by genes clustered in the so-called "epidermal differentiation complex" on human chromosome 1q21 (36–38) and mouse chromosome 3 (39,40), respectively (Fig. 4). Involucrin, SPRRPs, XP-5/LEP, and loricrin also share amino acid sequence homologies in their carboxyl-terminal domains, indicating a common origin of these genes [(32,41); Fig. 5].

Interestingly, the protein composition of the CE varies between tissues and body sites. Loricrin is the major component of the CE in the interfollicular epidermis, where as much as 70% of the CE mass is derived from this protein (14,42–44). In human foreskin epidermis, for example, two-thirds of the inner (cytoplasmic) CE consists of more than 85% loricrin (13). On the other hand, loricrin is absent in most internal epithelia (one notable exception is the mouse forestomach) (45). Furthermore, the molar ratio of the CE components may vary between tissues. A comparison of mouse epidermal and forestomach CEs, for example, showed that the ratio of loricrin to small proline-rich proteins was 100:1 in newborn epidermis and 3:1 in forestomach (14,15,43). SPRR proteins are co-expressed with loricrin and serve as molecular cross-linkers [see references in (17)]. It has been speculated that the relative molar ratio of loricrin and SPRR proteins may determine the biomechanical properties of the CE, i.e., CEs that are subject to mechanical stress may have a higher relative amount of SPRR proteins (14,15,43).

It has been proposed that the first step in epidermal CE formation in the stratum granulosum is the deposition of a monolayer of involucrin, envoplakin, and periplakin at the inner surface of the plasma membrane [(46) and references in (17); Fig. 2]. These proteins are thought to serve as a scaffold for the addition

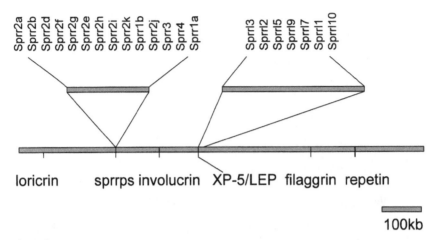

Figure 4 Gene arrangement within a small region of the epidermal differentiation complex on mouse chromosome 3. The genes for several CE components are located in this region. So far, approximately 40 genes have been identified in the mouse epidermal differentiation complex that encode known or putative CE components (own observation).

of other CE components. Loricrin (which initially accumulates in insoluble kerato-hyalin granules in human epidermis and L-granules in mouse epidermis), SPRRPs, and possibly other CE components are thought to be cross-linked in the cytoplasm by TGase 3, forming soluble multiprotein complexes that are transported to the cell periphery where they are integrated into the nascent CE, a reaction catalyzed by TGase 1 (Fig. 2); (24,47,48).

The CLE is formed by covalent linkage of ω-hydroxyceramides to the extracellular surface of the CE. Involucrin, envoplakin, and periplakin appear to be the major acceptor molecules for hydroxyceramides (12,49).

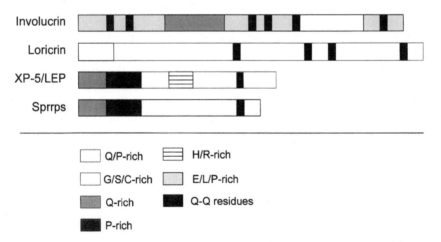

Figure 5 Schematic representation of the amino acid composition and domain structure of several CE components. Note the presence of similar domains in all proteins, suggesting that the corresponding genes were derived from a single ancestral gene. The Q-rich sequences are potential target sites for TGase-mediated cross-linking into the CE. Amino acids are given in single letter code.

At the same time, trans-Golgi network–derived lamellar bodies (LBs), which consist of lipid lamellae surrounded by a membrane, fuse with the apical membrane of granular cells (Fig. 2). These LBs contain lipids (free fatty acids, cholesterol, cholesterol ester, glucosylceramides) and enzymes (e.g., acid hydrolases) that are required to form the lamellar membrane sheets that provide the "mortar" in which the CE "bricks" are embedded (21,50–56). Proper lipid processing and the subsequent formation of intact lamellar lipid membrane sheets are required for barrier formation.

Mouse Models Designed to Determine "The Critical Component" of the CE

The development of skin barrier function during embryogenesis has been studied extensively in mice. A simple method to follow barrier formation is to extract embryos with an organic solvent and then stain with a histological dye (57). This procedure has revealed that the barrier is established late in mouse development, around embryonic day 17 (E17; gestation time of mice is approximately 20 days). It has been demonstrated that integration of loricrin into the nascent CE during embryogenesis coincides with the formation of a rudimentary barrier (57). This observation as well as the fact that loricrin is the major component of the CE in the interfollicular epidermis led to the hypothesis that this protein is required for barrier formation. To test this hypothesis, we have generated mice with a null mutation in the loricrin gene [Lor$^{-/-}$ mice (58)].

Lor$^{-/-}$ mice showed a delay in the formation of the skin barrier during embryonic development (Fig. 6). At birth, homozygous mutant mice weighed less than control littermates and showed skin abnormalities, i.e., congenital erythroderma with shiny, translucent skin. Nevertheless, we did not detect impaired epidermal barrier function in these mice, and the phenotype normalized within four to five days.

Although CEs isolated from Lor$^{-/-}$ mice had less regular shapes than wild-type CEs (example in Fig. 3), their thickness, as determined by electron microscopy, was essentially normal (59). Therefore, we suspected that other CE components substituted for loricrin in these mice. We confirmed that two members of the small proline-rich protein family, SPRRP2D and SPRRP2H, and repetin were upregulated in Lor$^{-/-}$ mice. Interestingly, these gene-expression studies revealed that the compensatory response was already triggered in utero.

Analysis of the amino acid composition of Lor$^{-/-}$ CEs indicated an approximately threefold increase in total SPRRP proteins compared with wild-type CEs (59) which was consistent with the observed increase in SPRRP2 transcripts. Surprisingly, Lor$^{-/-}$ CEs had high Gly/Ser contents like wild-type CEs, in which these amino acids are contributed mainly by loricrin. This suggested that novel loricrin-like proteins were integrated into the CE of Lor$^{-/-}$ mice. Subsequent studies revealed that increased expression of members of the XP-5/LEP protein family are likely to account for the high Gly/Ser content of Lor$^{-/-}$ CEs (own unpublished results).

The activation of compensatory mechanisms that maintain skin barrier function in the absence of a major CE protein does not appear to be unique to the loricrin knockout mouse. Mice with null mutations in the involucrin (60) and envoplakin (61) genes also did not show gross defects in barrier formation, suggesting the existence of compensatory mechanisms that maintain barrier function in the absence of these major CE components (see also below).

Although loricrin null mutations have not been reported in a human skin disease, a subset of patients with Vohwinkel's syndrome (VS) and one pedigree with

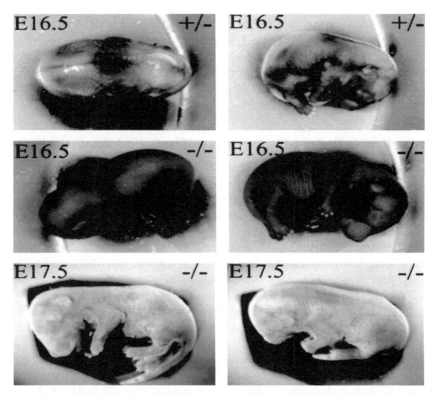

Figure 6 Dye penetration assay to follow skin barrier development in utero during embryonic development of loricrin null mice. Lor$^{+/-}$ and wild-type mice (not shown) begin to develop a rudimentary skin barrier by embryonic day 16.5 (E16.5). This becomes evident when these embryos are stained with a histological dye, which does not penetrate the skin in areas where the barrier has formed (back of E16.5 embryos). Lor$^{-/-}$ embryos are completely stained at this stage, indicating that the barrier has not formed yet. By E17.5, however, embryos of all genotypes (wild type, Lor$^{+/-}$, Lor$^{-/-}$) remain unstained. This indicates that the loricrin null mutation leads to a delay, not an elimination of barrier function. Nevertheless, Lor$^{-/-}$ mice are born with a mild skin phenotype, suggesting that the skin barrier is not completely formed in utero.

progressive symmetric erythrokeratodermia (PSEK) were shown to have mutations in the loricrin gene (11,62–69). These diseases are rare autosomal-dominant disorders that are clinically characterized by diffuse palmoplantar keratoderma (thickening of the stratum corneum of palms and soles) with a honeycomb appearance and the development of constricting bands around digits that can lead to auto-amputation. In pedigrees analyzed at the molecular level, mutations in gene sequence coding for the carboxyl-terminus of loricrin have been found. The mutations reported are single base pair insertions that lead to the synthesis of an aberrant protein in which carboxyl-terminal amino acid sequences are replaced by missense amino acids. These mutations also eliminate several glutamine and lysine residues that normally form isopeptide bonds (compare mutations reported in Refs. 63, 66–69 with cross-linking sites in Refs. 14, 26).

To establish a causative relationship between loricrin mutations and these diseases, we generated transgenic mice (ML.VS) expressing a carboxyl-terminally truncated form of loricrin that is similar to the protein expressed in VS and PSEK patients (70). At birth, ML.VS mutant mice exhibited erythrokeratodermia with an epidermal barrier dysfunction. Mice expressing high levels of the transgene exhibited a generalized scaling of the skin, as well as a constricting band encircling the tail and a thickening of footpads. The severe phenotype resulting from expression of the loricrin VS mutant, as compared to the mild $Lor^{-/-}$ phenotype, suggested that it is not functioning in a classic dominant-negative fashion, i.e., producing a functional knockout of loricrin. To test this prediction, we mated the loricrin VS mutation into the $Lor^{-/-}$ background. The severe phenotype resulting from this cross confirmed that the VS mutation did not require a direct interaction with wild-type loricrin.

The availability of the $ML.VS/Lor^{-/-}$ mice allowed us to further examine the molecular basis of the phenotype. Using immunoelectron microscopy, we were able to show that the VS mutant protein was almost exclusively present in the nucleus, with little, if any, incorporation into the CE. A survey of the missense amino acids created by the frameshift mutation revealed several putative nuclear localization signals (NLS). Transfection experiments confirmed that these sequences could function as an NLS. Taken together, these observations suggest that deposition of the mutant loricrin in the nucleus may interfere with late stages of epidermal differentiation.

CONCLUSIONS AND FUTURE DIRECTIONS

So far, loss-of-function studies in mice have not identified a single "critical" structural component that is required to establish and maintain barrier function. Recent results, including the completion of the mouse and human genome projects, revealed that mammals encode a large number of putative CE components. Elucidating the individual contributions of these genes in barrier formation using knockout approaches is therefore not feasible. Furthermore, the elaborate compensatory responses that establish barrier function in utero, even in the absence of major CE components, suggest that null mutations in most, if not all, of these genes would not result in obvious phenotypes.

How do we proceed to unravel the mechanisms that establish and maintain the barrier? One key question that needs to be addressed is how mammals regulate the genes that encode CE components and how these signal transduction mechanisms are used to repair barrier defects. Knowledge of these signaling pathways would help to identify therapeutic targets for drug intervention in cases of barrier loss. So far, however, little is known about CE gene regulation.

One key regulator of barrier formation, Klf4, was recently identified. A null mutation for this transcription factor in mice leads to neonatal lethality, with a loss of skin barrier function (71). Conversely, over-expression of Klf4 in the skin of transgenic mice induces premature barrier formation during embryonic development (72).

Is there a single "stress response" mechanism that is activated when the barrier fails? To address this question, we recently began to systematically compare the gene expression profiles of two genetically distinct mouse models with barrier defects, the $Lor^{-/-}$ line and the RXR403α transgenic line (unpublished results). The latter mouse strain expresses a dominant-negative retinoic acid receptor in the epidermis (73,74). These mice show defects in lipid processing and do not form lipid multilamellar structures between corneocytes. Newborn pups show increased TEWL and hypothermia. Most of these newborns die within 24 hours. The few transgenics that survive develop a scaly skin phenotype.

These two animal lines might serve as examples of mice with defects in either the "brick" ($Lor^{-/-}$) or "mortar" (RXR403α) component of the stratum corneum. Specifically, we analyzed the gene expression profiles of several CE protein components in both animal models (e.g., SPRRPs, XP-5/LEP genes). Although we did find overlapping gene induction patterns in both models, which might represent a common "stress-response" to a loss of barrier function, we also identified a distinct pattern of gene activation in each mouse model (data not shown). In summary, the examples given above suggest that general as well as context-specific compensatory mechanisms exist in vivo. The next challenge will be to characterize the transcription factors and signal transduction pathways that trigger both types of responses and use this information to identify new therapeutic targets for treatment of barrier defects.

REFERENCES

1. Kalia YN, Nonato LB, Lund CH, Guy RH. Development of skin barrier function in premature infants. J Invest Dermatol 1998; 111:320–326.
2. Getsios S, Huen AC, Green KJ. Working out the strength and flexibility of desmosomes. Nat Rev Mol Cell Biol 2004; 5:271–281.
3. Cheng X, Koch PJ. In vivo function of desmosomes. J Dermatol 2004; 31:171–187.
4. Elias PM, Matsuyoshi N, Wu H, Lin C, Wang ZH, Brown BE, Stanley JR. Desmoglein isoform distribution affects stratum corneum structure and function. J Cell Biol 2001; 153:243–249.
5. Brandner JM, Kief S, Grund C, Rendl M, Houdek P, Kuhn C, Tschachler E, Franke WW, Moll I. Organization and formation of the tight junction system in human epidermis and cultured keratinocytes. Eur J Cell Biol 2002; 81:253–263.
6. Langbein L, Pape UF, Grund C, Kuhn C, Praetzel S, Moll I, Moll R, Franke WW. Tight junction-related structures in the absence of a lumen: occludin, claudins and tight junction plaque proteins in densely packed cell formations of stratified epithelia and squamous cell carcinomas. Eur J Cell Biol 2003; 82:385–400.
7. Langbein L, Grund C, Kuhn C, Praetzel S, Kartenbeck J, Brandner JM, Moll I, Franke WW. Tight junctions and compositionally related junctional structures in mammalian stratified epithelia and cell cultures derived therefrom. Eur J Cell Biol 2002; 81:419–435.
8. Furuse M, Hata M, Furuse K, Yoshida Y, Haratake A, Sugitani Y, Noda T, Kubo A, Tsukita S. Claudin-based tight junctions are crucial for the mammalian epidermal barrier: a lesson from claudin-1-deficient mice. J Cell Biol 2002; 156:1099–1111.
9. Turksen K, Troy TC. Permeability barrier dysfunction in transgenic mice overexpressing claudin 6. Development 2002; 129:1775–1784.
10. Roop DR. Defects in the barrier. Science 1995; 267:474–475.
11. Ishida-Yamamoto A, Iizuka H. Structural organization of cornified cell envelopes and alterations in inherited skin disorders. Exp Dermatol 1998; 7:1–10.
12. Marekov LN, Steinert PM. Ceramides are bound to structural proteins of the human foreskin epidermal cornified cell envelope. J Biol Chem 1998; 273:17763–17770.
13. Steinert PM, Marekov LN. The proteins elafin, filaggrin, keratin intermediate filaments, loricrin, and small proline-rich proteins 1 and 2 are isodipeptide cross-linked components of the human epidermal cornified cell envelope. J Biol Chem 1995; 270:17702–17711.
14. Steinert PM, Kartasova T, Marekov LN. Biochemical evidence that small proline-rich proteins and trichohyalin function in epithelia by modulation of the biomechanical properties of their cornified cell envelopes. J Biol Chem 1998; 273:11758–11769.
15. Steinert PM, Candi E, Kartasova T, Marekov L. Small proline-rich proteins are cross-bridging proteins in the cornified cell envelopes of stratified squamous epithelia. J Struct Biol 1998; 122:76–85.
16. Wertz PW, Madison KC, Downing DT. Covalently bound lipids of human stratum corneum. J Invest Dermatol 1989; 92:109–111.
17. Kalinin AE, Kajava AV, Steinert PM. Epithelial barrier function: assembly and structural features of the cornified cell envelope. Bioessays 2002; 24:789–800.

18. Elias PM, Fartasch M, Crumrine D, Behne M, Uchida Y, Holleran WM. Origin of the corneocyte lipid envelope (CLE): observations in harlequin ichthyosis and cultured human keratinocytes. J Invest Dermatol 2000; 115:765–769.
19. Madison KC. Barrier function of the skin: "la raison d'etre" of the epidermis. J Invest Dermatol 2003; 121:231–241.
20. Behne M, Uchida Y, Seki T, de Montellano PO, Elias PM, Holleran WM. Omega-hydroxyceramides are required for corneocyte lipid envelope (CLE) formation and normal epidermal permeability barrier function. J Invest Dermatol 2000; 114:185–192.
21. Harding CR. The stratum corneum: structure and function in health and disease. Dermatol Therap 2004; 17:6–15.
22. Candi E, Tarcsa E, Digiovanna JJ, Compton JG, Elias PM, Marekov LN, Steinert PM. A highly conserved lysine residue on the head domain of type II keratins is essential for the attachment of keratin intermediate filaments to the cornified cell envelope through isopeptide crosslinking by transglutaminases. Proc Natl Acad Sci USA 1998; 95:2067–2072.
23. Steinert PM. Structural-mechanical integration of keratin intermediate filaments with cell peripheral structures in the cornified epidermal keratinocyte. Biol Bull 1998; 194:367–368.
24. Candi E, Tarcsa E, Idler WW, Kartasova T, Marekov LN, Steinert PM. Transglutaminase cross-linking properties of the small proline-rich 1 family of cornified cell envelope proteins. Integration with loricrin. J Biol Chem 1999; 274:7226–7237.
25. Candi E, Melino G, Lahm A, Ceci R, Rossi A, Kim IG, Ciani B, Steinert PM. Transglutaminase 1 mutations in lamellar ichthyosis. Loss of activity due to failure of activation by proteolytic processing. J Biol Chem 1998; 273:13693–13702.
26. Candi E, Melino G, Mei G, Tarcsa E, Chung SI, Marekov LN, Steinert PM. Biochemical, structural, and transglutaminase substrate properties of human loricrin, the major epidermal cornified cell envelope protein. J Biol Chem 1995; 270:26382–26390.
27. Elias PM, Schmuth M, Uchida Y, Rice RH, Behne M, Crumrine D, Feingold KR, Holleran WM, Pharm D. Basis for the permeability barrier abnormality in lamellar ichthyosis. Exp Dermatol 2002; 11:248–256.
28. Mauro T, Guitard M, Behne M, Oda Y, Crumrine D, Komuves L, Rassner U, Elias PM, Hummler E. The ENaC channel is required for normal epidermal differentiation. J Invest Dermatol 2002; 118:589–594.
29. Russell LJ, Digiovanna JJ, Rogers GR, Steinert PM, Hashem N, Compton JG, Bale SJ. Mutations in the gene for transglutaminase 1 in autosomal recessive lamellar ichthyosis. Nat Genet 1995; 9:279–283.
30. Jeon S, Djian P, Green H. Inability of keratinocytes lacking their specific transglutaminase to form cross-linked envelopes: absence of envelopes as a simple diagnostic test for lamellar ichthyosis. Proc Natl Acad Sci USA 1998; 95:687–690.
31. Matsuki M, Yamashita F, Ishida-Yamamoto A, Yamada K, Kinoshita C, Fushiki S, Ueda E, Morishima Y, Tabata K, Yasuno H, Hashida M, Iizuka H, Ikawa M, Okabe M, Kondoh G, Kinoshita T, Takeda J, Yamanishi K. Defective stratum corneum and early neonatal death in mice lacking the gene for transglutaminase 1 (keratinocyte transglutaminase). Proc Natl Acad Sci USA 1998; 95:1044–1049.
32. Krieg P, Schuppler M, Koesters R, Mincheva A, Lichter P, Marks F. Repetin (Rptn), a new member of the "fused gene" subgroup within the S100 gene family encoding a murine epidermal differentiation protein. Genomics 1997; 43:339–348.
33. Zhao XP, Elder JT. Positional cloning of novel skin-specific genes from the human epidermal differentiation complex. Genomics 1997; 45:250–258.
34. Wang A, Johnson DG, MacLeod MC. Molecular cloning and characterization of a novel mouse epidermal differentiation gene and its promoter. Genomics 2001; 73:284–290.
35. Marshall D, Hardman MJ, Nield KM, Byrne C. Differentially expressed late constituents of the epidermal cornified envelope. Proc Natl Acad Sci USA 2001; 98:13031–13036.

36. Marenholz I, Volz A, Ziegler A, Davies A, Ragoussis I, Korge BP, Mischke D. Genetic analysis of the epidermal differentiation complex (EDC) on human chromosome 1q21: chromosomal orientation, new markers, and a 6-Mb YAC contig. Genomics 1996; 37: 295–302.

37. Mischke D, Korge BP, Marenholz I, Volz A, Ziegler A. Genes encoding structural proteins of epidermal cornification and S100 calcium-binding proteins form a gene complex ("epidermal differentiation complex") on human chromosome 1q21. J Invest Dermatol 1996; 106:989–992.

38. Volz A, Korge BP, Compton JG, Ziegler A, Steinert PM, Mischke D. Physical mapping of a functional cluster of epidermal differentiation genes on chromosome 1q21. Genomics 1993; 18:92–99.

39. Rothnagel JA, Longley MA, Bundman DS, Naylor SL, Lalley PA, Jenkins NA, Gilbert DJ, Copeland NG, Roop DR. Characterization of the mouse loricrin gene: link-age with profilaggrin and the flaky tail and soft coat mutant loci on chromosome 3. Genomics 1994; 23:450–456.

40. Song HJ, Poy G, Darwiche N, Lichti U, Kuroki T, Steinert PM, Kartasova T. Mouse Sprr2 genes: a clustered family of genes showing differential expression in epithelial tissues. Genomics 1999; 55:28–42.

41. Backendorf C, Hohl D. A common origin for cornified envelope proteins? Nat Genet 1992; 2:91.

42. Hohl D, Mehrel T, Lichti U, Turner ML, Roop DR, Steinert PM. Characterization of human loricrin. Structure and function of a new class of epidermal cell envelope proteins. J Biol Chem 1991; 266:6626–6636.

43. Jarnik M, Kartasova T, Steinert PM, Lichti U, Steven AC. Differential expression and cell envelope incorporation of small proline-rich protein 1 in different cornified epithelia. J Cell Sci 1996; 109:1381–1391.

44. Steven AC, Steinert PM. Protein composition of cornified cell envelopes of epidermal keratinocytes. J Cell Sci 1994; 107:693–700.

45. Hohl D, Ruf OB, de Viragh PA, Huber M, Detrisac CJ, Schnyder UW, Roop DR. Expression patterns of loricrin in various species and tissues. Differentiation 1993; 54:25–34.

46. Steinert PM, Marekov LN. Direct evidence that involucrin is a major early isopeptide cross-linked component of the keratinocyte cornified cell envelope. J Biol Chem 1997; 272:2021–2030.

47. Steinert PM, Marekov LN. Initiation of assembly of the cell envelope barrier structure of stratified squamous epithelia. Mol Biol Cell 1999; 10:4247–4261.

48. Tarcsa E, Candi E, Kartasova T, Idler WW, Marekov LN, Steinert PM. Structural and transglutaminase substrate properties of the small proline-rich 2 family of cornified cell envelope proteins. J Biol Chem 1998; 273:23297–23303.

49. DiColandrea T, Karashima T, Maatta A, Watt FM. Subcellular distribution of envoplakin and periplakin: insights into their role as precursors of the epidermal cornified envelope. J Cell Biol 2000; 151:573–586.

50. Freinkel RK, Traczyk TN. Lipid composition and acid hydrolase content of lamellar granules of fetal rat epidermis. J Invest Dermatol 1985; 85:295–298.

51. Grayson S, Johnson-Winegar AG, Wintroub BU, Isseroff RR, Epstein EH Jr, Elias PM. Lamellar body-enriched fractions from neonatal mice: preparative techniques and partial characterization. J Invest Dermatol 1985; 85:289–294.

52. Madison KC, Swartzendruber DC, Wertz PW, Downing DT. Presence of intact intercel-lular lipid lamellae in the upper layers of the stratum corneum. J Invest Dermatol 1987; 88:714–718.

53. Forslind B. A domain mosaic model of the skin barrier. Acta Derm Venereol 1994; 74:1–6.

54. Bouwstra JA, Pilgram GS, Ponec M. Does the single gel phase exist in stratum corneum? J Invest Dermatol 2002; 118:897–898.

55. Bouwstra JA, Gooris GS, Dubbelaar FE, Ponec M. Phase behavior of stratum corneum lipid mixtures based on human ceramides: the role of natural and synthetic ceramide 1. J Invest Dermatol 2002; 118:606–617.

56. Chuong CM, Nickoloff BJ, Elias PM, Goldsmith LA, Macher E, Maderson PA, Sundberg JP, Tagami H, Plonka PM, Thestrup-Pederson K, Bernard BA, Schroder JM, Dotto P, Chang CM, Williams ML, Feingold KR, King LE, Kligman AM, Rees JL, Christophers E. What is the 'true' function of skin? Exp Dermatol 2002; 11:159–187.

57. Hardman MJ, Sisi P, Banbury DN, Byrne C. Patterned acquisition of skin barrier function during development. Development 1998; 125:1541–1552.

58. Koch PJ, de Viragh PA, Scharer E, Bundman D, Longley MA, Bickenbach J, Kawachi Y, Suga Y, Zhou Z, Huber M, Hohl D, Kartasova T, Jarnik M, Steven AC, Roop DR. Lessons from loricrin-deficient mice. Compensatory mechanisms maintaining skin barrier function in the absence of a major cornified envelope protein. J Cell Biol 2000; 151: 389–400.

59. Jarnik M, de Viragh PA, Scharer E, Bundman D, Simon MN, Roop DR, Steven AC. Quasi-normal cornified cell envelopes in loricrin knockout mice imply the existence of a loricrin backup system. J Invest Dermatol 2002; 118:102–109.

60. Djian P, Easley K, Green H. Targeted ablation of the murine involucrin gene. J Cell Biol 2000; 16:381–388.

61. Maatta A, DiColandrea T, Groot K, Watt FM. Gene targeting of envoplakin, a cytoskeletal linker protein and precursor of the epidermal cornified envelope. Mol Cell Biol 2001; 21:7047–7053.

62. Christiano AM. Frontiers in keratodermas—pushing the envelope. Trends Genet 1997; 13:227–233.

63. Armstrong DK, McKenna KE, Hughes AE. A novel insertional mutation in loricrin in Vohwinkel's Keratoderma. J Invest Dermatol 1998; 111:702–704.

64. Ishida-Yamamoto A, Kato H, Kiyama H, Armstrong DK, Munro CS, Eady RA, Nakamura S, Kinouchi M, Takahashi H, Iizuka H. Mutant loricrin is not crosslinked into the cornified cell envelope but is translocated into the nucleus in loricrin keratoderma. J Invest Dermatol 2000; 115:1088–1094.

65. Ishida-Yamamoto A, Takahashi H, Iizuka H. Loricrin and human skin diseases: molecular basis of loricrin keratodermas. Histol Histopathol 1998; 7:819–826.

66. Takahashi H, Ishida-Yamamoto A, Kishi A, Ohara K, Iizuka H. Loricrin gene mutation in a Japanese patient of Vohwinkel's syndrome. J Dermatol Sci 1999; 19:44–47.

67. Korge BP, Ishida-Yamamoto A, Punter C, Dopping-Hepenstal PJ, Iizuka H, Stephenson A, Eady RA, Munro CS. Loricrin mutation in Vohwinkel's keratoderma is unique to the variant with ichthyosis. J Invest Dermatol 1997; 109:604–610.

68. Maestrini E, Monaco AP, McGrath JA, Ishida-Yamamoto A, Camisa C, Hovnanian A, Weeks DE, Lathrop M, Uitto J, Christiano AM. A molecular defect in loricrin, the major component of the cornified cell envelope, underlies Vohwinkel's syndrome. Nat Genet 1996; 13:70–77.

69. Ishida-Yamamoto A, McGrath JA, Lam H, Iizuka H, Friedman RA, Christiano AM. The molecular pathology of progressive symmetric erythrokeratoderma: a frameshift mutation in the loricrin gene and perturbations in the cornified cell envelope. Am J Hum Genet 1997; 61:581–589.

70. Suga Y, Jarnik M, Attar PS, Longley MA, Bundman D, Steven AC, Koch PJ, Roop DR. Transgenic mice expressing a mutant form of loricrin reveal the molecular basis of the skin diseases, Vohwinkel syndrome and progressive symmetric erythrokeratoderma. J Cell Biol 2000; 151:401–412.

71. Segre JA, Bauer C, Fuchs E. Klf4 is a transcription factor required for establishing the barrier function of the skin. Nat Genet 1999; 22:356–360.

72. Jaubert J, Cheng J, Segre JA. Ectopic expression of kruppel like factor 4 (Klf4) accelerates formation of the epidermal permeability barrier. Development 2003; 130:2767–2777.

73. Attar PS, Wertz PW, McArthur M, Imakado S, Bickenbach JR, Roop DR. Inhibition of retinoid signaling in transgenic mice alters lipid processing and disrupts epidermal barrier function. Mol Endocrinol 1997; 11:792–800.
74. Imakado S, Bickenbach JR, Bundman DS, Rothnagel JA, Attar PS, Wang XJ, Walczak VR, Wisniewski S, Pote J, Gordon JS. Targeting expression of a dominant-negative retinoic acid receptor mutant in the epidermis of transgenic mice results in loss of barrier function. Genes Dev 1995; 9:317–329.

9

Profilaggrin and the Fused S100 Family of Calcium-Binding Proteins

Richard B. Presland
Departments of Oral Biology and Medicine (Dermatology), University of Washington, Seattle, Washington, U.S.A.

Joseph A. Rothnagel
Department of Biochemistry and Molecular Biology, and the Institute for Molecular Bioscience, University of Queensland, St. Lucia, Queensland, Australia

Owen T. Lawrence
Department of Oral Biology, University of Washington, Seattle, Washington, U.S.A.

INTRODUCTION

The mammalian epidermis forms a vital barrier between an organism and its environment. It is continuously replaced through the proliferation of basal keratinocytes, which migrate upwards and differentiate into spinous and granular cells, eventually forming the stratum corneum or anuclear squames that constitute the epidermal barrier. During the process of terminal differentiation, epidermal keratinocytes produce a large number of proteins that function either as structural components of the stratum corneum or are involved in its synthesis or assembly. One of the largest families of epidermally expressed genes is the S100 Ca^{2+}-binding proteins, which function as calcium-dependent sensors, modulating a diverse array of intracellular and extracellular processes. The S100 protein family can be regarded as a superfamily consisting of two related groups, namely the low molecular weight canonical S100 proteins of ~100 amino acids and the high molecular weight fused S100 family, which contains an N-terminal S100 domain, "fused" to other sequences. The S100 domain consists of two EF-hands with flanking α-helices that are critical for calcium binding and protein protein interactions (Fig. 1). The canonical S100 proteins form homodimers, and heterodimers with other S100 proteins. Upon calcium binding, these dimers associate with specific target proteins, which regulate their activity and/or subcellular distribution (1,2). This review will focus on the fused S100 family, with only limited discussion of the canonical S100 family, which have been the subject of several recent reviews (1–3).

One of the key regulators of epidermal differentiation is calcium, which regulates the expression of differentiation markers via protein kinase C and other signaling pathways. Calcium is also essential for the function of many enzymes involved in

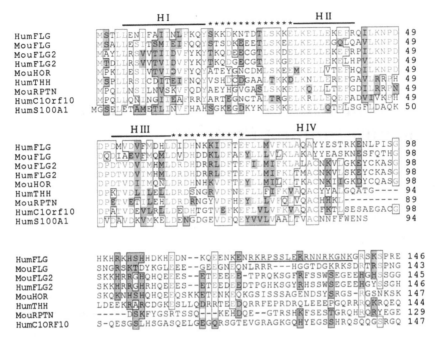

Figure 1 Amino acid similarity among the N-terminal domains of the fused S100 proteins. Shown are the S100 Ca^{2+}-binding domain (amino acids 1–92) and part of the downstream domains for HumFLG, MouFLG, MouFLG2, HumFLG-2, MouHOR, HumTHH, MouRPTN, HumC1orf10, and HumS100A1 analyzed for optimal alignment using ClustalW (150). The positions of the two Ca^{2+}-binding EF-hands are indicated by stars, and the four α-helices, HI–HIV, surrounding each EF-hand are indicated by lines above the sequence. Boxed amino acids in red show the identity and shaded blue residues indicate homology. The underlined sequence in humFLG indicates the position of the bipartite nuclear localization signal, which is not present at the same position in other fused S100 proteins (17). Numbers at right indicate the number of amino acids. *Abbreviations*: Hum FLG, human profilaggrin; MouFLG, mouse profilaggrin; MouFLG2, mouse Filaggrin-2; HumFLG-2, human Filaggrin-2; MouHOR, mouse hornerin; HumTHH, human trichohyalin; MouRPTN, mouse repetin; HumC1orf10, human C1orf10; and HumS100A1, human S100A1. (*See color insert.*)

cornified envelope (CE) assembly and barrier formation (4,5). Hence, the calcium gradient, which results in a high intracellular calcium concentration in the granular layer, is an essential element of normal barrier formation (6–8). As we will discuss in this review, the fused S100 proteins require this calcium gradient for their normal expression, Ca^{2+}-binding activity, and to carry out their individual function(s) in differentiating keratinocytes.

The fused S100 gene family consists of six known members: profilaggrin, Filaggrin-2 (Flg-2), hornerin, trichohyalin, repetin, and C1orf10 or cornulin. These proteins share a number of common features. Fused S100 proteins contain an N-terminal S100 Ca^{2+}-binding domain (Fig. 1), which is fused to a large downstream region that generally consists of multiple copies of one or more sequences. This downstream, repetitive domain imparts specific function(s) to the protein. Profilaggrin, Flg-2, and hornerin exhibit significant sequence homology in the repetitive central domain as well as in the S100 domain, suggesting that they represent a "profilaggrin-like" subfamily, which arose by gene duplication during the mammalian radiation (Fig. 2).

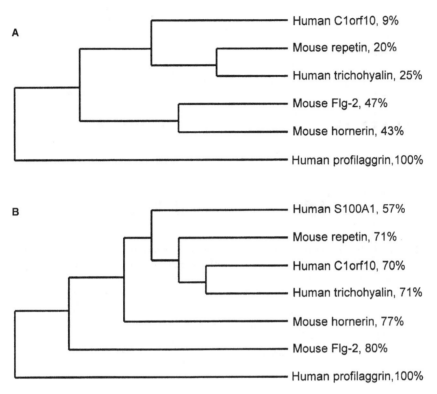

Figure 2 Phylogenetic tree of the fused S100 family. This unrooted phylogenetic tree was generated from an alignment of the complete protein sequences (A) and the S100 domains (amino acids 1–92) (B) of representative fused S100 protein sequences with the PHYLIP program using the Protein Sequence Parsimony method (Protpars, version 3.5 e; http://evolution.genetics.washington.edu/phylip/doc/protpars.html). It is noted that profilaggrin, Flg-2, and hornerin show significant amino acid sequence similarity (>30%), indicating homology beyond the S100 Ca^{2+}-binding domain (A). These three proteins also are the most closely related when examining only the S100 calcium-binding domain (B). Numbers at right indicate the percentage amino acid similarity of each protein to human profilaggrin. For Genbank accession numbers used in this analysis, see Table 4.

Trichohyalin, repetin, and C1orf10 show no significant homology to profilaggrin outside the conserved N-terminal S100 domain (Fig. 2). Another feature of this gene family is their expression in stratified keratinizing epithelia and the hair follicle. In addition, the fused S100 genes all map to the epidermal differentiation complex (EDC) on human chromosome 1q21. This 1.7 megabase region contains many genes expressed in epidermis, including the fused S100 family, most members of the canonical, low molecular weight S100 family, and many CE components, such as loricrin, involucrin, and the small proline-rich proteins (Fig. 3). A similar EDC is present on mouse chromosome 3 (9,10). The fused S100 genes have a similar genomic organization consisting of three exons, with introns that interrupt the 5′ untranslated region and the S100 domain, between the EF-hands. The conserved genomic organization is consistent with the evolution of this gene family by gene duplication of a single ancestral gene.

We will first discuss profilaggrin, the prototypical and best-studied member of the fused S100 family, followed by the related proteins Flg-2 and hornerin.

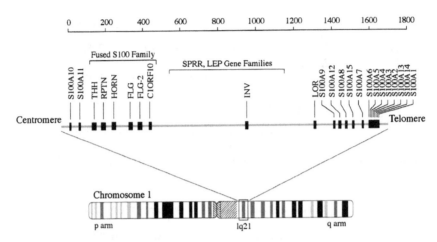

Figure 3 The EDC at chromosome 1q21. The organization of the fused S100 and S100 families within the EDC is shown, along with the position of the INV and LOR genes. The bracket shows where the SPRR and LEP gene families are located. It is noted that the fused S100 family is located as a clustered gene family spanning ~400 kb. This figure was developed from the NCBI Map Viewer of the Human Genome, Build 34 (http://www.ncbi.nlm.nih.gov/genome/guide/human). *Abbreviations*: EDC, epidermal differentiation complex; INV, involucrin; LEP, late envelope protein; LOR, loricrin; NCBI, National Center for Biotechnology Information; and SPRR, small proline-rich protein.

PROFILAGGRIN/FILAGGRIN

The Profilaggrin Pathway

An overview of the profilaggrin pathway showing its expression, proteolytic processing to filaggrin and the N-terminal peptide, and the intracellular location of these major end-products during epidermal terminal differentiation is shown in Figure 4. Profilaggrin is synthesized late in keratinocyte differentiation in the epidermal granular layer, where it is rapidly phosphorylated and packaged into keratohyalin granules (11–14). Profilaggrin consists of multiple filaggrin units (the polyfilaggrin domain) flanked by truncated filaggrin units and N- and C-terminal domains that differ from filaggrin. The N-terminal peptide includes the S100 Ca^{2+}-binding domain, which is located in the first 100 amino acids of the protein. During terminal differentiation, profilaggrin undergoes dephosphorylation and limited specific proteolysis to generate two major end-products, filaggrin and the N-terminal peptide (Fig. 4). Filaggrin functions as an intermediate filament–associated protein (IFAP) to aggregate keratin filaments into macrofibrils, the large filament bundles present in corneocytes. In the middle or upper layers of the epidermal stratum corneum, filaggrin is mostly degraded into free amino acids, which form a major component of the natural moisturizing factor (NMF) (see the section entitled "The Multiple Functions of Filaggrin: IFAP, Cornified Envelope Protein, and NMF"). These filaggrin-derived, hygroscopic amino acids are thought to have an important role in the maintenance of epidermal osmolarity and flexibility of skin (15,16). The other major product of profilaggrin processing, the N-terminal peptide, includes the S100 Ca^{2+}-binding domain and a downstream region (the B domain) that facilitates its nuclear transport (17). The N-terminal peptide localizes to the nuclei of granular and transition cells just prior to or coincident with nuclear destruction, suggesting that it may play a role in the program of terminal differentiation.

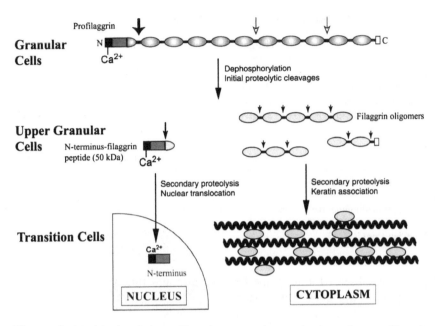

Granular Cells

Profilaggrin

N   Ca^{2+} C

Dephosphorylation
Initial proteolytic cleavages

Filaggrin oligomers

Upper Granular Cells

N-terminus-filaggrin peptide (50 kDa)   Ca^{2+}

Secondary proteolysis
Nuclear translocation

Secondary proteolysis
Keratin association

Transition Cells

Ca^{2+}

N-terminus

NUCLEUS   CYTOPLASM

Figure 4 Model showing profilaggrin expression and processing to filaggrin and the N-terminal peptide. Profilaggrin is expressed and phosphorylated by kinases in the granular layer of the epidermis and other keratinizing epithelia, and accumulates in keratohyalin granules. During the terminal differentiation (the granular to cornified cell transition), profilaggrin is dephosphorylated by phosphatases and processed by proteinases to generate filaggrin and the N-terminal S100 Ca^{2+}-binding peptide. Filaggrin aggregates keratin intermediate filaments in the cytoplasm of granular and transition cells, while the N-terminal Ca^{2+}-binding peptide accumulates in the nucleus of dying keratinocytes, where its function is unknown. For a list of enzymes involved in the post-translational modification of profilaggrin and processing to filaggrin, see Table 2. *Source*: From Ref. 17.

Thus, from a single polypeptide chain, keratohyalin-associated profilaggrin is processed into multiple products that display different intracellular localizations and functions in both living and cornified cells. Here we will summarize the recent findings relating to the function of these different profilaggrin-derived products, in particular the N-terminal S100 domain, and update the progress in other research areas, including the regulation of profilaggrin gene expression, the endoproteinases involved in its processing, and skin disorders associated with an altered profilaggrin expression and/or processing.

Profilaggrin Protein and Gene Structure

Profilaggrin consists of a central repetitive domain consisting of multiple filaggrin units (the polyfilaggrin domain) flanked by truncated filaggrin units and distinctive N- and C-termini [Fig. 4, Table 1; (18–22)]. In humans, profilaggrin contains either 10, 11, or 12 filaggrin units depending on the individual [Table 1; (23,24)]. The N-terminal domain consists of two distinct segments, an S100 Ca^{2+}-binding region, which is the A domain, and a cationic B domain that includes functional nuclear localization signals [Fig. 1; (17,25)]. The overall structure of profilaggrin is similar in other species, with the major differences being the size and the total number of filaggrin units (Table 1). These differences account for most of the variation in

Table 1 Interspecies Comparison of Mammalian Profilaggrins

Feature	Human	Rat	Mouse
Profilaggrin size	400 kDa[a]	≥800 kDa[a]	500 kDa[a]
Number of filaggrin units	10–12	20 ± 2	12–20
Size of filaggrin domain	324 aa	406 aa	250, 255 aa
Filaggrin size (SDS/PAGE)	37 kDa	42 kDa	26 kDa
Size of N-terminus[b] (A + B domains)	293 aa	283 aa	242 aa
mRNA size	13 kb[a]	27 kb[a]	17 kb[a]

[a]Actual size of protein and mRNA will vary, depending on the number of filaggrin units in the individual or rodent strain.
[b]Includes initiator methionine. Beyond the end of the B domain is the truncated filaggrin domain, which shows a significant similarity to filaggrin in the respective species.
Source: Modified from Ref. 13.

profilaggrin size observed among species. The fate and function of the unique C-terminal peptide is not known at present (18).

Filaggrin is a highly cationic (basic) protein that is unusually rich in histidine and arginine residues (21,26). The highly charged nature of filaggrin, and in particular its charge distribution, appears to be critical for its ionic interaction with keratin intermediate filaments (KIF) (27). Interspecies comparisons have shown that filaggrin is poorly conserved among mammals; for example, mouse and human filaggrin exhibit only 43% similarity (21). Even more remarkable is the sequence heterogeneity observed between the individual filaggrin units in human profilaggrin, which vary at almost 40% of amino acid positions (23,28). Taken together, these findings indicate that the charge and charge distribution, rather than the primary sequence, is the most critical determinant of KIF association. The most conserved regions of filaggrin are the sites involved in post–translational modification, including phosphorylation sites, and the linker peptide, which is the site of proteolytic processing of the polyfilaggrin domain [(13,21); see the sections "Profilaggrin Expression and Keratohyalin Granule Formation" and "Profilaggrin Processing to Filaggrin and the N-Terminal Peptide"].

The human and mouse profilaggrin genes consist of three exons, with one intron within the 5′ untranslated region and a second one within the S100 domain between the two EF-hands (18,19,25). A similarly located intron is present within the S100 domain of most, if not all, S100 family members (3,18). Rat profilaggrin appears to have a similar gene structure (17). Exon 3 encodes >95% of the profilaggrin mRNA and is unusually long for vertebrate genes.

Profilaggrin Expression and Keratohyalin Granule Formation

Profilaggrin is present in all mammalian species examined to date, including human, mouse, rat, rabbit, and guinea pig [Table 1; (11,14)]. It is expressed in the granular layer of epidermis and other orthokeratinizing epithelia, including the tongue, oral gingival, and rodent forestomach (21,29,30). Profilaggrin is rapidly phosphorylated by several kinases that have been partially characterized from rat epidermis, including casein kinase II (12,31). In rat profilaggrin, 21 serine and threonine residues are phosphorylated per filaggrin unit, with the majority of phosphorylation sites being conserved between humans and rodents (13,21). Phosphorylation may help fold profilaggrin into a compact, insoluble protein that can accumulate in keratohyalin granules. In vitro studies using profilaggrin and phosphorylated intermediates suggested that phosphorylation may also function to prevent the premature clumping of KIFs in the living epithelial layers (32,33). However, recent in vitro expression studies with various wild type, mutant, and truncated filaggrin proteins suggest that phosphorylation accounts only partially for the insolubility of profilaggrin and that the primary sequence of filaggrin and/or the size of the peptide is also an important determinant of solubility (34–36).

In rodent epidermis, there are two types of keratohyalin granules (KHGs) in the granular layer, termed F- (or P-F) granules and L-granules. F-granules or histidine-rich granules are large, irregularly shaped granules, which predominantly contain profilaggrin. In contrast, L-granules (or sulfur-rich granules) are small and round, and contain mostly loricrin, which becomes incorporated into the CE during terminal differentiation (13,37). Filaggrin was first identified as the histidine-rich protein of epidermis because of its unusually high histidine content (38–40). Tritiated histidine injected into newborn mouse skin readily labels the histidine-rich KHGs (41–43). In addition, an SDS/PAGE analysis of rodent skin radiolabeled with histidine demonstrated that profilaggrin, profilaggrin intermediates, and filaggrin are the predominant histidine-rich proteins of the epidermis (26). Thus, it is clear that profilaggrin is indeed localized to KHGs in the rodent epidermis. However, in the human epidermis studied by conventional electron microscopy, only profilaggrin was found to be localized to morphologically heterogenous keratohyalin granules (13,44). In a recent morphological study of cryoprocessed human skin prepared using high pressure freezing and freeze substitution, KHGs were completely absent, even though abundant profilaggrin immunoreactivity was detected in the upper living layers and in cornified cells under the same fixation conditions (45). These results suggest that the KHGs, seen in human skin using conventional processing, e.g., with Karnovsky's fixative (44), might be an artifact of strong tissue fixation. These studies, while intriguing, need to be reproduced by other laboratories; but they nevertheless point to species differences in the expression or solubility of profilaggrin in vivo.

Profilaggrin Processing to Filaggrin and the N-Terminal Peptide

Profilaggrin is rapidly processed, as keratinocytes undergo terminal differentiation during the granular to cornified cell transition. During this transition, there is a dramatic tissue transformation from living keratinocytes to dead, anuclear squames that contain a CE (46). Profilaggrin processing involves the action of two or more protein phosphatases that dephosphorylate profilaggrin, and specific proteolysis by endoproteinases to generate filaggrin and the N-terminal peptide (Fig. 4, Table 2).

Dephosphorylation of profilaggrin involves at least two enzymes. The best-characterized enzyme is the serine/threonine protein phosphatase type 2A (PP2A), which dephosphorylates profilaggrin and synthetic phosphofilaggrin substrates in vitro (47,48). It is abundantly expressed in the granular layer of newborn rat epidermis. PP2A expression and activity is markedly decreased in Harlequin ichthyosis (HI), a debilitating human skin disease characterized by severe hyperkeratosis, lack of profilaggrin processing, and abnormal or absent lipid-bearing lamellar granules (49,50). However, no mutations in the PP2A coding region were found in affected individuals, and the reduced PP2A levels appear to be a secondary rather than a primary effect in this disorder. As the catalytic subunit of PP2A removes only about half the labeled phosphate from mouse profilaggrin in vitro, other phosphatases are probably involved in profilaggrin dephosphorylation (35,36).

Table 2 Enzymes Involved in Profilaggrin Modification and Proteolytic Processing in Epidermis[a]

Event	Cell layer/stage of differentiation	Enzyme(s) involved
Phosphorylation	Granular layer (keratohyalin)	Casein kinase II
Dephosphorylation	Granular to cornified cell	PP2A
Proteolysis of polyfilaggrin domain to filaggrin	Granular to cornified cell	Profilaggrin endoproteinase I (PEP1) Calpain I Exoproteinase (trimming of filaggrin)
Cleavage of N-terminus	Granular to cornified cell	Proprotein convertase (PC)/furin Matriptase (MT-SP1)
Incorporation into cornified envelope	Granular to cornified cell	Transglutaminases
Amino acid modification	Middle layers of stratum corneum	Peptidyl arginine deiminase (PAD) Histidase
Proteolysis to free amino acids (NMF)	Middle to upper layers of stratum corneum	Cathepsins B, L, D

[a]This table is a summary of current data regarding enzymes involved in profilaggrin modification and proteolysis. Other enzymes are probably involved, particularly in phosphorylation, dephosphorylation, and conversion of filaggrin to free amino acids (see text for references).

Proteolytic processing of profilaggrin involves multiple proteinases that target either the polyfilaggrin region or the N-terminus (Fig. 4, Table 2). In mouse and rat epidermis, cleavage of the central polyfilaggrin domain is a two-stage process involving two endoproteinases, which are temporally separable in activity, initially yielding intermediates composed of two or more filaggrin domains, and then filaggrin (Fig. 4) (reviewed in Refs. 11–13,26). These processing events have been extensively studied in a rat epidermal cell line, in which the two-stage processing can be separated by manipulating the calcium concentration or by adding various inhibitors (36,51–53). The first stage endoproteinase is a chymotrypsin-like enzyme termed PEP1 (profilaggrin endoproteinase 1), which was partially purified from the rodent epidermis (36). The second stage protease is calcium-dependent. Processing to filaggrin occurs maximally in cultured keratinocytes at elevated calcium levels (5–10 mM) and is inhibited by nifedipine, a calcium channel blocker, and the calpain inhibitor leupeptin (53). In a separate study on cultured human keratinocytes, profilaggrin processing was preceded by the appearance of active μ-calpain, and the processing to filaggrin could be inhibited by calpastatin, a calpain inhibitor (54). The increased expression of calpain in granular cells (55) and confluent keratinocytes (53) suggests that calpain may be the second stage protease. Alternatively, calpain may activate the second stage protease.

Mouse profilaggrin contains two different types of linker sequence, which could provide the substrate for the two endoproteinases that process the polyfilaggrin region (20,51). Rat and human profilaggrin contain only one type of linker sequence between the filaggrin units, invoking a secondary structure and/or differential phosphorylation to explain the two-stage processing of profilaggrin observed in rat keratinocytes (56). Mass spectrometry analyses of human and rat epidermal filaggrin suggest that exopeptidase trimming of filaggrin occurs after processing, creating multiple N-termini (52,57).

Distinct endoproteinases are also involved in cleaving the N-terminus of profilaggrin (Table 2). The human and rodent profilaggrin N-termini are bounded by proprotein convertase (PC) cleavage sites, and both furin and PACE4 (members of the PC family) are able to release the profilaggrin N-terminus in vitro (58). Furin is expressed in the basal and granular layers of epidermis, and while furin and other related enzymes normally reside in the trans-Golgi secretory pathway, there is evidence for a novel cytoplasmic form of furin in keratinocytes that could cleave the profilaggrin N-terminus in vivo (58). Other non-secreted substrates of PC enzymes in keratinocytes include desmosomal cadherins (59), collagen XVII (60), and Notch-1/p300 (61). Recently, a second enzyme, the endoproteinase Matriptase/MT-SP1, has been implicated in the N-terminal processing of mouse profilaggrin. Matriptase-deficient mice lack the two end-products of profilaggrin processing, filaggrin and the N-terminal peptide, and the mutant mice exhibited a severe skin phenotype reminiscent of human HI (62). Matriptase is a member of the type II transmembrane endoproteinase family and plays an important role in the processing of cell surface receptors and adhesion molecules in the epidermis, hair follicle, and thymus (63). At present, it is unclear if matriptase is directly or indirectly involved in the profilaggrin N-terminal processing.

The Multiple Functions of Filaggrin: IFAP, Cornified Envelope Protein, and NMF Components

Filaggrin was originally identified as an IFAP based on its ability to rapidly aggregate keratins and other IFs in vitro to form macrofibrils (26,64,65). Filaggrin also causes a severe disruption of keratin and vimentin filaments when overexpressed in cultured epithelial cells, including keratinocytes (34,35,66). The close association between filaggrin and KIFs in the lower layers of the stratum corneum (67) is consistent with the hypothesis that filaggrin is important for the generation of macrofibrils that form the "keratin pattern," as originally proposed by Brody (68). However, in the filaggrin-deficient skin disease ichthyosis vulgaris (IV), the keratin pattern appears normal even though there is little or no filaggrin present (67,69). Similar findings have been reported in the hard palate of the oral cavity, which has a well-ordered keratin pattern despite an absence of immunologically detectable filaggrin (16). In transgenic mice that overexpress human filaggrin in the suprabasal layers, no KIF disruption was observed, and in fact there was a beneficial effect on barrier repair following an acute disruption (70). These findings suggest that the IFAP function of filaggrin can be substituted by other co-expressed epidermal IFAPs such as Flg-2 (see the section "Filaggrin-2: A Filaggrin-Related Protein") or trichohyalin (see the section "Trichohyalin").

In the middle to upper layers of the stratum corneum, filaggrin is degraded to free amino acids forming a major component of the natural moisturizing factor (NMF). NMF is important for maintaining the normal flexibility and osmolarity of skin, and may have an immune function (reviewed in Refs. 16,71,72). The degradative process begins after the keratins (primarily K1) and filaggrin undergo deimination by peptidyl arginine deiminase (PAD), which converts the peptide-bound arginine to citrulline (73–76). This chemical modification alters the charge of both the keratins and filaggrin, causing them to unfold and disassociate from one another (77,78). Filaggrin is subsequently hydrolyzed to free amino acids by proteinases such as cathepsins L and B in the acidic microenvironment of the stratum corneum (72,79–81). NMF is a complex mixture of low molecular weight humectants that includes pyrrolidone carboxylic acid (PCA), a cyclized derivative of glutamine, urocanic acid, derived from histidine by the action of histidase, and citrulline, produced from arginine by PAD (Table 2). These filaggrin-derived amino acids are highly hydroscopic and can absorb a large amount of water even at relatively low humidities (16,82). Urocanic acid may have several functions in the stratum corneum, including UV photoprotection, immune suppression, and as a scavenger of UV-generated hydroxyl radicals (reviewed in Ref. 16).

What is the evidence that filaggrin is a major precursor of NMF? There is a close correlation between the amino acid compositions of filaggrin and NMF under a number of different conditions (16,82). PCA was shown to be the N-terminal blocking group in human filaggrin, demonstrating that filaggrin is an important source of PCA in cornified cells (57). In the filaggrin-deficient human skin disease IV (44) and the flaky tail mutant mouse (83), the epidermis is dry and scaly, which could be readily explained by the lack of NMF components, including PCA that is normally produced by filaggrin proteolysis. In normal epidermis, the cornified cells appear to control the formation of NMF by regulating the activity of the filaggrin-degrading protease(s) in relation to the relative humidity (84). This filaggrin-degrading enzyme(s) is activated at birth when newborn animals are first exposed to a dry (low humidity) environment. Low humidity conditions cause an elevated expression of profilaggrin and CE proteins, presumably as a response to accelerated trans-epidermal water loss (8).

A small amount of filaggrin escapes complete proteolysis and is incorporated into CEs, where it is usually found crosslinked to loricrin (85–87). Thus, filaggrin has three functions, as 1) an IFAP; 2) a minor constituent of the CE; and 3) a major precursor of the NMF in the stratum corneum. The relative importance of these different functions probably varies between external and internal epithelia, which are subjected to different environmental stresses.

The Profilaggrin N-Terminal Peptide: Structure and Potential Functions

During terminal differentiation, the N-terminal peptide is cleaved from profilaggrin by furin or a related PC enzyme (58,88) and accumulates in the nuclei of epidermal granular and transition cells (25,89). The profilaggrin N-terminal peptide consists of two distinct subdomains, an A domain that contains the highly conserved S100 Ca^{2+}-binding region and a cationic B domain that contains one or more functional nuclear localization signals, which facilitate its nuclear translocation (Fig. 4) (17). Nuclear translocation is probably controlled by the endoproteinase(s) involved in cleaving the profilaggrin N-terminus (PC/furin and Matriptase/MT-SP1, Table 2) and perhaps by its association with the nuclear import machinery, as is the case for S100A11, which also localizes to the nuclei of differentiating keratinocytes (90).

Similar to the canonical or non-fused S100 proteins, the profilaggrin S100 domain contains two EF-hands, a non-conventional ("S100-specific") N-terminal EF-hand of 14 amino acids with a low affinity for Ca^{2+}, and a canonical C-terminal (calmodulin-like) EF-hand of 12 amino acids with a high affinity for Ca^{2+} (Fig. 1). Almost all canonical S100 proteins form homodimers or heterodimers with other co-expressed S100 proteins. Upon Ca^{2+} binding, these S100 dimers undergo a conformational change that exposes hydrophobic faces and allows specific target protein(s) to bind (1,2). Through this mechanism, S100 proteins regulate many intracellular and extracellular processes by altering the intracellular location and/ or activity of its target protein(s) in a Ca^{2+}-dependent manner (for recent examples, see Refs. 90,91). Hence, the S100 domain of profilaggrin could function presumably as both a Ca^{2+}-binding and a protein–protein interaction module like other S100 proteins.

Despite the close structural similarities of the profilaggrin N-terminus (indeed the N-terminus of all fused S100 proteins) with the canonical S100 family, little is known about the function of the fused S100 domain. Profilaggrin is a functional Ca^{2+}-binding protein in vitro, and probably binds Ca^{2+} in vivo, at least in keratohyalin granules (19,92). Calcium binding to the profilaggrin N-terminus in vitro induces a conformational change, which might allow it to bind other keratinocyte proteins (92). To directly address whether the profilaggrin N-terminus is capable of protein–protein interactions in vivo, we have utilized the yeast two-hybrid system developed by Fields and co-workers (93). The results, to date, demonstrate that the complete human profilaggrin N-terminus (A and B domains), expressed as Gal4 fusion proteins in yeast, formed homodimers in vivo (Fig. 5, Table 3). However, the human profilaggrin S100 domain, containing both EF-hands and all four α-helices deemed important for protein dimerization was non-functional in the two-hybrid assay (Fig. 5, Table 3). An altered version of the human profilaggrin N-terminus with mutated EF-hands that disrupt Ca^{2+} binding also formed homodimers in yeast. This result is consistent with studies of other S100 proteins, where Ca^{2+} binding is not required for homodimer formation, although it is necessary for the S100 dimer–target protein interaction (94,95). Analysis of the mouse profilaggrin N-terminus using the yeast two-hybrid assay demonstrated that the A domain could self-associate in vivo, while the complete mouse profilaggrin N-termi-

Histidine⁺ medium   Histidine⁻ medium

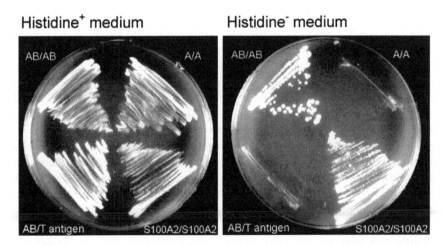

Figure 5 The human profilaggrin N-terminus forms homodimers in the yeast two-hybrid system. Either the complete human profilaggrin N-terminus (A + B domains, 293 amino acids) or only the S100 A domain (98 amino acids) were expressed as fusion proteins with Gal4 DNA binding domain (bait) and Gal4 activation domain (prey). Only the profilaggrin A + B bait and prey and the S100A2 bait and prey combinations can grow on histidine-deficient (His⁻) medium. The S100A2 plasmid was a gift of Dr J.T. Elder (151). For a summary of yeast two-hybrid data, see Table 3.

Table 3 Summary of Yeast Two-Hybrid Data Involving the Profilaggrin N-Terminus[a]

Bait	Prey	Interaction
Human profilaggrin A+B[b]	Human profilaggrin A+B	+
Human profilaggrin A+B (mutated EF-hands)	Human profilaggrin A+B (mutated EF-hands)	+
Human profilaggrin A+B[c]		−
Human profilaggrin A+B[c]	SV40 T-antigen	−
Human profilaggrin A[b]	Human profilaggrin A	−
Human profilaggrin B[b]	Human profilaggrin B	−
Mouse profilaggrin A+B[d]	Mouse profilaggrin A+B	−
Mouse profilaggrin A+B[c]		−
Mouse profilaggrin A[d]	Mouse profilaggrin A	+
p53[e]	SV40 T-antigen	+
p53[c]	Lamin C	−

[a]Baits, e.g., profilaggrin A+B, were cloned into the vector pOBD2 (148,149), encoding Gal 4 DNA binding protein fused to the bait protein. Preys, e.g., profilaggrin A+B, were cloned into the vector pOAD (148,149), encoding Gal4 activation domain fused to the prey protein. Bait and prey plasmids were transformed into yeast strain AH109, and tested for interaction by plating on histidine-deficient media (also lacking leucine and tryptophan) in the presence of 2.5 mM 3-amino-1,2-triazole. If a protein–protein interaction between bait and prey occurs, the His-3 gene will be expressed and the yeast will grow on the histidine-deficient media.
[b]Human profilaggrin A+B encodes a protein of 293 amino acids. Human profilaggrin A (the S100 domain) encodes a protein of 98 residues and includes both EF-hands and all four α-helices. The human B domain consists of residues 99–293.
[c]Negative controls.
[d]Mouse profilaggrin A+B encodes a protein of 283 amino acids. Mouse profilaggrin A is 99 amino acids in length.
[e]Positive control set provided by BD Biosciences/Clontech Inc, in the Matchmaker vector system.

nus was unable to form homodimers (Table 3). Overall, these results demonstrate that the profilaggrin N-terminus can form homodimers in vivo although the function of the downstream B domain may differ between the human and mouse proteins.

Potential functions for the profilaggrin N-terminal peptide include transcriptional regulation, or regulation of calcium-dependent nucleases or proteinases involved in nuclear destruction during the epidermal granular to cornified cell transition. Consistent with this hypothesis, the profilaggrin N-terminal domain co-localizes with the condensed chromatin in transition cells undergoing nuclear breakdown (89). The B domain shows significant homology to several transcription factors, and to other nuclear proteins such as helicases, suggesting that it might associate with the nuclear machinery. However, in vitro studies involving a transient expression in cultured epithelial cells have shown that the N-terminal peptide does not induce the nuclear destruction (17) directly. The identification of target proteins that interact with the profilaggrin N-terminus should provide important insights into its function during the epidermal terminal differentiation.

Regulation of Profilaggrin Gene Expression

Profilaggrin mRNA and protein are first detectable in the epidermal granular layer, implying that profilaggrin gene expression is largely controlled at the transcriptional level (12). This was confirmed by nuclear run-on studies, which demonstrated that nascent profilaggrin transcripts were present in epidermal keratinocytes, but not in Hela cells or dermal fibroblasts that do not express profilaggrin (96).

Similar to the case of many epidermally expressed genes, profilaggrin transcription is regulated by the Activator Protein 1 (AP1) family of transcription factors, principally c-jun, c-fos, and JunD, which are expressed in the suprabasal layers of epidermis [(96,97), and references therein]. An AP1 site is present in the proximal human profilaggrin promoter at −77, which, when abolished, severely abrogated gene transcription in cultured human keratinocytes (96). Other transcription factors implicated in the positive control of profilaggrin transcription include Dlx-3, a member of the distal-less family of Hox factors (98); Jen-1, a novel Ets family member that binds to both the Ets and HMG (high mobility group) recognition sites in DNA (99); and the POU domain protein Oct-1 (97). In the epidermis, Jen-1 and Dlx-3 are expressed in the granular layer as well as other tissues, emphasizing their importance in the regulation of late differentiation marker expression. Transcription factors involved in the repression of profilaggrin transcription include the POU domain proteins Skn1a/i, Oct6, and junB. Many of these transcription factors function by either cooperating with or antagonizing AP1 activity to activate or repress promoter function, respectively. For example, Jen-1 cooperates with AP1 to transactivate the profilaggrin promoter (99), while Skn1a and Oct-6 repress promoter activity in a jun-dependent manner (97). Binding sites for many of the same transcription factors are also present in the mouse profilaggrin promoter (25), as well as in the promoters of other late differentiation genes such as loricrin and caspase-14 (100–102).

Retinoids such as retinoic acid (RA) repress the expression of most epidermal differentiation markers in vitro, either directly through the binding of ligand-bound receptors (usually RAR–RXR heterodimers) to variant retinoic acid response elements (RAREs) or by antagonizing the AP1-mediated transcription (reviewed in Refs. 4,103). The profilaggrin promoter contains a number of RAREs that repress the promoter activity in cultured keratinocytes in the presence of RA and co-expressed receptors (104). These sequences are located in the region ~1 kb 5′ of the transcription start site. The RA receptors did not bind to this region of the profilaggrin promoter, and hence the mechanism by which these sequences function to antagonize transcription in the presence of RA is not understood (104).

Alteration of Profilaggrin/Filaggrin Expression in Disorders of Keratinization

In the normal epidermis, profilaggrin expression and processing to functional filaggrin units is tightly controlled and timed to coincide with terminal differentiation and barrier formation. This tight control over profilaggrin and filaggrin synthesis is altered in a number of disorders of keratinization, including ichthyosis vulgaris (IV) and Harlequin ichthyosis (HI) (105). In the common scaling disorder IV, profilaggrin and filaggrin expression is reduced or absent, and the relative reduction is correlated with the amount of keratohyalin and clinical severity (69). The defect in IV is specific to profilaggrin, as other markers of epidermal differentiation such as keratin 1 or loricrin are expressed normally, both in vivo and in cultured keratinocytes (24,106). In a subset of individuals with moderate to severe IV, the histological absence of a granular layer correlates completely with the absence of profilaggrin-containing KHGs. This form of the disease is referred to as IV with an absent granular layer (IV AGL) (44). While profilaggrin mRNA and protein levels are reduced or absent in IV keratinocytes, profilaggrin transcription measured by nuclear run-on assays is normal (106). These findings suggest that IV cells have a post–transcriptional defect involving profilaggrin. Consistent with this, profilaggrin mRNA from IV keratinocytes has a reduced half-life compared with that of control cells (24). The unstable profilaggrin mRNA in IV keratinocytes could result from a mutation in the profilaggrin gene, affecting mRNA stability and translation. Alternatively, the unstable mRNA could result from mutation in a gene located in the 1q21–22 region that regulates profilaggrin expression (107,108). Flaky tail mutant mice display a similar dry skin phenotype with an absence of normal F-granules and filaggrin in keratinizing epithelia (83). Biochemical data, including the expression of a truncated profilaggrin protein that lacks the normal C-terminal domain, point to a mutation in mouse profilaggrin; however, the mutation has not been identified to date (Presland and Fleckman, unpublished observations). In both IV and the flaky tail mice, it is hypothesized, though not proven, that the dry, flaky skin results from the absence of NMF components derived from filaggrin that bind water in the stratum corneum (see the section "The Multiple Functions of Filaggrin: IFAP, Cornified Envelope Protein, and NMF").

In the most common forms of the debilitating and often fatal disease HI, profilaggrin remains acidic in a thickened, plate-like scale and is not converted to filaggrin. Other features of this disease include abnormal or absent lipid-containing lamellar granules and decreased PP2A activity (49,50,109). A number of candidate genes have been examined and excluded as the cause of HI. The genes currently ruled out include the cysteine proteinase calpain 1, the NF-κB subunit relA/p65, and the cysteine proteinase inhibitor cystatin M/E (110,111). A recent case of HI was reported to have a chromosomal deletion at chromosome 18q, suggesting that one of the affected genes is located in this genomic region (112).

Profilaggrin and filaggrin expression is altered in many other skin disorders, where there is incomplete differentiation and parakeratosis, e.g., psoriasis vulgaris, or hyperkeratosis, e.g., epidermolytic hyperkeratosis (reviewed in Refs. 105,113). However, in most cases the altered expression is the result of a perturbed differentiation program and/or a dysfunctional permeability barrier. Nonetheless, altered profilaggrin expression or processing might impact epidermal function in either a negative or a positive way, for instance, by exacerbating skin diseases resulting from keratin mutations or accelerating barrier recovery (70,114).

Evolutionary Aspects

While profilaggrin has been identified in only mammals, the S100 Ca^{2+}-binding proteins are present in all vertebrates (1), and a gene with a filaggrin-like domain termed MUP-4 involved in intermediate filament association and epithelial cell adhesion is present in the invertebrate *C. elegans* (115). Proteins immunologically related to human filaggrin have been reported in amphibian epidermis, but have not been characterized (116). Keratohyalin-like granules have been reported in the monotreme and marsupial epidermis, suggesting that profilaggrin-like species may be present in other vertebrates (117). This is a reasonable hypothesis given the important and multiple roles of profilaggrin and filaggrin in epidermal terminal differentiation and permeability barrier function. The poor immunologic crossreactivity of profilaggrin/filaggrin antibodies among species will probably necessitate either protein isolation and microsequencing or whole genome sequencing to determine if profilaggrin-like proteins are present in lower vertebrates.

FILAGGRIN-2: A FILAGGRIN-RELATED PROTEIN

Filaggrin-2 (*Flg-2*) was recently identified as a novel profilaggrin-like gene that is expressed in the epidermal granular layer of mouse skin (Listwan, Karunaratne, Zhang and Rothnagel, in prep.). The *Flg-2* gene has a similar structural organization as other fused S100 genes and is located within the EDC on human chromosome 1q21 (Fig.3) and mouse chromosome 3. The Flg-2 protein shows a significant homology to profilaggrin and hornerin, suggesting the existence of a profilaggrin-like fused S100 gene subfamily (Fig. 2A). Mouse *Flg-2* encodes a 251 kDa protein of 2362 amino acids (Table 4).

Structure of Mouse *Flg-2*

The mouse *Flg-2* gene consists of three exons separated by introns of 2.9 and 0.5 kbp in size (Fig. 6; Listwan, Karunaratne, Zhang and Rothnagel, in preparation). The predicted open reading frame begins in exon 2 and contains two S100-like calcium-binding EF-hands at its N-terminus, followed by a unique sequence of 873 residues that is equivalent in position to the B domain of profilaggrin. The first intron interrupts the 5' untranslated region while the second intron separates the two S100-like EF-hands. The calcium-binding region shows a high sequence conservation with human and mouse profilaggrin, and with other S100 proteins (Fig. 1,2B). The Ca^{2+}-binding properties of Flg-2 have been experimentally verified by $^{45}Ca^{2+}$ binding assays (Listwan, Karunaratne, Zhang and Rothnagel, in prep.). This domain is unlikely to bind Zn^{2+} based on structural considerations.

The third and largest exon contains the B domain, which is about four times larger than the corresponding domain in profilaggrin. A potential recognition sequence for a proprotein convertase or furin-like protease is present at the end of the Flg-2 B domain, suggesting that it is processed in a similar manner to profilaggrin (58,88). The B domain is followed by several repetitive units (13 complete repeats in mouse, Fig. 6), which vary in size between 74 and 80 residues. The Flg-2 repeat unit has a basic p*I* and is rich in proline, glycine, serine, glutamine, arginine, and histidine. Each repeat unit is demarcated by a short stretch of hydrophobic residues that may be equivalent to the linker region found between filaggrin repeats, and is involved in the profilaggrin processing by endoproteinases (11,13). A long C-terminal domain of 338 residues follows the repetitive sequence domain of Flg-2.

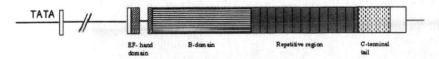

Figure 6 Organization of the mouse *Flg-2* gene. The mouse *Flg-2* gene consists of three exons and two introns. The two EF-hand domains are separated by intron II. The third, largest exon, encodes 2316 amino acids including the B domain, 13 complete repeats, one partial repeat, and the C-terminal tail domain. Open boxes represent 5' and 3' untranslated regions. The EF-hand domains, B domain, repetitive central region, and C-terminal tail domain are indicated.

Flg-2 Shows Epidermal-Specific Expression

Northern blot analysis revealed a single *Flg-2* mRNA species of >12 kb that is abundantly expressed in the epidermis but not in the tongue or other epithelial tissues. This was confirmed by RT–PCR, indicating that *Flg-2* has a more restricted expression pattern than profilaggrin, hornerin, and trichohyalin (Listwan, Karunaratne, Zhang and Rothnagel, in prep.). *Flg-2* transcripts are first detectable at day 15.5 of embryonic mouse development, which precedes the appearance of profilaggrin mRNA by 12–24 hours (118,119). A polyclonal Flg-2 antibody, against a synthetic peptide derived from the repeat region, localized the protein to the granular and cornified layers of the epidermis. Immunofluorescence staining was localized to small keratohyalin granules that could be distinguished from the larger profilaggrin (F or PF) granules (Fig. 7). Western blot analysis using the same antibody revealed both high (>500 kDa) and low (<30 kDa) molecular weight products in epidermal extracts, consistent with the processing of a polypeptide precursor as seen for profilaggrin.

The *Flg-2* Repeats Function as a Keratin-Aggregating Protein

The high percentage of basic amino acids present in the Flg-2 repeats presages an ability to bind to and aggregate keratin filaments. Indeed, when a purified recombinant protein containing Flg-2 repeats was added to keratin filaments extracted from the bovine tongue, there was a marked increase in turbidity, indicative of keratin aggregation (65). This was not seen when the control protein, bovine serum albumin, was added to the keratin filaments (Listwan, Karunaratne, Zhang and Rothnagel, in prep.). Analysis of these mixtures by transmission electron microscopy revealed that the Flg-2 repeat, but not albumin, organized the keratin filaments into almost parallel bundles that were similar to those produced by filaggrin (26,65). These studies indicate that Flg-2 is both a structural and functional homologue of profilaggrin.

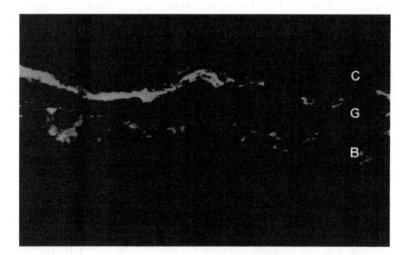

Figure 7 Immunofluorescence microscopy of newborn mouse epidermis with Flg-2 antibody. Sections were double-labeled with antibodies against Flg-2 (red) and K14 (green). Flg-2 is restricted to the granular and cornified layers (red cells). B, basal layer; G, granular layer; C, cornified layer. Total magnification, 300×. (*See color insert.*)

The structural and functional similarity of Flg-2 to profilaggrin suggests a significant degree of redundancy in the fused S100 protein family, although each of these proteins is likely to play unique roles in differentiating keratinocytes.

HORNERIN

Hornerin was first isolated by RNA differential display as a gene that is expressed during mouse embryonic development during epidermal stratification and barrier formation (120). Mouse hornerin encodes a protein of 2496 amino acids consisting of an N-terminal S100 domain followed by a spacer sequence and a series of ~170 amino acid repeat units that were classified into two groups, A and B. The basic organization of the protein and the amino acid composition closely resembles profilaggrin, although there is limited sequence similarity outside of the S100 domain (Fig. 2). Hornerin and profilaggrin exhibit a similar expression pattern during embryonic development, where they are expressed at embryonic day 16. Both genes are also expressed in the differentiating layers of epidermis, tongue, esophagus, and forestomach of the adult mouse, although at quantitatively different levels (119,120). Lastly, hornerin localizes to KHGs like a number of other fused S100 proteins, including profilaggrin, Flg-2, and trichohyalin (119). Hornerin appears to undergo proteolytic processing in vivo, though not to a readily distinguishable product like filaggrin. Whether the hornerin protein or a proteolytic fragment can function as an IFAP is not known. In this respect, immunoreactive hornerin is present in the lower cornified layers where filaggrin localizes.

The human homologue of mouse hornerin is located in the EDC on chromosome 1q21, adjacent to the profilaggrin gene (Fig. 3). The human gene encodes a predicted protein of 2850 residues with a structure broadly similar to that of mouse hornerin (Table 4).

TRICHOHYALIN

Structure and Function of Trichohyalin

Trichohyalin is a fused S100 protein of approximately 200 kDa that consists of an S100 Ca^{2+}-binding domain fused to a highly charged region comprising short tandem repeats that are predicted to form a single-stranded α-helical rod (121–123). It functions as an IFAP in the inner root sheath (IRS) of hair follicles, and as a structural component of CEs in the medulla of coarse hairs and in epithelial tissues subject to severe mechanical stress.

Trichohyalin was originally characterized from sheep and guinea pig hair follicles and is abundantly expressed in the IRS and medulla of hair follicles (124,125). It is also present in lower quantities in most keratinized epithelia, such as the filiform papillae of the tongue, the nail bed, the hard palate, the epithelial cells lining the sheep rumen, and in newborn human foreskin epidermis (30,121,126–128). In IRS cells, trichohyalin, like profilaggrin, initially accumulates in cytoplasmic electron dense granules termed trichohyalin granules. Later, as these cells terminally differentiate, the granules disperse and trichohyalin forms an interfilamentous matrix closely associated with KIFs in differentiated IRS cells (124,129,130). These studies demonstrate that trichohyalin functions as an IFAP in the IRS, which forms a rigid structure that supports the growing hair. In the filiform ridges of the tongue, the nail bed, and some hyperplastic skin conditions, trichohyalin co-localizes with profilaggrin in hybrid granules where the two proteins are often physically separated (30,128,131).

In hair follicles, trichohyalin is chemically modified by two Ca^{2+}-dependent enzymes, namely PAD, which converts the peptide-bound arginine residues to citrulline, and transglutaminases, which form ε-(γ-glutamyl) isodipeptide crosslinks between glutamine and lysine residues. Trichohyalin, like filaggrin, is unfolded by deimination, which allows an association with IRS keratins and crosslinking by transglutaminases (76,78,132). Recent studies demonstrate that transglutaminase 3 is particularly important in the crosslinking process in IRS tissue, which renders the trichohyalin extremely resistant to chemical extraction (132,133). Trichohyalin is crosslinked to multiple proteins in the IRS, including itself, keratins, small proline-rich proteins (SPRRs), involucrin, and other CE proteins, providing a rigid structure that encases the growing hair. A similar structural role for trichohyalin has been demonstrated in the rodent forestomach, where it forms abundant crossbridges with SPRRs, loricrin, and other CE proteins (134). The increased expression of trichohyalin and SPRRs, which are extensively crosslinked by transglutaminases, is thought to enhance the rigidity of the crosslinked CEs, allowing tissues to withstand severe mechanical abrasions.

Trichohyalin is a functional Ca^{2+}-binding protein in vitro (122). The role of the S100 domain of trichohyalin is unknown, but it may play a role in sequestering Ca^{2+} and regulating the calcium-dependent enzymes PAD and transglutaminase that chemically modify trichohyalin in terminally differentiating cells. Trichohyalin does not appear to undergo proteolytic processing prior to its transglutaminase-mediated crosslinking (124).

Trichohyalin and Disease

Trichohyalin exhibits an increased expression in a wide variety of hyperproliferative skin disorders, including lichen planus, EHK, psoriasis, molluscum contagiosa, and some epidermal and hair follicle–derived carcinomas (30,135,136). Expression of the "hyperproliferative" keratins K6 and K16 and loss of filaggrin expression are also common features of hyperplastic skin diseases, which led to the proposal (30) that trichohyalin may associate specifically or preferentially with K6/K16, thereby stabilizing the KIF networks in the absence of filaggrin. Autoantibodies to trichohyalin, as well as to other hair proteins, have been reported in the autoimmune disorder alopecia areata (137). At present, it is not known if trichohyalin (or other hair proteins) represent autoantigens that have a role in the pathogenesis of this complex disease.

REPETIN

Mouse repetin is a protein of 130 kDa (1130 amino acids) that contains an N-terminal S100 domain followed by 49 highly homologous glutamine-rich repeats of 12 amino acids, with an amino acid composition similar to that of involucrin (138). A similar protein is predicted to exist within the human genome but has not yet been characterized (Fig. 3, Table 4). Repetin is expressed in the epidermal granular layer where it localizes in granules, possibly keratohyalin (139). It is also found in tongue and forestomach and is overexpressed in certain mouse tumors, including papillomas and squamous cell carcinomas. Recent biochemical studies demonstrate that repetin, like trichohyalin, is a CE component of mouse IRS tissue (133), confirming that it is a transglutaminase substrate. Repetin is upregulated in both lor-icrin- and kruppel-like factor 4 (Klf4)-null mice that exhibit skin barrier abnormal-ities (139,140). The increased expression of one or more CE proteins in the knockout animals probably reflects a compensatory or "backup" mechanism, which allows the organism to produce a functional epidermal barrier (141). The function of the S100 domain in repetin is unknown, but, like trichohyalin, it may facilitate the transport of repetin to the plasma membrane and crosslinking into CEs.

C1ORF10 (CORNULIN)

C1Orf10 (Chromosome 1 open reading frame 10) was first reported as an esophageal-expressed gene that exhibits reduced or absent expression in human esophageal cancer (142). It is also expressed in a variety of other epithelia, including bladder, scalp, and epidermis, where it localizes to the granular layer (143). It is also induced in vitro in response to heat shock (144). Human cornulin encodes a protein of 495 amino acids (57 kDa on SDS protein gels), making it the smallest known member of the fused S100 family (Table 4). It contains an N-terminal S100 Ca^{2+}-binding domain followed by two consecutive repeats of 60 amino acids (142,143). It has a similar genomic organization to other fused S100 genes and localizes to the human EDC at chromosome 1q21 (Fig. 3).

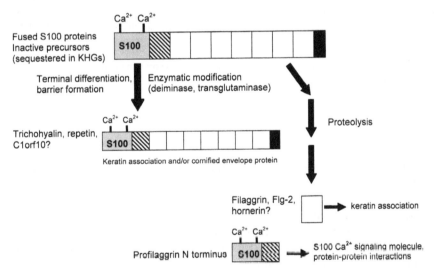

Figure 8 Model summarizing the structural features and functions of the fused S100 proteins. Most fused S100 proteins are synthesized as inactive precursors, and are sequestered in storage granules, e.g., KHGs or trichohyalin granules. During terminal differentiation and formation of the epithelial barrier, they undergo post-translational modification to generate their biologically active forms that function as IFAPs in keratin association, as CE components, or in other pathways. Some proteins are active as intact proteins, after modification by PAD and/or transglutaminases, while others require specific proteolysis. The proteolysis of filaggrin to hygroscopic amino acids and their role in water retention in the stratum corneum are not shown. *Abbreviations*: CE, cornified envelope; IFAP, intermediate fila-ment–associated protein; KHGs, keratohyalin granules; PAD, peptidyl arginine deiminase.

Table 4 Biochemical Properties and Possible Functions of the Fused S100 Protein Family

Gene/protein	Predicted mol. wt.[a]	Tissues expressed[b]	Function(s)[b]
Human profilaggrin	435 kDa (4061)	Keratinizing epithelia, especially epidermis, tongue, oral mucosa, forestomach (mouse)	IFAP; CE protein; NMF component; calcium-regulated nuclear signaling molecule[c]
Flg-2	251 kDa (2362)[d] 248 kDa (2391)[e]	Keratinizing epithelia, especially epidermis	IFAP
Hornerin	248 kDa (2496)[d] 282 kDa (2850)[e]	Keratinizing epithelia, especially epidermis, forestomach (mouse)	Unknown
Human trichohyalin	247 kDa (1898)	Hair follicle IRS and medulla, mouse forestomach; limited expression in other keratinizing epithelia	CE protein; IFAP (IRS tissue, hair follicle)
Repetin	130 kDa (1130)[d] 91 kDa (784)[e]	Keratinizing epithelia, especially tongue and forestomach	CE protein
Human C1orf10 (cornulin)	53.5 kDa (495)	Esophagus, epidermis, bladder	Unknown

[a]Molecular weights were based on predicted amino acid sequences derived from the gene sequences of: human profilaggrin (assembled from Genbank accession number AL356504); mouse Flg-2, Listwan, Karunaratne, Zhang and Rothnagel, in preparation; mouse hornerin, accession number AAK15791; human hornerin, accession number XP_352327; human trichohyalin, accession number NP_009044; mouse repetin, accession number X99251; human repetin, accession number AY219924; and human C1orf10, accession number NP_057274. Number in brackets is the number of amino acids in the predicted protein sequence. Molecular weights were predicted from the protein sequences using the program Compute pI/Mw (us.expasy.org).
[b]See text for references.
[c]Includes functions of both filaggrin and processed N-terminal peptide.
[d]Mouse.
[e]Human.

In addition to C1orf10 (cornulin), a number of canonical S100 genes that regulate cell proliferation display an altered expression or function in human cancers (3,145). These include S100A2, S100A4, and C1orf10, which along with HSP70 and transglutaminase 3, are induced in esophageal epithelium in vitro in response to heat shock, suggesting that C1orf10 is a stress-regulated gene (144). Further studies are required to determine its function(s) in normal epithelial differentiation and its possible role in the stress response.

SUMMARY AND CONCLUDING REMARKS

In this chapter, we have summarized current knowledge of the fused S100 family, a family of high molecular weight Ca^{2+}-binding proteins that function in epithelial differentiation and keratinization. They vary in molecular weight from 54 to > 400 kDa and are expressed in a variety of external and internal stratified epithelia, as well as the hair follicle (Table 4). They function primarily as structural components of epithelial tissues, either as CE components, or as IFAPs that aggregate the keratin IFs into macrofibrils, enabling them to survive the terminal differentiation process and form the cytoskeleton of cornified cells.

While the fused S100 genes share only a limited amino acid homology outside of the S100 domain, they have a number of common features, which are summarized in Figure 8. Most, if not all, of these proteins are expressed in stratified epithelia as inactive precursors that are functionally sequestered, e.g., in keratohyalin granules. They are then activated by post-translational modification, including specific proteolysis, deimination, and/or transglutaminase crosslinking (Fig. 8). The S100 domain may be important for sequestering these proteins in an inactive, insoluble form prior to the formation of the stratum corneum. The S100 domain might also regulate the activity of the calcium-dependent enzymes that modify profilaggrin and other fused S100 proteins (Table 2). The Ca^{2+}-binding domain of the fused S100 proteins may also be necessary for protein–protein interactions, or their transport and assembly into the CE during keratinocyte differentiation (146,147).

While a number of fused S100 proteins, or their proteolytic products, are involved in protein–protein interactions (e.g., filaggrin-keratin, trichohyalin-keratin, Flg-2 repeat unit-keratin), only the profilaggrin N-terminus has been shown to form homodimers in a manner analogous to the canonical S100 proteins (Fig. 8). It remains to be seen if the profilaggrin S100 domain, or other family members, is involved in Ca^{2+}-dependent or -independent protein–protein interactions. Future studies on the fused S100 gene family should provide intriguing insights into how calcium and calcium-binding proteins regulate the epidermal differentiation and the formation of the epidermal barrier.

ACKNOWLEDGMENTS

We thank Dr. Beverly Dale for a critical reading of the manuscript. The work in the authors' laboratories described in this review was supported by grants R01 AR49183 and R29 AR45276 from the National Institutes of Health (to R. B. Presland), and by a Wellcome Trust Senior Research Fellowship in Medical Research and the NHMRC (to J. A. Rothnagel). We thank Pawel Listwan, Seetha Karunaratne, and Dana Zhang (University of Queensland) for allowing us to discuss the Flg-2 data.

NOTE ADDED IN PROOF

Since this manuscript was submitted, Contzler et al (2005) have reported an analysis of the expression pattern and intracellular localization of human cornulin (C1orf10) (R Contzler, B Favre, M Huber, D Hohl. Cornulin, a new memer of the "fused gene" family, is expressed during epidermal differentiation. J Invest Dermatol 2005; 124:990-997). Human cornulin was shown to be expressed in the upper layers of stratified epithelia including the epidermis and to be a functional calcium-binding protein. A companion paper from the same group reported the sequence analysis and characterization of human repetin (M Huber, G Siegenthaler, N Mirancea, I Marenholz, D Nizetic, D Breitkreutz, D Mischke, D Hohl. Isolation and characterization of human repetin, a member of the fused gene family of the epidermal differentiation complex. J Invest Dermatol 2005; 124:998-1007). They demonstrated that

human repetin is also a functional calcium-binding protein and is localized to keratohyalin granules in human epidermis.

Finally, Kelsell et al. (2005) identified mutations in the ABCA12 gene is a number of Harlequin ichthyosis patients (DP Kelsell, EE Norgett, H Unsworth, MT
Tech, et al. Mutations in ABCA12 underlie the severe congenital skin disease Harlequin Ichthyosis. Am. J. Hum. Gen. 2005; 76:794-803). ABCA12 is a member of the
ABC family of transmembrane proteins that transport various substances across cell
membranes. The function of ABCA12 is unknown, but the authors suggested that
ABCA12 may play a role in lipid transport and metabolism in the epidermis and
other epithelia that are affected in this disorder.

REFERENCES

1. Donato R. S100: a multigenic family of calcium-modulated proteins of the EF-hand type with intracellular and extracellular functional roles. Int J Biochem Cell Biol 2001; 33:637–668.
2. Donato R. Intracellular and extracellular roles of S100 proteins. Microsc Res Tech 2003; 60:540–551.
3. Heizmann CW, Fritz G, Schafer BW. S100 proteins: structure, functions and pathology. Front Biosci 2002; 7:d1356–d1368.
4. Presland RB, Dale BA. Epithelial structural proteins of the skin and oral cavity: function in health and disease. Crit Rev Oral Biol Med 2000; 11:383–408.
5. Kalinin AE, Kajava AV, Steinert PM. Epithelial barrier function: assembly and structural features of the cornified cell envelope. Bioessays 2002; 24:789–800.
6. Menon GK, Elias PM. Ultrastructural localization of calcium in psoriatic and normal human epidermis. Arch Dermatol 1991; 127:57–63.
7. Menon GK, Elias PM, Feingold KR. Integrity of the permeability barrier is crucial for maintenance of the epidermal calcium gradient. Br J Dermatol 1994; 130:139–147.
8. Elias PM, Ahn SK, Denda M, Brown BE, Crumrine D, Kimutai LK, Komuves L, Lee SH, Feingold KR. Modulations in epidermal calcium regulate the expression of differentiation-specific markers. J Invest Dermatol 2002; 119:1128–1136.
9. Ridinger K, Ilg EC, Niggli FK, Heizmann CW, Schafer BW. Clustered organization of S100 genes in human and mouse. Biochim Biophys Acta 1998; 1448:254–263.
10. Waterston RH, Lindblad-Toh K, Birney E, Rogers J, Abril JF, Agarwal P, Agarwala R, Ainscough R, Alexandersson M An P, Antonarakis SE, et al. Initial sequencing and comparative analysis of the mouse genome. Nature 2002; 420:520–562.
11. Resing KA, Dale BA. Proteins of keratohyalin. In: Goldsmith LA, ed. Physiology, Biochemistry, and Molecular Biology of the Skin. New York: Oxford University Press, 1991:148–167.
12. Dale BA, Presland RB, Fleckman P, Kam E, Resing KA. Phenotypic expression and processing of filaggrin in epidermal differentiation. In: Darmon M, Blumenberg M, eds. Molecular Biology of the Skin: The Keratinocyte. San Diego: Academic Press, 1993:79–106.
13. Dale BA, Resing KA, Presland RB. Keratohyalin granule proteins. In: Leigh IM, Lane EB, Watt FM, eds. The Keratinocyte Handbook. Cambridge: Cambridge University Press, 1994:323–350.
14. Dale BA, Presland RB. Filaggrins. In: Kreis T, Vale R, eds. Guidebook to the Cytoskeletal and Motor Proteins. New York: Oxford University Press, 1999:333–337.
15. Rawlings AV, Harding CR. Moisturization and skin barrier function. Dermatol Ther 2004; 17(suppl 1):43–48.
16. Harding CR, Scott IR. Stratum corneum moisturizing factors. In: Leyden JJ, Rawlings AV, eds. Skin Moisturization. Weimar: Culinary and Hospitality Industry Publication Services, pp. 61–80.

17. Pearton DJ, Dale BA, Presland RB. Functional analysis of the profilaggrin N-terminal peptide: identification of domains that regulate nuclear and cytoplasmic distribution. J Invest Dermatol 2002; 119;661–669.
18. Presland RB, Haydock PV, Fleckman P, Nirunsuksiri W, Dale BA. Characterization of the human epidermal profilaggrin gene. Genomic organization and identification of an S-100-like calcium binding domain at the amino terminus. J Biol Chem 1992; 267: 23772–23781.
19. Markova NG, Marekov LN, Chipev CC, Gan SQ, Idler WW, Steinert PM. Profilaggrin is a major epidermal calcium-binding protein. Mol Cell Biol 1993; 13:613–625.
20. Rothnagel JA, Steinert PM. The structure of the gene for mouse filaggrin and a comparison of the repeating units. J Biol Chem 1990; 265:1862–1865.
21. Haydock PV, Dale BA. Filaggrin, an intermediate filament-associated protein: structural and functional implications from the sequence of a cDNA from rat. DNA Cell Biol 1990; 9:251–261.
22. Rothnagel JA, Mehrel T, Idler WW, Roop DR, Steinert PM. The gene for mouse epidermal filaggrin precursor. Its partial characterization, expression, and sequence of a repeating filaggrin unit. J Biol Chem 1987; 262:15643–15648.
23. Gan SQ, McBride OW, Idler WW, Markova N, Steinert PM. Organization, structure, and polymorphisms of the human profilaggrin gene. Biochemistry 1990; 29:9432–9440.
24. Nirunsuksiri W, Zhang SH, Fleckman P. Reduced stability and bi-allelic, coequal expression of profilaggrin mRNA in keratinocytes cultured from subjects with ichthyosis vulgaris. J Invest Dermatol 1998; 110:854–861.
25. Zhang D, Karunaratne S, Kessler M, Mahony D, Rothnagel JA. Characterization of mouse profilaggrin: evidence for nuclear engulfment and translocation of the profilaggrin B-domain during epidermal differentiation. J Invest Dermatol 2002; 119: 905–912.
26. Dale BA, Resing KA, Lonsdale-Eccles JD. Filaggrin: a keratin filament associated protein. Ann NY Acad Sci 1985; 455:330–342.
27. Mack JW, Steven AC, Steinert PM. The mechanism of interaction of filaggrin with intermediate filaments. The ionic zipper hypothesis. J Mol Biol 1993; 232:50–66.
28. Thulin CD, Taylor JA, Walsh KA. Microheterogeneity of human filaggrin: analysis of a complex peptide mixture using mass spectrometry. Protein Sci 1996; 5:1157–1164.
29. Dale BA, Gown AM, Fleckman P, Kimball JR, Resing KA. Characterization of two monoclonal antibodies to human epidermal keratohyalin: reactivity with filaggrin and related proteins. J Invest Dermatol 1987; 88:306–313.
30. Manabe M, O'Guin WM. Existence of trichohyalin-keratohyalin hybrid granules: co-localization of two major intermediate filament-associated proteins in non-follicular epithelia. Differentiation 1994; 58:65–75.
31. Resing KA, Dale BA, Walsh KA. Multiple copies of phosphorylated filaggrin in epidermal profilaggrin demonstrated by analysis of tryptic peptides. Biochemistry 1985; 24:4167–4175.
32. Lonsdale-Eccles JD, Teller DC, Dale BA. Characterization of a phosphorylated form of the intermediate filament-aggregating protein filaggrin. Biochemistry 1982; 21:5940–5948.
33. Harding CR, Scott IR. Histidine-rich proteins (filaggrins): structural and functional heterogeneity during epidermal differentiation. J Mol Biol 1983; 170:651–673.
34. Dale BA, Presland RB, Lewis SP, Underwood RA, Fleckman P. Transient expression of epidermal filaggrin in cultured cells causes collapse of intermediate filament networks with alteration of cell shape and nuclear integrity. J Invest Dermatol 1997; 108:179–187.
35. Kuechle MK, Thulin CD, Presland RB, Dale BA. Profilaggrin requires both linker and filaggrin peptide sequences to form granules: implications for profilaggrin processing in vivo. J Invest Dermatol 1999; 112:843–852.
36. Resing KA, Thulin C, Whiting K, al-Alawi N, Mostad S. Characterization of profilaggrin endoproteinase 1. A regulated cytoplasmic endoproteinase of epidermis. J Biol Chem 1995; 270:28193–28198.

37. Steven AC, Bisher ME, Roop DR, Steinert PM. Biosynthetic pathways of filaggrin and loricrin—two major proteins expressed by terminally differentiated epidermal keratinocytes. J Struct Biol 1990; 104:150–162.

38. Ball RD, Walker GK, Bernstein IA. Histidine-rich proteins as molecular markers of epidermal differentiation. J Biol Chem 1978; 253:5861–5868.

39. Dale BA. Purification and characterization of a basic protein from the stratum corneum of mammalian epidermis. Biochim Biophys Acta 1977; 491:193–204.

40. Dale BA, Vadlamudi B, DeLap LW, Bernstein IA. Similarities between stratum corneum basic protein and histidine-rich protein II from newborn rat epidermis. Biochim Biophys Acta 1981; 668:98–106.

41. Fukuyama K, Epstein WL. Sulfur-containing proteins and epidermal keratinization. J Cell Biol 1969; 40:830–838.

42. Fukuyama K, Epstein WL. Heterogenous proteins in keratohyaline granules studied by quantitative autoradiography. J Invest Dermatol 1975; 65:113–117.

43. Fukuyama K, Epstein WL. A comparative autoradiographic study of keratogyalin granules containing cystine and histidine. J Ultrastruct Res 1975; 51:314–325.

44. Fleckman P, Brumbaugh S. Absence of the granular layer and keratohyalin define a morphologically distinct subset of individuals with ichthyosis vulgaris. Exp Dermatol 2002; 11:327–336.

45. Pfeiffer S, Vielhaber G, Vietzke JP, Wittern KP, Hintze U, Wepf R. High-pressure freezing provides new information on human epidermis: simultaneous protein antigen and lamellar lipid structure preservation. Study on human epidermis by cryoimmobilization. J Invest Dermatol 2000; 114:1030–1038.

46. Nemes Z, Steinert PM. Bricks and mortar of the epidermal barrier. Exp Mol Med 1999; 31:5–19.

47. Haugen-Scofield J, Resing KA, Dale BA. Characterization of an epidermal phosphatase specific for filaggrin phosphorylated by casein kinase II. J Invest Dermatol 1988; 91:553–559.

48. Kam E, Resing KA, Lim SK, Dale BA. Identification of rat epidermal profilaggrin phosphatase as a member of the protein phosphatase 2A family. J Cell Sci 1993; 106(Pt 1):219–226.

49. Dale BA, Kam E. Harlequin ichthyosis. Variability in expression and hypothesis for disease mechanism. Arch Dermatol 1993; 129:1471–1477.

50. Kam E, Nirunsuksiri W, Hager B, Fleckman P, Dale BA. Protein phosphatase activity in human keratinocytes cultured from normal epidermis and epidermis from patients with harlequin ichthyosis. Br J Dermatol 1997; 137:874–882.

51. Resing KA, Walsh KA, Haugen-Scofield J, Dale BA. Identification of proteolytic cleavage sites in the conversion of profilaggrin to filaggrin in mammalian epidermis. J Biol Chem 1989; 264:1837–1845.

52. Resing KA, Johnson RS, Walsh KA. Characterization of protease processing sites during conversion of rat profilaggrin to filaggrin. Biochemistry 1993; 32:10036–10045.

53. Resing KA, al-Alawi N, Blomquist C, Fleckman P, Dale BA. Independent regulation of two cytoplasmic processing stages of the intermediate filament-associated protein filaggrin and role of Ca^{2+} in the second stage. J Biol Chem 1993; 268:25139–25145.

54. Yamazaki M, Ishidoh K, Suga Y, Saido TC, Kawashima S, Suzuki K, Kominami E, Ogawa H. Cytoplasmic processing of human profilaggrin by active mu-calpain. Biochem Biophys Res Commun 1997; 235:652–656.

55. Miyachi Y, Yoshimura N, Suzuki S, Hamakubo T, Kannagi R, Imamura S, Murachi T. Biochemical demonstration and immunohistochemical localization of calpain in human skin. J Invest Dermatol 1986; 86:346–349.

56. Resing KA, Johnson RS, Walsh KA. Mass spectrometric analysis of 21 phosphorylation sites in the internal repeat of rat profilaggrin, precursor of an intermediate filament associated protein. Biochemistry 1995; 34:9477–9487.

57. Thulin CD, Walsh KA. Identification of the amino terminus of human filaggrin using differential LC/MS techniques: implications for profilaggrin processing. Biochemistry 1995; 34:8687–8692.

58. Pearton DJ, Nirunsuksiri W, Rehemtulla A, Lewis SP, Presland RB, Dale BA. Proprotein convertase expression and localization in epidermis: evidence for multiple roles and substrates. Exp Dermatol 2001; 10:193–203.

59. Posthaus H, Dubois CM, Muller E. Novel insights into cadherin processing by subtilisin-like convertases. FEBS Lett 2003; 536:203–208.

60. Schacke H, Schumann H, Hammami-Hauasli N, Raghunath M, Bruckner-Tuderman L. Two forms of collagen XVII in keratinocytes. A full-length transmembrane protein and a soluble ectodomain. J Biol Chem 1998; 273:25937–25943.

61. Logeat F, Bessia C, Brou C, LeBail O, Jarriault S, Seidah NG, Israel A. The Notch1 receptor is cleaved constitutively by a furin-like convertase. Proc Natl Acad Sci USA 1998; 95:8108–8112.

62. List K, Szabo R, Wertz PW, Segre J, Haudenschild CC, Kim SY, Bugge TH. Loss of proteolytically processed filaggrin caused by epidermal deletion of Matriptase/MT-SP1. J Cell Biol 2003; 163:901–910.

63. List K, Haudenschild CC, Szabo R, Chen W, Wahl SM, Swaim W, Engelholm LH, Behrendt N, Bugge TH. Matriptase/MT-SP1 is required for postnatal survival, epidermal barrier function, hair follicle development, and thymic homeostasis. Oncogene 2002; 21:3765–3779.

64. Dale BA, Holbrook KA, Steinert PM. Assembly of stratum corneum basic protein and keratin filaments in macrofibrils. Nature 1978; 276:729–731.

65. Steinert PM, Cantieri JS, Teller DC, Lonsdale-Eccles JD, Dale BA. Characterization of a class of cationic proteins that specifically interact with intermediate filaments. Proc Natl Acad Sci USA 1981; 78:4097–4101.

66. Presland RB, Kuechle MK, Lewis SP, Fleckman P, Dale BA. Regulated expression of human filaggrin in keratinocytes results in cytoskeletal disruption, loss of cell–cell adhesion, and cell cycle arrest. Exp Cell Res 2001; 270:199–213.

67. Manabe M, Sanchez M, Sun TT, Dale BA. Interaction of filaggrin with keratin filaments during advanced stages of normal human epidermal differentiation and in ichthyosis vulgaris. Differentiation 1991; 48:43–50.

68. Brody I. An ultrastructural study on the role of the keratohyalin granules in the keratinization process. J Ultrastruct Res 1959; 3:84–104.

69. Sybert VP, Dale BA, Holbrook KA. Ichthyosis vulgaris: identification of a defect in synthesis of filaggrin correlated with an absence of keratohyaline granules. J Invest Dermatol 1985; 84:191–194.

70. Presland RB, Coulombe PA, Eckert RL, Mao-Qiang M, Feingold KR, Elias PM. Barrier function in transgenic mice overexpressing K16, involucrin, and filaggrin in the suprabasal epidermis. J Invest Dermatol 2004; 123:603–606.

71. Rawlings AV, Scott IR, Harding CR, Bowser PA. Stratum corneum moisturization at the molecular level. J Invest Dermatol 1994; 103:731–741.

72. Elias PM. The epidermal permeability barrier: from the early days at Harvard to emerging concepts. J Invest Dermatol 2004; 122:xxxvi–xxxix.

73. Senshu T, Akiyama K, Kan S, Asaga H, Ishigami A, Manabe M. Detection of deiminated proteins in rat skin: probing with a monospecific antibody after modification of citrulline residues. J Invest Dermatol 1995; 105:163–169.

74. Senshu T, Kan S, Ogawa H, Manabe M, Asaga H. Preferential deimination of keratin K1 and filaggrin during the terminal differentiation of human epidermis. Biochem Biophys Res Commun 1996; 225:712–719.

75. Kanno T, Kawada A, Yamanouchi J, Yosida-Noro C, Yoshiki A, Shiraiwa M, Kusakabe M, Manabe M, Tezuka T, Takahara H. Human peptidylarginine deiminase type III: molecular cloning and nucleotide sequence of the cDNA, properties of the

recombinant enzyme, and immunohistochemical localization in human skin. J Invest Dermatol 2000; 115:813–823.

76. Rogers G, Winter B, McLaughlan C, Powell B, Nesci T. Peptidylarginine deiminase of the hair follicle: characterization, localization, and function in keratinizing tissues. J Invest Dermatol 1997; 108:700–707.

77. Ishida-Yamamoto A, Senshu T, Eady RA, Takahashi H, Shimizu H, Akiyama M, Iizuka H. Sequential reorganization of cornified cell keratin filaments involving filaggrin-mediated compaction and keratin 1 deimination. J Invest Dermatol 2002; 118:282–287.

78. Tarcsa E, Marekov LN, Mei G, Melino G, Lee SC, Steinert PM. Protein unfolding by peptidylarginine deiminase. Substrate specificity and structural relationships of the natural substrates trichohyalin and filaggrin. J Biol Chem 1996; 271:30709–30716.

79. Kawada A, Hara K, Hiruma M, Noguchi H, Ishibashi A. Rat epidermal cathepsin L-like proteinase: purification and some hydrolytic properties toward filaggrin and synthetic substrates. J Biochem (Tokyo) 1995; 118:332–337.

80. Kawada A, Hara K, Morimoto K, Hiruma M, Ishibashi A. Rat epidermal cathepsin B: purification and characterization of proteolytic properties toward filaggrin and synthetic substrates. Int J Biochem Cell Biol 1995; 27:175–183.

81. Benavides F, Starost MF, Flores M, Gimenez-Conti IB, Guenet JL, Conti CJ. Impaired hair follicle morphogenesis and cycling with abnormal epidermal differentiation in nackt mice, a cathepsin L-deficient mutation. Am J Pathol 2002; 161:693–703.

82. Scott IR, Harding CR, Barrett JG. Histidine-rich protein of the keratohyalin granules. Source of the free amino acids, urocanic acid and pyrrolidone carboxylic acid in the stratum corneum. Biochim Biophys Acta 1982; 719:110–117.

83. Presland RB, Boggess D, Lewis SP, Hull C, Fleckman P, Sundberg JP. Loss of normal profilaggrin and filaggrin in flaky tail (ft/ft) mice: an animal model for the filaggrin-deficient skin disease ichthyosis vulgaris. J Invest Dermatol 2000; 115:1072–1081.

84. Scott IR, Harding CR. Filaggrin breakdown to water binding compounds during development of the rat stratum corneum is controlled by the water activity of the environment. Dev Biol 1986; 115:84–92.

85. Steinert PM, Marekov LN. The proteins elafin, filaggrin, keratin intermediate filaments, loricrin, and small proline-rich proteins 1 and 2 are isodipeptide cross-linked components of the human epidermal cornified cell envelope. J Biol Chem 1995; 270: 17702–17711.

86. Richards S, Scott IR, Harding CR, Liddell JE, Powell GM, Curtis CG. Evidence for filaggrin as a component of the cell envelope of the newborn rat. Biochem J 1988; 253:153–160.

87. Simon M, Haftek M, Sebbag M, Montezin M, Girbal-Neuhauser E, Schmitt D, Serre G. Evidence that filaggrin is a component of cornified cell envelopes in human plantar epidermis. Biochem J 1996; 317(Pt 1):173–177.

88. Presland RB, Kimball JR, Kautsky MB, Lewis SP, Lo CY, Dale BA. Evidence for specific proteolytic cleavage of the N-terminal domain of human profilaggrin during epidermal differentiation. J Invest Dermatol 1997; 108:170–178.

89. Ishida-Yamamoto A, Takahashi H, Presland RB, Dale BA, Iizuka H. Translocation of profilaggrin N-terminal domain into keratinocyte nuclei with fragmented DNA in normal human skin and loricrin keratoderma. Lab Invest 1998; 78:1245–1253.

90. Sakaguchi M, Miyazaki M, Takaishi M, Sakaguchi Y, Makino E, Kataoka N, Yamada H, Namba M, Huh NH. S100C/A11 is a key mediator of Ca^{2+}-induced growth inhibition of human epidermal keratinocytes. J Cell Biol 2003; 163:825–835.

91. Benaud C, Gentil BJ, Assard N, Court M, Garin J, Delphin C, Baudier J. AHNAK interaction with the annexin 2/S100A10 complex regulates cell membrane cytoarchitecture. J Cell Biol 2004; 164:133–144.

92. Presland RB, Bassuk JA, Kimball JR, Dale BA. Characterization of two distinct calcium-binding sites in the amino-terminus of human profilaggrin. J Invest Dermatol 1995; 104:218–223.

93. Bartel PL, Fields S. The Yeast Two-hybrid System. New York, NY: Oxford University Press, 1997.
94. Deloulme JC, Gentil BJ, Baudier J. Monitoring of S100 homodimerization and hetero-dimeric interactions by the yeast two-hybrid system. Microsc Res Tech 2003; 60:560–568.
95. Kim EJ, Helfman DM. Characterization of the metastasis-associated protein, S100A4. Roles of calcium binding and dimerization in cellular localization and interaction with myosin. J Biol Chem 2003; 278:30063–30073.
96. Jang SI, Steinert PM, Markova NG. Activator protein 1 activity is involved in the regulation of the cell type-specific expression from the proximal promoter of the human profilaggrin gene. J Biol Chem 1996; 271:24105–24114.
97. Jang SI, Karaman-Jurukovska N, Morasso MI, Steinert PM, Markova NG. Complex interactions between epidermal POU domain and activator protein 1 transcription factors regulate the expression of the profilaggrin gene in normal human epidermal keratinocytes. J Biol Chem 2000; 275:15295–15304.
98. Morasso MI, Markova NG, Sargent TD. Regulation of epidermal differentiation by a Distal-less homeodomain gene. J Cell Biol 1996; 135:1879–1887.
99. Andreoli JM, Jang SI, Chung E, Coticchia CM, Steinert PM, Markova NG. The expression of a novel, epithelium-specific Ets transcription factor is restricted to the most differentiated layers in the epidermis. Nucleic Acids Res 1997; 25:4287–4295.
100. Jang SI, Steinert PM. Loricrin expression in cultured human keratinocytes is controlled by a complex interplay between transcription factors of the Sp1, CREB, AP1, and AP2 families. J Biol Chem 2002; 277:42268–42279.
101. DiSepio D, Bickenbach JR, Longley MA, Bundman DS, Rothnagel JA, Roop DR. Characterization of loricrin regulation in vitro and in transgenic mice. Differentiation 1999; 64:225–235.
102. Eckhart L, Ban J, Fischer H, Tschachler E. Caspase-14: analysis of gene structure and mRNA expression during keratinocyte differentiation. Biochem Biophys Res Commun 2000; 277:655–659.
103. Fisher C, Blumenberg M, Tomic-Canic M. Retinoid receptors and keratinocytes. Crit Rev Oral Biol Med 1995; 6:284–301.
104. Presland RB, Tomic-Canic M, Lewis SP, Dale BA. Regulation of human profilaggrin promoter activity in cultured epithelial cells by retinoic acid and glucocorticoids. J Dermatol Sci 2001; 27:192–205.
105. Fleckman P, Dale BA. Structural protein expression in the ichthyoses. In: Shroot B, Schaefer H, eds. Pharmacology and the Skin. Basel: Karger, 1993:1–15.
106. Nirunsuksiri W, Presland RB, Brumbaugh SG, Dale BA, Fleckman P. Decreased profilaggrin expression in ichthyosis vulgaris is a result of selectively impaired post-transcriptional control. J Biol Chem 1995; 270:871–876.
107. Compton JG, DiGiovanna JJ, Johnston KA, Fleckman P, Bale SJ. Mapping of the associated phenotype of an absent granular layer in ichthyosis vulgaris to the epidermal differentiation complex on chromosome 1. Exp Dermatol 2002; 11:518–526.
108. Zhong W, Cui B, Zhang Y, Jiang H, Wei S, Bu L, Zhao G, Hu L, Kong X. Linkage analysis suggests a locus of ichthyosis vulgaris on 1q22. J Hum Genet 2003; 48:390–392.
109. Dale BA, Holbrook KA, Fleckman P, Kimball JR, Brumbaugh S, Sybert VP. Hetero-geneity in harlequin ichthyosis, an inborn error of epidermal keratinization: variable morphology and structural protein expression and a defect in lamellar granules. J Invest Dermatol 1990; 94:6–18.
110. Dunnwald M, Zuberi AR, Stephens K, Le R, Sundberg JP, Fleckman P, Dale BA. The ichq mutant mouse, a model for the human skin disorder harlequin ichthyosis: mapping, keratinocyte culture, and consideration of candidate genes involved in epidermal growth regulation. Exp Dermatol 2003; 12:245–254.
111. Zeeuwen PL, Dale BA, de Jongh GJ, van Vlijmen-Willems IM, Fleckman P, Kimball JR, Stephens K, Schalkwijk J. The human cystatin M/E gene (CST6): exclusion candidate gene for harlequin ichthyosis. J Invest Dermatol 2003; 121:65–68.

112. Stewart H, Smith PT, Gaunt L, Moore L, Tarpey P, Andrew S, Dady I, Rifkin R, Clayton-Smith J. De novo deletion of chromosome 18q in a baby with harlequin ichthyosis. Am J Med Genet 2001; 102:342–345.

113. Ishida-Yamamoto A, Takahashi H, Iizuka H. Immunoelectron microscopy links molecules and morphology in the studies of keratinization. Eur J Dermatol 2000; 10:429–435.

114. Ishida-Yamamoto A, Eady RA, Underwood RA, Dale BA, Holbrook KA. Filaggrin expression in epidermolytic ichthyosis (epidermolytic hyperkeratosis). Br J Dermatol 1994; 131:767–779.

115. Hong L, Elbl T, Ward J, Franzini-Armstrong C, Rybicka KK, Gatewood BK, Baillie DL, Bucher EA. MUP-4 is a novel transmembrane protein with functions in epithelial cell adhesion in *Caenorhabditis elegans*. J Cell Biol 2001; 154:403–414.

116. Alibardi L. Adaptation to the land: the skin of reptiles in comparison to that of amphibians and endotherm amniotes. J Exp Zoolog Part B Mol Dev Evol 2002; 298:12–41.

117. Alibardi L, Maderson PF. Distribution of keratin and associated proteins in the epidermis of monotreme, marsupial, and placental mammals. J Morphol 2003; 258:49–66.

118. Bickenbach JR, Greer JM, Bundman DS, Rothnagel JA, Roop DR. Loricrin expression is coordinated with other epidermal proteins and the appearance of lipid lamellar granules in development. J Invest Dermatol 1995; 104:405–410.

119. Makino T, Takaishi M, Toyoda M, Morohashi M, Huh NH. Expression of hornerin in stratified squamous epithelium in the mouse: a comparative analysis with profilaggrin. J Histochem Cytochem 2003; 51:485–492.

120. Makino T, Takaishi M, Morohashi M, Huh NH. Hornerin, a novel profilaggrin-like protein and differentiation-specific marker isolated from mouse skin. J Biol Chem 2001; 276:47445–47452.

121. Fietz MJ, McLaughlan CJ, Campbell MT, Rogers GE. Analysis of the sheep trichohyalin gene: potential structural and calcium-binding roles of trichohyalin in the hair follicle. J Cell Biol 1993; 121:855–865.

122. Lee SC, Kim IG, Marekov LN, O'Keefe EJ, Parry DA, Steinert PM. The structure of human trichohyalin. Potential multiple roles as a functional EF-hand-like calcium-binding protein, a cornified cell envelope precursor, and an intermediate filament-associated (cross-linking) protein. J Biol Chem 1993; 268:12164–12176.

123. Rogers GE, Fietz MJ, Fratini A. Trichohyalin and matrix proteins. Ann N Y Acad Sci 1991; 642:64–80; discussion 80–61.

124. Rothnagel JA, Rogers GE. Trichohyalin, an intermediate filament-associated protein of the hair follicle. J Cell Biol 1986; 102:1419–1429.

125. Rogers GE, Harding HW, Llewellyn-Smith IJ. The origin of citrulline-containing proteins in the hair follicle and the chemical nature of trichohyalin, an intracellular precursor. Biochim Biophys Acta 1977; 495:159–175.

126. Hamilton EH, Payne RE Jr, O'Keefe EJ. Trichohyalin: presence in the granular layer and stratum corneum of normal human epidermis. J Invest Dermatol 1991; 96:666–672.

127. Hamilton EH, Sealock R, Wallace NR, O'Keefe EJ. Trichohyalin: purification from porcine tongue epithelium and characterization of the native protein. J Invest Dermatol 1992; 98:881–889.

128. O'Keefe EJ, Hamilton EH, Lee SC, Steinert P. Trichohyalin: a structural protein of hair, tongue, nail, and epidermis. J Invest Dermatol 1993; 101:65S–71S.

129. Rogers GE. Isolation and properties of inner sheath cells of hair follicles. Exp Cell Res 1964; 33:264–276.

130. O'Guin WM, Sun TT, Manabe M. Interaction of trichohyalin with intermediate filaments: three immunologically defined stages of trichohyalin maturation. J Invest Dermatol 1992; 98:24–32.

131. Manabe M, O'Guin WM. Keratohyalin, trichohyalin and keratohyalin-trichohyalin hybrid granules: an overview. J Dermatol 1992; 19:749–755.

132. Tarcsa E, Marekov LN, Andreoli J, Idler WW, Candi E, Chung SI, Steinert PM. The fate of trichohyalin. Sequential post-translational modifications by peptidyl-arginine deiminase and transglutaminases. J Biol Chem 1997; 272:27893–27901.

133. Steinert PM, Parry DA, Marekov LN. Trichohyalin mechanically strengthens the hair follicle: multiple cross-bridging roles in the inner root sheath. J Biol Chem 2003; 278:41409–41419.

134. Steinert PM, Kartasova T, Marekov LN. Biochemical evidence that small proline-rich proteins and trichohyalin function in epithelia by modulation of the biomechanical properties of their cornified cell envelopes. J Biol Chem 1998; 273:11758–11769.

135. Lee SC, Lee JB, Seo JJ, Kim YP. Expression of trichohyalin in dermatological disorders: a comparative study with involucrin and filaggrin by immunohistochemical staining. Acta Derm Venereol 1999; 79:122–126.

136. Manabe M, Yaguchi H, Iqbal Butt K, O'Guin WM, Loomis CA, Sung TT, Ogawa H. Trichohyalin expression in skin tumors: retrieval of trichohyalin antigenicity in tissues by microwave irradiation. Int J Dermatol 1996; 35:325–329.

137. Tobin DJ. Characterization of hair follicle antigens targeted by the anti-hair follicle immune response. J Invest Dermatol Symp Proc 2003; 8:176–181.

138. Krieg P, Schuppler M, Koesters R, Mincheva A, Lichter P, Marks F. Repetin (Rptn), a new member of the "fused gene" subgroup within the S100 gene family encoding a murine epidermal differentiation protein. Genomics 1997; 43:339–348.

139. Koch PJ, de Viragh PA, Scharer E, Bundman D, Longley MA, Bickenbach J, Kawachi Y, Suga Y, Zhou Z, Huber M, et al. Lessons from loricrin-deficient mice: compensatory mechanisms maintaining skin barrier function in the absence of a major cornified envelope protein. J Cell Biol 2000; 151:389–400.

140. Segre JA, Bauer C, Fuchs E. Klf4 is a transcription factor required for establishing the barrier function of the skin. Nat Genet 1999; 22:356–360.

141. Jarnik M, de Viragh PA, Scharer E, Bundman D, Simon MN, Roop DR, Steven AC. Quasi-normal cornified cell envelopes in loricrin knockout mice imply the existence of a loricrin backup system. J Invest Dermatol 2002; 118:102–109.

142. Xu Z, Wang MR, Xu X, Cai Y, Han YL, Wu KM, Wang J, Chen BS, Wang XQ, Wu M. Novel human esophagus-specific gene c1orf10: cDNA cloning, gene structure, and frequent loss of expression in esophageal cancer. Genomics 2000; 69:322–330.

143. Contzler C, Uhlmann M, Panizzon R, Huber M, Hohl D. C1orf10, a novel marker of late terminal keratinocyte differentiation. J Invest Dermatol 121:Abstract #479, Society of Investigative Dermatology meeting, 2003.

144. Yagui-Beltran A, Craig AL, Lawrie L, Thompson D, Pospisilova S, Johnston D, Kernohan N, Hopwood D, Dillon JF, Hupp TR. The human oesophageal squamous epithelium exhibits a novel type of heat shock protein response. Eur J Biochem 2001; 268:5343–5355.

145. Donato R. Functional roles of S100 proteins, calcium-binding proteins of the EF-hand type. Biochim Biophys Acta 1999; 1450:191–231.

146. Robinson NA, Lapic S, Welter JF, Eckert RL. S100A11, S100A10, annexin I, desmosomal proteins, small proline rich proteins, plasminogen activator inhibitor-2, and involucrin are components of the cornified envelope of cultured human epidermal keratinocytes. J Biol Chem 1997; 272:12035–12046.

147. Eckert RL, Broome AM, Ruse M, Robinson N, Ryan D, Lee K. S100 proteins in the epidermis. J Invest Dermatol 2004; 123:23–33.

148. Hudson JR Jr, Dawson EP, Rushing KL, Jackson CH, Lockshon D, Conover D, Lanciault C, Harris JR, Simmons SJ, Rothstein R, Fields S. The complete set of predicted genes from Saccharomyces cerevisiae in a readily usable form. Genome Res 1997; 7:1169–1173.

149. McCraith S, Holtzman T, Moss B, Fields S. Genome-wide analysis of vaccinia virus protein–protein interactions. Proc Natl Acad Sci USA 2000; 97:4879–4884.

150. Thompson JD, Higgins DG, Gibson TJ. CLUSTAL W: improving the sensitivity of progressive multiple sequence alignment through sequence weighting, position-specific gap penalties and weight matrix choice. Nucleic Acids Res 1994; 22:4673–4680.

151. Deshpande R, Woods TL, Fu J, Zhang T, Stoll SW, Elder JT. Biochemical characterization of S100A2 in human keratinocytes: subcellular localization, dimerization, and oxidative cross-linking. J Invest Dermatol 2000; 115:477–485.

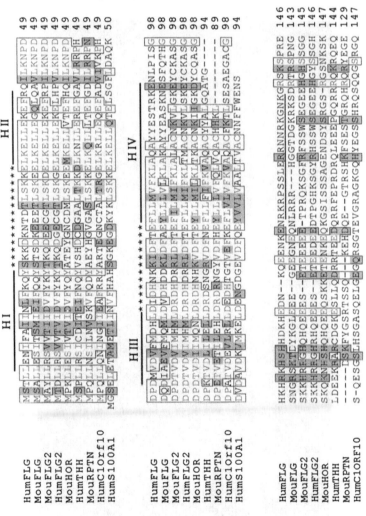

Figure 1 Amino acid similarity among the N-terminal domains of the fused S100 proteins. Shown are the S100 Ca^{2+}-binding domain (amino acids 1–92) and part of the downstream domains for HumFLG, MouFLG, MouFLG2, HumFLG-2, MouHOR, HumTHH, MouRPTN, HumC1orf10, and HumS100A1 analyzed for optimal alignment using ClustalW (150). The positions of the two Ca^{2+}-binding EF-hands are indicated by stars, and the four α-helices, HI–HIV, surrounding each EF-hand are indicated by lines above the sequence. Boxed amino acids in red show the identity and shaded blue residues indicate homology. The underlined sequence in humFLG indicates the position of the bipartite nuclear localization signal, which is not present at the same position in other fused S100 proteins (17). Numbers at right indicate the number of amino acids. *Abbreviations*: Hum FLG, human profilaggrin; MouFLG, mouse profilaggrin; MouFLG2, mouse Filaggrin-2; HumFLG-2, human Filaggrin-2; MouHOR, mouse hornerin; HumTHH, human trichohyalin; MouRPTN, mouse repetin; HumC1orf10, human C1orf10; and HumS100A1, human S100A1.

1

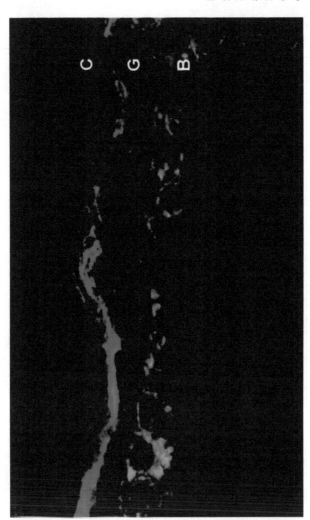

Figure 7 Immunofluorescence microscopy of newborn mouse epidermis with Flg-2 antibody. Sections were double-labeled with antibodies against Flg-2 (red) and K14 (green). Flg-2 is restricted to the granular and cornified layers (red cells). B, basal layer; G, granular layer; C, cornified layer. Total magnification, 300×.

10

The Role of Keratins in Epithelial Homeostasis

Thomas M. Magin, Julia Reichelt, and Jian Chen
Institut für Physiologische Chemie, Abteilung für Zellbiochemie, Bonner Forum Biomedizin and LIMES, Universitätsklinikum Bonn, Nussallee, Bonn, Germany

INTRODUCTION

Among all cytoskeletal proteins, keratins have evolved into the most divergent group in mammals, reflecting the functional needs of diverse epithelial cell types and tissues. The assembly and regulation of the actin and the microtubule cytoskeleton, and their predominant function in cell adhesion, polarity, intracellular transport, migration, and cell division are relatively well known. The subcellular architecture and the cell- and tissue-specific function of 6 human actins and 13 α- and β-tubulins is mainly regulated by a very large number of well-characterized associated protein families. This does not appear to be the case for keratins, for which only a very limited number of bona fide associated proteins, mainly plakins and cornified envelope proteins, are presently known (1,2). These provide membrane attachment sites and mediate the transient interaction of keratins with the actin and the microtubule cytoskeleton. The prevailing principle responsible for tissue-specific keratin function and regulation appears to result from the transcriptional regulation of their genes and the intrinsic property of the >50 different protein sequences. The former gives rise to exquisite, cell type–specific keratin profiles, which are responsible for the micromechanical properties of epithelial cells and their distinct cytoskeletal architecture. The latter has endowed them with distinct assembly properties and half-life times, and provides unique target sites for a large number of kinases and phosphatases (1,3). These principles govern the scaffolding function of keratins, which is their predominant function as underscored by keratinopathies (4–6) and experiments in knockout mice (1,2,7,8).

KERATIN COMPLEXITY, NOMENCLATURE, AND GENOME ORGANIZATION

Keratins are structural proteins that form the intermediate filament (IF) cytoskeleton in all epithelia. They assemble into long filaments built from obligate heterodimeric double-stranded coiled-coils, which consist of a type I and a type II protein.

Keratins are encoded by a large and well-conserved gene family with 54 members in humans and in mice (9,10). Of these, 15 type I and 10 type II proteins are hair and/or inner root sheath keratins (10–13). In humans, all type I keratin genes, except for *K18* (14), cluster on chromosome 17q21 and type II genes cluster on 12q13 (Int. Human Genome Seq. Cons., 2001). In the mouse, the orthologs are similarly clustered on chromosomes 11D and 15F, respectively (15). Among the 70 known IF genes, keratins represent by far the most complex family. In any given epithelium, at least one type I and one type II keratin are present to form tissue-type and differentiation-specific "expression pairs." Up to now, neither the regulatory mechanisms nor the functional significance of this diverse keratin expression has been understood.

NOMENCLATURE OF KERATINS

The present nomenclature of keratins is based on their position in 2D gels or their primary site of expression. This has resulted in a complex numbering system, which in some cases does not reflect sequence relatedness (Table 1). We have recently proposed a new nomenclature for all keratins based on established principles (10). All type I keratin genes are named *Ka9* to *Ka41* and all type II keratin genes are named *Kb1* to *Kb40*. The species is indicated by a prefix (H, human; M, mouse). Table 1 lists known human and mouse keratins in the previous and the new nomenclature. The nomenclature proposed is an open system, allowing the addition of novel keratins in other species by additional numbers. The nomenclature principles proposed by the "HUGO Gene Nomenclature Committee" (HGNC) were followed. Pseudogenes that are not derived from a functional keratin gene have their own number and are indicated by a "P." Pseudogenes derived from keratin genes by duplication or retrotransposition are numbered, starting with P1 if more than one pseudogene exists. Orthologs share the same numbers, but genes unique to a species are individually numbered (Table 1).

THE MAMMALIAN KERATIN TYPE I CLUSTERS

The human keratin I gene cluster located on chromosome 17q21.2 is completely sequenced (NCBI Build 34, July 2003) and its mouse counterpart on chromosome 11D is essentially known (release, February 2003). The human keratin type I gene cluster consists of 27 keratin type I genes and four keratin type I pseudogenes, which are all arranged in the same orientation. Inserted into this cluster is a domain of a large number of genes encoding the high and ultrahigh sulfur keratin-associated proteins (KAPs) (16). These KAP genes show both orientations and divide the keratin cluster into two subclusters. For most human and mouse type I genes, cDNA accession numbers are available. The size of the human type I keratin cluster is 977 kb including the KAP-cluster. The gene density in the telomeric part of the keratin cluster is 14.4 kb. The centromeric part has a gene density of 25.2 kb. In the mouse, the telomeric part has a size of 260 kb with a gene density of 16.2 kb and the centromeric part a has size of 309 kb with a gene density of 25.8 kb.

The first part of the mammalian type I cluster contains several genes encoding the keratins of the inner root sheath of hair follicles (17). Past the gene for *Ka23* (*K23*) lie two newly defined hair keratin genes (*Ka34* and *Ka35*) and the genes encoding

Table 1 Keratin Nomenclature

Old name Type I	New names Human	Acc.No.	Mouse	Acc.No.	Old name Type II	New names Human	Acc.No.	Mouse	Acc.No.
K9	Ka9	NM_000226	Ka9	AK028845	K1	Kb1	NM_006121	Kb1	M10937
K10	Ka10	J04029	Ka10	AK076508	K1b	Kb39	AJ564104	Kb39	BK003993
Ka11*[a]	–	–	Ka11P	BK004024	K2e	Kb2	AF019084	Kb2	X74784
K12	Ka12	D78367	Ka12	NM_010661	K2p	Kb9	M99063	Kb9	AK009075
K13	Ka13	X52426	Ka13	NM_010662	K3	Kb3	NM_057088	–	
K14	Ka14	NM_000526	Ka14	BC011074	K4	Kb4	NM_002272	Kb4	X03491
K15	Ka15	NM_002275	Ka15	NM_008469	K5	Kb5	NM_000424	Kb5	BC006780
K16	Ka16	NM_005557	Ka16	NM_008470	K5b	Kb40	AK096419	Kb40	BK004080
K17	Ka17	NM_000422	Ka17	NM_010663	K6a	Kb6	NM_005554	Kb6	NM_008476
K18	Ka18	NM_000224	Ka18	NM_010664	K6b	Kb10	NM_005555	–	
K19	Ka19	NM_002276	Ka19	NM_008471	mK6b	–	–	Kb11	NM_010669
K20	Ka20	BC031559	Ka20	AK018567	mK6d	–	–	Kb15	AK028791
Ka21P*[a]	Ka21P	BK004052	Ka21P	AK031954	K6e	Kb12	NM_173086	Kb18	NM_133357
Ka22P*[a]	Ka22P	BK004056	Ka22	BK004025	K6hf	Kb18	NM_004693	Kb34	NM_019956
K23	Ka23	BC028356	Ka23	AF102849	K6irs1,K6i	Kb34	AJ308599	Kb35	BK001584
K24, K10B	Ka24	AK000268	Ka24	AK010165	K6irs2,K6k	Kb35	NM_080747	Kb36	BK003988
K25A, K10C	Ka38	NM_181534	Ka38	BC018391	K6irs3	Kb36	AJ508776	Kb37	BK003986
K25B, K10D	Ka39	NM_181539	Ka39	AK028591	K6irs4,K5c	Kb37	AJ508777	Kb38	BC031593
K25C, K12b	Ka40	NM_181537	Ka40	AK077384	K6l	Kb38	BC039148	Kb7	NM_033073
K25D	Ka41	NM_181535	Ka41	AK014642	K7	Kb7	NM_005556	Kb8	NM_031170
KRTHA1	Ka25	X86570	Ka25	NM_010659	K8	Kb8	X74929	Kb13	BC046626
KRTHA2	Ka26	NM_002278	Ka26	NM_010665	Kb13*	–	–	Kb14	BK003987
KRTHA3A	Ka27	NM_004138	Ka27	BC029257	Kb14*[a]	–	–	Kb16P	BK003992
KRTHA3B	Ka28	X82634	Ka28	X75650	mK6ψ1	–	–	Kb17P	BK003991
KRTHA4	Ka29	NM_021013	Ka29	NM_027563	mK6ψ2	–	–	–	
KRTHA5	Ka30	NM_002280	Ka30	AF020790	Kb19P*[a]	Kb19P	BK003989	–	

(Continued)

Table 1 Keratin Nomenclature (*Continued*)

Old name Type I	New names Human	Acc.No.	Mouse	Acc.No.	Old name Type II	New names Human	Acc.No.	Mouse	Acc.No.
KRTHA6	Ka31	NM_003771	Ka31	AK028845	Kb20*[a]	Kb20	BC047308	Kb20	AK004811
KRTHA7	Ka32	NM_003770	–	–	KRTHB1	Kb21	NM_002281	Kb21	AF312018
KRTHA8	Ka33	NM_006771	–	–	KRTHB2	Kb22	NM_033033	Kb22	AY028606
ψ KRTHAA	Ka34P	Y16795			KRTHB3	Kb23	NM_002282	Kb23	M92088
Ka35*[a]	Ka35	BK004054	Ka35	BK004022	KRTHB4	Kb24	NM_033045	Kb24	AY028607
Ka36*[a]	Ka36	BK004055	Ka36	BK004023	KRTHB5	Kb25	NM_002283	Kb25	BK001583
Ka37P*[a]	Ka37P	BK004053	–		KRTHB6	Kb26	NM_002284	Kb26	X99143
					Kb27*[a]	–	–	gap	
					ψHbA	Kb28P	Y19213	–	–
					ψHbB	Kb29P	Y19214	–	–
					ψHbC	Kb30P	Y19215	–	–
					ψHbD	Kb31P	Y19216	–	–
					Kb32P*[a]	–	–	Kb32P	BK003990
					Kb33P*[a]	–	–	Kb33P	NM_025487

[a]Newly identified in this work; P, pseudogene; m, mouse; h, human; n.p., no reliable prediction.

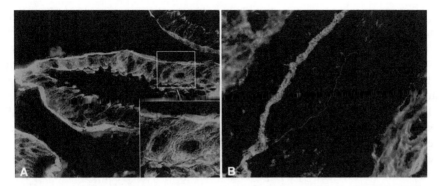

Figure 1 Cell type-specific localization of Ka20 in the mouse. (A) In intestinal epithelial cells, Ka20 forms a cytoskeleton with Kb8 throughout the cell. Inset shows higher magnification. (B) In bladder umbrella cells, Ka20 is highly enriched toward the luminal aspect. The basolateral membrane domain is demarcated by a white line.

the high/ultrahigh sulfur KAPs. The KAP domain is flanked by the hair keratin gene *Ka27* (*KRTHA3A*), which is followed in the rodent clusters by six additional hair keratin genes. There are 9 and 11 hair keratin I genes in rodents and man, respectively (Fig. 1).

The KAP subdomain comprises about 362 kb in humans and 466 kb in mice. In human, it contains 29 genes of high/ultrahigh sulfur hair KAPs, which can be divided into seven individual gene families. Their respective mRNAs are localized in the upper cortex of the hair shaft (16). These KAPs have cysteine contents either below (high sulfur) or above (ultrahigh) 30%. The entire KAP region is inserted into the hair keratin domain. Interestingly, seven other human genes encoding high sulfur KAPs lie together with 17 genes for high glycine–tyrosine KAPs on human chromosome 21q22.1 (18).

Beyond the hair keratin region, the three mammalian type I clusters remain very similar with very good conservation of synteny. The type I cluster ends with a novel rodent gene (*Ka22*) related to keratins 14 and 17. In man, this gene was converted into a pseudogene (*Ka22P*). It is remarkable that cytokeratins (*Ka9–Ka24*), hair keratins (*Ka25–Ka36*), and inner root sheath keratins (*Ka38–Ka41*) are clustered together in small subdomains. The gene for K11, identified previously by 2D gel electrophoresis (19,20), is undetectable in the human or mouse genomes and therefore must be considered a variant of an existing keratin, such as *Ka10* (*K10*), in agreement with former studies (21).

THE MAMMALIAN KERATIN TYPE II CLUSTERS

The sequence of the human keratin II gene cluster located on chromosome 12q13.13 (size 783 kb) is now completely known. The corresponding murine gene cluster, located on chromosome 15F3 (size 699 kb) still shows a variety of gaps (release February 2003), but most of the genes in the cluster are unambiguously located versus their human orthologs. Nearly all type II genes have the same orientation. Notable exceptions are for instance *Kb7* (*K7*) and the terminal type I *Ka18* (*K18*).

The human keratin II cluster (size 783 kb) consists of 26 type II genes, five type II pseudogenes, three keratin-unrelated pseudogenes and ends with the type I keratin

Ka18 (*K18*) gene. The gene density for the cluster is 22.4 kb. In the murine genome, there are at least 27 functional type II genes resulting in a gene density of 21.9 kb, and a further type II gene past *Kb7* present in the rat cluster may be obscured by a gap in the murine sequence. Among the cDNA accession numbers for the murine genes there is also one for *Kb33P*, indicating that this hair keratin pseudogene may be transcribed.

The human gene for keratin *Kb39* (*K1b*) describes a novel keratin II gene (9) with 66% identity to *Kb1* (K1) on the protein level. A human cDNA and accession number of an EST-sequence for the murine ortholog indicates that *Kb39* (*K1b*) is expressed in the skin. Past the three non-keratin genes, the human type II cluster continues with another six type II genes for *Kb9* (*K2p*), *Kb3* (*K3*), *Kb4* (*K4*), *Kb38* (*K6l*), *Kb40* (*K5b*), and *Kb8* (*K8*) before the end position, occupied by the type I keratin *Ka18* (*K18*) gene, is reached. Keratins *Kb8* (*K8*) and *Ka18* (*K18*) are typical of inner epithelia and represent the earliest IF expression pair in embryogenesis. Unexpectedly, the gene for human cornea *Kb3* (*K3*) situated between genes *Kb9* (*K2p*) and *Kb4* (*K4*) lacks a murine counterpart. Thus, the human *Kb3* (*K3*) gene may be the result of a recent gene duplication or an older mammalian *Kb3* (*K3*) gene was lost on the lineage leading to mice. Using RT–PCR, the *Kb5* (*K5*) was determined as the major type II keratin expressed in the murine cornea. Therefore, the concept of keratin pairs is less rigorous than thought in the past.

DOMAIN STRUCTURE, ASSEMBLY, AND PROTEIN MODIFICATIONS

All keratins possess the same tripartite secondary structure with a central, largely α-helical "rod" domain, flanked by non-α-helical amino-terminal and carboxy-terminal domains forcing the molecules into double-stranded and parallel coiled-coils (22–24). At each end of the rod, 15–20 amino acids are highly conserved among keratins and all other IF proteins. The rod is built from four consecutive domains of highly conserved amino acid numbers: segment 1A accounting for 35, segment 1B for 101, segment 2A for 19, and segment 2B for 121 amino acids. The non-α-helical "linker" domains between these segments are variable in length (8–22 amino acids). The individual α-helical segments exhibit a heptad substructure (abcdefg)$_n$, where a and d positions are occupied by apolar amino acids (23,25). These hydrophobic amino acids generate a hydrophobic seam that is wound around the axis of a single right-handed α-helix, ultimately forming coiled-coils of two such molecules (for details, see Ref. 2 and references therein).

The phasing of the heptads is broken in the middle of segment 2B giving rise to a "stutter." This represents an α-helical segment not engaged in coiled-coil formation but running in parallel with the corresponding part of the second molecule of the parallel coiled-coil dimer. The evolutionarily conserved end of segment 2B is not entirely part of the coiled-coil structure; the last 10 amino acids bend away from the coiled-coil axis (26,27).

Keratin filament formation in vitro is a self-assembly process, resulting from the intrinsic sequence features of polypeptides. The building block of all keratin filaments is a heterodimer, built from one type I and one type II protein, whose assembly is initiated through "trigger motifs" in the coil 1B and 2B (28,29). Parallel dimers assemble to antiparallel, half-staggered tetramers (with different overlap modes possible), which laterally associate to unit-length-filaments (ULFs). These anneal longitudinally into long and non-polar filaments, which finally compact into IF with a diameter of ~11 nm width (22,23,27). In vitro, any heterotypic keratin combination is possible (30) and there is mounting evidence from knockout mice and in vitro studies that indicate at least some keratins can replace each other, supporting functional redundancy (8,31,32).

Several motifs along the head domain are essential for IF formation, while the tail is dispensable (33). Tail sequences regulate filament diameter (2,34) and in the case of Kb5 and Ka14 at least, the tail of Ka14 might contribute to filament bundling (35). In general, bundling of keratin IF—if it is not an artifact of fixation procedures—appears to be an intrinsic property of some keratins, as convincingly shown by the ectopic coexpression and bundle formation of Kb1 and Ka10 in the mouse pancreas (36). Mutations that alter tail sequences of Kb1 and Kb5 have most recently been shown to cause ichthyosis hystrix and epidermolysis bullosa simplex (EBS) with migrating erythema, respectively, possibly by changing binding sites for associated proteins (37–42).

When mutations in Ka14 and Kb5 were recognized to cause EBS (43–45), it was assumed that at least those mutations, which led to severe disease, abolished IF formation. It is now clear, however, that even the most widespread $Ka14R_{125}C/H$ mutation that causes extensive keratin clumping in men and mice has no effect on filament assembly or length in vitro (22). The mechanical properties of these filaments were not analyzed in that study, however. Differential interference contrast microscopy and rheological measurements of in vitro formed keratin filaments containing keratins with the same mutation, revealed a greatly reduced resilience of filaments against large deformations (46). These authors concluded that EBS-type mutations impair the ability of keratin polymers to form bundles, which appear to be a prerequisite to withstand mechanical stress. Upon transfection in cultured cells and in vivo, however, the above Ka14 mutation leads to filament aggregation, depending on the stoichiometry of mutant to wild-type protein [(44,47) and references therein].

Filament formation in vivo, under steady-state conditions in tissues, is not well understood and involves the existence of soluble tetramers, representing ~1–5% of total cellular keratin (1,48,49). At present, there is little known about the subcellular organization of keratin cytoskeletons. In early embryonic development, the first IF appear in nascent desmosomes (50), suggesting a role for desmosomes in IF assembly and organization. Thorough studies using live cell imaging of GFP-tagged keratins transfected in epithelial cells have provided very good evidence that filament formation is initiated close to the plasma membrane and proceeds through the formation of small particles, which on their transport toward the cell center become incorporated into existing IF (51,52).

It was assumed for sometime that Kb1 and Ka10 require a Kb5 and Ka14 "scaffold" to form IF (53). The formation of intact Kb1 and Ka10-containing IF in Kb5 null mice, which lack IF in their basal compartment altogether, has answered that question (54). Clearly, most if not all combinations of type I and type II keratins form IF in cells and tissues. What determines their subcellular organization and distribution, which can be very different, is not known. Ka20, for example, is evenly distributed in intestinal epithelial cells but restricted to the apical domain of umbrella cells in the mouse bladder (Hesse and Magin, unpublished, see Fig. 1). Another unresolved issue is how the >10 different keratins that can be present in the same cell are organized. At which level of assembly do they mix? Do the final IF contain an equal mixture and distribution of all subunits? What are the regulatory principles determining their organization? Given that in vitro, complexes between different keratins show a distinct stability, it would be surprising if cells did not make use of these properties (30,55).

One way to orchestrate keratin organization in cells is by using phosphorylation. It affects the organization of filaments, either by increasing the exchange between the soluble and the cytoskeletal fractions or by regulating the binding sites of associated proteins, e.g., 14-3-3 (1,56,57). All phosphorylation sites identified so far involve distinct serine residues in the head domains of Kb1, Kb8, Ka18, and Ka19, most of which are unique (1). Hyperphosphorylation of keratins is observed under conditions of tissue injury or stress, and the consequences depend on the serine residue phosphorylated and the tissue analyzed. It can be protective or increase tissue damage (1). How phosphorylation of keratins affects epithelial integrity is not known. Among the candidate kinases are p38 and Jun kinase for which recognition sites are present on Kb8 (57,58).

Human Kb8, Ka13, and Ka18 are modified by O-linked N-acetylglucosamines in their head domains. As for many other glycosylated cytoplasmic proteins, significance of this modification is unknown but appears to be independent of phosphorylation (1). In addition, human Kb8, Ka18, and Ka19, isolated from cultured tumor cells, contain GalNac–glycan chains which might provide binding sites for galectin-3 (59).

The major modifications of epidermal keratins are transglutamination and deamination of arginine residues. The former covalently attaches predominantly type II keratins to cornified envelope proteins; in the case of Kb1, a lysine residue in the head domain is involved (60,61). The latter occurs during the transition of granular cells to corneocytes and involves preferentially an arginine residue in the V1 and V2 subdomains, respectively (62). While its role is not clear, it is worth noting that modifying arginine residues in the head domain of vimentin using canavanine interferes with its polymer state (63).

Like many other cytosolic proteins, keratins are modified by ubiquitination. For Kb8 and Ka18, hyperphosphorylation has been shown to inhibit ubiquitination and subsequent degradation (64). Most recently, it was reported that mutant Ka14 forms keratin aggregates typical of EBS and, despite being ubiquitinated, prevented keratin degradation via proteasomal pathways in cultured human keratinocytes (65). Protein aggregation appears to be a general mechanism by which protein degradation via the proteasome is impaired (66). Most type I keratins are processed by caspases through recognition of the VEMD or VEVD amino acid motifs in the L12 linker region. In type II keratins, which appear not to be cleaved by caspases, these motifs are absent in the L12 region but present in other domains (1). The significance of keratin targeting by caspases in the orchestration of cell death has not been resolved.

GENE REGULATION AND EXPRESSION

The expression of most, if not all, keratins is regulated at the transcriptional level. However, the principles governing the pair-wise and tissue-specific activity of keratin genes remain unknown. A recent search based on available algorithms has failed to reveal common regulatory sequences in promoters of co-expressed genes (10). The reported activity of Kb8 and Ka18 in several non-epithelial tissues (67) argues that whatever governs non-epithelial repression of the type II gene cluster can be overcome by transcriptional activation of Kb8 and Ka18.

It has been shown that the regulatory elements responsible for the transcription control of the human Ka18 gene are contained in a 10 kb genomic fragment. Flanked by 2.5 kb of 5'- and 3.5 kb of 3'-regulatory sequences, it reproduced quite faithfully the expression pattern of mouse Ka18 in a copy-number-dependent and position-independent manner. Involved in the regulation are conserved Alu sequences and four potential SP1 binding sites in the proximal promoter and a regulatory element in exon 6 with an additional AP-1 consensus site (68). This element seems to cooperate with the intron 1 sites, which also harbor Ets-1 elements (69,70). Moreover, the *Ka18* gene harbors two differentially methylated CpGs in the Ka18 first intron enhancer (70).

Keratinocyte-specific expression of the human *Kb5* and *Ka14* genes appears to rely on an array of five DNaseI-hypersensitive sites located in the 6 kb 5'-upstream region of the *Kb5* and ~2.1 kb of the *Ka14* gene (71,72). These sites contain binding sites for general and tissue-specific transcription factors of the AP-1, AP-2, SP-1, SP-3, NF-1, and Skn-1 families (73) in addition to motifs for yet unknown transcription factors. Most of our current knowledge about the regulation of other epidermal keratin genes has been recently reviewed (74). It is noteworthy that the promoter of the *Kb6* (former *K6a*) gene was found to contain an antioxidant response element (ARE), which binds the transcription factor Nrf-2 (75). This places at least Kb6 on a comprehensive list of genes induced following oxidative stress and offers a new view to explain the expression and diversity of keratins.

Jave-Suarez et al. have identified HOXC13 consensus binding sites of the sequence TT(A/T) ATNPuPu in several human hair keratin genes (76) and, most recently, demonstrated that the hair keratin gene Ka32 (former hHa7) promoter is a direct target for the androgen receptor (77). This might provide a link for the study of androgen-linked hair disorders.

The predominant expression pair of embryonic and internal, "simple" epithelia is Kb8 and Ka18, present from embryonic day (E) 2.5 onwards (77a). This basic keratin set can be complemented by Kb7, Ka19, Ka20, and Ka23 in most epithelia with the expression of Kb7 and Ka19 starting around E3.5 (77a). Kb7 and Ka19 are widely expressed in most internal and ductal epithelia, and appear to be capable of replacing Kb8 and Ka18, provided they are present in the same cell type and in appropriate amounts (8,78). Ka23 was originally identified by RT–PCR in a human pancreas carcinoma cell line (79); and is also present in lung, vagina, and glandular stomach, at least in the mouse (Magin and Reichelt, unpublished).

Stratified epithelia express predominantly Kb5 and Ka14, with varying amounts of Ka15 and Ka17 in their basal layer (54,80–82). Ka17 expression is not only largely correlated with formation of epidermal appendages (83–85) but is also induced upon wound healing and other types of epidermal injury, both in humans and in mice (86–88). In addition, it is present in low amounts in the interfollicular epidermis, the epidermis of palms/soles, and in the esophagus [(81,85,89), Reichelt and Magin, unpublished, Fig. 2] The newly identified gene *Ka22*, also named *K17n*, is preferentially expressed in nail tissue, but also in filiform and fungiform papillae of oral mucosa (10,81). The upper strata of epidermis maintain keratins Kb5 and Ka14, due to the long half-life time of the proteins, but as soon as keratinocytes begin to differentiate, they express large quantities of Kb1 and Ka10. In addition, Kb39 (former K1b), Kb2 (former K2e), and Ka9 are present in upper spinous and granular keratinocytes at locations exposed to particular stress, e.g., palms (89,90). In the soft palate, Kb2 is replaced by its close relative Kb9 (former K2p) (91). Other non-cornifying human epithelia, e.g., esophagus, express Kb4 and Ka13 in the upper cell layers instead of the above keratins. In human cornea, the differentiated layers are characterized by Kb3 and Ka12. In the mouse, however,

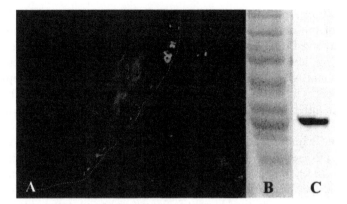

Figure 2 Constitutive expression of Ka17 in mouse esophagus. In esophagus of adult mice, Ka17 is expressed in individual basal cells, using an antiserum kindly provided by P. Coulombe. (A) Immunofluorescence, (B) and (C) Coomasie-stained blot and corresponding K17 Western blot.

the *Kb3* gene is absent from the genome (10,92), forcing its replacement by *Kb5*. Therefore, the concept of "keratin expression pairs" is not universal. In settings of an altered proliferation and differentiation, like keratinocyte migration and wound healing, the reinforcement keratins Kb6, Kb10, Kb12, Kb18 (former K6a, b, e, and hf, respectively), and Ka16 are transiently or constitutively expressed and often replace Kb1, Kb2, Ka9, and Ka10 (85). Under those conditions, Kb6 is present in basal and suprabasal epidermis, whereas Kb10 is expressed in suprabasal keratinocytes (93–95).

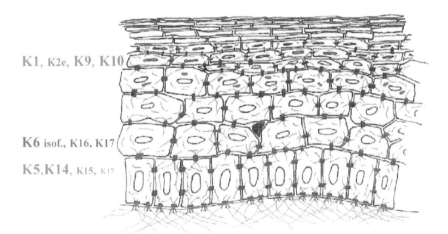

Figure 3 Keratin expression in epidermis and other stratified epithelia. All basal cells express Kb5 and Ka14 with low and variable amounts of Ka15 and Ka17. Spinous and granular cells express large amounts of Kb1 and Ka10. Kb2 and Ka9 expression starts in the upper spinous and granular layers. Ka9 is restricted to palmoplantar epidermis, whereas Kb2 is present in many stratified epithelia, at least in humans. In activated keratinocytes (following wounding, UV light, psoriasis, hyperproliferation), "K6 isoforms," Ka16 and Ka17 are switched on in suprabasal cells, whereas Kb5, Ka14, Kb1, and Ka10 are down regulated. Kb6 is also present in basal keratinocytes.

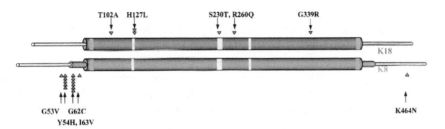

Figure 4 Mutations in human *Kb8* and *Ka18* genes accompanying liver, intestinal and pancreatic disorders. Mutations in liver-specific disorders, inflammatory bowel disorders, and pancreatic disorders are labeled. Mutations also occur outside the conserved helical end domains. The numbering of amino acid positions includes the start methionine. Note that the same mutation at position 62 is found in liver and bowel disease.

Embryonic expression of epidermal keratins is initiated well before the onset of stratification when the embryo is covered by a single layered surface ectoderm, specified by Kb8 and Ka18 (96). It is noted that the Kb5 protein expression starts in the surface ectoderm of the hind limb as early as E9.25, while the expression of its partner, Ka14, begins at E9.75. From E9.25 to E9.75, Kb5 is able to form filaments without Ka14 because of the expression of the simple epithelial Ka18 (77a). Very early expression has also been reported for Kb1 and Ka10, the mRNAs of which were identified by RNase protection at E10.5 in the mouse (97,98). In keeping, the induction of Kb6 (former K6a), Kb10 (former K6b), Ka16, and Ka17 was reported to occur as early as E11.5, well before the onset of stratification, which starts at ~E13.5 in the mouse (99). The early onset of epidermal keratin expression, before the onset of epidermal stratification, raises the issue as to what specifies the regional differentiation of the surface epithelium and what functions keratins play in this process.

One other example, which highlights potentially new avenues to explore keratin function is the stem cell connection. The *Ka15* gene shows a regional and developmentally regulated expression in the basal layer of interfollicular epidermis and other stratified epithelia, and becomes lost upon wound healing. There is good evidence that Ka15 is predominantly expressed in label-retaining cells, the putative epidermal stem cells (80,82,100,101). Most notably, Cotsarelis and coworkers were able to strongly enrich for bulge region-derived label-retaining mouse keratinocytes, using ~4 kb of Ka15 promoter sequences (102,103). As the authors point out, there is no evidence at present for an involvement of Ka15 or any other keratin in stem cell function. Nevertheless, in line with emerging data from keratinocyte explant cultures and from Ka10 knockout mice, one might hypothesize that a certain keratin composition renders cells more or less motile (1,95,103a). For the expression of keratins in hair, we refer to Refs. (11–13).

KERATINOPATHIES

The major function of keratins and their mutations in epidermal diseases has been extensively reviewed (5,6,104–106) and will not be covered here. Among the issues remaining open for investigation are: (a) how actually do mutations lead to cell fragility, (b) why does the same mutation lead to a range of pathologies, and (c) what do diseases tell us about keratin function? An electronic database is located at www.interfil.org. Recent cell-culture studies have provided some evidence that in addition to IF being less resilient to mechanical forces due to mutations (46), other mechanisms contribute to EBS. The appearance of EBS-type keratin aggregates was accompanied by a TNF increase in cell-culture supernatant of the transiently transfected keratinocytes, and interestingly, the most prominent $Ka14R_{125}C$ mutation was found to weaken binding to the TNF-α receptor-associated death domain (TRADD). Also, transfectants were susceptible to caspase-3 and -8–mediated apoptosis. The authors hypothesized that the susceptibility of keratinocytes to caspase-8–mediated apoptosis is increased in mutated Ka14 because of impairment of the cytoprotective mechanism mediated by Ka14–TRADD interaction (65). Another study used live cell imaging of stable cell transfectants, expressing the same Ka14 mutant as a YFP fusion protein. It reported that, unlike expected from the analysis of EBS tissue sections, keratin aggregates were in dynamic equilibrium with soluble subunits at a half-life time of less than 15 minutes. The authors suggested that dominant-negative mutations act by altering cytoskeletal dynamics and solubility. Moreover, they showed that the dominance of mutations is limited and strictly depends on the ratio of mutant to wild-type protein, offering one explanation why the conditions of some EBS patients may improve with age (47). As one might suspect, keratin mutations render keratinocytes more susceptible to osmotic shock and lead to activation of the SAPK/JNK pathway (47,107).

In contrast to epidermal keratins in which point mutations cause monogenic keratinopathies, the role of embryonic and internal epithelial keratins is still controversial. Mutations in *Kb8* and *Ka18* genes have been associated with cryptogenic cirrhosis and additional liver disorders, at least in the American population (108–110). These mutations occur at gene positions different from those in epidermal keratins and do neither disrupt IF nor cause tissue fragility. Two European studies focusing on similar populations have not detected the above mutations (10,110a), suggesting that population differences contribute to the complexity of polygenic keratinopathies. One of the above Kb8 mutations, G62C, was also associated with chronic pancreatitis (111). Most recently, four mutations, G62C, I63V, and K464N in Kb8 and S230T in Ka18 were found in a subset of patients suffering from ulcerative colitis and Crohn's disease (112). One of these Kb8 mutations, G62C is also associated with various liver and pancreatic disorders (110,111).

Based on in vitro filament assembly and cell transfection studies, it has been suggested that some of the "mild" Kb8 and Ka18 mutations may increase the soluble keratin fraction and render cells more susceptible to oxidative stress (112). To what extent this contributes to intestinal pathology has to await the development of appropriate transgenic mouse models. Why are mutations analogous to those in EBS and other monogenic disorders apparently absent from *Kb8* and *Ka18* genes? The embryonic lethality of mice deficient for Kb8/Ka19 or Ka18/Ka19 strongly suggests that such mutations, which compromise cell integrity, are likely to be lethal. This is supported by findings in mice, where an EBS-type mutation in K18 causes embryo lethality (112a).

KERATINS AND SIGNALING

Recent studies have provided evidence for a role of certain keratins in cell signaling events. Three studies point to a modulation of the apoptotic response through death receptor signaling. A first clue came from Caulin et al. (113), showing that epithelial cells with disrupted Kb8/Ka18 filaments were significantly more sensitive to TNF-mediated apoptosis. These findings were accompanied by an increase of JNK- and NFκB-protein levels, both being downstream targets of the TNF signaling pathway. Also, Kb8$^{-/-}$- and Ka18$^{-/-}$-mice were much more sensitive to concanavalin A (ConA)-induced liver damage. ConA mediates an immune response through activated T cells, which in turn secrete TNF-α, thus causing apoptosis. But how is the interaction between keratin IFs and this signaling pathway established? The authors suppose a direct interaction between the TNFR2 (TNF receptor 2) and the N-terminal parts of Kb8 and Ka18 supported by a GST-fusion protein-binding assay. Another clue came from Inada et al. (114), who demonstrated a direct interaction between the TRADD (TNFR1-associated death domain protein) protein and the coil 1a domain of Ka18 and Ka14 by co-immunoprecipitation. TRADD is an adaptor protein vital for TNFR-1 mediated apoptosis and links TNFR1 to FADD and RIP. Binding of TRADD to Ka18 could therefore withhold TRADD from operating as a mediator of apoptosis. Overexpression of Kb8/Ka18 in immortalized SW13 cells confirmed this scenario by procuring some resistance to TNF treatment. In this setting, Ka18 seemed to sequester TRADD, thereby modulating TNFR1-signaling.

Similar findings were made with primary hepatocytes derived from Kb8$^{-/-}$ mice (115). These hepatocytes were more sensitive to Fas-mediated apoptosis. Interestingly, the number of Fas receptors at the cell surface was increased, possibly due to an increased rate of traffic to the cell membrane. However, the transport of Fas is dependent on microtubules and it must be investigated whether IF-associated proteins of the plakin family like plectin can connect the two cytoskeletal compartments thereby mediating protein transport. Provided that a modulating role of keratins in the apoptotic response can be confirmed in future experiments, this will be of great importance for inflammatory diseases of intestine and liver. The role of keratins in apoptosis has been reviewed recently (115a).

KERATIN KNOCKOUT MICE AND OTHER FUNCTIONAL STUDIES
Simple and Embryonic Epithelia

So far, 13 keratin genes have been inactivated or mutated by gene targeting. With the possible exception of Ka19 null mice, gene knockouts of all other keratins have provided a range of pathologies [(1,2,7,116,117); and Table 2]. The apparent lack of obvious defects in Ka19 null mice underlines that functional redundancy is an important principle in keratin biology. In those mice, Ka18 is present in Ka19-deficient cells and tissues in sufficient amounts, providing compensation. Conversely, Ka18 null mice form perfect IF between Kb8 and the tailless Ka19 in most tissues and develop a mild liver pathology, due to the absence of Ka19 in hepatocytes (8). One might predict that the absence of Kb7 may not cause pathology, for all cells expressing Kb7 represent a subset of Ka8-positive cells.

The function of keratins during embryonic development and in simple epithelia is less clear than in epidermis. Mice deficient for Kb8 die from placental failure at E12.5 in the C57Bl/6 strain of mice and display colonic hyperplasia in adult FVB/N mice (118,119). In colonic epithelia, mistargeting of several apical membrane proteins was observed (78). A reason for the observed diarrhea could be the net Na$^+$-absorption associated with Cl$^-$-secretion in jejunal epithelia, which displayed partial loss of H$^+$/K$^+$-ATPase-beta, and redistributed anion exchanger AE1/2 and Na$^+$-transporter ENaC-gamma (120). It is not clear how the loss of Kb8 affects those proteins.

Table 2 Keratin Knockout Mice

Kzeratin	Predominant expression	Phenotype	Comment	Related human pathology	References
Kb4	Stratified, non-cornified epithelia	Mild cell fragility, acanthosis	Induction of Kb6 might compensate	White sponge nevus	161
Kb5	Basal epidermis	Extensive skin blistering, cytolysis of basal cells	No compensation; neonates die	Epidermolysis bullosa simplex	54
Kb5	Hair follicles and activated keratinocytes	None	Compensation by Kb10	Not known	93
Kb6/Kb10	Hair follicles and activated keratinocytes	Tongue lesions	Pups die before P10	Pachyonychia congenita	94
		Cell lysis upon migration during wound healing			95
		75% die within 2 weeks postnatally; 25% survive	Survivors show compensation by Kb18 in hair follicles and nails	Not known	148
Kb8	Simple epithelia	Embryonically lethal (E12.5), trophoblast giant cell fragility (C57/Bl6; 129X1/SvJ)	Strain dependent	Not known	119,122
		Colorectal hyperplasia, colitis, rectal prolapse, predisposition to liver injury (FVB/N)			118
Ka10	Suprabasal epidermis	Acanthosis, hyperproliferation of basal cells, hyperkeratosis	Compensation by Ka14	Non-epidermolytic hyperkeratosis	31,144
Ka12	Cornea	Cell fragility		Meesmann's corneal dystrophy	162

Ka14	Basal epidermis	Skin blistering, cytolysis of basal cells	Most neonates die within 3–4 days	Epidermolysis bullosa simplex	80
Ka17	Hair follicles, oesophagus, activated keratinocytes	Alopecia	Compensation by Ka14 and Ka16	Pachyonychia congenita	84
Ka18	Simple epithelia	Mild liver pathology		Not known	8
Ka19	Simple epithelia	None	Might be compensated by Ka18 and/or Ka20	Not known	117,163
Ka18/Ka19	Simple epithelia	Embryonic lethal (E9.5); trophoblast giant cell fragility		Not known	163
Kb8/Ka19	Simple epithelia	Embryonic lethal (E10); trophoblast/placental defect		Not known	117

Note: E, embryonic developmental day; P, postnatal developmental day; C57/Bl6, 129X1/SvJ and FVB/N are mouse strains.

In order to clarify whether embryonic development requires keratins, the combined deletion of Ka18/Ka19 or of Kb8/Ka19 was carried out. As Ka18 and Ka19 represent the only type I keratins during early development, no filaments should form in K18 and K19 null mice. In fact, all double-deficient mice died at E9.5–E10 from trophoblast fragility. The latter was accompanied by the deposition of Kb7/Kb8 aggregates in trophoblast cells, reminiscent of the deletion of the chaperone hsp40, which resulted in a similar keratin aggregate phenotype (121). At this time of development, the embryo proper appeared normal in the absence of keratin filaments. The pathology was interpreted by our laboratory as a result of mechanical fragility similar to keratinocyte fragility in EBS. Given the potential toxicity of Kb7/Kb8 aggregates in the Ka18/Ka19 double-deficient embryos, the precise function of keratins in development is still unclear and requires deletion of all embryonic keratin genes. Unfortunately, *Kb8* and *Ka18* genes are closely linked with less than 30 kb separating them, which precludes mating of available mice (10). Another interpretation for the trophoblast fragility and embryonic death was provided by Oshima and colleagues. They argued that the absence of keratin filaments rendered trophoblast giant cells more susceptible to maternal TNF, which would trigger an apoptotic response. This was based on the finding that Kb8 and Ka18 can moderate apoptosis by sequestering TNFR1 and TRADD (122). It appears that the protective role of Kb8 and Ka18 in apoptosis is independent of them being soluble, aggregated, or assembled into a cytoskeleton.

Stratified Epithelia

In basal epidermal keratinocytes, where keratins Kb5, Ka14, and Ka15 are co-expressed (19,54,80), keratin IF are organized in loose filament bundles. They are attached to hemidesmosomes via plectin and BPAG-1 (123–125) and to desmosomes via desmoplakin (126,127) and plakophilin (128,129). The interaction between keratin IF and junctional proteins, which is vital for cell integrity, is mediated most likely via the keratin rod domain (130). The strongly bundled Kb1/Ka10-containing IF are oriented parallel to the surface of flattened keratinocytes and are covalently cross-linked to cornified envelope (CE) proteins, predominantly through type II keratins (reviewed in Ref. 31). In support, Ka10 mutations that cause epidermolytic hyperkeratosis (EHK) do not affect CE integrity (132). The function of keratins in CE formation is not yet resolved and the most likely genetic alterations to affect CE integrity are those in Kb1. CE proteins of the plakin-type were originally considered as epidermis-restricted proteins. It is clear now that at least periplakin, envoplakin, and Macf2 are present in other tissues and associate with type I, II, and III IF proteins, which could help to investigate their interaction and regulation (133–136).

Three mouse models affecting basal epidermal keratinocytes showed cytolysis with slightly distinct phenotypes. Kb5$^{-/-}$ mice were most severely affected, as the complete absence of a basal keratin cytoskeleton resulted in cytolysis and the mice died immediately after birth (54). Although the majority of Ka14$^{-/-}$ mice exhibited generalized blistering of the skin accompanied by an increased mortality, some mice survived the first three months of life, possibly because of a partial compensation of the Ka14 loss by endogenous Ka15 (80). In contrast to Ka14$^{-/-}$ mice, Kb5$^{-/-}$ mice showed a strong induction of the wound-healing keratins Kb6 and Kb10 in the suprabasal epidermis of cytolysed areas. In embryonic Kb5 knockout mice, Kb8 is able to compensate for Kb5 until E14.5, the time at which Kb8 expression ceases (77a). This suggests that an "embryonic" type keratin might be able to replace an epidermal one, providing the use of an appropriate promoter.

Roop and co-workers utilized the Cre/lox recombination system to produce a mouse model for epidermolysis bullosa simplex in which the expression of a point mutation in codon 131 (equivalent to the "hotspot" mutation of R125 in human Ka14) in the mouse *Ka14* gene was spatially and temporally controlled (137). Upon expression of the mutant keratin, blister formation was initiated. When expression of the mutant was switched off, blistered areas healed and a normal epidermis continued to form, probably due to the migration of normal keratinocytes into the blister sites, where they gave rise to a new epithelium (137).

Targeted expression of dominant-negative forms of Ka10 produced skin lesions resembling severe forms of EHK (138,139). Moreover, those mice displayed changes in the composition of epidermal lipids and barrier function (140,141). Mice with an inducible Ka10 mutation (R154C, equivalent to R156C in the human) produced local blisters and scaling at the sites of induction. The blisters persisted later in life together with unaffected epidermis. This suggested that epidermal stem cells were targeted. In agreement with mosaic form of EHK in humans, which is due to post-zygotic somatic mutations, this shows that in the absence of selective pressure—the mutant Ka10 is silent in presumptive stem cells—mutant and wild-type stem cells can coexist. If considering therapy approaches of EHK, they must include either ablation or correction of mutant stem cells (142).

Unexpectedly, the generation of Ka10$^{-/-}$ mice revealed that K10 appeared not to be essential for the stability of the epidermis. This was probably due to the persistence of Kb5/Ka14 and the concomitant induction of Kb6, Kb10, and Ka16 IF in suprabasal keratinocytes. Together, these formed sufficient IF to maintain epidermal stability and integrity in the absence of Ka10 (31). Paramio et al. (143) have proposed a direct role for Ka10 in the suppression of cell proliferation. However, the analysis of Ka10$^{-/-}$ mice did not support their view. If Ka10 was directly involved in the regulation of cell proliferation, one would have expected an increase in suprabasal cell proliferation in K10 null mice. This was not observed, however. In adult animals, the lack of Ka10 led to a novel phenotype, characterized by a more than five-fold increase in basal cell proliferation, the induction of keratins Kb6, Kb10, Ka16, and Ka17, and a mild hyperkeratosis. Most remarkably, an induction of cyclin D1 and of c-myc in basal cells as well as that of the cell-cycle regulator 14-3-3sigma in post-mitotic keratinocytes was noted. The elevated expression of cyclin D1 and of c-myc in Ka10$^{-/-}$ mice was in agreement with an increase in wnt-4 mRNA (144). It is probably mediated by an increase in MAP kinase activity (103a). Most recently, we found that Ka10$^{-/-}$ mice treated with 7,12-dimethylbenz[a]anthracene (DMBA)/12-*O*-tetradecanoylphorbol-13-acetate (TPA) developed far less papillomas than wild-type mice. BrdU-labeling revealed a strongly accelerated keratinocyte turnover in Ka10$^{-/-}$ epidermis, suggesting an increased elimination of initiated keratinocytes at early stages of developing tumors. This was further supported by the absence of label-retaining cells 18 days after the pulse whereas in wild-type mice label-retaining cells were still present. The concomitant increase in keratins Kb6, Kb10, Ka16, and Ka17 in Ka10 null epidermis and the increased motility of keratinocytes is in agreement with the view that Ka10 and Kb1 render cells more stable and static (95).

The identification of Kb1 frameshift mutations in the dominant inherited skin disorder ichthyosis hystrix not only represented the first tail domain mutation causing disease but also indicated novel functions for this keratin (39,40,42). Due to the frameshift, the glycine-rich V$_2$ tail domain of Kb1 was shortened, and resulting IF were not bundled. It is notable that the distribution of the CE protein loricrin was altered. In contrast to its typical localization underneath the plasma membrane and around des-mosomes, where its incorporation into the cornified envelope may start (145), loricrin was irregularly distributed throughout the cytoplasm of keratinocytes. This observa-tion points to a novel and functionally important role of the Kb1 tail domain. It should be noted that the other two CE proteins, involucrin and filaggrin, were not altered in their distribution, arguing for the specificity of the Kb1–loricrin interaction.

Ka17 is predominantly expressed not only in epidermal appendages [(81,85) and references therein] but also in basal cells of stratified epithelia (Reichelt and Magin, unpublished, Fig. 2). It forms IF with Kb5 and any of the "K6 proteins" pre-sent (54,84,146). In humans, Ka17 mutations give rise to the nail disorder pachyony-chia congenita (PC) type 2 and to the sebaceous gland disorder steatocystoma multiplex (5,6). Ka17 null mice lacked a proper coat during the first postnatal week. The alopecia probably resulted from hair shaft fragility and apoptosis in hair matrix cells. This pathology reverted to normalcy along with the first postnatal hair cycle at three weeks of age. This was correlated with the upregulation of Ka16, able to form normal IF with type II keratins (84). Therefore, Ka16 can compensate for the absence of other keratins, as suggested before (147). The alopecia noted in Ka17 null animals was restricted to the mouse strain C57/Bl6. The unexpected lack of a nail pathology in Ka17 null mice was most recently explained by the expression of K17n (81), renamed Ka22 recently, which in humans is a pseudogene (10).

Of the nine "*K6*" genes expressed in mouse epidermis, its appendages and hair (10), *Kb6* and *Kb10* have been deleted. The majority of double-deficient mice died after birth, resulting from extensive cell fragility in oral mucosa (94,148). Mice sur-viving did so due to compensation by Kb18 (former K6hf) expressed in lingual epithelia, in a strain-dependent fashion (148). Extending their in vivo observations, Wong and Coulombe used a keratin explant assay to investigate the contribution of Kb6 and Kb10 in wound healing. Following thorough experimentation, they arrived at the conclusion that the lack of the above "K6 isoforms" rendered keratinocytes more motile, involving changes in actin organization. While this supports a more rapid wound healing, they also noted an increased fragility of Kb6/Kb10 null keratinocytes in cell culture and in vivo (95). They put forward the hypothesis that alterations in IF composition enable epithelial cells to adapt to environmental needs with a more pliable cytoskeleton in migrating and a more resilient one in stress-exposed, terminally differentiated keratinocytes. This view fits well with obser-vations from Ka10 null mice in which keratinocytes turn over much faster (103a,144).

Live Cell Imaging

Keratinopathies and keratin knockout mice have nourished the view that of all cytoskeletal systems, keratins represent static structures. Live cell imaging, using GFP-tagged wild-type and mutant keratins are recently beginning to reveal that keratins, like other cytoskeletal proteins, are highly dynamic. Given that all IF are non-polar due to the antiparallel arrangement of dimers, their assembly and intracel-lular re/organization must rely on microtubule- and actin-based mechanisms and the signal transduction pathways governing their organization. Unlike one might expect from the embryonic co-localization of keratin IF with desmosomes (50), photo-bleaching studies have revealed that the keratin–desmoplakin connection is very stable and most likely is not the site of keratin assembly (149). A present view from the analysis of stably transfected cells supports the concept that assembly and reorganization of keratin IF under steady state conditions starts close to the actin-enriched cell cortex. Here, <100 nm sized keratin particles form and are transported toward existing keratin IF in an actin- and microtubule-dependent mechanism (47,52). Remarkably, this transport is unilateral toward the cell center where the more stable keratin IF reside. Whether these particles are unit length filaments identified in vitro (2) cannot be answered at present owing to the limits of resolution. During their inward transport at speeds of ~100 nm/min, particles grow to short filaments by longitudinal bilateral annealing of subunits. Through their ends, they finally insert into or merge with existing IF (52). Particle growth appears to be regulated by phosphorylation (150) and could also involve associated proteins (for discussion, see Ref. 52). It is noted that EBS-type keratin mutations halt keratin assembly at the particle state (47). These particles aggregate but are highly dynamic. Small keratin particles are also present at low concentrations in normal cells and may represent soluble intermediates transported via microtubule-based mechanisms (151). Fluorescence recovery after photobleaching showed that keratin IF in the cell center recovered with $t_{1/2}$ of ~100 min (152). The same study showed that individual IF are able to move and bend, pointing toward a role for associated proteins and/or protein modification. In view of their propensity to assemble into IF in vitro, even at concentrations of 20 µg/ml, which is far below that of cells and tissues (2), it is surprising that keratins do not assemble everywhere in the cytoplasm. Where type I and type II subunits meet and what regulates their assembly remains a challenge for future investigations.

CONCLUSIONS AND PERSPECTIVES

Work by a number of groups has shown that there are more than 50 different keratins present in mammals (10,13,81,153,154). In a recent review, keratin functions were classified according to "hard" and "soft" principles. The "hard" principle of keratin function is to maintain epithelial integrity under conditions of mechanical stress (1). We predict that in those tissues in which gene deletions of individual keratins have not caused fragility, it will require the deletion of all keratins present in that particular cell type to reveal their role. This is supported by the comprehensive analysis on *C. elegans* IF proteins carried out in Klaus Weber's laboratory (155–157) and might lead to some surprises in mammals. Among the "hard" principles are: (i) The amount of keratins can vary from less than 0.1% to more than 50% of total protein per cell (158,159). (ii) The expression patterns of many keratins overlap. This can lead to various degrees of compensation in some, but not all cells (8,84,148). Very few cells (adult hepatocytes and enterocytes in the mouse) express only one keratin pair (19,78). (iii) Those keratin complexes analyzed have distinct stabilities and assembly properties in vitro (2,30,55,160). Taken together, these principles endow epithelial cells with distinct mechanical and other properties. Unfortunately, these have not been rigorously explored up to now, but cells cultured from knockout mice are beginning to support this principle. The "hard" question arises whether keratins have an important function only in those tissues, namely epidermis and trophoblasts, in which they are highly expressed and where gene ablations and disease mutations reveal this function.

The absence of cell fragility in mice or the presence of subtle pathological changes in patients carrying keratin gene mutations has been regarded as support for "soft" keratin principles, e.g., roles in signal transduction and participation in protein targeting. Clearly, genetic approaches in model organisms with shorter generation times than the mouse will resolve this issue.

At present, we have no concept of how the subcellular organization of keratin IF is regulated and organized to sustain mechanical stress. With respect to gene regulation and assembly, we are still lacking an understanding how regulation and assembly of keratin pairs in vivo are controlled.

The major challenge remains, whether individual keratins have distinct functions. Can embryonic development proceed with Kb5/Ka14 instead of Kb8/Ka18 IF? Would label-retaining cells and epidermal regeneration be different in the absence of Ka15 in those but not other cells? How much is cell migration and stress resilience affected if the keratin composition is altered? Answering these and additional issues will have a profound impact on epithelial biology.

ACKNOWLEDGMENTS

We thank Ursula Reuter for excellent technical assistance. Work in the authors laboratory is supported by the DFG, the BMBF, and the Thyssen foundation. We dedicate this work to Klaus Weber on the occasion of his 68th birthday. We apologize to those colleagues whose work has not been cited for space constraint.

REFERENCES

1. Coulombe PA, Omary MB. 'Hard' and 'soft' principles defining the structure, function and regulation of keratin intermediate filaments. Curr Opin Cell Biol 2002; 14: 110–122.
2. Herrmann H, Hesse M, Reichenzeller M, Aebi U, Magin TM. Functional complexity of intermediate filament cytoskeletons: from structure to assembly to gene ablation. Int Rev Cytol 2003; 223:83–175.
3. Omary MB, Ku NO, Liao J, Price D. Keratin modifications and solubility properties in epithelial cells and in vitro. Subcell Biochem 1998; 31:105–140.
4. Freedberg IM. Keratin: a journey of three decades. J Dermatol 1993; 20:321–328.
5. Irvine AD, McLean WH. Human keratin diseases: the increasing spectrum of disease and subtlety of the phenotype–genotype correlation. Br J Dermatol 1999; 140:815–828.
6. Smith F. The molecular genetics of keratin disorders. Am J Clin Dermatol 2003; 4: 347–364.
7. Kirfel J, Magin TM, Reichelt J. Keratins: a structural scaffold with emerging functions. Cell Mol Life Sci 2003; 60:56–71.
8. Magin TM, Schroder R, Leitgeb S, Wanninger F, Zatloukal K, Grund C, Melton DW. Lessons from keratin 18 knockout mice: formation of novel keratin filaments, secondary loss of keratin 7 and accumulation of liver-specific keratin 8-positive aggregates. J Cell Biol 1998; 140:1441–1451.
9. Hesse M, Magin TM, Weber K. Genes for intermediate filament proteins and the draft sequence of the human genome: novel keratin genes and a surprisingly high number of pseudogenes related to keratin genes 8 and 18. J Cell Sci 2001; 114:2569–2575.
10. Hesse M, Zimek A, Weber K, Magin TM. Comprehensive analysis of keratin gene clusters in humans and rodents. Eur J Cell Biol 2004; 83:19–26.
11. Langbein L, Rogers MA, Winter H, Praetzel S, Beckhaus U, Rackwitz HR, Schweizer J. The catalog of human hair keratins. I. Expression of the nine type I members in the hair follicle. J Biol Chem 1999; 274:19874–19884.

12. Langbein L, Rogers MA, Winter H, Praetzel S, Schweizer J. The catalog of human hair keratins. II. Expression of the six type II members in the hair follicle and the combined catalog of human type I and II keratins. J Biol Chem 2001; 276:35123–35132.

13. Porter RM, Gandhi M, Wilson NJ, Wood P, McLean WH, Lane EB. Functional analysis of keratin components in the mouse hair follicle inner root sheath. Br J Dermatol 2004; 150:195–204.

14. Waseem A, Gough AC, Spurr NK, Lane EB. Localization of the gene for human simple epithelial keratin 18 to chromosome 12 using polymerase chain reaction. Genomics 1990; 7:188–194.

15. Waterston RH, Lindblad-Toh K, Birney E, Rogers J, Abril JF, Agarwal P, Agarwala R, Ainscough R, Alexandersson M AnP, Antonarakis SE, et al. Initial sequencing and comparative analysis of the mouse genome. Nature 2002; 420:520–562.

16. Rogers MA, Langbein L, Winter H, Ehmann C, Praetzel S, Korn B, Schweizer J. Characterization of a cluster of human high/ultrahigh sulfur keratin-associated protein genes embedded in the type I keratin gene domain on chromosome 17q12–21. J Biol Chem 2001; 276:19440–19451.

17. Bawden CS, McLaughlan C, Nesci A, Rogers G. A unique type I keratin intermediate filament gene family is abundantly expressed in the inner root sheaths of sheep and human hair follicles. J Invest Dermatol 2001; 116:157–166.

18. Rogers MA, Langbein L, Winter H, Ehmann C, Praetzel S, Schweizer J. Characterization of a first domain of human high glycine–tyrosine and high sulfur keratin-associated protein (KAP) genes on chromosome 21q22.1. J Biol Chem 2002; 277: 48993–49002.

19. Moll R, Franke WW, Schiller DL, Geiger B, Krepler R. The catalog of human cytokeratins: patterns of expression in normal epithelia, tumors and cultured cells. Cell 1982; 31:11–24.

20. Rieger M, Franke WW. Identification of an orthologous mammalian cytokeratin gene. High degree of intron sequence conservation during evolution of human cytokeratin 10. J Mol Biol 1988; 204:841–856.

21. Mischke D. The complexity of gene families involved in epithewlial differentiation. Keratin genes and the epidermal differentiation complex. Subcell Biochem 1998; 31:71–104.

22. Herrmann H, Wedig T, Porter RM, Lane EB, Aebi U. Characterization of early assembly intermediates of recombinant human keratins. J Struct Biol 2002; 137:82–96.

23. Parry DA, Steinert PM. Intermediate filaments: molecular architecture, assembly, dynamics and polymorphism. Q Rev Biophys 1999; 32:99–187.

24. Weber K, Geisler N. Intermediate filaments: structural conservation and divergence. Ann NY Acad Sci 1985; 455:126–143.

25. Parry DA. Protein chains in hair and epidermal keratin IF: structural features and spatial arrangements. EXS 1997; 78:177–207.

26. Herrmann H, Strelkov SV, Feja B, Rogers KR, Brettel M, Lustig A, Haner M, Parry DA, Steinert PM, Burkhard P, et al. The intermediate filament protein consensus motif of helix 2B: its atomic structure and contribution to assembly. J Mol Biol 2000; 298:817–832.

27. Strelkov SV, Herrmann H, Geisler N, Wedig T, Zimbelmann R, Aebi U, Burkhard P. Conserved segments 1A and 2B of the intermediate filament dimer: their atomic structures and role in filament assembly. EMBO J 2002; 21:1255–1266.

28. Kammerer RA, Schulthess T, Landwehr R, Lustig A, Engel J, Aebi U, Steinmetz MO. An autonomous folding unit mediates the assembly of two-stranded coiled coils. Proc Natl Acad Sci USA 1998; 95:13419–13424.

29. Wu KC, Bryan JT, Morasso MI, Jang SI, Lee JH, Yang JM, Marekov LN, Parry DA, Steinert PM. Coiled-coil trigger motifs in the 1B and 2B rod domain segments are required for the stability of keratin intermediate filaments. Mol Biol Cell 2000; 11:3539–3558.

30. Hatzfeld M, Franke WW. Pair formation and promiscuity of cytokeratins: formation in vitro of heterotypic complexes and intermediate-sized filaments by homologous and heterologous recombinations of purified polypeptides. J Cell Biol 1985; 101: 1826–1841.

31. Reichelt J, Bussow H, Grund C, Magin TM. Formation of a normal epidermis supported by increased stability of keratins 5 and 14 in keratin 10 null mice. Mol Biol Cell 2001; 12:1557–1568.

32. Yamada S, Wirtz D, Coulombe PA. Pairwise assembly determines the intrinsic potential for self-organization and mechanical properties of keratin filaments. Mol Biol Cell 2002; 13:382–391.

33. Bader BL, Magin TM, Freudenmann M, Stumpp S, Franke WW. Intermediate filaments formed de novo from tail-less cytokeratins in the cytoplasm and in the nucleus. J Cell Biol 1991; 115:1293–1307.

34. Heins S, Wong PC, Muller S, Goldie K, Cleveland DW, Aebi U. The rod domain of NF-L determines neurofilament architecture, whereas the end domains specify filament assembly and network formation. J Cell Biol 1993; 123:1517–1533.

35. Bousquet O, Ma L, Yamada S, Gu C, Idei T, Takahashi K, Wirtz D, Coulombe PA. The nonhelical tail domain of keratin 14 promotes filament bundling and enhances the mechanical properties of keratin intermediate filaments in vitro. J Cell Biol 2001; 155:747–754.

36. Blessing M, Ruther U, Franke WW. Ectopic synthesis of epidermal cytokeratins in pancreatic islet cells of transgenic mice interferes with cytoskeletal order and insulin production. J Cell Biol 1993; 120:743–755.

37. Gu LH, Kim SC, Ichiki Y, Park J, Nagai M, Kitajima Y. A usual frameshift and delayed termination codon mutation in keratin 5 causes a novel type of epidermolysis bullosa simplex with migratory circinate erythema. J Invest Dermatol 2003; 121: 482–485.

38. Ishida-Yamamoto A, Richard G, Takahashi H, Iizuka H. In vivo studies of mutant keratin 1 in ichthyosis hystrix Curth-Macklin. J Invest Dermatol 2003; 120:498–500.

39. Sprecher E, Ishida-Yamamoto A, Becker OM, Marekov L, Miller CJ, Steinert PM, Neldner K, Richard G. Evidence for novel functions of the keratin tail emerging from a mutation causing ichthyosis hystrix. J Invest Dermatol 2001; 116:511–519.

40. Sprecher E, Yosipovitch G, Bergman R, Ciubutaro D, Indelman M, Pfendner E, Goh LC, Miller CJ, Uitto J, Richard G. Epidermolytic hyperkeratosis and epidermolysis bullosa simplex caused by frameshift mutations altering the v2 tail domains of keratin 1 and keratin 5. J Invest Dermatol 2003; 120:623–626.

41. Whittock NV, Ashton GH, Griffiths WA, Eady RA, McGrath JA. New mutations in keratin 1 that cause bullous congenital ichthyosiform erythroderma and keratin 2e that cause ichthyosis bullosa of Siemens. Br J Dermatol 2001; 145:330–335.

42. Whittock NV, Smith FJ, Wan H, Mallipeddi R, Griffiths WA, Dopping-Hepenstal P, Ashton GH, Eady RA, McLean WH, McGrath JA. Frameshift mutation in the V2 domain of human keratin 1 results in striate palmoplantar keratoderma. J Invest Dermatol 2002; 118:838–844.

43. Bonifas JM, Rothman AL, Epstein EH Jr. Epidermolysis bullosa simplex: evidence in two families for keratin gene abnormalities. Science 1991; 254:1202–1205.

44. Coulombe PA, Hutton ME, Letai A, Hebert A, Paller AS, Fuchs E. Point mutations in human keratin 14 genes of epidermolysis bullosa simplex patients: genetic and functional analyses. Cell 1991; 66:1301–1311.

45. Lane EB, Rugg EL, Navsaria H, Leigh IM, Heagerty AH, Ishida-Yamamoto A, Eady RA. A mutation in the conserved helix termination peptide of keratin 5 in hereditary skin blistering. Nature 1992; 356:244–246.

46. Ma L, Yamada S, Wirtz D, Coulombe PA. A 'hot-spot' mutation alters the mechanical properties of keratin filament networks. Nat Cell Biol 2002; 3:503–506.

47. Werner NS, Windoffer R, Strnad P, Grund C, Leube RE, Magin TM. Epidermolysis bullosa simplex-type mutations alter the dynamics of the keratin cytoskeleton and reveal a contribution of actin to the transport of keratin subunits. Mol Biol Cell 2004; 15:990–1002.

48. Bachant JB, Klymkowsky MW. A nontetrameric species is the major soluble form of keratin in Xenopus oocytes and rabbit reticulocyte lysates. J Cell Biol 1996; 132: 153–165.

49. Soellner P, Quinlan RA, Franke WW. Identification of a distinct soluble subunit of an intermediate filament protein: tetrameric vimentin from living cells. Proc Natl Acad Sci USA 1985; 82:7929–7933.

50. Jackson BW, Grund C, Schmid E, Burki K, Franke WW, Illmensee K. Formation of cytoskeletal elements during mouse embryogenesis. Intermeediate filaments of the cyto-keratin type and desmosomes in preimplantation embryos. Differentiation 1980; 17: 161–179.

51. Windoffer R, Leube RE. De novo formation of cytokeratin filament networks origi-nates from the cell cortex in A-431 cells. Cell Motil Cytoskeleton 2001; 50:33–44.

52. Windoffer R, Woll S, Strnad P, Leube RE. Identification of novel principles of keratin filament network turnover in living cells. Mol Biol Cell 2004; 15:2436–2448.

53. Kartasova T, Roop DR, Holbrook KA, Yuspa SH. Mouse differentiation-specific keratins 1 and 10 require a preexisting keratin scaffold to form a filament network. J Cell Biol 1993; 120:1251–1261.

54. Peters B, Kirfel J, Bussow H, Vidal M, Magin TM. Complete cytolysis and neonatal lethality in keratin 5 knockout mice reveal its fundamental role in skin integrity and in epidermolysis bullosa simplex. Mol Biol Cell 2001; 12:1775–1789.

55. FrankeWW, Schiller DL, Hatzfeld M, Winter S. Protein complexes of intermediate-sized filaments: melting of cytokeratin complexes in urea reveals different polypeptide separation characteristics. Proc Natl Acad Sci USA 1983; 80:7113–7117.

56. Ku NO, Liao J, Omary MB. Phosphorylation of human keratin 18 serine 33 regulates binding to 14-3-3 proteins. EMBO J 1998; 17:1892–1906.

57. Ku NO, Azhar S, Omary MB. Keratin 8 phosphorylation by p38 kinase regulates cellular keratin filament reorganization: modulation by a keratin 1-like disease causing mutation. J Biol Chem 2002; 277:10775–10782.

58. He T, Stepulak A, Holmstrom TH, Omary MB, Eriksson JE. The intermediate filament protein keratin 8 is a novel cytoplasmic substrate for c-Jun N-terminal kinase. J Biol Chem 2002; 277:10767–10774.

59. Goletz S, Hanisch FG, Karsten U. Novel alphaGalNAc containing glycans on cytoker-atins are recognized invitro by galectins with type II carbohydrate recognition domains. J Cell Sci 1997; 110(Pt 14):1585–1596.

60. Candi E, Tarcsa E, Digiovanna JJ, Compton JG, Elias PM, Marekov LN, Steinert PM. A highly conserved lysine residue on the head domain of type II keratins is essential for the attachment of keratin intermediate filaments to the cornified cell envelope through isopeptide crosslinking by transglutaminases. Proc Natl Acad Sci USA 1998; 95: 2067–2072.

61. Steinert PM, Marekov LN. The proteins elafin, filaggrin, keratin intermediate filaments, loricrin, and small proline-rich proteins 1 and 2 are isodipeptide cross-linked com-ponents of the human epidermal cornified cell envelope. J Biol Chem 1995; 270: 17702–17711.

62. Ishida-Yamamoto A, Takahashi H, Iizuka H. Lessons from disorders of epidermal differentiation-associated keratins. Histol Histopathol 2002; 17:331–338.

63. Moon RT, Lazarides E. Canavanine inhibits vimentin assembly but not its synthesis in chicken embryo erythroid cells. J Cell Biol 1983; 97:1309–1314.

64. Ku NO, Omary MB. Keratins turn over by ubiquitination in a phosphorylation-modulated fashion. J Cell Biol 2000; 149:547–552.

65. Yoneda K, Furukawa T, Zheng YJ, Momoi T, Izawa I, Inagaki M, Manabe M, Inagaki N. An autocrine/paracrine loop linking keratin 14 aggregates to tumor necrosis factor alpha-mediated cytotoxicity in a keratinocyte model of epidermolysis bullosa simplex. J Biol Chem 2004; 279:7296–7303.

66. Bence NF, Sampat RM, Kopito RR. Impairment of the ubiquitin–proteasome system by protein aggregation. Science 2001; 292:1552–1555.

67. Bader BL, Jahn L, Franke WW. Low level expression of cytokeratins 8, 18 and 19 in vascular smooth muscle cells of human umbilical cord and in cultured cells derived therefrom, with an analysis of the chromosomal locus containing the cytokeratin 19 gene. Eur J Cell Biol 1988; 47:300–319.

68. Neznanov N, Umezawa A, Oshima RG. A regulatory element within a coding exon modulates keratin 18 gene expression in transgenic mice. J Biol Chem 1997; 272: 27549–27557.

69. Oshima RG, Abrams L, Kulesh D. Activation of an intron enhancer within the keratin 18 gene by expression of c-fos and c-jun in undifferentiated F9 embryonal carcinoma cells. Genes Dev 1990; 4:835–848.

70. Oshima RG, Baribault H, Caulin C. Oncogenic regulation and function of keratins 8 and 18. Cancer Metastasis Rev 1996; 15:445–471.

71. Kaufman CK, Sinha S, Bolotin D, Fan J, Fuchs E. Dissection of a complex enhancer element: maintenance of keratinocyte specificity but loss of differentiation specificity. Mol Cell Biol 2002; 22:4293–4308.

72. Sinha S, Degenstein L, Copenhaver C, Fuchs E. Defining the regulatory factors required for epidermal gene expression. Mol Cell Biol 2000; 20:2543–2555.

73. Sugihara TM, Kudryavtseva EI, Kumar V, Horridge JJ, Andersen B. The POU domain factor Skin-1a represses the keratin 14 promoter independent of DNA binding. A possible role for interactions between Skn-1a and CREB-binding protein/p300. J Biol Chem 2001; 276:33036–33044.

74. Magin TM. Lessons from keratin transgenic and knockout mice. Subcell Biochem 1998; 31:141–172.

75. Wakabayashi N, Itoh K, Wakabayashi J, Motohashi H, Noda S, Takahashi S, Imakado S, Kotsuji T, Otsuka F, Roop DR, et al. Keap1-null mutation leads to post-natal lethality due to constitutive Nrf2 activation. Nat Genet 2003; 35:238–245.

76. Jave-Suarez LF, Winter H, Langbein L, Rogers MA, Schweizer J. HOXC13 is involved in the regulation of human hair keratin gene expression. J Biol Chem 2002; 277: 3718–3726.

77. Jave-Suarez LF, Langbein L, Winter H, Praetzel S, Rogers MA, Schweizer J. Androgen regulation of the human hair follicle: the type I hair keratin hHa7 is a direct target gene in trichocytes. J Invest Dermatol 2004; 122:555–564.

77a. Lu H, Hesse M, Peters B, Magin TM. Type II keratins precede type I keratins during early embryonic development. Eur J Cell Biol. In press.

78. Ameen NA, Figueroa Y, Salas PJ. Anomalous apical plasma membrane phenotype in CK8-deficient mice indicates a novel role for intermediate filaments in the polarization of simple epithelia. J Cell Sci 2001; 114:563–575.

79. Zhang JS, Wang L, Huang H, Nelson M, Smith DI. Keratin 23 (K23), a novel acidic keratin, is highly induced by histone deacetylase inhibitors during differentiation of pancreatic cancer cells. Genes Chromosomes Cancer 2001; 30:123–135.

80. Lloyd C, Yu QC, Cheng J, Turksen K, Degenstein L, Hutton E, Fuchs E. The basal keratin network of stratified squamous epithelia: defining K15 function in the absence of K14. J Cell Biol 1995; 129:1329–1344.

81. Tong X, Coulombe PA. A novel mouse type I intermediate filament gene, keratin 17n (k17n), exhibits preferred expression in nail tissue. J Invest Dermatol 2004; 122: 965–970.

82. Waseem A, Dogan B, Tidman N, Alam Y, Purkis P, Jackson S, Lalli A, Machesney M, Leigh IM. Keratin 15 expression in stratified epithelia: downregulation in activated keratinocytes. J Invest Dermatol 1999; 112:362–369.
83. McGowan KM, Coulombe PA. Keratin 17 expression in the hard epithelial context of the hair and nail, and its relevance for the pachyonychia congenita phenotype. J Invest Dermatol 2000; 114:1101–1107.
84. McGowan KM, Tong X, Colucci-Guyon E, Langa F, Babinet C, Coulombe PA. Keratin 17 null mice exhibit age- and strain-dependent alopecia. Genes Dev 2002; 16: 1412–1422.
85. McGowan KM, Coulombe PA. Onset of keratin 17 expression coincides with the definition of major epithelial lineages during skin development. J Cell Biol 1998; 143:469–486.
86. Freedberg IM, Tomic-Canic M, Komine M, Blumenberg M. Keratins and the keratinocyte activation cycle. J Invest Dermatol 2001; 116:633–640.
87. Panteleyev AA, Paus R, Wanner R, Nurnberg W, Eichmuller S, Thiel R, Zhang J, Henz BM, Rosenbach T. Keratin 17 gene expression during the murine hair cycle. J Invest Dermatol 1997; 108:324–329.
88. Troyanovsky SM, Leube RE, Franke WW. Characterization of the human gene encoding cytokeratin 17 and its expression pattern. Eur J Cell Biol 1992; 59:127–137.
89. Swensson O, Langbein L, McMillan JR, Stevens HP, Leigh IM, McLean WH, Lane EB, Eady RA. Specialized keratin expression pattern in human ridged skin as an adaptation to high physical stress. Br J Dermatol 1998; 139:767–775.
90. Herzog F, Winter H, Schweizer J. The large type II 70-kDa keratin of mouse epidermis is the ortholog of human keratin K2e. J Invest Dermatol 1994; 102:165–170.
91. Collin C, Ouhayoun JP, Grund C, Franke WW. Suprabasal marker proteins distinguishing keratinizing squamous epithelia: cytokeratin 2 polypeptides of oral masticatory epithelium and epidermis are different. Differentiation 1992; 51:137–148.
92. Kasper M. Patterns of cytokeratins and vimentin in guinea pig and mouse eye tissue: evidence for regional variations in intermediate filament expression in limbal epithelium. Acta Histochem 1992; 93:319–332.
93. Wojcik SM, Bundman DS, Roop DR. Delayed wound healing in keratin 6a knockout mice. Mol Cell Biol 2000; 20:5248–5255.
94. Wong P, Colucci-Guyon E, Takahashi K, Gu C, Babinet C, Coulombe PA. Introducing a null mutation in the mouse K6alpha and K6beta genes reveals their essential structural role in the oral mucosa. J Cell Biol 2000; 150:921–928.
95. Wong P, Coulombe PA. Loss of keratin 6 (K6) proteins reveals a function for intermediate filaments during wound repair. J Cell Biol 2003; 163:327–337.
96. Brock J, McCluskey J, Baribault H, Martin P. Perfect wound healing in the keratin 8 deficient mouse embryo. Cell Motil Cytoskeleton 1996; 35:358–366.
97. Ouellet T, Lussier M, Babai F, Lapointe L, Royal A. Differential expression of the epidermal K1 and K10 keratin genes during mouse embryo development. Biochem Cell Biol 1990; 68:448–453.
98. Ouellet T, Lussier M, Belanger C, Kessous A, Royal A. Differential expression of keratin genes during mouse development. Dev Biol 1986; 113:282–287.
99. Mazzalupo S, Wong P, Martin P, Coulombe PA. Role for keratins 6 and 17 during wound closure in embryonic mouse skin. Dev Dyn 2003; 226:356–365.
100. Leube RE, Bader BL, Bosch FX, Zimbelmann R, Achtstaetter T, Franke WW. Molecular characterization and expression of the stratification-related cytokeratins 4 and 15. J Cell Biol 1988; 106:1249–1261.
101. Porter RM, Lunny DP, Ogden PH, Morley SM, McLean WH, Evans A, Harrison DL, Rugg EL, Lane EB. K15 expression implies lateral differentiation within stratified epithelial basal cells. Lab Invest 2000; 80:1701–1710.
102. Liu Y, Lyle S, Yang Z, Cotsarelis G. Keratin 15 promoter targets putative epithelial stem cells in the hair follicle bulge. J Invest Dermatol 2003; 121:963–968.

103. Morris RJ, Liu Y, Marles L, Yang Z, Trempus C, Li S, Lin JS, Sawicki JA, Cotsarelis G. Capturing and profiling adult hair follicle stem cells. Nat Biotechnol 2004; 22:411–417.

103a. Reichelt J, Furstenberger G, Magin TM. Loss of keratine 10 leads to mitogen-activated protein kinase (MAPK) activation, increased keratinocyte turnover, and decreased tumor formation in mice. J Invest Dermatol 2004; 123:973–981.

104. Corden LD, McLean WH. Human keratin diseases: hereditary fragility of specific epithelial tissues. Exp Dermatol 1996; 5:297–307.

105. Fuchs E, Cleveland DW. A structural scaffolding of intermediate filaments in health and disease. Science 1998; 279:514–519.

106. Irvine AD, McLean WH. The molecular genetics of the genodermatoses: progress to date and future directions. Br J Dermatol 2003; 148:1–13.

107. D'Alessandro M, Russell D, Morley SM, Davies AM, Lane EB. Keratin mutations of epidermolysis bullosa simplex alter the kinetics of stress response to osmotic shock. J Cell Sci 2002; 115:4341–4351.

108. Ku NO, Wright TL, Terrault NA, Gish R, Omary MB. Mutation of human keratin 18 in association with cryptogenic cirrhosis. J Clin Invest 1997; 99:19–23.

109. Ku NO, Gish R, Wright TL, Omary MB. Keratin 8 mutations in patients with cryptogenic liver disease. N Engl J Med 2001; 344:1580–1587.

110. Ku NO, Darling JM, Krams SM, Esquivel CO, Keeffe EB, Sibley RK, Lee YM, Wright TL, Omary MB. Keratin 8 and 18 mutations are risk factors for developing liver disease of multiple etiologies. Proc Natl Acad Sci USA 2003; 100:6063–6068.

110a. Halangk J, Berg T, Pulh G, Mueller T, Nickel R, Kage A, Landt O, Luck W, Wiedenmann B, Neuhaus P, Witt H. Keratin 8 Y54H and G62C mutations are not associated with liver disease. J Med Genet 2004; 41:e92–94.

111. Cavestro GM, Frulloni L, Nouvenne A, Neri TM, Calore B, Ferri B, Bovo P, Okolicsanyi L, Di Mario F, Cavallini G. Association of keratin 8 gene mutation with chronic pancreatitis. Dig Liver Dis 2003; 35:416–420.

112. Owens DW, Wilson NJ, Hill AJ, Rugg EL, Porter RM, Hutcheson AM, Quinlan RA, Van Heel D, Parkes M, Jewell DP, et al. Human keratin 8 mutations that disturb filament assembly observed in inflammatory bowel disease patients. J Cell Sci 2004; 117:1989–1999.

112a. Hesse M, Berg T, Wiedenmann B, Spengler U, Woitas RP, Magin TM. A frequent keratine 8p. L227L polymorphism, but no point mutations in keratine 8 and 18 genes, in patients with various livers disorders. J Med Genet 2004; 41:e42–45.

113. Caulin C, Salvesen GS, Oshima RG. Caspase cleavage of keratin 18 and reorganization of intermediate filaments during epithelial cell apoptosis. J Cell Biol 1997; 138:1379–1394.

114. Inada H, Izawa I, Nishizawa M, Fujita E, Kiyono T, Takahashi T, Momoi T, Inagaki M. Keratin attenuates tumor necrosis factor-induced cytotoxicity through association with TRADD. J Cell Biol 2001; 155:415–426.

115. Gilbert S, Loranger A, Daigle N, Marceau N. Simple epithelium keratins 8 and 18 provide resistance to Fas-mediated apoptosis. The protection occurs through a receptor-targeting modulation. J Cell Biol 2001; 154:763–773.

115a. Oshima RG. Apoptosis and keratine intermediate filaments. Cell Death Differ 2002; 9:486–492.

116. Magin TM, Kaiser HW, Leitgeb S, Grund C, Leigh IM, Morley SM, Lane EB. Supplementation of a mutant keratin by stable expression of desmin in cultured human EBS keratinocytes. J Cell Sci 2000; 113 Pt 23:4231–4239.

117. Tamai Y, Ishikawa T, Bosl MR, Mori M, Nozaki M, Baribault H, Oshima RG, Taketo MM. Cytokeratins 8 and 19 in the mouse placental development. J Cell Biol 2000; 151:563–572.

118. Baribault H, Penner J, Iozzo RV, Wilson-Heiner M. Colorectal hyperplasia and inflammation in keratin 8-deficient FVB/N mice. Genes Dev 1994; 8:2964–2973.

119. Baribault H, Price J, Miyai K, Oshima RG. Mid-gestational lethality in mice lacking keratin 8. Genes Dev 1993; 7:1191–1202.

120. Toivola DM, Krishnan S, Binder HJ, Singh SK, Omary MB. Keratins modulate colonocyte electrolyte transport via protein mistargeting. J Cell Biol 2004; 164: 911–921.

121. Izawa I, Nishizawa M, Ohtakara K, Ohtsuka K, Inada H, Inagaki M. Identification of Mrj, a DnaJ/Hsp40 family protein, as a keratin 8/18 filament regulatory protein. J Biol Chem 2000; 275:34521–34527.

122. Jaquemar D, Kupriyanov S, Wankell M, Avis J, Benirschke K, Baribault H, Oshima RG. Keratin 8 protection of placental barrier function. J Cell Biol 2003; 161: 749–756.

123. Andra K, Lassmann H, Bittner R, Shorny S, Fassler R, Propst F, Wiche G. Targeted inactivation of plectin reveals essential function in maintaining the integrity of skin, muscle, and heart cytoarchitecture. Genes Dev 1997; 11:3143–3156.

124. Geerts D, Fontao L, Nievers MG, Schaapveld RQ, Purkis PE, Wheeler GN, Lane EB, Leigh IM, Sonnenberg A. Binding of integrin alpha6beta4 to plectin prevents plectin association with F-actin but does not interfere with intermediate filament binding. J Cell Biol 1999; 147:417–434.

125. Guo L, Degenstein L, Dowling J, Yu QC, Wollmann R, Perman B, Fuchs E. Gene targeting of BPAG1: abnormalities in mechanical strength and cell migration in stratified epithelia and neurologic degeneration. Cell 1995; 81:233–243.

126. Kowalczyk AP, Bornslaeger EA, Norvell SM, Palka HL, Green KJ. Desmosomes: intercellular adhesive junctions specialized for attachment of intermediate filaments. Int Rev Cytol 1999; 185:237–302.

127. Stappenbeck TS, Green KJ. The desmoplakin carboxyl terminus coaligns with and specifically disrupts intermediate filament networks when expressed in cultured cells. J Cell Biol 1992; 116:1197–1209.

128. McGrath JA, McMillan JR, Shemanko CS, Runswick SK, Leigh IM, Lane EB, Garrod DR, Eady RA. Mutations in the plakophilin 1 gene result in ectodermal dysplasia/skin fragility syndrome. Nat Genet 1997; 17:240–244.

129. Smith EA, Fuchs E. Defining the interactions between intermediate filaments and desmosomes. J Cell Biol 1998; 141:1229–1241.

130. Fontao L, Favre B, Riou S, Geerts D, Jaunin F, Saurat JH, Green KJ, Sonnenberg A, Borradori L. Interaction of the bullous pemphigoid antigen 1 (BP230) and desmoplakin with intermediate filaments is mediated by distinct sequences within their COOH terminus. Mol Biol Cell 2003; 14:1978–1992.

131. Steinert PM, Marekov LN. Initiation of assembly of the cell envelope barrier structure of stratified squamous epithelia. Mol Biol Cell 1999; 10:4247–4261.

132. Akiyama M, Takizawa Y, Sawamura D, Matsuo I, Shimizu H. Disruption of the suprabasal keratin network by mutation M150T in the helix initiation motif of keratin 10 does not affect cornified cell envelope formation in human epidermis. Exp Dermatol 2003; 12:638–645.

133. Aho S. Many faces of periplakin: domain-specific antibodies detect the protein throughout the epidermis, explaining the multiple protein-protein interactions. Cell Tissue Res 2004; 316:87–97.

134. Karashima T, Watt FM. Interaction of periplakin and envoplakin with intermediate filaments. J Cell Sci 2002; 115:5027–5037.

135. Leonova EV, Lomax MI. Expression of the mouse Macf2 gene during inner ear development. Brain Res Mol Brain Res 2002; 105:67–78.

136. Leung CL, Green KJ, Liem RK. Plakins: a family of versatile cytolinker proteins. Trends Cell Biol 2002; 12:37–45.

137. Cao T, Longley MA, Wang XJ, Roop DR. An inducible mouse model for epidermolysis bullosa simplex: implications for gene therapy. J Cell Biol 2001; 152:651–656.

138. Porter RM, Leitgeb S, Melton DW, Swensson O, Eady RA, Magin TM. Gene targeting at the mouse cytokeratin 10 locus: severe skin fragility and changes of cytokeratin expression in the epidermis. J Cell Biol 1996; 132:925–936.

139. Reichelt J, Bauer C, Porter R, Lane E, Magin V. Out of balance: consequences of a partial keratin 10 knockout. J Cell Sci 1997; 110(Pt 18):2175–2186.

140. Elias P, Man MQ, Williams ML, Feingold KR, Magin T. Barrier function in K-10 heterozygote knockout mice. J Invest Dermatol 2000; 114:396–397.

141. Reichelt J, Doering T, Schnetz E, Fartasch M, Sandhoff K, Magin AM. Normal ultra-structure, but altered stratum corneum lipid and protein composition in a mouse model for epidermolytic hyperkeratosis. J Invest Dermatol 1999; 113:329–334.

142. Arin MJ, Longley MA, Wang XJ, Roop DR. Focal activation of a mutant allele defines the role of stem cells in mosaic skin disorders. J Cell Biol 2001; 152:645–649.

143. Paramio JM, Casanova ML, Segrelles C, Mittnacht S, Lane EB, Jorcano JL. Modula-tion of cell proliferation by cytokeratins K10 and K16. Mol Cell Biol 1999; 19:3086–3094.

144. Reichelt J, Magin TM. Hyperproliferation, induction of c-Myc and 14-3-3sigma, but no cell fragility in keratin-10-null mice. J Cell Sci 2002; 115:2639–2650.

145. Kalinin A, Marekov LN, Steinert PM. Assembly of the epidermal cornified cell envelope. J Cell Sci 2001; 114:3069–3070.

146. Troy TC, Turksen K. In vitro characteristics of early epidermal progenitors isolated from keratin 14 (K14)-deficient mice: insights into the role of keratin 17 in mouse keratinocytes. J Cell Physiol 1999; 180:409–421.

147. Porter RM, Hutcheson AM, Rugg EL, Quinlan RA, Lane EB. cDNA cloning, expres-sion, and assembly characteristics of mouse keratin 16. J Biol Chem 1998; 273:32265–32272.

148. Wojcik SM, Longley MA, Roop DR. Discovery of a novel murine keratin 6 (K6) isoform explains the absence of hair and nail defects in mice deficient for K6a and K6b. J Cell Biol 2001; 154:619–630.

149. Windoffer R, Borchert-Stuhltrager M, Leube RE. Desmosomes: interconnected calcium-dependent structures of remarkable stability with significant integral membrane protein turnover. J Cell Sci 2002; 115:1717–1732.

150. Strnad P, Windoffer R, Leube RE. In vivo detection of cytokeratin filament network breakdown in cells treated with the phosphatase inhibitor okadaic acid. Cell Tissue Res 2001; 306:277–293.

151. Liovic M, Mogensen MM, Prescott AR, Lane EB. Observation of keratin particles showing fast bidirectional movement colocalized with microtubules. J Cell Sci 2003; 116:1417–1427.

152. Yoon KH, Yoon M, Moir RD, Khuon S, Flitney FW, Goldman RD. Insights into the dynamic properties of keratin intermediate filaments in living epithelial cells. J Cell Biol 2001; 153:503–516.

153. Rogers MA, Winter H, Wolf C, Heck M, Schweizer J. Characterization of a 190-kilobase pair domain of human type I hair keratin genes. J Biol Chem 1998; 273:26683–26691.

154. Rogers MA, Winter H, Langbein L, Wolf C, Schweizer J. Characterization of a 300 kbp region of human DNA containing the type II hair keratin gene domain. J Invest Dermatol 2000; 114:464–472.

155. Karabinos A, Wang J, Wenzel D, Panopoulou G, Lehrach H, Weber K. Developmen-tally controlled expression patterns of intermediate filament proteins in the cephalo-chordate Branchiostoma. Mech Dev 2001; 101:283–288.

156. Karabinos A, Schulze E, Schunemann J, Parry DA, Weber K. In vivo and in vitro evidence that the four essential intermediate filament (IF) proteins A1, A2, A3 and B1 of the nematode Caenorhabditis elegans form an obligate heteropolymeric IF system. J Mol Biol 2003; 333:307–319.

157. Karabinos A, Schunemann J, Meyer M, Aebi U, Weber K. The single nuclear lamin of Caenorhabditis elegans forms in vitro stable intermediate filaments and paracrystals with a reduced axial periodicity. J Mol Biol 2003; 325:241–247.

158. Fuchs E, Green H. Changes in keratin gene expression during terminal differentiation of the keratinocyte. Cell 1980; 19:1033–1042.

159. Zhong B, Zhou Q, Toivola DM, Tao GZ, Resurreccion EZ, Omary MB. Organ-specific stress induces mouse pancreatic keratin overexpression in association with NF-[kappa]B activation. J Cell Sci 2004; 117:1709–1719.

160. Hofmann I, Franke WW. Heterotypic interactions and filament assembly of type I and type II cytokeratins in vitro: viscometry and determinations of relative affinities. Eur J Cell Biol 1997; 72:122–132.

161. Ness SL, Edelmann W, Jenkins TD, Liedtke W, Rustgi AK, Kucherlapati R. Mouse keratin 4 is necessary for internal epithelial integrity. J Biol Chem 1998; 273: 23904–23911.

162. Kao WW, Liu CY, Converse RL, Shiraishi A, Kao CW, Ishizaki M, Doetschman T, Duffy J. Keratin 12-deficient mice have fragile corneal epithelia. Invest Ophthalmol Vis Sci 1996; 37:2572–2584.

163. Hesse M, Franz T, Tamai Y, Taketo MM, Magin TM. Targeted deletion of keratins 18 and 19 leads to trophoblast fragility and early embryonic lethality. EMBO J 2000; 19:5060–5070.

11

Corneodesmosomes: Pivotal Actors in the Stratum Corneum Cohesion and Desquamation

Marek Haftek
Department of Dermatology, Hôpital E. Herriot, Université Lyon I, Lyon, France

Michel Simon and Guy Serre
Différenciation Épidermique et Autoimmunité Rhumatoïde, CNRS-UPS UMR5165, Toulouse, France

STRUCTURAL ASPECTS

Cell–Cell Junctions in the Human Epidermis

One of the fundamental functions of epithelial tissues, such as the epidermis, is separation and thus protection of the underlying tissues from the potentially hostile "environment." To assist in such a role, a sophisticated network of cell–cell junctions has been developed by the epidermal cells, keeping them close together and coordinating their behavior. Intercellular junctions are classically subdivided into (i) communication junctions, allowing direct connection between cytosols of adjacent interacting cells; (ii) mechanical junctions, establishing intercellular connections stabilized by actin or keratin cytoskeletons; and (iii) tight junctions, which seal off paracellular transport within the epithelia. Regardless of the primary function of any type of junction, all the cell–cell contacts are involved in some sort of transmission or perception of the information which helps each cell to "keep in touch" with the others, within the same epithelium, both literally and metaphorically.

The specialized communication junctions are commonly called "gap" junctions and are involved in "electrical coupling" of the cells. They are formed by an array of transmembrane half-channels, called connexons, elaborated by each cell, which connect across the extracellular spaces with homologous structures on neighboring cells, thereby forming a continuous channel for the passage of small molecules. The connexons meet at a distance that results in minute spacing between the aligned cell membranes. This gap of approximately 2 to 4 nm can be visualized on standard electron microscopic examination with appropriate counterstaining. Each connexon is composed of six proteins called connexins, which span the cell membrane four times and keep both N- and C-terminals in the cytosol. The cells are able to regulate the flow of ions and small cytosolic molecules up to 1 kDa by opening and closing the connexons. This results in a very interactive and extremely rapid form of communication.

The overall structural design of the remaining types of cell–cell junctions is based on the common sequence of transmembrane proteins that interact within the intercellular space and connect to the cytoskeleton through a series of intracellular molecules. Tight junctions, which play a crucial role in non-stratified epithelia by sealing the intercellular spaces between the apical portions of the cells lining body lumens, e.g., in the jejunum, are described in detail elsewhere in this book.

The "mechanical" junctions, involved primarily in cell cohesion, can be most expeditiously subdivided into those connected to the actin microfilament network and those interacting with keratin intermediate filaments. Both families express variants involved in the attachment of keratinocytes to the basement membrane, i.e., focal adhesions and hemidesmosomes, respectively, as well as junctions riveting adjacent cells together, i.e., adherens junctions and desmosomes. Epidermal actin-associated adherens junctions are composed of classic transmembrane cadherins which first establish labile interactions between keratinocytes entering into physical contact. Subsequent stacking of additional cadherin molecules at the site of contact reinforces attachment, and the intracellular portions of the proteins become stabilized by intracellular elements called catenins α, β, and γ. The whole intracellular cadherin–catenin complex is subject to phosphorylation, which modulates its susceptibility to bind F-actin filaments via vinculin and β-actinin, and which may influence the conformation of the extracellular portions of cadherins. Sequestration of β-catenin at the cell periphery, by binding to E-cadherin involved in cell–cell adhesion, prevents its translocation to the nucleus. When the latter occurs, as in some junction-deficient cancer cells, β-catenin signals cell proliferation. This example illustrates eloquently the manner in which the structural components of intercellular junctions can also function as signaling molecules. Extracellular calcium is also necessary for the adequate conformation of the extracellular parts of cadherins. In its absence, the formation of cadherin-mediated cell–cell junctions is compromised. In human epidermis, adherens junctions can be visualized using immunocytochemistry. Their morphological appearance being inconspicuous under standard electron microscopy investigation, it is the focal expression of β-catenin on both sides of alignments of keratinocyte membranes which allowed the confirmation of the existence of such interkeratinocyte junctions. Interestingly, structures of the adherens junction type are most frequently observed at the periphery of desmosomes or in their close vicinity, suggesting that the dynamically formed adherens junctions may serve as a template for establishing more stable and physically stronger desmosome structures. This assumption is also supported by the fact that plakoglobin, a desmosomal plaque protein identical to γ-catenin and binding to the intracellular portions of desmosomal cadherins, desmocollins, and desmogleins, can also be found in adherens junctions, where it uses the same binding sites for interactions with E-cadherin and α-catenin (1). Interestingly, desmogleins are able to bind to plakoglobin with a much higher affinity than E-cadherin does. Reciprocal steric hindrance may thus be a mechanism leading to the segregation of protein complexes typical for one or other type of junction. In the adherens junction, plakoglobin may compete with β-catenin for association with E-cadherin, as they are highly homologous (66% identity). The transfer of plakoglobin molecules from the classical to desmosomal cadherins, if it really occurs, could be involved in the recruitment of the latter into the pre-existing adherens junctions and, additionally, it would be susceptible to influencing cell signaling through the modulation of cytosolic and perhaps nuclear pools of β-catenin and plakoglobin.

The number and composition of cell–cell junctions change during epidermal differentiation. Although the basic molecular composition of the various types of junctions is already known, it must be kept in mind that the list is probably not yet closed, that the exact set of interacting molecules may depend on the actual functional state of a cell, and that the simple presence of a given protein at the cell periphery by no means signifies the existence of a fully functional cell–cell junction.

Desmosomes

A particular type of "mechanical" junction, the desmosome, is the most distinctive junctional structure in the epidermis (2). It is a symmetrical structure built according to the same scheme as the adherens junction. Desmosomal cadherins, desmocollins and desmogleins, occupy the central, intercellular part of the junction. It has been demonstrated that desmocollin 1 and desmoglein 2 expressed on adjacent cells may form stable heterodimers, but it is not clear yet whether such molecules undergo lateral dimerization at the cell surface, as is the case for classical cadherins. The intracellular portions of the cadherins interact with plakoglobin and desmoplakins, which in turn mediate the association of the junctions with the keratin bundles. Several other plakins, desmocalmin, and pinin are also present in these intermediate, button-like structures called desmosomal plaques, but their precise function is not yet fully understood. Desmosomes join the individual cytoskeletons of epidermal keratinocytes into a tissue-wide suprastructure that is quite resistant physically, yet sufficiently flexible to allow adaptive responses. During the process of epidermal differentiation, the number, size, and composition of desmosomes change considerably. In the basal layer of human epidermis, desmosomes are large but not numerous. Their number increases very significantly in the lower spinous cell layers. In the upper layers of the stratum spinosum, desmosomes appear to slightly diminish in number and show a significant reduction in size (3). This situation stabilizes in the upper epidermal layers where desmosomes begin to be cross-linked within the newly forming cornified envelopes.

Constant formation and withdrawal of desmosomes is required to allow the keratinocytes to change their shape while they move from the basal to the horny layer. Two different mechanisms of desmosome recycling are currently being studied. One relies on the internalization of the entire symmetric desmosomal structures, and the other on the removal from the cell surface of half-desmosomes subsequent to their dissociation along the extracellular middle line. Both mechanisms are apparently possible, depending on the physiological or pathological stimulus leading to desmosome removal or replacement and on the state of differentiation of the responding keratinocyte. As cornified envelopes arise beneath the cell membranes of keratinocytes in the upper spinous and granular layers, the cross-linking of proteins, mediated by transglutaminase 1, immobilizes structures present at the cell periphery. Therefore, desmosome turnover is partially reduced in terminally differentiating keratinocytes, and then stops at the upper faces of the granular layer keratinocytes, just before their transition to the horny layer.

Partial autolysis of keratinocytes during cornification results in cell collapse and flattening. It is associated with extensive convolution of the cell outline, especially at the periphery of the corneocyte "discs," due to the persistence of solid desmosomal attachments maintaining association with rigidified keratin bundles.

Corneodesmosomes: Specialized and Reorganized Desmosomes of the Stratum Corneum

Unlike the "living" part of the epidermis, the corneocytes of the stratum corneum (SC) are no longer able to synthesize new proteins or build new cellular structures. However, several dynamic processes continue or even start to occur in the horny layer, due to the presence of numerous enzymes and their substrates produced before the cornification. The extent of the changes and their speed are autoregulated and rather constant under physiological conditions, but the environment still has some influence, e.g., through modification of the SC hydration or a rupture of the SC barrier with the subsequent repair-related changes (see other chapters in this volume).

As observed in standard electron microscopy, the morphology of desmosomes changes dramatically during the transition from the stratum granulosum (SG) to the SC (Fig. 1). The intercellular portion of the junction loses its electron-dense central band flanked by symmetric light bands and becomes homogeneous, whereas the intracellular plaque becomes embedded within the cross-linked cornified envelope. Products resulting from proteolysis and from the dispersion of keratohyalin granules fill the interior of corneocytes tightly and make the remnants of the keratin cytoskeleton disappear, so even the points of insertion of keratin bundles into desmosomal plaques become invisible.

Such a drastic modification of the desmosome structure once made the desmosomal "plugs" between corneocytes to be considered as non-functional remnants.

However, several, more recent lines of evidence lead to a quite different conclusion. In particular, it has been observed that cohesion of the SC in the pig skin

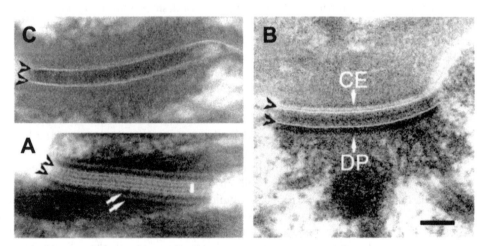

Figure 1 Comparison of the ultrastructure of a spinous layer desmosome (A) and a corneodesmosome (C). Transition from the granular to the horny layer is shown in (B) with a corneodesmosome showing asymmetrical intracellular features. Arrowheads point to the cell membranes or lipid cell envelopes in the living and cornified keratinocytes, respectively. White arrows in (A) point to the internal and external desmosomal plaques, the latter being associated with keratin filaments. The white rectangle spans the extracellular portion of the junction—the desmosome core. The junctions have been photographed in uranyl acetate–counterstained sections of a normal human epidermis embedded at −35°C in an acrylic resin after 3% paraformaldehyde fixation. Bar 100 nm. *Abbreviations*: DP, desmosomal plaque; CE, protein cell envelope.

depends on the number of modified desmosomes present, and that desquamation can be induced by proteolysis which leads to desmosome degradation (4,5). In fact, desmosomes from the SC are functional and because they morphologically differ from the regular desmosomes, we proposed calling them "corneodesmosomes."

A closer examination of electron microscopy images of the upper SC cells, where advancing proteolysis has led to clarification of a once homogeneous interior, reveals that a significant proportion of the keratin filaments remain organized in bundles and that often such cytoskeletal structures are still attached to the corneodesmosomes at the cell periphery. Moreover, immunolabeling of cornified envelopes isolated from the SC shows the persistence of desmosome proteins embedded periodically in the cross-linked structure (6).

Corneodesmosomes in the lower SC, called the SC compactum, are frequent and evenly distributed on the corneocyte surface, just like desmosomes in the SG. Degradation of these plug-like structures occurs first within the flat, straight spaces between the superimposed corneocyte discs. As the vertical cohesion diminishes, the

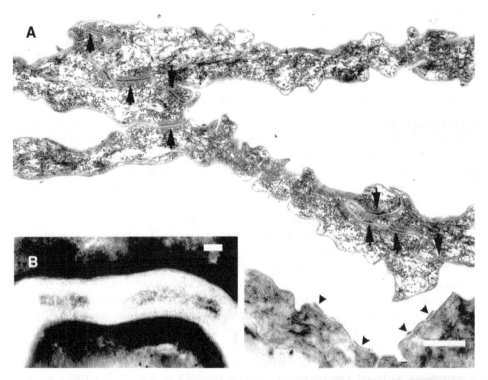

Figure 2 Preferential dissociation of the SC along the flat surfaces of corneocyte "discs," with corneodesmosomes (short arrows) persisting at the lateral portions of the cells (A). The splitting of the upper SC has been enhanced by a treatment with topically applied propylene glycol. The asymmetrically split corneodesmosome "plugs" (arrowheads) can be focally seen. In (B), mechanically stretched corneodesmosomes display partially degraded, irregular "cores," attached to the cell membranes with perpendicular, uniformly spaced fibrils. It is this kind of transmembrane protein attachment which is apparently ruptured in the case of an asymmetrical "plug" splitting. The corneocyte interior is labeled with an anti-filaggrin immunogold, 15 nm size. Bars in (A) 500 nm and (B) 100 nm. *Source of (B):* From Ref. 6.

SC starts to display a looser arrangement and is called, from this point on, the SC disjunctum. On standard histological sections of the skin, from which SC lipids are largely extracted during the paraffin-embedding procedure, this part of the tissue shows a typical "basket-weave" pattern, related to the persistence of the junctions at the periphery of the corneocyte discs (Fig. 2). The fragilized tissue is more susceptible to the action of mechanical forces and to further degradation by endogenous enzymes. Eventually, the lateral/peripheral corneodesmosomes cease to resist as well and the corneocytes are gradually shed. Disappearance of the junctions is preceded by fine morphological modifications in the structure of their intercellular plug, namely irregular clarification of its central part. In contrast, mechanical disruption of apparently intact corneodesmosomes occurs along one or the other side of the plug facing the corneocyte lipid envelope. Both phenomena exist in normal SC, but their proportions may vary according to the "environmental" conditions (Fig. 2). The reasons for the preferential loss of corneodesmosomes from the relatively flat surfaces on the upper and lower faces of corneocytes are so far unknown, but they may include, e.g., (i) easier access for the enzymes, displaced by self-organizing lipid bilayers, when compared to the convoluted lateral intercorneocyte spaces; (ii) an additional protection of the peripheral/lateral junctions by putative supplementary structures, like poorly organized and difficult-to-observe tight junctions; or (iii) a higher impact of shearing forces on junctions between flat rigid surfaces, when they are applied to the skin or when they simply occur during changes of the corneocyte volume due to variations in the water content.

Corneodesmosomes in the Hair Follicle

Just as in every other epithelial tissue, desmosomal junctions are established by keratinocytes from various parts of the hair follicle (7). The number and size of desmosomes vary between the layers, and they carry out different functions and display marked differences in cell morphology. These junctions are less pronounced between the keratinocytes of the outer root sheath (ORS), but they become better structured at the limit between the ORS and inner root sheath (IRS). In fact, the single outer cell layer of the IRS, called Henle's layer, has a homogeneous hyalinated appearance, very much like the first cornified layer of the SC. The keratinocytes of Henle's layer are attached to neighboring cells by desmosomes that resemble SC corneodesmosomes. On the outer surface of Henle's layer these corneodesmosomes mediate adhesion with the innermost flattened keratinocytes of the ORS and on the other, internal side, with the Huxley's layer of the IRS. Keratinocytes from the SG-like Huxley's layer express rounded, electron-dense cytoplasmic granules containing trichohyalin. The size and number of the trichohyalin granules increase in the cells situated closest to Henle's layer and more distally along the longitudinal hair axis. The cells in Huxley's layer are separated from the hair shaft by a narrow zone of extremely flattened keratinocytes forming the IRS cuticle. This latter layer and a similar cuticle of the hair shaft remain connected in the deeper portions of the hair follicle. As the hair moves outwards, the two cuticles part and the IRS cells are progressively shed into the infundibulum.

All three layers of the IRS undergo differentiation and cornification at different rates. These changes occur first within Henle's layer, then within the cuticle, and finally within Huxley's layer. They are observed in the IRS before hardening of the hair shaft is completed. In such a way the mature IRS forms a rigid cylindrical tube that surrounds and shapes the ascending hair structure (8).

BIOCHEMICAL ANALYSIS

Components of Corneodesmosomes

Corneodesmosomes have been noted for many years, but their components were not definitively identified, mainly because of difficulties in purifying them, since they are covalently bound to the cornified cell envelopes. They consist of desmosomal cadherins, desmogleins, and desmocollins, of desmosomal plaque proteins, and of an extracellular protein—corneodesmosin (Cdsn). Three desmocollin genes (DSC 1–3) have been described, while the number of desmoglein genes varies depending upon the species: four in man (DSG 1–4) and six in mouse (DSG 1—α, β, γ, and DSG 2–4). Their expression is tissue-specific and differentiation-dependent, the terminally differentiating keratinocytes of human epidermis expressing Dsg1, Dsg4, and Dsc1 (9,10). While Dsg1 and Dsc1 have been shown to be components

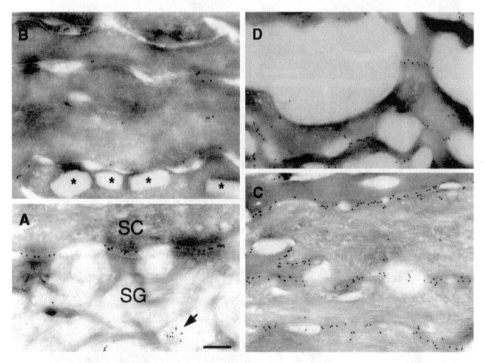

Figure 3 Immunogold detection of corneodesmosin on ultrahin sections of Lowicryl K4M–embedded human skin. (A) Normal epidermis: the protein is secreted through vesicles of the lamellar body size and structure (arrow) and incorporated into desmosomes at the limit between the stratum granulosum (SG) and stratum corneum (SC). The labeling with the G36–19 monoclonal antibody, which is directed to the central portion of corneodesmosin, persists in the corneodesmosome "plugs" until their complete degradation in the upper SC. An irregular proteolysis of the protein in the SC of non-bullous ichthyosis congenita (B) may be related to the flaky desquamation observed in this genodermatosis (intracorneocyte crystals of cholesterol are marked with asterisks). In X-linked ichthyosis (C and D), the corneodesmosome degradation is highly impaired due to accumulation of the cholesterol sulfate, not converted into cholesterol by deficient steroid sulfatase. In this case, the corneodesmosin labeling remains extremely strong throughout the compact ichthyotic squame (C) and up to the last corneocytes, stripped off mechanically at the epidermal surface (D). Bar 100 nm.

of corneodesmosomes, it is not yet known whether Dsg4 is present. As is the case with desmosomes, the cytoplasmic tails of corneodesmosomal Dsg1 and Dsc1 are linked to intermediate filaments of keratins 1 and 10 via the desmosomal plaque proteins, including plakoglobin, desmoplakins, and probably other plakins. However, corneodesmosomal cadherins and plaque proteins are also covalently cross-linked to the other components of the cornified cell envelopes (6,11,12), thereby anchoring them in place. Synthesized and secreted by the granular layer keratinocytes, Cdsn is an adhesive protein too. It was shown to associate with desmosomes just before their transformation into corneodesmosomes, and above that point, Cdsn can be detected in the extracellular parts of these junctions up to the skin surface (13,14) (Fig. 3).

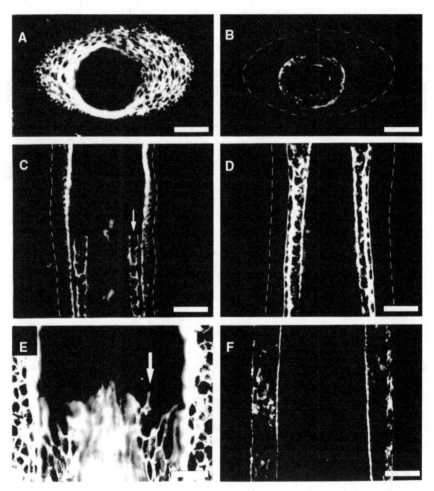

Figure 4 Indirect immunofluorescence study of the Cdsn expression pattern (B, D, F; labeling with G36–19 MAb), compared with plakoglobin (A, E; PG5.1 MAb) and desmoglein 1&2 (C; DG3.10 MAb) on the cryosections of human scalp hair follicles. Desmosome antigens are detected in the outer root sheath and in the inner root sheath up to the keratogenous zone (C, E; arrows). The Cdsn labeling, restricted to the inner root sheath, persists up to the isthmus level (B). Only the outer root sheath keratinocytes express plakoglobin and desmogleins at the isthmus (A). The broken lines in B, C, D highlight the outer limits of the outer root sheath. Bars: A–D 45 μm; E and F 25 μm. *Source*: From Ref. 8.

It is also worth noting that Cdsn is expressed in the three epithelial components of the IRS of hair in a pattern following the sequence of terminal differentiation of these layers (8,13) (Fig. 4).

Corneodesmosin: Structure and Function

Cdsn is mainly expressed in the epidermis, hard palate epithelium, and hair follicles. In the epidermis, Cdsn is synthesized by keratinocytes in the upper spinous and granular layers as a 52- to 56-kDa glycoprotein phosphorylated on serine residues. It is secreted via lamellar bodies from granular layer keratinocytes. In the SG, Cdsn is found not only in the lamellar bodies but also in the extracellular "cores" of desmosomes. In the normal SC, the protein is detected exclusively in the corneodesmosome core. However, in certain pathologic situations, such as harlequin ichthyosis, where lamellar bodies are defective and remain partially non-extruded, Cdsn can be used to identify these organelles inside the corneocytes, despite the absence of typical lamellar internal structures (15). Cdsn was shown to be covalently bound, by disulfide bonds and perhaps other covalent linkages of unknown chemical nature, to the external side of the cornified envelopes in discrete regions corresponding to corneodesmosomes (6,13,16–18). Its presence in the corneodesmosome plug, and the close

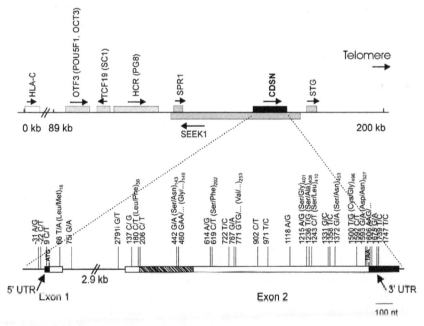

Figure 5 Genomic organization and polymorphisms of human *CDSN*. Genomic structure of PSORS1 locus (top) on chromosome 6p21.3, and schematic representation of *CDSN* gene (bottom). The genes on the locus are represented by boxes. Their transcription orientations are shown by arrowheads. Exon 1 (non-coding + 82 bp) and exon 2 (1503 bp + non-coding) of *CDSN* are separated by a 2.9-kb intron. Untranslated transcribed regions (UTR) at both the 5′ and 3′ ends are indicated by black boxes. All known polymorphic sites are given, with the corresponding amino acid exchange. The region of *CDSN* exon 2 encoding the N-terminal glycine loop domain is shown by a hatched box.

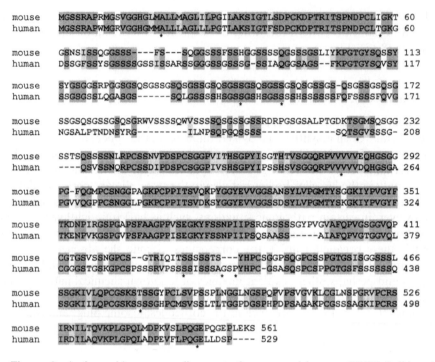

```
mouse   MGSSRAPRMGSVGGHGLMALLMAGLILPGILAKSIGTLSDPCKDPTRITSPNDPCLIGKT 60
human   MGSSRAPWMGRVGGHGMMALLLAGLLLPGTLAKSIGTFSDPCKDPTRITSPNDPCLTGKG 60

mouse   GSNSISSQGGSSS----FS---SQGGSSSFSSHGGSSSSQGSSSGSLIYKPGTGYSQSSY 113
human   DSSGFSSYSGSSSSGSSISSARSSGGGSSGSSSG-SSIAQGGSAGS--FKPGTGYSQVSY 117

mouse   SYGSGGSRPGGSGSQSGSSGSQSGSSGSGSQSGSSSGSQSGSSSGSQSGSSSGS-QSGSSGSQSG 172
human   SSGSGSSLQGASGS------SQLGSSSSHSGSSGSHSGSSSSHSSSSSSFQFSSSSFQVG 171

mouse   SSGSQSGSSSGSQSGRWVSSSSQWVSSSSQSGSSGSSRDRPGSGSALPTGDKTSGMSQSGG 232
human   NGSALPTNDNSYRG---------ILNPSQPGQSSSS------------SQTSGVSSSG- 208

mouse   SSTSQSSSSNLRPCSSNVPDSPCSGGPVITHSGPYISGTHTVSGGQRPVVVVVEQHGSGG 292
human   ----QSVSSNQRPCSSDIPDSPCSGGPIVSHSGPYIPSSHSVSGGQRPVVVVVDQHGSGA 264

mouse   PG-FQGMPCSNGGPAGKPCPPITSVQKPYGGYEVVGGSANSYLVPGMTYSGGKIYPVGYF 351
human   PGVVQGPPCSNGGLPGKPCPPITSVDKSYGGYEVVGGSSDSYLVPGMTYSKGKIYPVGYF 324

mouse   TKDNPIRGSPGAPSFAAGPPVSEGKYFSSNPIIPSRGSSSSSGYPVGVAFQPVGSGGVQP 411
human   TKENPVKGSPGVPSFAAGPPISEGKYFSSNPIIPSQSAASS-----AIAFQPVGTGGVQL 379

mouse   CGTGSVSSNGPCS--GTRIQITSSSSSTS---YHPCSGGPSQGPCSSPGTGSISGGSSSL 466
human   CGGGSTGSKGPCSPSSSRVPSSSSISSSAGSPYHPC-GSASQSPCSPPGTGSFSSSSSSQ 438

mouse   SSGKIVLQPCGSKSTSSGYPCLSVPSSPLNGGLNGSPQPVPSVGVKLCGLNSPGRVPCRS 526
human   SSGKIILQPCGSKSSSSGHPCMSVSSLTLTGGPDGSPHPDPSAGAKPCGSSSAGKIPCRS 498

mouse   IRNILTQVKPLGPQLMDPKVSLPQGEPQGEPLEKS 561
human   IRDILAQVKPLGPQLADPEVFLPQGELLDSP---- 529
```

Figure 6 Amino acid sequence alignment of mouse and human *CDSN*. Solid and shaded backgrounds indicate identical or similar (R/K/H, A/S/T, I/L/V/M/C/F/Y/W, G/P and E/D/Q/N) amino acids, respectively. For each sequence, the number of amino acids is shown on the right. Stars indicate polymorphic amino acids described in humans.

association observed between Cdsn degradation at the epidermal surface and corneocyte shedding suggest that the protein plays a major role in reinforcing cell cohesion in the SC. The demonstration that Cdsn displays homophilic adhesive properties in an aggregation assay of fibroblasts expressing a chimeric protein comprising extracellular Cdsn and the transmembrane and cytoplasmic domains of E-cadherin supports this hypothesis (19). An alternative proposal suggesting a possible protective role of Cdsn against premature proteolysis of the junction proteins has also been advanced but remains unverified (14,20).

The *CDSN* gene is located on 6p21.3 in the Major Histocompatibility Complex region. It consists of two exons separated by a single 2.9-kb intron (17). The gene is amazingly polymorphic (more than one polymorphism every 100 bp), with 12 known coding single nucleotide polymorphisms (cSNPs) leading to amino acid exchanges (Fig. 5). In contrast, *CDSN* is conserved across species: only two amino acids differ between the chimpanzee and human *CDSN* sequences (GenBank accession numbers AB100083 and AF030130, respectively); mouse Cdsn shows 63% identity and 71% homology with the human protein (Fig. 6). Secondary structure prediction algorithms indicate for Cdsn a high content of beta-turns, and a high degree of flexibility. The main characteristic of Cdsn composition is that serine and glycine constitute almost half of its 529 amino acids, with proline also being particularly abundant (10% of total amino acids). In particular, in one domain of the protein, from amino acid 60 to 171, repetitions of serine- and glycine-rich sequences are separated by aromatic or aliphatic residues (17). According to a structural model proposed by Steinert et al. (21), these are likely to associate and force the intervening serine and glycine residues to fold up into flexible loop-like motifs called "glycine loops." Glycine loops in a given molecule may interact with similar motifs on neighboring proteins, mediating adhesive properties. In the epidermis, glycine loops were first identified in cytokeratins and loricrin. Mutations in the glycine loop domains of keratins K1, K5, and K16 result in various cutaneous diseases with intermediate filament abnormalities and tissular fragility, e.g., ichthyosis hystrix and palmoplantar keratoderma (22–25). In agreement with the model, when tested using overlay binding assays and surface plasmon resonance, the glycine loop domain of Cdsn is able to bind the entire Cdsn (19,26). Deletion of the domain dramatically reduces the Cdsn homophilic interactions. We also demonstrated that the domain mediates homo-oligomerization of Cdsn. The dissociation constant (K_D) was calculated to be around 10^{-5} M (26). This moderate strength of interaction probably allows dynamic regulation of the Cdsn–Cdsn association to occur in vivo, the glycine loops being able to stick and detach in a reversible manner. In this way, Cdsn reinforces SC cohesion while respecting the elastic properties of the epidermis.

Cdsn is progressively proteolysed as corneodesmosomes evolve toward the SC surface. Immunoblotting, immunohistochemistry, and immunoelectron microscopy experiments using monoclonal antibodies and affinity-purified anti-peptide antibodies directed against various domains of Cdsn showed that both extremities of the protein are cleaved in a first step of the processing, probably before its incorporation into desmosomes. Then, the N-terminal glycine loop domain is cleaved. Finally, just the central portion of the molecule of approximately 15 kDa, containing only part of the C-terminal glycine loop domain and probably lacking the adhesive properties, is detectable on exfoliated corneocytes (18).

FUNCTIONAL CORRELATES

The Role of Corneodesmosomes in SC Cohesion and Their Orderly Degradation During SC Desquamation

Several studies have demonstrated the importance of corneodesmosomes in SC cohesion.

In the SC compactum of normal human epidermis, and also in the entire SC of palmoplantar epidermis and hard palate epithelium, corneodesmosomes are present over the entire surface of corneocytes. However, in the stratum disjunctum, where cohesion is weaker, they are located only at the overlapping edges of the corneocytes, in cell–cell interdigitation zones. Moreover, there is a clear direct relationship between the number of corneodesmosomes and the strength of cellular cohesion (13,27,28). Corneodesmosomes form strong attachments between interacting cornified cell envelopes that remain cross-linked on their internal face to the keratin-filaggrin–containing corneocyte matrix. Such links result in a supracellular network contributing to the SC integrity and its physical barrier function (Fig. 7).

Exfoliation of corneocytes from the skin surface is the result of a tightly regulated multi-step proteolytic process. It begins with the degradation of non-peripheral corneodesmosomes at the interface between the SC compactum and SC disjunctum and finally results in the breakdown of the persistent "peripheral" corneodesmosomes at the epidermis surface (4) (Fig. 7). An experimental in vitro model allowing semi-quantitative studies of desquamation was used to demonstrate

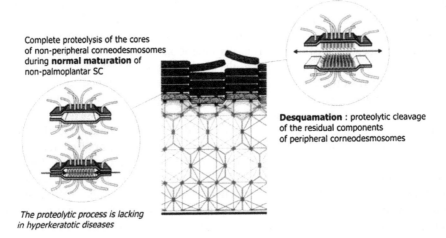

Complete proteolysis of the cores
of non-peripheral corneodesmosomes
during **normal maturation** of
non-palmoplantar SC

Desquamation : proteolytic cleavage
of the residual components
of peripheral corneodesmosomes

*The proteolytic process is lacking
in hyperkeratotic diseases*

Figure 7 Involvement of corneodesmosomes in the SC cohesion, and their proteolysis in desquamation: a model. From the stratum basale (SB) to the stratum granulosum (SG), tissue cohesion is provided by the desmosome-intermediate filament network which is anchored on the basal membrane via hemidesmosomes. The SC cohesion is provided by corneodesmosomes which link together cornified cell envelopes. In normal non-palmoplantar SC, corneodesmosomes have to be degraded in two proteolysis waves for desquamation to occur.

that SC cohesion is impaired by corneodesmosome degradation following treatments with proteolytic enzymes (29). This is consistent with the effect of topical applications of protease inhibitors on mouse skin resulting in ichthyosiform hyperkeratosis (30).

Protease-dependent dissociation of human plantar SC was shown to occur upon complete degradation of Dsg1 (31). Additionally, biochemical investigation of a tapestripped human non-plantar SC indicated that the disappearance of Dsg1 from the uppermost horny layers coincides with the enzymatic processing of Cdsn (20). Furthermore, the partial degradation of corneodesmosomes during transition between the SC compactum and disjunctum seems to occur when the N-terminal glycine loop domain of Cdsn becomes eliminated (18).

Several proteases are believed to take part in the process of SC desquamation: two serine proteases of the kallikrein family (stratum corneum chymotryptic enzyme/kallikrein 7, SCCE/KLK7 and stratum corneum tryptic enzyme/kallikrein 5, SCTE/KLK5), and four cathepsins — two cysteine proteases (stratum corneum thiol protease, SCTP/cathepsin L2, and a cathepsin L-like enzyme) and two aspartic proteases (cathepsin D and cathepsin E-like) (32–35). Indeed, SCCE, either recombinant or purified from human epidermis, is able to degrade Dsc1 and Cdsn but not Dsg1 at pH 5.6, a pH close to that of the SC. After incubation of an extract of epidermis in the presence of an enriched fraction of SCTE in the same acidic conditions, we observed degradation of Cdsn, Dsc1, and also Dsg1 (36). Dsc1 is also degraded by partially purified SCTP, and Cdsn is a substrate of cathepsin L-like enzyme (34,35). Identification of missense and nonsense mutations in the cathepsin C gene resulting in undetectable activity of the enzyme in the Papillon–Lefèvre syndrome, a periodontal disease associated with palmoplantar hyperkeratosis, suggests that this cathepsin may be also involved in desquamation (37). Synthesized as proenzymes, all these proteases undergo proteolytic maturation, but the enzymes involved have not been clearly identified. Our preliminary results seem to indicate that SCTE activates SCCE (38).

Several protease inhibitors are present in the extracellular spaces of the SC and potentially regulate desquamation. Elafin, a member of the trappin protein family formerly known as skin-derived antileukoprotease, has been shown to inhibit SCCE and to significantly reduce the shedding of corneocytes in vitro (39). It is covalently bound to the corneocyte envelopes and its expression is upregulated in psoriasis and other inflammatory processes in the skin. Antileukoproteinase (ALP), also called secretory leukocyte protease inhibitor (SLPI), was shown to prevent the detachment of corneocytes from human plantar epidermis in vitro and to strongly inhibit SCCE (39). The SPINK-5–encoded protein, the lymphoepithelial Kazal-type 5 serine protease inhibitor (LEKTI), could also target SCCE and SCTE. Indeed, trypsin and chymotrypsin activities are increased in the SC of patients suffering from a linear migratory type of congenital ichthyosis caused by mutations of SPINK-5, the Netherthon syndrome (40). In this dermatosis, the squames are apparently due to the abnormal desquamation, irritation, and compensatory hyperactivity of the underlying epidermis. The impaired SC desquamation in X-linked ichthyosis may be due to the protease inhibition by accumulating cholesterol sulfate (41). Indeed, the latter is not converted into cholesterol due to a mutation in the gene encoding cholesterol sulfatase, located on chromosome X.

Two cysteine protease inhibitors also present in the SC, namely cystatin α and cystatin M/E, may also be involved in the regulation of desquamation (42). Although mice with a null mutation of the cystatin M/E gene present with a severe ichthyosis and do not survive after birth, the corresponding human phenotype, harlequin ichthyosis, is not related to the absence of such inhibitor (43).

In addition to their potential role in the degradation of corneodesmosomes, some cathepsins are able to cleave and inactivate ALP, thereby removing inhibition of SCCE (44).

Besides the structural proteins of corneodesmosomes, proteases, and their inhibitors, other molecules and factors are also able to influence SC cohesion and desquamation. Detergent-induced unipolar cell shedding from the non-plantar SC occurs only in the presence of EDTA, which strongly suggests that depletion of extracellular calcium fragilizes corneodesmosomes rendering them susceptible to proteolysis (45). Pre-treatment of skin samples with glycosidases enhances protease-dependent shedding of corneocytes, indicating that cell surface sugars protect junctions from enzymatic degradation (46).

Clearly, SC pH and water content affect the rate of proteolytic reactions leading to desquamation. When the SC pH is increased, after topic applications of either superbases or inhibitors of secreted phospholipase A2 (sPLA2, involved in hydrolysis of lipids to fatty acids), corneodesmosome degradation is increased and corneocyte cohesion is altered (47). On the other hand, the impaired proteolysis of corneodesmosomes in winter xerosis may be due to reduced hydration of the SC (48). Corneodesmosomes remain highly hydrophilic structures within the intercorneocyte spaces occupied by self-organizing lamellar lipids. Various enzymes which are brought to the extracellular spaces by keratinosomes have to segregate with the hydrophilic compartments, compatible with the proteinaceous content. Indeed, hydrophilic lacunae are present within the extracellular lamellar lipids and their fusion with corneodesmosomes is often observed in the upper part of the SC compactum (49). It is tempting to speculate that the self-organization of the extracellular lipids into multilamellar hydrophobic structures helps to bring

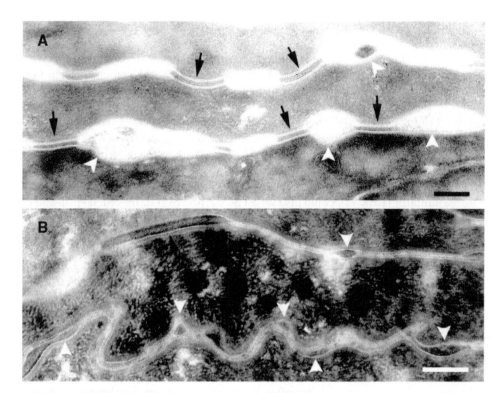

Figure 8 Hydration of the SC promotes the lateral displacements, coalescence and increase in volume of the extracellular hydrophilic microdomains, leading to the increased frequency of their association with corneodesmosomes. Such hydrophilic compartments may be visualized within the intercellular lipids of a normal human stratum corneum with RuO$_4$ staining. (A) In the occluded skin, the well hydrated SC shows voluminous hydrophilic lacunae (white arrowheads) in the proximity of corneodesmosomes (black arrows). Both structures are easily revealed with RuO$_4$, well before the staining visualizes the multilamellar lipid organization of the remaining portions of the intercellular compartment. (B) The non-occluded SC also contains hydro-

the enzyme-rich lacunae into contact with the corneodesmosomes. Both the lacunae size and mobility increase within the highly hydrated SC showing enhanced desquamation (Fig. 8).

Corneodesmosomes in Skin Pathology

As we have seen, corneodesmosome degradation is required for orderly desquamation. During such a process, corneocytes detach individually and their loss is invisible macroscopically, unlike the situation in which whole clusters of several irregularly attached cells form squames.

Accordingly, in psoriasis, winter xerosis, and various ichthyoses, all characterized by varying degrees of scaly skin, the number of corneodesmosomes in the outer SC does not decrease and both the marginal and non-marginal junctions are retained (14,48). In the same hyperkeratotic conditions, Cdsn can be found in corneodesmosomes through the whole thickness of the SC (Fig. 3).

Corneodesmosomes persisting in the pathologic scales express, besides Cdsn, other desmosomal antigens, e.g., Dsg1, Dsc1, and plakoglobin, indicating their reduced degradation (28,48,50). Indeed, an impaired cleavage of Dsg1 was reported in the hyperkeratotic SC (51,52). In contrast, an uneven distribution of Cdsn and irregular proteolysis of corneodesmosomes were observed in the parakeratotic SC of non-bullous congenital ichthyotic erythroderma. It may contribute to the mechanism of detachment of whole SC fragments corresponding to the fine scales observed in this disease (14).

The fact that none of the diseases is associated with the absence of Cdsn suggests that the protein is essential for the formation of the SC barrier and, therefore, for survival. No CDSN knockout animals have been produced so far to confirm this hypothesis.

There exist two human pathologies in which the CDSN gene is apparently involved. In the first place, Cdsn appears to play an important role in scalp hair physiology. Indeed, we have identified nonsense mutations of CDSN in three families with hypotrichosis simplex of the scalp (OMIM 146520), an autosomal dominant form of isolated alopecia. The mutations result in premature stop codons (Gln200- or Gln215-to-ter). Aggregates of SDS- and boiling-resistant dimers, trimers, and larger oligomers of truncated Cdsn were detected in the superficial dermis of patients' scalp and at the periphery of remaining hair follicles deeper in the dermis. In the epidermis, the truncated Cdsn was not detected, whereas the wild-type form seemed to be abnormally proteolysed (53). The aggregates observed may be toxic to the hair follicle cells. Alternatively, a dominant negative interaction between the mutated and wild-type Cdsn may account for loss of cohesion of the IRS of the hair follicles.

Although environmental factors, including infections and stress, affect the onset and clinical presentation of psoriasis (OMIM *177900), family studies indicated a strong genetic background of the disease. Genome-wide scans have identified several susceptibility regions, the major locus, namely PSORS1, being mapped to chromosome 6p21. Linkage disequilibrium studies using microsatellite markers have refined PSORS1 to a 160-kb interval harboring at least eight genes, including CDSN and three pseudogenes in the intervening region between HLA-C and OTF3. Among them, three genes carry coding polymorphisms repeatedly associated with familial psoriasis: HLA-Cw*0602, HCR*WWCC, and CDSN*5 (54,55, and references therein). In the recent analyses of both UK and Gujarati Indian family cohorts, Trembath et al. have observed a susceptibility haplotype which loses the HCR risk alleles while keeping HLA-C and CDSN disease-associated cSNPs. This suggests that particular CDSN alleles confer psoriasis susceptibility when expressed in an appropriate HLA context. Furthermore, the same group identified a CDSN risk haplotype significantly over-transmitted in UK and Gujarati patients, and suggested the existence of a CDSN protective haplotype (56). The two haplotypes differ at 10 SNPs, 7 of which are localized in potential expression regulatory regions, and 3 which induce amino acid exchanges that may influence the protein properties and/or function. We showed that Cdsn expression in psoriasis lesions differs from that in normal skin. There is an increase in Cdsn expression in the psoriatic plaques, and the protein is expressed and secreted earlier during the epidermis' differentiation program (14,57). However, no modifications of Cdsn expression can be found in non-involved psoriatic skin. Nonetheless, we observed alterations and a reduction in the proteolytic processing of Cdsn in the epidermis of both involved and uninvolved skin of psoriatic patients (58). Further functional studies are now necessary to precisely determine the role of Cdsn in the pathogenesis of psoriasis.

REFERENCES

1. Cowin P, Burke B. Cytoskeleton—membrane interactions. Curr Opin Cell Biol 1996; 8:56–65.
2. Kowalczyk AP, Bornslaeger EA, Norvell SM, Palka HL, Green KJ. Desmosomes: intercellular adhesive junctions specialized for attachment of intermediate filaments. Int Rev Cytol 1999; 185:237–302.
3. McMillan JR, Haftek M, Akiyama M, South AP, Perrot H, McGrath JA, Eady RAJ, Shimizu H. Alterations in desmosome size and number coincide with loss of keratinocyte cohesion in skin with homozygous and heterozygous defects in the desmosomal protein plakophilin 1. J Invest Dermatol 2003; 121:96–103.
4. Chapman SJ, Walsh A. Desmosomes, corneosomes, and desquamation: an ultrastructural study of adult pig epidermis. Arch Dermatol Res 1990; 282:304–310.
5. Chapman SJ, Walsh A, Jackson SM, Friedmann PS. Lipids, proteins and corneocyte adhesion. Arch Dermatol Res 1991; 283:167–173.
6. Haftek M, Serre G, Mils V, Thivolet J. Immunocytochemical evidence for a possible role of cross-linked keratinocyte envelopes in stratum corneum cohesion. J Histochem Cytochem 1991; 39:1531–1538.
7. Sperling LC. Hair anatomy for the clinician. JAAD 1991; 25:1–17.
8. Mils V, Vincent C, Croute F, Serre G. The expression of desmosomal and corneodesmosomal antigens shows specific variations during the terminal differentiation of epidermis and hair follicle epithelia. J Histochem Cytochem 1992; 40:1329–1337.
9. Garrod DR, Merritr AJ, Nie Z. Desmosomal cadherins. Curr Opin Cell Biol 2002; 14: 537–545.
10. Kljuic A, Bazzi H, Sundberg JP, Martinez-Mir A, O'Shaughnessy R, Mahoney MG, Levy X, Montagutelli M, Ahmad W, Aita VM, Gordon D, Uitto J, Whiting D, Ott J, Fischer S, Gilliam TC, Jahoda CA, Morris RJ, Panteleyev AA, Nguyen VT, Christiano AM. Desmoglein 4 in hair follicle differentiation and epidermal adhesion: evidence from inherited hypotrichosis and acquired pemphigus vulgaris. Cell 2003; 113:249–260.
11. Robinson NA, Lapic S, Welter JF, Eckert RL. S100A11, S100A10, annexin I, desmosomal proteins, small proline-rich proteins, plasminogen activator inhibitor-2, and involucrin are components of the cornified envelope of cultured human epidermal keratinocytes. J Biol Chem 1997; 272:12035–12046.
12. Kalinin AE, Kajava AV, Steinert PM. Epithelial barrier function: assembly and structural features of the cornified cell envelope. Bioessays 2002; 24:789–800.
13. Serre G, Mils V, Haftek M, Vincent C, Croute F, Réano A, Ouhayoun J-P, Bettinger S, Soleilhavoup J-P. Identification of late differentiation antigens of human cornified epithelia, expressed in re-organized desmosomes and bound to cross-linked envelope. J Invest Dermatol 1991; 97:1061–1072.
14. Haftek M, Simon M, Kanitakis J, Maréchal S, Claudy A, Serre G, Schmitt D. Expression of corneodesmosin in the granular layer and stratum corneum of normal and diseased epidermis. Br J Dermatol 1997; 137:864–873.
15. Haftek M, Cambazard F, Dhouailly D, Réano A, Lachaux A, Simon M, Serre G, Claudy A, Schmitt D. A longitudinal study of harlequin infant presenting clinically as non-bullous congenital ichthyosiform erythroderma. Br J Dermatol 1996; 135:448–453.
16. Simon M, Montézin M, Guerrin M, Durieux J-J, Serre G. Characterization and purification of human corneodesmosin, an epidermal basic glycoprotein associated with corneocyte-specific modified desmosomes. J Biol Chem 1997; 272:31770–31776.
17. Guerrin M, Simon M, Montézin M, Haftek M, Vincent C, Serre G. Expression cloning of human corneodesmosin proves its identity with the product of the S gene and allows improved characterization of its processing during keratinocyte differentiation. J Biol Chem 1998; 273:22640–22647.

18. Simon M, Jonca N, Guerrin M, Haftck M, Bernard D, Caubet C, Egelrud T, Schmidt R, Serre G. Refined characterization of corneodesmosin proteolysis during terminal differentiation of human epidermis and its relationship to desquamation. J Biol Chem 2001; 276:20292–20299 (and errata in J Biol Chem 2001, 276:47742).

19. Jonca N, Guerrin M, Hadjiolova K, Caubet C, Gallinaro H, Simon M, Serre G. Corneodesmosin, a component of epidermal corneocyte desmosomes, displays homophilic adhesive properties. J Biol Chem 2002; 277:5024–5029.

20. Lundström A, Serre G, Haftek M, Egelrud T. Evidence for a role of corneodesmosin, a protein which may serve to modify desmosomes during cornification, in stratum corneum cell cohesion and desquamation. Arch Dermatol Res 1994; 286:369–389.

21. Steinert PM, Mack JW, Korge BP, Gan S-Q. Glycine loops in proteins: their occurrence in certain intermediate filament chains, loricrins and single-stranded RNA binding proteins. Int J Biol Macromol 1991; 13:130–136.

22. Sprecher E, Yosipovitch G, Bergman R, Ciubutaro D, Indelman M, Pfendner E, Goh LC, Miller CJ, Uitto J, Richard G. Epidermolytic hyperkeratosis and epidermolysis bullosa simplex caused by frameshift mutations altering the v2 tail domains of keratin 1 and keratin 5. J Invest Dermatol 2003; 120:623–626.

23. Terrinoni A, Puddu P, Didona B, De Laurenzi V, Candi E, Smith FJ, McLean WH, Melino G. A mutation in the V1 domain of K16 is responsible for unilateral palmoplantar verrucous nevus. J Invest Dermatol 2000; 114:1136–1140.

24. Sprecher E, Ishida-Yamamoto AM, Becker OM, Marekov L, Miller CJ, Steinert PM, Neldner K, Richard G. Evidence for novel functions of the keratin tail emerging from a mutation causing ichthyosis hystrix. J Invest Dermatol 2001; 116:511–519.

25. Whittock NV, Smith FJ, Wan H, Mallipeddi R, Griffiths WA, Dopping-Hepenstal P, Ashton GH, Eady RA, McLean WH, McGrath JA. Frameshift mutation in the V2 domain of human keratin 1 results in striate palmoplantar keratoderma. J Invest Dermatol 2002; 118:838–844.

26. Caubet C, Jonca N, Lopez F, Estève J-P, Simon M, Serre G. Homo-oligomerization of human corneodesmosin is mediated by its N-terminal glycine loop domain. J Invest Dermatol 2004; 122:747–754.

27. Allen TD, Potten CS. Desmosomal form, fate, and function in mammalian differentiation epidermis. J Ultrastruct Res 1975; 51:94–105.

28. Skerrow CJ, Clelland DG, Skerrow D. Changes to desmosomal antigens and lectin-binding sites during differentiation in normal human epidermis: a quantitative ultrastructural study. J Cell Sci 1989; 92:667–677.

29. Egelrud T, Hofer P-A, Lundström A. Proteolytic degradation of desmosomes in plantar stratum corneum leads to cell dissociation in vitro. Acta Derm Venereol (Stockh) 1988; 68:93–97.

30. Sato J, Denda M, Nakanishi J, Nomura J, Koyama J. Cholesterol sulfate inhibits proteases that are involved in desquamation of stratum corneum. J Invest Dermatol 1998; 111: 189–193.

31. Lundström A, Egelrud T. Evidence that cell shedding from plantar stratum corneum in vitro involves endogenous proteolysis of the desmosomal protein desmoglein 1. J Invest Dermatol 1990; 94:216–220.

32. Ekholm E, Brattsand M, Egelrud T. Stratum corneum tryptic enzyme in normal epidermis: a missing link in the desquamation process. J Invest Dermatol 2000; 114: 56–63.

33. Hansson L, Strömqvist M, Bäckman A, Wallbrandt P. Cloning, expression, and characterization of stratum corneum chymotryptic enzyme. J Biol Chem 1994; 269: 19420–19426.

34. Bernard D, Mehul B, Thomas-Collignon A, Simonetti L, Remy V, Bernard MA, Schmidt R. Analysis of proteins with caseinolytic activity in a human stratum corneum extract revealed a yet unidentified cysteine protease and identified the so-called "stratum corneum thiol protease" as cathepsin L2. J Invest Dermatol 2003; 120:592–600.

35. Horikoshi T, Arany I, Rajaraman S, Chen SH, Brysk H, Lei G, Tyring SK, Brysk MM. Isoforms of cathepsin D and human epidermal differentiation. Biochimie 1998; 80:605–612.

36. Simon M, Bernard D, Guerrin M, Egelrud T, Schmidt R, Serre G. Corneodesmosomal proteins are proteolyzed in vitro by SCTE and SCCE—two proteases which are thought to be involved in desquamation. In: Marks R, Lévêque J-L, Voegeli R, eds. Stratum Corneum. London: Martin Dunitz Limited Edition, 2002:81–83.

37. Toomes C, James J, Wood AJ, Wu CL, McCormick D, Lench N, Hewitt C, Moynihan L, Roberts E, Woods CG, Markham A, Wong M, Widmer R, Ghaffar KA, Pemberton M, Hussein IR, Temtamy SA, Davies R, Read AP, Sloan P, Dixon MJ, Thakker NS. Loss-of-function mutations in the cathepsin C gene result in periodontal disease and palmoplantar keratosis. Nat Genet 1999; 23:421–424.

38. Caubet C, Jonca N, Brattsand M, Guerrin M, Bernard D, Schmidt R, Egelrud T, Simon M, Serre G. Degradation of corneodesmosome proteins by two serine proteases of the kallikrein family, SCTE/KLK5/hK5 and SCCE/KLK7/hK7. J Invest Dermatol 2004; 122:1235–1244.

39. C-W Franzke, Baici A, Bartels J, Christophers E, Wiedow O. Antileukoprotease inhibits stratum corneum chymotryptic enzyme. Evidence for a regulating function in desquamation. J Biol Chem 1996; 271:21886–21890.

40. Chavanas S, Bodemer C, Rochat A, Hamel-Teillac D, Ali M, Irvine AD, Bonafé JL, Wilkinson J, Taïeb A, Barrandon Y, Harper JI, de Prost Y, Hovnanian A. Mutations in SPINK5, encoding a serine protease inhibitor, cause Netherton syndrome. Nat Genet 2000; 25:141–142.

41. Sato J, Denda M, Nakanishi J, Nomura J, Koyama J. Cholesterol sulfate inhibits proteases that are involved in desquamation of stratum corneum. J Invest Dermatol 1998; 111:189–193.

42. Zeeuwen PLJM, Van Vlijmen-Willems IM, Jansen BJ, Sotiropoulou G, Curfs JH, Meis JF, Janssen JJ, Van Ruissen F, Schalkwijk J. Cystatin M/E expression is restricted to differentiated epidermal keratinocytes and sweat glands: a new skin-specific proteinase inhibitor that is a target for cross-linking by transglutaminase. J Invest Dermatol 2001; 116:693–701.

43. Zeeuwen PL, Dale BA, de Jongh GJ, van Vlijmen-Willems IM, Fleckman P, Kimball JR, Stephens K, Schalkwijk J. The human cystatin M/E gene (CST6): exclusion candidate gene for harlequin ichthyosis. J Invest Dermatol 2003; 121:65–68.

44. Taggart CC, Lowe GJ, Greene CM, Mulgrew AT, O'Neill SJ, Levine RL, McElvaney NG. Cathepsin B, L, and S cleave and inactivate secretory leukoprotease inhibitor. J Biol Chem 2001; 276:33345–33352.

45. Egelrud T, Lundström A. The dependence of detergent-induced cell dissociation in non-palmo-plantar stratum corneum on endogenous proteolysis. J Invest Dermatol 1990; 95:456–459.

46. Walsh A, Chapman SJ. Sugars protect desmosome and corneosome glycoproteins from proteolysis. Arch Dermatol Res 1991; 283:174–179.

47. Hachem JP, Crumrinc D, Fluhr J, Brown BE, Feingold KR, Elias PM. pH directly regulates epidermal permeability barrier homeostasis, and stratum corneum integrity/cohesion. J Invest Dermatol 2003; 121:345–353.

48. Simon M, Bernard D, Minondo A-M, Camus C, Fiat F, Corcuff P, Schmidt R, Serre G. Persistence of both peripheral and non-peripheral corneodesmosomes in the upper stratum corneum of winter xerosis skin versus only peripheral in normal skin. J Invest Dermatol 2001; 116:23–31.

49. Haftek M, Teillon MH, Schmitt D. Stratum corneum, corneodesmosomes, and ex-vivo percutaneous penetration. Microsc Res Tech 1998; 43:1–8.

50. Haftek M, Serre G, Roche P, Mils V, Thivolet J. Immunocytochemical evidence of preservation of desmosome proteins in the cohesive keratinocytes from normal and pathological stratum corneum [abstr]. J Invest Dermatol 1990; 95:470.

51. Lundström A, Egelrud T. Evidence that cell shedding from plantar stratum corneum in vitro involves endogeneous proteolysis of the desmosomal protein desmoglein 1. J Invest Dermatol 1990; 94:216–220.

52. Suzuki Y, Koyama J, Horo O, Horii I, Kikuchi K, Tanida M, Tagami H. The role of two endogeneous proteases of the stratum corneum in degradation of desmoglein-1 and their reduced activity in the skin of ichthyotic patients. Br J Dermatol 1996; 134: 460–464.

53. Levy-Nissenbaum E, Betz R, Frydman M, Simon M, Lahat H, Bakhan T, Goldman B, Bygum A, Pierick M, Hillmer AM, Jonca N, Toribio J, Kruse R, Dewald G, Cichon S, Kubisch C, Guerrin M, Serre G, Nothen MM, Pras E. Hypotrichosis simplex of the scalp is associated with nonsense mutations in CDSN encoding corneodesmosin. Nat Genet 2003; 34:151–153.

54. Tazi-Ahnini R. Novel genetic association between the corneodesmosin (MHC/S) gene and susceptibility to psoriasis. Hum Mol Genet 1999; 8:1135–1140.

55. Capon F, Munro M, Barker J, Trembath R. Searching for the major histocompatibility complex psoriasis susceptibility gene. J Invest Dermatol 2002; 118:745–751.

56. Capon F, Toal IK, Evans JC, Allen MH, Patel S, Tillman D, Burden D, Barker JN, Trembath RC. Haplotype analysis of distantly related populations implicates corneodesmosin in psoriasis susceptibility. J Med Genet 2003; 40:447–452.

57. Allen M, Ishida-Yamamoto A, McGrath J, Davison S, Iizuka H, Simon M, Guerrin M, Hayday A, Vaughan R, Serre G, Trembath R, Barker J. Corneodesmosin expression in psoriasis vulgaris differs from normal skin and other inflammatory skin disorders. Lab Invest 2001; 81:969–976.

58. Simon M, Tazi-Ahnini R, Cork M, Serre G. Abnormal proteolysis of corneodesmosin in psoriatic skin [abstr]. Br J Dermatol 2002; 147:1053.

12

Epidermal Barrier Function: Role of Tight Junctions

Johanna M. Brandner
Department of Dermatology and Venerology, University Hospital Hamburg Eppendorf, Hamburg, Germany

Ehrhardt Proksch
Department of Dermatology, University of Kiel, Kiel, Germany

INTRODUCTION

The skin's permeability barrier prevents excessive water loss and protects against the entry of harmful substances into the skin, such as chemicals and microbes. Although the stratum corneum, the outermost layer, is recognized as the most important physical barrier, the lower epidermal layers are also significant in barrier function. After tape stripping in mouse and human skin, increase in transepidermal water loss (TEWL) can be measured by the Meeco® Water Analyzer. Loss of nucleated epidermal layers through induction of suction blisters results in a tremendous increase in TEWL which can no longer be measured with the Meeco® Water Analyzer. Measurements with the TEWA-meter® or the Evaporimeter® reach water vapor saturation even earlier. This suggests that the nucleated epidermal layers are important for water retention.

Observations of human skin diseases further support the role of the lower epidermal layers in barrier function. Loss of the stratum corneum and parts of the granular layers, typical components of childhood and adult staphylococcal scaled skin syndrome, are not usually life-threatening (1–3). In contrast, suprabasal bulla in the epidermis and loss of bulla cover including stratum corneum, granular, and spinous layers, as seen in pemphigus vulgaris, is life-threatening when large areas of the body are involved. Sufficient treatment has been possible only since the 1950s, when corticosteroids were introduced to modulate disease immunopathogenesis (4,5). Drug-induced toxic epidermal necrolysis [TEN, Lyell syndrome (6)] is also a life-threatening disease due to loss of the complete epidermis. Loss of the epidermis over large areas of the body is also seen in patients with burn injury. Patients with extensive pemphigus vulgaris, TEN, or severe burns may die because of extensive water loss or sepsis induced by external bacterial infection—outcomes directly resulting from perturbed barrier function. Survival rates can be greatly improved with application of an artificial barrier in the form of a foil or a grease ointment, often containing active antimicrobial substances. These clinical observations confirm the importance of the nucleated epidermal layers in skin barrier function in both directions, both in preventing excessive water loss and the entry of harmful substances into the skin.

TIGHT JUNCTIONS (TJ) IN SIMPLE EPITHELIA

Most research on TJ has been gathered from simple epithelia and endothelia. Since, still only little data are available from mammalian skin, this sub-chapter describes the structure, composition, and function of TJ based on the research on simple epithelia and endothelia.

Tight junctions are cell–cell junctions sealing neighboring cells and controlling the paracellular pathway of molecules ("barrier function"). Moreover, they separate the molecular components of the apical from the basolateral portions of the plasma membrane ["fence function," for reviews (7–13)]. At the molecular level, it appears that TJ molecules from neighboring cells associate and form paired strands or fibrils that tightly connect the cells (14) and thereby seal the paracellular pathway (Fig. 1). There is evidence that aqueous pores or paracellular channels exist within paired strands, explaining the ion- and size selectivity for passaging molecules in TJ [(15–18); for reviews (14,19,20); Fig. 1]. In freeze–fracture electron microscopy, typical TJ structures appear as continuous anastomosing ridges or fibrils in the P-face fracture (21) (Fig. 2).

In thin-section electron microscopy, TJ are seen as small subapical regions of direct contact between the plasma membranes of two adjacent cells without extracellular gaps or intermembranous material ["kissing points" or "sites of fusion" (22)] (Fig. 3).

The molecular composition of TJ is highly complex and varies according to the cell type and degree of differentiation. The TJ proteins can be divided into transmembrane and plaque proteins.

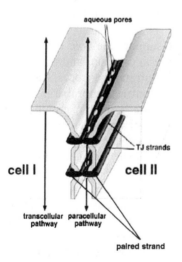

Figure 1 Schematic drawing of tight junctions. TJ proteins from neighboring cells form paired TJ strands which are thought to contain aqueous pores or paracellular channels. *Source*: From Ref. 8.

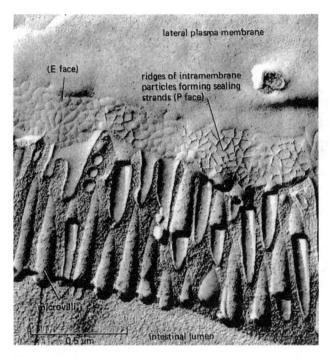

Figure 2 Freeze–fracture electron micrograph showing the structure of tight junctions between epithelial cells of the small intestine. Cells are oriented with their apical ends down. TJ consist of a band of anastomosing sealing strands. The strands are seen as ridges of intramembrane particles on the cytoplasmic fracture face of the membrane (P face) and as complementary grooves on the external face of the membrane (E face). *Source*: From Ref. 157.

Occludin, a protein with putatively four transmembrane domains, was the first TJ integral membrane protein identified [(23,24); for review see Ref. 8]. It is important for both barrier and fence functions of TJ. This was shown, for example, by the introduction of COOH-terminally truncated occludin into MDCK (canine kidney epithelial) cells, which resulted in an increased paracellular permeability of small molecular tracers and affected the TJ fence (25). Overexpression of occludin in MDCK cells leads to an increase of transepithelial resistance (TER) as a sign of TJ tightness, while the TER of Xenopus epithelial cells decreased after incubation with a synthetic peptide corresponding to the second extracellular loop of occludin [(26,27); for review see Ref. 8]. Moreover, occludin is a target for various intracellular signaling pathways and might be important for the dynamics of TJ [for reviews see Refs. 8,10,28]. However, occludin deficient visceral endoderm cells still have a well-developed network of TJ strands (29) and occludin-deficient mice showed normal morphology and barrier function in intestinal epithelial cells, even though there were changes, e.g., in the gastric mucosa resulting in chronic gastritis and hyperplasia, and in the brain, resulting in calcification (30).

As evidence increased that occludin was not the only TJ transmembrane protein, Tsukita and coworkers discovered the family of claudins. Claudins, like occludin, have putatively four transmembrane spanning regions, but otherwise do not show sequence similarities to occludin. Up to now at least 24 claudin types have been identified in mouse and human, with specific expression based on cell type and degree of differentiation [(31–33); for reviews see Refs. 10,14,20]. In fibroblasts

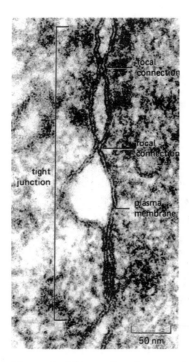

Figure 3 Thin-section electron micrograph of a tight junction between epithelial cells of the small intestine. TJ are seen as direct contacts between the plasma membranes of two adjacent cells without extracellular gaps or intermembranous material ("kissing points" "sites of fusion"). *Source*: From Ref. 157.

lacking TJ, claudin expression produces well-developed networks of TJ strands (31,34). Often two or more claudin isoforms are coexpressed in cells, where they may subsequently polymerize to form heteropolymeric TJ strands. The TJ strands from two cells can adhere in homotypic and heterotypic bonds depending on the claudins involved (35,36). Various studies provide evidence for the influence of claudin combinations and mixing ratios in the tightness and selectivity of TJ. In MDCK II cells, which have a much lower TER than MDCK I cells, claudins 1, 2, and 4 are present. Claudin 2 is notably absent in MDCK I cells. The additional expression of claudin 2 in MDCK I cells results in a decrease of TER on the level of MDCK II cells (37). The importance of claudins for barrier function in simple epithelia was also demonstrated by removing claudin 4 from MDCK I cells with *Clostridium perfringens* enterotoxin, which resulted in a significant increase of TJ permeability and a decrease in the number of TJ strands (38).

A third group of TJ transmembrane proteins are junctional adhesion molecules (JAM). These single transmembrane spanning TJ proteins belong to the immunoglobulin superfamily and are involved in homotypic and heterotypic cell–cell interactions (39–43). It was suggested that JAM-1 (JAM-A) interacts by homophilic adhesion (44,45) and regulates monocyte transmigration across endothelia (39,46). The VEJAM/JAM-2/ JAM-B is considered important for the interaction of endothelial cells with T-, NK-, and dendritic-cells, partly supported by JAM-3 (JAM-C), which is a receptor for JAM-2, and for promotion of lymphocyte transendothelial migration (47–49).

In addition to the TJ transmembrane proteins, a growing number of cytoplasmatic TJ plaque proteins have been identified, the first of them being protein

ZO-1 [for various examples, (Table 1); for reviews see (28,50,51)]. It is suggested that cytoplasmic TJ proteins are involved in scaffolding, intracellular signaling, and vesicle transport/membrane trafficking. Moreover, they are responsible for the connection of TJ to the actin filament cytoskeleton.

Interestingly, the cytoplasmatic TJ plaque proteins ZO-1 and ZO-2, as well as symplekin, show dual localization at TJ and in the nucleus. This and the identification of nuclear interaction partners further suggest functions of TJ (or TJ proteins)

Table 1 TJ Plaque Proteins

Protein	Known binding partners in TJ	Putative function/special features	References
4.1.R	ZO-2		114
7H6		Regulation of paracellular barrier function of TJ	115,116
AF-6	ZO-1, JAM, Ras, cingulin	Scaffold protein; cell polarity	117–120
ASIP/Par3-Par6	JAM-1, -2, -3	Signaling molecule; regulation of TJ formation, cell polarity	121–127
Cingulin	ZO-1, ZO-2, ZO-3. actin, myosin, AF-6 JAM1, occludin	Coiled-coil rod domain Linker between TJ plaque and cytoskeleton	128–134
JEAP			135
MAGI 1	JAM-4	Scaffold protein, guanylate kinase	43,136
MUPP1	Claudin 1, JAM1	Scaffold protein	137
PILT			138
Rab 3b		TJ assembly/membrane trafficking/vesicle transport; GTPase	139,140
Rab 8			141–143
Rab 13		TJ assembly/membrane trafficking/vesicle transport GTPase	140,144–146
Symplekin		Nuclear localization	53,55
Sec6/8		Vesicle transport	143
ZA-1TJ			147
ZO-1	Occludin, claudins, JAM, ZO-2, ZO-3, cingulin, actin, ZONAB	Scaffold protein, signaling molecule member of the MAGUK-family, nuclear localization	54,57,130,134,148–153
ZO-2	ZO-1, actin, occludin, claudins, 4.1R	Scaffold protein, member of the MAGUK-family, nuclear localization	150,151,154,155
ZO-3	ZO-1, occludin, claudins, cingulin	Scaffold protein, member of the MAGUK-family	130,150,151,156

in signal transduction and, subsequently, proliferation and differentiation of cells [(52–58); for reviews see Refs. 28,59].

Several diseases have been linked to TJ. Mutations in the gene coding for claudin 14 result in human hereditary deafness, putatively by increasing the permeability of the Corti organ, which influences the compartmentalization in the cochlea (60). Patients with hereditary hypomagnesaemia have mutations in the gene coding for claudin 16/paracellin 1. In these patients, the normal resorption of Mg^{2+} ions in the thick ascending limb of Henle in the kidney is disturbed and, therefore, the loss of Mg^{2+} ions is higher than in normal persons [(61,62); for bovine see (63)]. Furthermore, several examples of interactions among TJ and pathogens and allergens exist. The toxins of *Clostridium difficile*, causing severe diarrhea and colitis, lead to a dissociation of occludin and proteins ZO-1 and ZO-2 from the lateral plasma membrane of epithelial cells, and a reduced interaction of F-actin and protein ZO-1. The mechanisms of this TJ alteration include the inactivation of members of the Rho-family of GTPases by monoglucosylation via *C. difficile* toxins and a subsequent alteration of the actin-cytoskeleton (64–66). The enterotoxin of *Clostridium perfringens*, also causing severe diarrhea, directly binds to claudins 3 and 4 (originally identified as "*Clostridium perfringens* enterotoxin-receptors") and separates claudin 4 from TJ (38,67). However, the importance of TJ binding via the C-terminal region to the clinical symptoms must be clarified, as the NH_2-terminal region of the enterotoxin increases membrane permeability by forming small pores in the plasma membrane (68,69). The RTX toxin and the zonula occludens toxin (ZOT) of *Vibrio cholerae* lead to a depolymerization of actin and a breakdown of the barrier function of TJ via different, but not yet completely understood, mechanisms (70–74). *Helicobacter pylori* infections are accompanied by the disruption of the paracellular barrier of the gastric mucosa and an alteration of the distribution of the TJ proteins 7H6 and occludin, as well as cortical actin. The increase in transepithelial permeability can be inhibited by the protein kinase C (PKC) activator phorbol myristate-acetate, arguing for an involvement of the PKC-pathway (75,76). JAM-1 is a receptor for reovirus and permits its infection in non-permissive cells (77). Allergens with proteolytic activity can disrupt TJ and might thereby facilitate the accessibility of epithelia to the allergens (78–80).

In addition to bacteria and their toxins, inflammatory cells attracted by the bacterial infection may also influence TJ (46,81–85) and contribute to changes in epithelial permeability.

In summary, TJ are dynamic and highly complex structures involved in several functions, most importantly the provision of a permeability barrier for simple epithelia and endothelia, and the formation of a fence for molecular diffusion in plasma membranes. TJ are targets for various exogenous and endogenous stimuli.

TIGHT JUNCTIONS IN THE SKIN

In adult human skin (including hair follicles), several mRNAs coding for TJ proteins have been identified, including claudins 1, 3, 4, 5, 7, 8, 10, 11, 12, 16, and 17, occludin, and protein ZO-1 (86–88). At the protein level, the existence of claudins 1, 4, 5, 7, 12, occludin, proteins ZO-1 and ZO-2, cingulin, and symplekin in the skin has been shown by immunofluorescence microscopy using specific antibodies [(86–91); for mouse (92,93)]. Localization of TJ proteins in the skin varies considerably (Fig. 4). Localization of occludin and cingulin is restricted to the cell–cell borders of the stratum granulosum and partly to the transitional layer. Protein ZO-1, claudin 4, and symplekin are found in several suprabasal layers, and claudins 1 and 7 are found in all epidermal layers (86,90–93). Localization of claudin 5 is, as in other tissues, restricted to endothelia (94). Claudin 12 is found in hair follicles (87). All TJ proteins in the epidermis show apparently continuous zonula occludens–like immunostainings at the cell borders of the stratum granulosum/transition layer, especially at the lateral plasma membranes that can clearly be seen in horizontal sections through the epidermis (Fig. 5) (86,91).

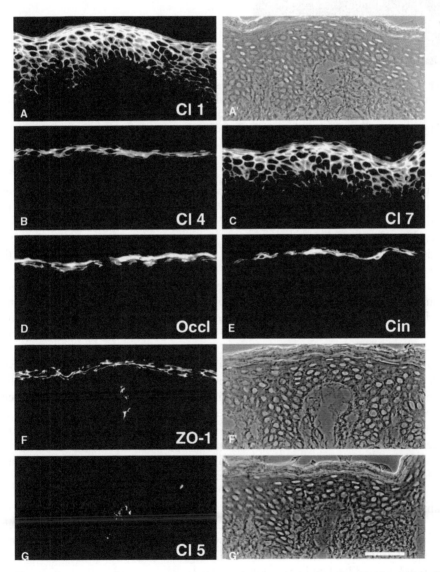

Figure 4 Immunoflurorescence microscopy showing the immunolocalization of (A) claudin-1, (B) claudin-4, (C) claudin-7, (D) occludin (E) cingulin, (F) protein ZO-1, and (G) claudin-5 in vertical sections through adult human epidermis. Same regions of A, F, and G are shown by phase contrast optics in A′, F′, and G′. Note the heterogeneous localization of the various TJ proteins. (Bar: 50 μm.)

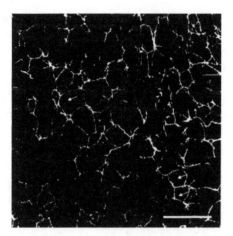

Figure 5 Laser-scanning confocal microscopy, showing immunofluroescence localization of occludin in near-horizontal cryostat sections of adult human skin. Arrows denote examples of cell circumferences completely positive for occludin, suggesting that there exists a continuous zonula occludens. (Bar: 50 μm.) *Source*: From Ref. 86.

After decades of discussion about the existence of typical TJ structures in the epidermis (92,95–104), their existence has finally been demonstrated in thin sections of both human and mouse epidermis (86,89,90,93). The successful identification of TJ structures is attributable to the use of antibodies recognizing TJ proteins as markers, allowing a more specific search for the structures. Previous reports denying the existence of typical TJ structures mostly did not have the benefit of these antibodies in their studies (97–100).

Typical TJ structures show the same ultrastructural morphology in cross-sections of human and mouse skin as in simple epithelia and endothelia, i.e., "kissing points" or "sites of fusion" (Fig. 6). (86,89,90,93; Fig. 8 in 99). TJ structures are often interspersed with desmosomes (86,91,93). Typical anastomosing fibrils in freeze–fracture replica have been found in the specialized skin of amphibians (105), cultured human skin keratinocytes (101), human gingival keratinocytes in vivo and in vitro (106), vitamin-A or humid milieu–treated skin (98,99), and occasionally in human fetal skin (102). In normal neonatal and adult skin, they have been described as absent or too fragmentary and of too limited extension for barrier formation ("maculae occludentes"; 97,99,100). The difficulties in identification of zonulae occludentes in freeze–fracture electron microscopy may be due to their restricted localization in mammalian skin. Technical improvements will lead to more precise descriptions of TJ in skin in the near future.

In addition to the typical TJ structures ("kissing points") various other occludin-containing structures have been identified in the stratum granulosum, including occludens junctions, lamellated junctions (coniunctiones laminosae), and sandwich junctions (iuncturae structae) (91). In the lower epidermal layers, occludin is absent, but other TJ proteins have been identified. Therefore, there are indications that more, hitherto unknown TJ-related structures may exist.

Percutaneous absorption of substances occurs not only by diffusion through the lipid domains of the stratum corneum, but also may involve skin appendages, specifically hair follicles and sweat glands. For example, Otberg et al. (107) recently showed that variations in hair follicle size and distribution influence skin penetration (107).

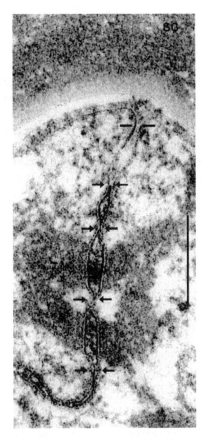

Figure 6 Electron micrograph of an ultrathin section through fetal plantar epidermis at the apical portion of the lateral membranes of outer stratum granulosum [transition of stratum granulosum to stratum corneum (sc)]. Note the numerous intercellular contact sites (kissing points; *arrows*). The horizontal bar denotes a close, but not tight contact site. (Bar: 0.2 μm.) *Source*: From Ref. 86.

Interestingly, co-expression of various TJ proteins, suggesting typical TJ or TJ-like structures, is not restricted to the stratum granulosum/transition layer of the epidermis but is also found in hair follicles (87,91,92). TJ are found in cell layers facing the hair shaft and the stratum corneum, suggesting a continuous TJ system in the skin, which extends from the epidermis into the skin appendages (87).

TJ proteins and TJ-related structures are also found in tumors derived from epidermal cells, such as squamous cell carcinoma and Merkel cell carcinoma (108,109), even though these tumors do not border on luminal or body surfaces. One might speculate that the formation of a TJ-related barrier within the tumors limits the effects of cytostatic drugs in tumor therapy.

In various diseases, e.g., psoriasis vulgaris, lichen ruber planus, eczema, and ichthyosis vulgaris, a broadened co-localization of TJ proteins has been found. While in normal epidermis, the co-localization is restricted to the stratum granulosum/transition layer, in these diseases it is also found in subjacent spinous layers [(90,104), Brandner et al., in prep.]. Interestingly enough, the broadened co-localization of TJ proteins is also found in stratified squamous epithelia bordering on moist surroundings, for example, in gingival, tongue, exocervical, and vaginal epithelia (91; for an increased number of TJ strands in freeze–fracture electron microscopy, 99).

A co-localization of adherens junction (AJ) and TJ proteins has been demonstrated in the lower granular and uppermost spinous cell layer of the epidermis and at the border of companian cell layer and Henle's layer in the lower portion of hair follicles (87,90). In simple epithelial (MDCK) cells, it has been described that TJ assembly begins with the formation of preliminary cell–cell junctions containing AJ and TJ components, which then mature into distinct AJ and TJ (for review, 28). It is possible that the areas with co-localizing TJ and AJ proteins in the epidermis and hair follicles represent these preliminary cell–cell junctions. However, it cannot be excluded that AJ and TJ are so tightly grouped together in these areas that they cannot be separated on the light microscopic level. Alternatively, a special skin structure containing TJ and AJ proteins may exist.

BARRIER FUNCTION OF TJ IN THE SKIN

It is well accepted that the stratum corneum plays a significant role in the physical barrier of the skin. There are, however, several experimental results indicating a role for TJ in barrier function, as well.

In healthy neonatal or adult skin with normal barrier function and normal stratum corneum, a co-localization of all known epidermal TJ proteins is found in the stratum granulosum/transition layer (86–93,109). However, as soon as the barrier of the skin is perturbed, the area of co-localization of TJ proteins is altered. In various diseases with perturbed stratum corneum barrier function, for example, psoriasis vulgaris, lichen ruber planus, acute and chronic eczema, and ichthyosis vulgaris, TJ proteins that were formerly restricted to the stratum granulosum/upper stratum spinosum (e.g., occludin, protein ZO-1, and claudin 4) were also found in deeper layers of the epidermis (90,104; Brandner et al., in prep.). After wounding of the skin where the stratum corneum barrier function is completely lost, a co-localization of TJ proteins is found in suprabasal layers of the regenerating epidermis as well as in the wound borders (86,110). The broadened synthesis of TJ proteins can be observed until wound healing is complete and a functional stratum corneum is formed (86). Also in tape-stripped skin, a model system for the impairment of barrier function of the skin, a broadened synthesis, and upregulation of TJ mRNA and TJ proteins can be observed (Brandner et al., in prep.). These results agree with observations made in other experimental systems for investigation of stratification. Previously, Elias and Friend (98) showed the induction of TJ formation in vitamin-A–treated embryonal chicken skin, which is characterized by the absence of cornification, mucous metaplasia, and because of these conditions, impaired barrier function. Moreover, it was shown that during the stratification of human skin equivalents the TJ proteins are synthesized early and that, in particular, occludin is not restricted to the uppermost living cell layer but is also found in deeper layers. Again, the early and broadened synthesis of TJ proteins precedes the formation of the stratum corneum (86). Therefore, TJ and TJ proteins might be especially involved in barrier formation, serving as a "rescue system" when the stratum corneum is missing or impaired.

However, TJ and TJ proteins are not only involved in skin (re)-generation but also seem to play an important role in basal permeability barrier function. Claudin-1–deficient mice die within one day of birth due to tremendous water loss

(93), although no morphological abnormalities in the living epidermal layers and TJ structures on light- and electron microscopic levels have been found in these mice. Permeability assays show that the diffusion of subcutaneously injected tracers (ca. 600 Da) is stopped at the TJ in the stratum granulosum in wild type mice, while the tracers pass freely in claudin-1–deficient mice. Tracer stops at TJ have also been demonstrated by Hashimoto (96) using lanthanum, but the results have not been confirmed (97,99). In claudin-1–deficient mice, the stratum corneum was altered, thickness increased, and the layers seemed to be more compact indicating a potential compensatory mechanism. Due to altered TJ permeability, ion gradients in the epidermis may be altered, influencing the synthesis and processing of proteins and lipids involved in maintaining the stratum corneum. Moreover, TJ could regulate the fluidity of apical versus basolateral membrane surfaces, restricting certain receptors and signaling mechanisms to specific sites. By regulating fluidity, they could also stipulate that lamellar body (LB) secretion is directed apically. And TJ could contain secreted LB contents, ensuring that tracers do not diffuse basally. It still must be clarified whether the impressive increase in TEWL seen in claudin-1–deficient animals is only due to increased TJ permeability or whether it is secondary to the altered stratum corneum structure. Nevertheless, either possibility demonstrates the importance of TJ for barrier function of the epidermis.

Even though tracer experiments showed a stop of tracers at the apical part of lateral plasma membranes in the stratum granulosum/transition layer—an area where typical TJ structures are found—it cannot be excluded that the frequently identified maculae occludentes as well as other TJ-related structures may also play a role for the barrier function of the epidermis. One could, for example, suppose that both zonulae and maculae occludentes could provide an initial line of defense against water loss. Moreover, maculae occludentes could also serve in receptor restriction and LB control as mentioned above. In addition, TJ-related structures may fulfill barrier functions in deeper layers of the epidermis.

Altered barrier function of the skin has also been demonstrated in mice overexpressing claudin-6 in the epidermis (111). Claudin-6 is weakly expressed in the upper layers of newborn (111) and is absent in adult mouse epidermis (112). During embryogenesis claudin-6 is clearly present in the periderm (112). The overexpression of claudin-6 in the upper layers of the epidermis resulted in a thicker and disorganized epidermis, a moderately thicker and frequently fragmented stratum corneum and, a fragile and poorly formed cornified envelope (111). The transgenic mice died within two days of birth and showed elevated TEWL and dye (X-gal) permeability. As various epidermal differentiation markers, such as cytokeratin K1, filaggrin, loricrin, transglutaminase 3, involucrin, repetin, and SPRRs, as well as various TJ proteins and transcription factor Klf4 are altered in these mice (111, Turksen and Troy 2002), it becomes difficult to define which of the described effects are responsible for the loss of barrier function. Electron microscopy studies in claudin-6 transgenic mice have not yet been published.

Interestingly, a perturbation in stratum corneum barrier function has also been found after the alteration of desmosomal proteins (113). An aberrant expression of desmoglein 3 in the upper epidermal layers of the skin via the involucrin promoter in addition to the normal expression in the lower layers, resulted in a thinner stratum corneum with a compact lamellar pattern and a reduced adherence of corneocytes resembling the morphology of oral mucosa. The transgenic mice died within 7–10 days of birth due to an elevated TEWL (113).

FUTURE ASPECTS

Several reports have been published in recent years that TJ are present in the epidermis and significant in barrier function. Many questions remain unanswered regarding the role of TJ in barrier function and the functions of various TJ-related structures. It is not yet understood why TJ proteins are heterogeneously distributed in the various layers of epidermis and hair follicles, how and where TJ assemble in the epidermis, and which signal transduction pathways are connected to TJ in the skin. Future research should examine whether TJ in the skin are influenced by similar substances as in simple epithelia, for example, bacterial toxins and allergens, and whether it is possible to use TJ structures to specifically deliver drugs to selected epidermal layers. Answers to these questions will significantly increase our knowledge of the skin barrier.

ACKNOWLEDGMENTS

We thank Dr. Ingrid Moll for stimulating discussions and Katherine Houghton, Dr. Jens-Michael Jensen, and Germar Schüring for careful manuscript work.

NOTE ADDED IN PROOF

Recently, an extended system integrating transmembraneous ridge configurations with desmosomes have been identified by using freeze fracture electron microscopy in the stratum granulosum/stratum corneum of the human epidermis (158). Moreover, a mutation of human claudin-1 was described in NISCH (neonatal ichthyosis and sclerosing cholangitis) syndrome (159) and the influence of E-cadherin on epidermal tight junctions has been shown very nicely in a mouse model (160).

REFERENCES

1. Elias PM, Fritsch P, Epstein EH. Staphylococcal scalded skin syndrome. Clinical features, pathogenesis, and recent microbiological and biochemical developments. Arch Dermatol 1977; 113:207–219.
2. Hanakawa Y, Schechter NM, Lin C, Garza L, Li H, Yamaguchi T, Fudaba Y, Nishifuji K, Sugai M, Amagai M, Stanley JR. Molecular mechanisms of blister formation in bullous impetigo and staphylococcal scalded skin syndrome. J Clin Invest 2002; 110:53–60.
3. Patel GK, Finlay AY. Staphylococcal scalded skin syndrome: diagnosis and management. Am J Clin Dermatol 2003; 4:165–175.
4. Stanley JR. Pathophysiology and therapy of pemphigus in the 21st century. J Dermatol 2001; 28:645–646.
5. Amagai M. Desmoglein as a target in autoimmunity and infection. J Am Acad Dermatol 2003; 48:244–252.
6. Prendiville J. Stevens-Johnson syndrome and toxic epidermal necrolysis. Adv Dermatol 2002; 18:151–173.
7. van Meer G, Simons K. The function of tight junctions in maintaining differences in lipid composition between the apical and the basolateral cell surface domains of MDCK cells. EMBO J 1986; 5:1455–1464.
8. Matter K, Balda MS. Occludin and the functions of tight junctions. Int Rev Cytol 1999; 186:117–146.
9. Matter K, Balda MS. Holey barrier: claudins and the regulation of brain endothelial permeability. J Cell Biol 2003; 161:459–460.

10. Tsukita Sh, Itoh M, Furuse M. Structural and signalling molecules come together at tight junctions. Curr Opin Cell Biol 1999; 11:628–633.

11. Tsukita Sh, Furuse M, Itoh M. Multifunctional strands in tight junctions. Nat Rev Mol Cell Biol 2001; 2:285–293.

12. Anderson JM. Molecular structure of tight junctions and their role in epithelial transport. News Physiol Sci 2001; 16:126–130.

13. D'Atri F, Citi S. Molecular complexity of vertebrate tight junctions. Mol Membr Biol 2002; 19:103–112.

14. Tsukita Sh, Furuse M. Pores in the wall: claudins constitute tight junction strands containing aqueous pores. J Cell Biol 2000; 149:13–16.

15. Lindemann B, Solomon AK. Permeability of luminal surface of intestinal mucosal cells. J Gen Physiol 1962; 54:801–810.

16. Moreno JH, Diamond JM. Cation permeation mechanisms and cation selectivity in "tight junctions" of gallbladder epithelium. In: Eisenman G, ed. Membranes: A Series Of Advances. Vol. 3. New York: Dekker, 1975:383–497.

17. Cereijido M, Robbins ES, Dolan WJ, Rotunno CA, Sabatini DD. Polarized monolayers formed by epithelial cells on a permeable and translucent support. J Cell Biol 1978: 853–880.

18. Reuss L. Tight junction permeability to ions and water. In: Cereijido M, ed. Tight Junctions. Boca Raton: CRC Press, 1992:49–66.

19. Gumbiner BM. Breaking through the tight junction barrier. J Cell Biol 1993; 123: 1631–1633.

20. Tsukita Sh, Furuse M. Claudin-based barrier in simple and stratified cellular sheets. Curr Opin Cell Biol 2002; 14:531–536.

21. Staehelin LA. Further observations on the fine structure of freeze-cleaved tight junctions. J Cell Sci 1973; 13:763–786.

22. Farquhar MG, Palade GE. Junctional complexes in various epithelia. J Cell Biol 1963; 17:375–412.

23. Furuse M, Hirase T, Itoh M, Nagafuchi A, Yonemura S, Tsukita Sh. Occludin: a novel integral membrane protein localizing at tight junctions. J Cell Biol 1993; 123: 1777–1788.

24. Ando-Akatsuka Y, Saitou M, Hirase T, Kishi M, Sakakibara A, Itoh M, Onemura S, Furuse M, Tsukita Sh. Interspecies diversity of the occludin sequence: cDNA cloning of human, mouse, dog, and rat-kangaroo homologues. J Cell Biol 1996; 133:43–47.

25. Balda MS, Whitney JA, Flores C, Gonzalez S, Cereijido M, Matter K. Functional dissociation of the paracellular permeability and transepithelial electrical resistance and disruption of the apical-basolateral intramembrane diffusion barrier by expression of a mutant tight junction membrane protein. J Cell Biol 1996; 134:1031–1049.

26. McCarthy KM, Skare IB, Stankewich MC, Furuse M, Tsukita Sh, Rogers RA, Lynch RD, Schneeberger EE. Occludin is a functional component of the tight junction. J Cell Sci 1996; 109:2287–2298.

27. Wong V, Gumbiner BM. A synthetic peptide corresponding to the extracellular domain of occludin perturbs the tight junction permeability barrier. J Cell Biol 1997; 136:399 409.

28. Matter K, Balda MS. Signalling to and from tight junctions. Nat Rev Mol Cell Biol 2003; 4:225–236.

29. Saitou M, Fujimoto K, Doi Y, Itoh M, Fujimoto T, Furuse M, Takano H, Noda T, Tsukita Sh. Occludin-deficient embryonic stem cells can differentiate into polarized epithelial cells bearing tight junctions. J Cell Biol 1998; 141:397–408.

30. Saitou M, Furue M, Sasaki H, Schulzke J-D, Fromm M, Takano H, Toda T, Tsukita Sh. Complex phenotype of mice lacking occludin, a component of tight junction strands. Mol Biol Cell 2000; 11:4131–4142.

31. Furuse M, Fujita K, Hiiragi T, Fujimoto K, Tsukita Sh. Claudin-1 and -2: novel integral membrane proteins localizing at tight junctions with no sequence similarity to occludin. J Cell Biol 1998; 141:1539–1550.

32. Furuse M, Sasaki H, Fujimoto K, Tsukita Sh. A single gene product, claudin-1 or -2 reconstitutes tight junction strands and recruits occludin in fibroblasts. J Cell Biol 1998; 143:391–401.

33. Morita K, Furuse M, Fujimoto K, Tsukita Sh. Claudin multigene family encoding four-transmembrane domain protein components of tight junction strands. Proc Natl Acad Sci USA 1999; 96:511–516.

34. Morita K, Sasaki H, Furuse M, Tsukita Sh. Endothelial claudin: claudin-5/TMVCF constitutes tight junction strands in endothelial cells. J Cell Biol 1999; 147:185–194.

35. Furuse M, Sasaki H, Tsukita Sh. Manner of interaction of heterogeneous claudin species within and between tight junction strands. J Cell Biol 1999; 147:891–903.

36. Kubota K, Furuse M, Sasaki H, Sonoda N, Fujita K, Nagafuchi A, Tsukita Sh. Ca^{2+}-independent cell-adhesion activity of claudins, a family of integral membrane proteins localized at tight junctions. Curr Biol 1999; 9:1035–1038.

37. Furuse M, Furuse K, Sasaki H, Tsukita Sh. Conversion of zonulae occludentes from tight to leaky strand type by introducing claudin-2 into Madin–Darby canine kidney I cells. J Cell Biol 2001; 153:263–272.

38. Sonoda N, Furuse M, Sasaki H, Yonemura S, Katahira J, Horiguchi Y, Tsukita Sh. Clostridium perfringens enterotoxin fragment removes specific claudins from tight junction strands: evidence for direct involvement of claudins in tight junction barrier. J Cell Biol 1999; 147:195–204.

39. Martin-Padura I, Lostaglio S, Schneemann M, Williams L, Romano M, Fruscella P, Panzeri C, Stoppacciaro A, Ruco L, Villa A, Simmons D, Dejana E. Junctional adhesion molecule, a novel member of the immunoglobulin superfamily that distributes at intercellular junctions and modulates monocyte transmigration. J Cell Biol 1998; 142:117–127.

40. Palmeri D, van Zante A, Huang CC, Hemmerich S, Rosen SD. Vascular endothelial junction-associated molecule, a novel member of the immunoglobulin superfamily, is localized to intercellular boundaries of endothelial cells. J Biol Chem 2000; 275: 1939–1945.

41. Arrate MP, Rodriguez JM, Tran TM, Brock TA, Cunningham SA. Cloning of human junctional adhesion molecule 3 (JAM3) and its identification as the JAM2 counter-receptor. J Biol Chem 2001; 276:45826–45832.

42. Aurrand-Lions M, Duncan L, Ballestrem C, Imhof BA. JAM-2, a novel immunoglobulin superfamily molecule, expressed by endothelial and lymphatic cells. J Biol Chem 2001; 276:2733–2741.

43. Hirabayashi S, Tajima M, Yao I, Nishimura W, Mori H, Hata Y. JAM4, a junctional cell adhesion molecule interacting with a tight junction protein, MAGI-1. Mol Cell Biol 2003; 23:4267–4282.

44. Bazzoni G, Martinez-Estrada OM, Müller F, Nelböck P, Schmid G, Bartfai T, Dejana E, Brockhaus M. Homophilic interaction of junctional adhesion molecule. J Biol Chem 2000; 275:30970–30976.

45. Kostrewa D, Brockhaus M, D'Arcy A, Dale GE, Nelböck P, Schmid G, Müller F, Bazzoni G, Dejana E, Bartfai T, Winkler FK, Henning M. X-ray structure of junctional adhesion molecule: structural basis for homophilic adhesion via a novel dimerization motif. EMBO J 2001; 20:4391–4398.

46. Ostermann G, Weber KS, Zernecke A, Schroder A, Weber C. JAM-1 is a ligand of the beta(2) integrin LFA-1 involved in transendothelial migration of leukocytes. Nat Immunol 2002; 3:151–158.

47. Cunningham SA, Rodriguez JM, Arrate MP, Tran TM, Brock TA. JAM2 interacts with alpha4beta1. Facilitation by JAM3. J Biol Chem 2002; 277:27589–27592.

48. Johnson-Leger CA, Aurrand-Lions M, Beltraminelli N, Fasel N, Imhof BA. Junctional adhesion molecule-2 (JAM-2) promotes lymphocyte transendothelial migration. Blood 2002; 100:2479–2486.

49. Liang TW, Chiu HH, Gurney A, Sidle A, Tumas DB, Schow P, Foster J, Klassen T, Dennis K, DeMarco RA, Pham T, Frantz G, Fong S. Vascular endothelial-junctional adhesion molecule (VE-JAM)/JAM 2 interacts with T, NK, and dendritic cells through JAM 3. J Immunol 2002; 168:1618–1626.

50. Stevenson BT, Keon BH. The tight junctions: morphology to molecules. Annu Rev Cell Dev Biol 1998; 119:89–109.

51. Mitic LL, Van Itallie CM, Anderson JM. Molecular physiology and pathophysiology of tight junctions. I. Tight junction structure and function: lessons from mutant animals and proteins. Am J Physiol Gastrointest Liver Physiol 2000; 279:G250–G254.

52. Gottardi CJ, Arpin M, Fanning AS, Louvard D. The junction-associated protein zonula occludens-1, localizes to the nucleus before the maturation and during the remodelling of cell-cell contacts. Proc Natl Acad Sci USA 1996; 93:10779–10784.

53. Keon BH, Schäfer S, Kuhn C, Grund C, Franke WW. Symplekin, a novel type of tight junction plaque protein. J Cell Biol 1996; 134:1003–1018.

54. Balda MS, Matter K. The tight junction protein ZO-1 and an interacting transcription factor regulate ErbB-2 expression. EMBO J 2000; 19:2024–2033.

55. Hofmann I, Schnölzer M, Kaufmann I, Franke WW. Symplekin, a constitute protein of karyo- and cytoplasmic particles involved in mRNA biogenesis in Xenopus laevis oocytes. Mol Biol Cell 2002; 13:1665–1678.

56. Islas S, Vega J, Ponce L, Gonzalez-Mariscal L. Nuclear localization of the tight junction protein ZO-2 in epithelial cells. Exp Cell Res 2002; 274:138–148.

57. Balda MS, Garrett MD, Matter K. The ZO-1-associated Y-box factor ZONAB regulates epithelial cell proliferation and cell density. J Cell Biol 2003; 160:423–432.

58. Traweger A, Fuchts R, Krizbai IA, Weiger TM, Bauer HC, Bauer H. The tight junction protein ZO-2 localizes to the nucleus and interacts with the heterogeneous nuclear ribonucleoprotein scaffold attachment factor-B. J Biol Chem 2003; 278:2692–2700.

59. Zahraoui A, Louvard D, Galli T. Tight Junction, a platform for trafficking and signalling protein complexes. J Cell Biol 2000; 151:F31–F36.

60. Wilcox ER, Burton QL, Naz S, Riazuddin S, Smith TN, Ploplis B, Belyantseva I, Ben-Yosef T, Liburd NA, Morell RJ, Kachar B, Wu DK, Griffith AJ, Riazuddin S, Friedman TB. Mutations in the gene encoding tight junction claudin-14 cause autosomal recessive deafness DFNB29. Cell 2001; 104:165–172.

61. Simon DB, Lu Y, Choate KA, Velazquez H, Al-Sabban E, Praga M, Casiri G, Bettinelli A, Colussi G, Rodriguez-Soriano J, McCredie D, Milford D, Danjad S, Lifton RP. Paracellin-1, a renal tight junction protein required for paracellular Mg^{2+} resorption. Science 1999; 285:103–106.

62. Weber S, Schneider L, Peters M, Misselwitz J, Ronnefarth G, Boswald M, Bonzel KE, Seeman T, Sulakova T, Kuwertz-Broking E, Gregoric A, Palcoux JB, Tasic V, Manz F, Scharer K, Seyberth HW, Konrad M. Novel paracellin-1 mutations in 25 families with familial hypomagnesaemia with hypercalciuria and nephrocalcinosis. J Am Soc Nephrol 2001; 12:1872–1881.

63. Hirano T, Kobayashi N, Itoh T, Takasuga A, Nakamura T, Hirotsune S, Sugimoto Y. Null mutation of PCLN-1/claudin-16 results in bovine chronic interstitial nephritis. Genome Res 2000; 10:659–663.

64. Hecht G, Pothoulakis C, LaMont JT, Madara JL. Clostridium difficile toxin A perturbs cytoskeletal structure and tight junction permeability of cultured human intestinal epithelial monolayers. J Clin Invest 1988; 82:1516–1524.

65. Nusrat A, von Eichel-Streiber C, Turner JR, Verkade P, Madara JL, Parkos CA. Clostridium difficile toxins disrupt epithelial barrier function by altering membrane microdomain localization of tight junction proteins. Infect Immun 2001; 69:1329–1336.

66. Pothoulakis C, Lamont JT. Microbes and microbial toxins: Paradigms for microbial-mucosal interactions. II. The integrated response of the intestine to Clostridium difficile toxins. Am J Physiol Gastrointest Liver Physiol 2001; 280:G178–G183.

67. Katahira J, Inoue N, Horiguchi Y, Matsuda M, Sugimoto N. Molecular cloning and functional characterization of the receptor for Clostridium perfringens enterotoxin. J Cell Biol 1997; 136:1239–1247.
68. Matsuda M, Sugimoto N. Calcium-independent and dependent steps in action of Clostridium perfringens enterotoxin on Hela and vero cells. Biochem Biophys Res Commun 1979; 91:629–636.
69. Hanna PC, Wieckowski EH, Mietzner TA, McClane BA. Mapping of functional regions of Clostridium perfringens type A enterotoxin. Infect Immun 1992; 60:2110–2114.
70. Fasano A, Fiorentini G, Donelli G, Uzzau S, Kaper JB, Margaretten K, Ding X, Guandalini S, Comstock L, Goldblum SE. Zonula occludens toxin modulates tight junctions through PKC-dependent actin reorganization in vitro. J Clin Invest 1995; 96: 710–720.
71. Fasano A, Uzzau S, Fiore C, Margaretten K. The enterotoxic effect of zonula occludens toxin (Zot) on rabbit small intestine involves the paracellular pathway. Gastroenterology 1997; 112:839–846.
72. Fullner JK, Mekalanos JJ. In vivo covalent crosslinking of actin by the RTX toxin of *Vibrio cholerae*. EMBO J 2000; 19:5315–5323.
73. DiPierro M, Lu R, Uzzau S, Wang W, Margaretten K, Pazzani C, Maimone F, Fasano A. Zonula occludens toxin structure-function analysis. J Biol Chem 2001; 276:19160–19165.
74. Fullner KJ, Lencer WI, Mekalanos JJ. Vibrio cholerae-induced cellular responses of polarized T84 intestinal epithelial cells are dependent on production of cholera toxin and the RTX toxin. Infect Immun 2001; 69:6310–6317.
75. Terres AM, Pajares JM, Hopkins AM, Murphy A, Moran A, Baird AW, Kelleher D. Helicobacter pylori disrupts epithelial barrier function in a process inhibited by protein kinase C activators. Infect Immun 1998; 66:2943–2950.
76. Suzuki K, Kokai Y, Sawada N, Taktkuwa R, Kuwahara K, Isogai E, Isogai H, Mori M. SS1 Helicobacter pylori disrupts the paracellular barrier of the gastric mucosa and leads to neutrophilic gastritis in mice. Virchows Arch 2002; 440:318–324.
77. Barton ES, Forrest JC, Connolly JL, Chappell JD, Liu Y, Schnell FJ, Nusrat A, Parkos CA, Dermody TS. Junction adhesion molecule is a receptor for reovirus. Cell 2001; 104:441–451.
78. Wan H, Winton HL, Soeller C, Tovey ER, Gruenert DC, Thompson PJ, Stewart GA, Taylor GW, Garrod DR, Cannell MB, Robinson C. Der p 1 facilitates transepithelial allergen delivery by disruption of tight junctions. J Clin Invest 1999; 104:123–133.
79. Wan H, Winton HL, Söller C, Taylor GW, Gründer DC, Thompson PJ, Cannell MB, Stewart GA, Garrod DR, Robinson C. The transmembrane protein occludin of epithelial tight junctions is a functional target for serine peptidases from faecal pellets of Dermatophagoides pteronyssinus. Clin Exp Allergy 2001; 31:186–192.
80. Robinson C, Baker SF, Garrod DR. Peptidase allergens, occludin and claudins. Do their interactions facilitate the development of hypersensitivity reactions at mucosal surfaces? Clin Exp Allergy 2001; 31:186–192.
81. Pollard JD, Westland KW, Harvey GK, Jung S, Bonner J, Spies JM, Toka KV, Hartung HP. Activated T cells of nonneural specificity open the blood-nerve barrier to circulating antibody. Ann Neurol 1995; 37:467–475.
82. Parkos CA. Molecular events in neutrophil transepithelial migration. Bioessays 1997; 19:865–873.
83. Bolton SJ, Anthony DC, Perr VH. Loss of the tight junction proteins occludin and zonula occludines-1 from cerebral vascular endothelium during neutrophil-induced blood-brain barrier breakdown in vivo. Neuroscience 1998; 86:1245–1257.
84. Huber D, Balda MS, Matter K. Occludin modulates transepithelial migration of neutrophils. J Biol Chem 2000; 275:5773–5778.
85. Rescigno M, Urbano M, Valzasina B, Francolini M, Rotta G, Bonasio R, Granucci F, Kraehenbuhl JP, Ricciardi-Castagnoli P. Dendritic cells express tight junction proteins and penetrate gut epithelial monolayers to sample bacteria. Nat Immunol 2001; 2:361–367.

86. Brandner JM, Kief S, Grund C, Rendl M, Houdek P, Kuhn C, Tschachler E, Franke WW, Moll I. Organization and formation of the tight junction system in human epidermis and cultured keratinocytes. Eur J Cell Biol 2002; 81:253–263.

87. Brandner JM, McIntyre M, Kief S, Wladykowski E, Moll I. Expression and localization of tight junction-associated proteins in human hair follicles. Arch Dermatol Res 2003; 295:211–221.

88. Tebbe B, Mankertz J, Schwarz C, Amasheh S, Fromm M, Assaf C, Schultz-Ehrnburg U, Sánchez Ruderisch H, Schulzke J-D, Orfanos CE. Tight junction proteins: a novel class of integral membrane proteins. Expression in human epidermis and in HaCaT keratinocytes . Arch Dermatol Res 2002; 294:14–18.

89. Brandner JM, Houdek P, Kuhn C, Grund C, Kief S, Franke WW. Tight-junction systems in mammalian squamous stratified epithelia. DGZ/SBCF: first German/French cell biology congress, Strassbourg. Biol Cell 2001; 93:247.

90. Pummi K, Malminen M, Aho H, Karvonen S-L, Peltonen J, Peltonen S. Epidermal tight junctions: ZO-1 and occludin are expressed in mature, developing, and affected skin and in vitro differentiating keratinocytes. J Invest Dermatol 2001; 117:1050–1058.

91. Langbein L, Grund C, Kuhn C, Prätzel S, Kartenbeck J, Brandner JM, Moll I, Franke WW. Tight junctions and compositionally related junctional structures in mammalian stratified epithelia and cell cultures derived there from. Eur J Cell Biol 2002; 81:419–435.

92. Morita K, Itoh M, Saitou M, Ando-Akatsuka Y, Furuse M, Yoneda K, Imamura S, Fujimoto K, Tsukita Sh. Subcellular distribution of tight junction-associated proteins (occludin, ZO-1, ZO-2) in rodent skin. J Invest Dermatol 1998; 110:862–866.

93. Furuse M, Hata M, Furuse K, Yoshida Y, Haratake A, Sugitani Y, Noda T, Kubo A, Tsukita Sh. Claudin-based tight junctions are crucial for the mammalian epidermal barrier: a lesson from claudin-1-deficient mice. J Cell Biol 2002; 156:1099–1111.

94. Morita K, Sasaki H, Furuse K, Furuse M, Tsukita Sh, Miyachi Y. Expression of claudin-5 in dermal vascular endothelia. Exp Dermatol 2003; 12:289–295.

95. Breathnach AS. An Atlas of the Ultrastructure of Human Skin. 1st ed. London: J&A Churchill, 1971.

96. Hashimoto K. Intercellular spaces of the human epidermis as demonstrated with lanthanum. J Invest Dermatol 1971; 57:17–31.

97. Elias PM, Friend DS. The permeability barrier and pathways in mammalian epidermis. J Cell Biol 1975; 65:180–191.

98. Elias PM, Friend DS. Vitamin-A induced mucous metaplasia. J Cell Biol 1976; 68: 173–188.

99. Elias PM, Scott McNutt N, Friend DS. Membrane alterations during cornification of mammalian squamous epithelia: a freeze-fracture, tracer, and thin-section study. Anat Rec 1977; 189:557–594.

100. Caputo R, Peluchetti D. The junctions of normal human Epidermis. J Ultrastruct Res 1977; 61:44–61.

101. Kitajima Y, Eguchi K, Ohno T, Mori S, Yaoita H. Tight junctions of human keratinocytes in primary culture: a freeze-fracture study. J Ultrastruct Res 1983; 82:309–313.

102. Fleck RM, Barnadas M, Schulz WW, Roberts LJ, Freeman RG. Harlquin ichthyosis: an ultrastructural study. J Am Acad Dermatol 1989; 21:999–1006.

103. Fawcett DW. A Textbook of Histology. New York: Chapman & Hall, 1994, p69.

104. Yoshida Y, Morita K, Mizoguchi A, Ide C, Miyachi Y. Altered expression of occludin and tight junction formation in psoriasis. Arch Dermatol Res 2001; 293:239–244.

105. Farquhar MG, Palade GE. Cell junctions in amphibian skin. J Cell Biol 1965; 26: 263–291.

106. Meyle J, Gültig K, Rascher G, Wolburg H. Transepithelial resistance and tight junctions of human gingival keratinocytes. J Peridont Res 1999; 34:214–222.

107. Otberg N, Richter H, Schaefer H, Blume-Peytave U, Sterry W, Lademann J. Variations of hair follicle size and distribution in different body sites. J Invest Dermatol 2004; 122: 14–19.

108. Haass NK, Houdek P, Wladykowski E, Moll I, Brandner JM. Expression pattern of tight junction proteins in Merkel cell carcinoma. In: Baumann KI, Halata Z, Moll I, eds. The Merkel Cell: Structure–Development–Function–Cancerogenesis. Berlin: Springer, 2003:23–226.

109. Langbein L, Pape U-F, Grund C, Kuhn C, Prätzel S, Moll I, Moll R, Franke WW. Tight junction-related structures in the absence of a lumen: occludin, claudins and tight junction plaque proteins in densely packed cell formations of stratified epithelia and squamous cell carcinomas. Eur J Cell Biol 2003; 82:385–400.

110. Malminen M, Koivukangas V, Peltoen J, Karvonen S-L, Oikarinen A, Peltonen S. Immunohistological distribution of the tight junction components ZO-1 and occludin in regenerating human epidermis. Br J Dermatol 2003; 149:255–260.

111. Turksen K, Troy TC. Permeability barrier dysfunction in transgenic mice overexpressing claudin 6. Development 2002; 129:1775–1784.

112. Morita K, Furuse M, Yoshida Y, Itoh M, Sasaki H, Tsukita Sh, Miyachi Y. Molecular architecture of tight junctions of periderm differs from that of the maculae occludentes of epidermis. J Invest Dermatol 2002; 118:1073–1079.

113. Elias PM, Matsuyoshi N, Wu H, Lin C, Wang ZH, Brown BE, Stanley JR. Desmoglein isoform distribution affects stratum corneum structure and function. J Cell Biol 2001; 153:243–249.

114. Mattagajasingh SN, Huang SC, Hartenstein JS, Benz EJ Jr. Characterization of the interaction between protein 4.1R and ZO-2. A possible link between the tight junction and the actin cytoskeleton. J Biol Chem 2000; 275:30573–30585.

115. Zhong YT, Saitoh T, Minase T, Sawada N, Enomoto K, Mori M. Monoclonal antibody 7H6 reacts with a novel tight junction-associated protein distinct from ZO-1, cingulin and ZO-2. J Cell Biol 1993; 120:477–483.

116. Satoh H, Zhong Y, Isomura H, Saitoh M, Enomoto K, Sawada N, Mori M. Localization of 7H6 tight junction-associated antigen along the cell border of vascular endothelial cells correlates with paracellular barrier function against ions, large molecules, and cancer cells. Exp Cell Res 1996; 222:269–274.

117. Prasad R, Gu Y, Alder H, Nakamura T, Canaani O, Saito H, Hübner K, Gale RP, Nowell PC, Kuriyama K. Cloning of the ALL-1 fusion partner, the AF-6 gene, involved in acute myeloid leukemias with the t(6;11) chromosome translocation. Cancer Res 1993; 53:5624–5628.

118. Yamamoto T, Harada N, Kano S, Taya E, Canaani E, Matsuura Y, Mizoguchi A, Ide C, Kaibuchi K. The Ras target AF-6 interacts with ZO-1 and serves as a peripheral component of tight junctions in epithelial cells. J Cell Biol 1997; 139:785–795.

119. Zhadanov AB, Provance DW Jr, Speer CA, Coffin JD, Goss D, Blixt JA, Reichert CM, Mercer JA. Absence of the tight junctional protein AF-6 disrupts epithelial cell–cell junctions and cell polarity during mouse development. Curr Biol 1999; 9:880–888.

120. Ebnet K, Schulz CU, Meyer zu Brickwedde, MK, Pendl GG, Vestweber D. Junctional adhesion molecule interacts with the PDZ domain-containing proteins AF-6 and ZO-1. J Biol Chem 2000; 275:27979–27988.

121. Izumi Y, Hirose T, Tamai Y, Hirai S, Nagashima Y, Fujimoto T, Tabuse Y, Kemphues KJ, Ohno D. An atypical PKC directly associates and colocalizes at the epithelial tight junction with ASIP, a mammalian homologue of Caenorhabditis elegans polarity protein PAR-3. J Cell Biol 1998; 143:95–106.

122. Joberty G, Peterson C, Gao L, Macara IG. The cell polarity protein Par6 links Par3 and an atypical protein kinase C to Cdc42. Nat Cell Biol 2000; 2:531–539.

123. Lin D, Edwards AS, Fawcett JP, Mbamalu G, Scott JD, Pawson T. A mammalian Par3–Par6 complex implicated in Cxc42/Rac1 and aPKC signalling an cell polarity. Nat Cell Biol 2000; 2:540–547.

124. Ebnet K, Suzuki A, Horikoshi Y, Hirose T, Meyer zu Brickwedde MK, Ohno S, Vestweber D. The cell polarity protein ASIP/PAR-3 directly associates with junctional adhesion molecule (JAM). EMBO J 2001; 20:3738–3748.

125. Ebnet K, Aurrand-Lions M, Kuhn A, Kiefer F, Butz S, Zander K, Brickwedde MK, Suzuki A, Imhof BA, Vestweber D. The junctional adhesion molecule (JAM) family members JAM-2 and JAM-3 associate with the cell polarity protein PAR-3: a possible role for JAMs in endothelial cell polarity. J Cell Sci 2003; 116:3879–3891.

126. Itoh M, Sasaki H, Furuse M, Ozaki H, Kita T, Tsukita S. Junctional adhesion molecule (JAM) binds to PAR-3: a possible mechanism for the recruitment of PAR-3 to tight junctions. J Cell Biol 2001; 154:1351–1363.

127. Hirose T, Izumi Y, Nagashima Y, Tamai-Nagai Y, Kurihara H, Sakai T, Suzuki Y, Yamanaka T, Suzuki A, Mizuno K, Ohno S. Involvement of ASIP/PAR-3 in the promotion of epithelial tight junction formation. J Cell Sci 2002; 115:2485–2495.

128. Citi S, Sabanay H, Jakes R, Geiger B, Kendrick-Jones J. Cingulin, a new peripheral component of tight junctions. Nature 1988; 333:272–276.

129. Citi S, D'Atri F, Parry DAD. Human and Xenopus cingulin share a modular organization of the coiled-coil rod domain: predictions for intra- and inter-molecular assembly. J Struct Biology 2000; 131:135–145.

130. Cordenonsi M, D'Atri F, Hammar E, Parry DA, Kendrick-Jones J, Shore D, Citi S. Cingulin contains globular and coiled-coil domains and interacts with ZO-1, ZO-2, ZO-3 and myosin. J Cell Biol 1999; 147:1569–1582.

131. Cordenonsi M, Turco F, D'Atri F, Hammar E, Martinucci G, Meggio F, Citi S. Xenopus laevis occludin. Identification of in vitro phosphorylation sites by protein kinase CK2 and association with cingulin. Eur J Biochem 1999; 264:374–384.

132. Bazzoni G, Martinez-Estrada OM, Orsenigo F, Cordenonsi M, Citi S, Dejana E. Interaction of junctional adhesion molecule with the tight junction components ZO-1, cingulin, and occludin. J Biol Chem 2000; 275:20520–20526.

133. D'Atri F, Citi S. Cingulin interacts with F-actin in vitro. FEBS Lett 2001; 507:21–24.

134. D'Atri F, Nadalutti F, Citi S. Evidence for a functional interaction between cingulin and ZO-1 in cultured cells. J Biol Chem 2002; 277:27757–27764.

135. Nishimura M, Kakizaki M, Ono Y, Morimoto K, Takeuchi M, Inoue Y, Imai T, Takai Y. JEAP, a novel component of tight junctions in exocrine cells. J Biol Chem 2002; 277:5583–5587.

136. Laura RP, Ross S, Koeppen H, Lasky LA. MAGI-1: a widely expressed, alternatively spliced tight junction protein. Exp Cell Res 2002; 275:155–170.

137. Hamazaki Y, Itoh M, Sasaki H, Furuse M, Tsukita S. Multi-PDZ domain protein 1 (MUPP1) is concentrated at tight junctions through its possible interaction with claudin-1 and junctional adhesion molecule. J Biol Chem 2002; 277:455–461.

138. Kawabe H, Nakanishi H, Asada M, Fukuhara A, Morimoto K, Takeuchi M, Takai Y. Pilt, a novel peripheral membrane protein at tight junctions in epithelial cells. J Biol Chem 2001; 276:48350–48355.

139. Weber E, Berta G, Tousson A, St John P, Green MW, Gopalokrishnan U, Jilling T, Sorscer EJ, Elton TS, Abrahamson DR, Kirk KL. Expression and polarized targeting of a rab3 isoform in epithelial cells. J Cell Biol 1994; 125:583–594.

140. Yamamoto Y, Nishimura N, Morimoto S, Kitamura H, Manabe S, Kanayama HO, Kagawa S, Sasaki T. Distinct roles of Rab3B and Rab13 in the polarized transport of apical, basolateral, and tight junctional membrane proteins to the plasma membrane. Biochem Biophys Res Commun 2003; 308:270–275.

141. Huber LA, Pimplikar S, Parton RG, Virta H, Zerial M, Simmons K. Rab8, a small GTPase involved in vesicular traffic between the TGN and the basolateral plasma membrane. J Cell Biol 1993; 123:35–45.

142. Ren M, Zeng J, De L, Chiarandini C, Rosenfeld M, Adesnik M, Sabatini DD. In its active form, the TRP-binding protein rab8 interacts with a stress-activated protein kinase. Proc Natl Acad Sci USA 1996; 93:5151–5155.

143. Grindstaff K, Yeaman C, Anandasabapathy N, Hus SC, Rodriguez-Boulan E, Scheller RH, Nelson WJ. Sec6/8 complex is recruited to cell–cell contacts and specifies transport vesicle deliver to the basal-lateral membrane in epithelial cells. Cell 1998; 93:731–740.

144. Zahraoui A, Joberty G, Arpin M, Fontaine JJ, Hellio R, Tavitian A, Louvard D. A small rab GTPase is distributed in cytoplasmic vesicles in nonpolarized cells but colocalizes with the tight junction marker ZO-1 in polarized epithelial cells. J Cell Biol 1994; 124:101–115.

145. Marzesco AM, Galli T, Louvard D, Zahraoui A. The rod cGMP phosphodiesterase subunit dissociates the small GTPase Rab13 from membranes. J Biol Chem 1998; 273:22340–22345.

146. Marzesco AM, Dunia I, Pandjaitan R, Recouvreur M, Dauzonne D, Benedetti EL, Louvard D, Zahraoui A. The small GTPase Rab13 regulates assembly of functional tight junctions in epithelial cells. Mol Biol Cell 2002; 13:1819–1831.

147. Kapprel H, Duden R, Owaribe K, Schmelz M, Franke WW. Subplasmalemmal plaques of intercellular junctions: common and distinguishing proteins. In: Edelman GM, Cunningham BA, Thiery JP, eds. Morphoregulatory Molecules. New York: Wiley, 1990:285–314.

148. Stevenson B, Silicano JD, Mooseker M, Goodenough DA. Identification of ZO-1: a high molecular weight polypeptide associated with the tight junction (zonula occludens) in a variety of epithelia. J Cell Biol 1986; 103:755–766.

149. Itoh M, Nagafuchi A, Yonemura S, Kitani-yasuda T, Tsukita S, Tsukita Sh. The 220 kDa protein colocalizing with cadherins in non-epithelial cells is identical to ZO-1, a tight junction associated protein in epithelial cells: cDNA cloning and immuno-localization. J Cell Biol 1993; 124:491–502.

150. Itoh M, Furuse M, Morita K, Kubota K, Saitou M, Tsukita S. Direct binding of three tight junction-associated MAGUKs, ZO-1, ZO-2, and ZO-3, with the COOH termini of claudins. J Cell Biol 1999; 147:1351–1363.

151. Wittchen ES, Haskins J, Stevenson BR. Protein interactions at the tight junction. J Biol Chem 1999; 274:35179–35185.

152. Fanning AS, Ma TY, Anderson JM. Isolation and functional characterization of the actin binding region in the tight junction protein ZO-1. FASEB J 2002; 16:1835–1837.

153. Fukuhara A, Irie K, Nakanishi H, Takekuni K, Kawakatsu T, Ikeda W, Yamada A, Katata T, Honda T, Sato T, Shimizu K, Ozaki H, Horiuchi H, Kita T, Takai Y. Involvement of nectin in the localization of junctional adhesion molecule at tight junctions. Oncogene 2002; 21:7642–7655.

154. Gumbiner B, Lowenkopf T, Apatira D. Identification of a 160 kDa polypeptide that binds to the tight junction protein ZO-1. Proc Natl Acad Sci 1991; 88:3460–3464.

155. Beatch M, Jesaitis LA, Gallin WJ, Goodenough DA, Stevenson BR. The tight junction protein ZO-2 contains three PDZ (PSD-95/Discs-Large/ZO-1) domains and an alternatively spliced region. J Biol Chem 1996; 271:25723–25726.

156. Haskins J, Gu L, Wittchen ES, Hibbard J, Stevenson BR. ZO-3, a novel member of the MAGUK protein family found at the tight junction, interacts with ZO-1 and occludin. J Cell Biol 1998; 141:199–208.

157. Alberts B, Bray D, Lewis J, Raff M, Roberts K, Watson JD. Molecular Biology of the Cell. 2nd ed. New York: Taylor & Francis Books Inc., 1989:794.

158. Schlüter H, Wepf R, Moll I, Franke WW. Sealing the live part of the skin: The integrated meshwork of demsosomes, tight junctions and curvilinear ridge structures in the cells of the uppermost granular layer of the human epidermis. Eur J Cell Biol 2004; 83:655–665.

159. Hadj-Rabia S, Baala L, Vabres P, Hamel-Teillac D, Jacquemin E, Fabre M, Lyonnet S, De-Prost Y, Munnich A, Hadchouel M, Smahi A. Claudin-1 gene mutations in neonatal sclerosing cholangitis associated with ichthyosis: a tight junction disease. Gastroenterology 2004; 127:1386–1390.

160. Tunggal JA, Helfrich I, Schmitz A, Schwarz H, Gunzel D, Fromm M, Kemler R, Krieg T, Niessen CM. E-cadherin is essential for in vivo epidermal barrier function by regulating tight junctions. EMBO J 2005; 24:1146–1156.

13

What Makes a Good Barrier? Adaptive Features of Vertebrate Integument

Gopinathan K. Menon
Global Research and Development, Avon Products, Inc., Suffern, New York, U.S.A.

INTRODUCTION

Barrier functions of skin have different meanings to different investigators, depending on their focus of investigation or subspecialty within skin biology. To the majority of investigators in dermatology and the field of transdermal drug delivery, it is synonymous with the permeability barrier, primarily located in the stratum corneum (SC). This paper-thin tissue, which in humans, ranges from 15 to 18 layers of corneocytes embedded in a matrix of hydrophobic lipids (a brick-and-mortar organization), is a composite material with unique functional properties (1). Investigators from multiple disciplines continue to explore this fascinating tissue, which permits the survival of almost all vertebrates on land and in water. Most studies contributing to our present day understanding of the formation and homeostasis of the permeability barrier come from studies on the epidermis of two mammalian species: laboratory mice and humans. However, extrapolating from these models to arrive at a global rationale for how this tissue allows for survival (i.e., when the barrier is good enough) is fraught with hazard. To begin a discussion on this topic, it is appropriate to consider the many different kinds of barriers that exist in the vertebrate integument: from physical barriers (impact resistance, barriers to ultraviolet radiation, ice crystal propagation), chemical barriers (antimicrobial, metabolic defenses, anti-oxidant), immune barriers (initiation of cytokine cascade, immunoglobulins, dendritic cell–mediated), barriers to biofowling (cetacean mammals), to psychological barriers to human relations (xenophobia based on skin color). Adaptations to specific ecological challenges and seasonal changes in habitats add another layer of complexity, where survival depends on the skin's capacity for "facultative barrier upregulation," documented in experimental acclimation studies on the lower vertebrates. An overview of the barrier functions of lower vertebrates, as well as homeotherms living under different environments, provides us with a broader understanding of the multifaceted barrier that we often overlook due to our primary focus on the permeability barrier.

So the answer to the question, "When is barrier good enough?" depends on a lot of variables, such as: barrier to what, under which environmental conditions (aquatic, terrestrial, xeric, mesic, etc.) and even, what specific developmental stages of the individual life cycle (premature, neonatal, juvenal, senile, etc.) that are under investigation? Although trans-epidermal water loss (TEWL) values are good indicators of its functional status, the skin barrier encompasses a number of integumentary functions (Table 1). In this brief review, I will attempt to highlight the fact that higher TEWL values may not necessarily reflect a defect, and may even have an adaptive significance of great survival value. The correlation between TEWL values, measured by a variety of techniques and instruments, and the multilamellar organization of barrier lipids of the SC has been well established during the past two decades (2). The origin of the barrier lipids from epidermal lamellar bodies (LBs), the significance of the post-secretory processing of these pro-barrier lipids (3,4), and an accelerated LB secretion following a barrier abrogation (and increased TEWL) that results in the restoration of the barrier (5) have all been well documented. Figure 1 demonstrates the morphological features of the secretion of the epidermal LB at the stratum granulosum–stratum corneum (SG–SC) interface. As the outermost cell of the SG transforms into a corneocyte, subjacent granulocytes take their place at the SG–SC interface. This is the typical pattern in the mammalian epidermis, where the morphological appearance and contents of LBs can be altered by experimental manipulations (inhibitors of lipogenic enzymes, exposure to cold, etc.). The altered lipid composition results in an abnormal morphology of the LBs and SC lipid lamellae, an increased permeability of the SC, and an abnormal pattern of desquamation. The abnormal desquamation leads to a "scaly" appearance and hence the tendency to view scaly skin as barrier-compromised, which is true for the mammalian skin. Creative advertising for products that treat dry skin and moisturize it often include a "dry, scaly"

Table 1 Barriers in Integument

Type	Function	Basis	Location
Physical barrier	Impact resistance	Structural organization/ collagen	Epidermis and dermis
	Shear resistance	Desmosomes	Epidermis
Permeability barrier	Keep water in/out	Lipids	SC
UV/Radiation barrier	Prevent photodamage to DNA, dermis, etc.	Melanin	Melanocytes
		DNA repair enzymes	Epidermis
		Carotenoids and other pigments (lower vertebrates)	Dermal chromatophores
Oxidant barrier	Prevent peroxidation/ free radical damage	Antioxidants (Vitamin C, E, etc.)	Epidermis
			Sebaceous glands
Thermal barrier	Protection from heat/ cold injury	HSPs	Epidermis
		Anti-freeze proteins	Dermis
Immune barrier	Provide immunity	LCs	Epidermis
		Dendritic cells	Sweat glands
		Immunoglobulins	
Microbial barrier	Protection from pathogens	Defensins	SC
		Sphingosine Symbiotic microflora	Epidermis

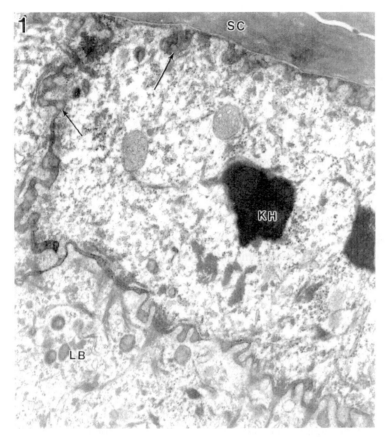

Figure 1 Ultrastructural profile of murine epidermis showing nascent LBs, and secreted LBs between cells of SG and at the SG–SC interface.

skin of a reptile, which is presumed to have an inferior barrier! The truth is far from it: they have excellent barrier properties, and an enviable ability to acclimate to changing ambient humidity, as will be discussed later.

IMPACT RESISTANCE OF THE INTEGUMENT

From the tough, calcified exoskeleton of invertebrates (crustaceans and mollusks), to the armor-like skin of specialized mammals (armadillos, rhinoceros), the outermost barrier provides varying degrees of impact resistance and physical protection. Interestingly, the oyster shell and the SC share a brick-and-mortar organization. In other words, both of them are functional composite materials, i.e., made of two or more dissimilar materials, having functional properties that are more than the sum of its components (6). This organization is exploited for a biomimetic application in material sciences, such as superior ceramics, based on the microstructure of oyster shell. While the impact resistance of the skin of a rhinoceros is mainly due to the highly developed collagen in the dermis that provide resistance to compressive forces, as seen in the horns of competing males, the SC also shows an extraordinary abundance of specialized desmosomes, providing resistance to shear. Even the human SC provides

a formidable barrier to particles delivered under pressures up to 350 psi from a gene
gun (7).

PERMEABILITY BARRIER

This is perhaps the most intensely studied aspect of the SC. As terrestrial life depends
on retaining the body fluids, environmental biologists have long been interested in
the water barrier. Dermatologists and surgeons, especially those treating widespread
burns, and neonatologists caring for premature infants, in particular, have focused
on the permeability barrier of skin as critical to patient survival. For industries with
an active interest in transdermal drug delivery, the permeability barrier has been a
formidable problem to be overcome. All these factors have contributed to several
multidisciplinary studies in this area, and innumerable publications that continue
to grow daily. Several excellent reviews and books on this topic are available (8–10).
Only a brief account of the formation and maintenance of the permeability barrier is
given below, mainly for the purpose of comparison of the barrier structures of mammals with other vertebrates and further addressing the question of when the barrier
becomes good enough.

     In higher vertebrates, ultrastructural studies have identified the epidermal
production and secretion of specialized lipid–enriched organelles (variously named
as membrane coating granules, mesos granules, multi-granular bodies (MGBs), keratinosomes, Odland bodies, or LBs), and sequestration of these lipids in the SC
extracellular domains as the basis of the permeability barrier formation (8,9). A
minimal description of the sequence of events is as follows: as the basal keratinocytes
proliferate and move up or outward into the stratum spinosum, they embark on a
path of progressive differentiation that involves the synthesis of specific proteins
(keratins, filaggrin, cornified envelope proteins, etc.) and lipids (for packaging in
LBs). In the outermost cells of the SG (2–3 cells thick), about 20% of the cytosol
is occupied by LBs, which remain interconnected by a trans-Golgi-like membrane
system (11); the rest of the cytoplasm is predominantly occupied by keratohyalin
granules, keratin filaments, ribosomes, and mitochondria. When appropriate cellular
signals are received, the granulocyte (i) begins to assemble a cornified envelope from
the cross-linking of the envelope proteins (involucrin, loricrin, cornifin), catalyzed by
transglutaminase; (ii) secretes the LBs into the SG–SC interface; and (iii) transforms
into a transitional cell that matures into a terminally differentiated corneocyte within
a few hours (12). Upon secretion, the contents of LBs unfurl, fuse end to end with
each other, anchor onto the desmosomes, and by a series of metabolic processing
events mediated by a battery of enzymes (co-secreted with LB lipids), are converted
to multiple lamellar structures composed of non-polar barrier lipids that fill the
intercellular domains of the SC. This imparts the brick-and-mortar organization
to this tissue. The extracellular lipid mortar occluding the tortuous extracellular
spaces of the SC is the physical location of the permeability barrier, as shown by
a tracer permeation at the ultrastructural level of observation (13), as well as by
increased TEWL values that follow lipid extraction and/or disruption of the multiple lamellar organization of the SC lipids (reviewed in Ref. 14). A "pore-pathway"
for the permeation of hydrophilic molecules across the SC had been postulated (15),
and much debated. Ultrastructural evidence that the pore-pathway is transiently
formed from a "lacunar system" (partly derived from degradation of corneodesmosomes) embedded within the lamellar lipids was presented by Menon and Elias (16).

FACULTATIVE WATERPROOFING

Although the permeability barrier resides in similar locations in other vertebrates, and is also based on the secretion of LB (Fig. 1) or their analogues, deviations from this model are seen as the norm in many sub-mammalian species, as well as in certain aquatic mammals. Aves (birds) show high TEWL values compared with mammals, even with their complete absence of sweat glands. They also lack discreet sebaceous glands except for the large uropygial gland at the base of the tail and the ceruminous glands of the ear canal (17). Although the basic sequence of epidermal proliferation and differentiation is similar to that of mammals, the highly lipogenic nature is a distinguishing hallmark of the avian epidermis (18). The whole epidermis is composed of hybrid sebo-keratinocytes, which produce "lamellar body"–like organelles (multi-granular bodies or MGBs), as well as non-membrane bound lipid droplets (19,20). MGBs differ from the typical LBs of mammalian epidermis in several features: they are much larger and polymorphic, ranging from circular membrane bound packets of several LB-like organelles, co-mingled with non-lamellar phases to long, sometimes crescent shaped structures having a lamellar substructure (Figs. 2A and 2B). The fate of MGBs, whether secreted or retained, is determined largely by environmental challenges. Under basal conditions, most of the MGBs are transformed in situ into electron lucent lipid droplets, which coalesce to form a lipid filled core within the corneocyte (Fig. 2A), from which they later escape to the extracellular domains via porosities in the corneocyte envelope (19). Despite an abundance of lipids, no lamellar organization of the lipids is observed in the avian SC (Fig. 2A), where high TEWL values are recorded (21,22). This "imperfect barrier" is actually of considerable survival value to birds, whose only avenue for evaporative cooling without energy expenditure (the other mode, panting, is energetically expensive) is through cutaneous evaporation. Their lack of sweat glands, and a higher metabolic rate and body temperature compared with mammals, further necessitate the high TEWL. However, unsecreted lamellar lipids are often seen trapped within the corneocyte cytosol, the significance of which became clear during the investigations on avian response to xeric stress. Newly hatched (featherless) chicks, as well as adult captive Zebra finches (*Taeniopygia guttata castanotis*) deprived of drinking water, decrease their TEWL overnight by secreting the lamellar contents of MGBs, and organizing these into tight lamellar arrays (Fig. 2B) as in mammals (23). The chicks, as they fledge, and adults when water is replenished, begin to increase their TEWL, by degrading the nascent MGBs into lipid droplets, and secreting non-lamellar neutral lipids into the SC domains; this displays not only an ability for facultative waterproofing, but also reverses the trend within a few days of being provided with drinking water (23,24). This adaptability helps the Zebra finch survive their arid Australian habitat, where rainfall is rather unpredictable. Another family of birds that have a distribution pattern covering a wide variety of geography and climates, the pigeons, display high TEWL values when acclimated to desert heat (up to 60°C); but when cold-acclimated, they form multiple lipid lamellae within the SC (similar to the finches), waterproofing the skin and preventing heat loss by evaporative cooling (25). Ostriches, native to deserts, also show ultrastructural features of an epidermal barrier that denotes a relatively high TEWL. However, no TEWL measurements are available on this species, and no information with respect to the barrier lipid organization under xerically stressed conditions has been reported.

The ability for facultative modulation of skin permeability is not unique to birds, and can in fact be traced back to reptiles and even certain tree frogs. Reptiles

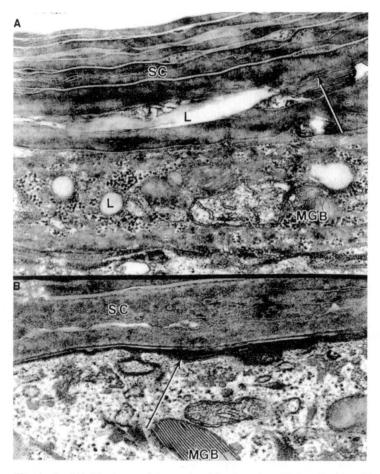

Figure 2 (A) Electron micrograph of basic avian (Zebra finch) epidermal differentiation results in most MGBs being degraded in situ into lipid droplets, and not secreted into SC extracellular domains. Lipid droplets coalesce to form the core of corneocytes, which also retain unsecreted lamellar lipids (*arrow*). OSO4 post-fixation. (B) Epidermis of newly hatched nestlings, in dire need for conserving body water, shows lipid bilayers (*arrow*) within the SC domains, following secretion of MGBs. Xeric-stressed adults (not shown) display similar morphology. OSO4 post-fixation. *Source*: Reproduced from Ref. 21; with kind permission from the Korean Society for Skin Barrier Research.

have a complicated epidermal structure, and an even more complex cycle of epidermal shedding and renewal. The histology of a "typical" reptilian skin is difficult to describe, as lizards, snakes, crocodiles, and turtles all differ in their epidermal organization; however, the skin of snakes can be used to illustrate the complexity and adaptive responses of an integument functioning in locomotion, as well as a permeability barrier. Although it has a stratified epithelium like other amniotes, snake skin has certain unique features. The skin is covered with overlapping scales, with flexible hinge regions between scales. The thick cornified tissues on the outer surface make the scales thick and inflexible, but the inner scale surface and the hinge regions with thinner cornified tissues permit flexibility and distensibility of the integument, which is needed for locomotion and feeding. Cells derived from the basal keratinocytes do not result in a single type of terminally differentiated corneocyte; rather, they form a complex "epidermal generation" comprising six morphologically distinct layers and represent the alternate pathways of beta and alpha keratinization (26). The typical scale shows an outermost *oberhautchen*, followed by a B layer filled with B-keratin and occasional pigment granules, but lacks any evidence of lipids. In this layer, cell boundaries are obliterated, forming a syncytium. In the inner scale surface and hinge region, the B-keratin is limited to the *oberhautchen* alone, permitting flexibility. Subjacent to the B layer is the mesos layer, where the permeability barrier is located. The extracellular domains of the alpha keratinizing mesos layer contain lipid bilayers (Fig. 3, Inset) derived from mesos granules. Below the mesos layer is the alpha layer, synthesizing alpha keratin and lipids, which are often in the form of MGBs. Beneath

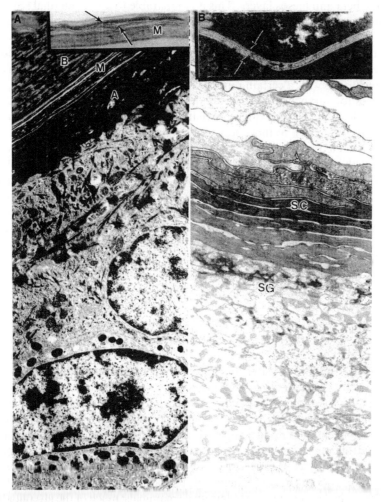

Figure 3 Comparison of snake epidermis (A) with (B) mammalian (human) epidermis. Four distinct strata (beta, mesos, alpha, and viable cells) reflect specific terminal differentiation paths of keratinocytes in snakes. In contrast, the human SC with monomorphic corneocytes shows a stratum compactum and stratum disjunctum; the latter shows ongoing desquamation (absent in the snakes). OSO4 post-fixation. Inset (B): The lamellar organization of typical mammalian SC lipids is shown. Inset (A): A similar organization exists only in the mesos layer of snakes. *Source*: Reproduced from Ref. 21; with kind permission from the Korean Society for Skin Barrier Research.

the alpha layer (and above the germinal/basal layer) may be seen the lacunar layer (the clear layer), or undifferentiated viable cells, depending on the stage of skin shedding (i.e., resting, renewal, or shedding phase). The periodic skin shedding renews the entire epidermal generation, and there is no ongoing desquamation from the SC as in mammals. As the skin is intimately associated with locomotion, the brunt of wear and tear of the scales is borne by the tough beta layer.

The rather delicate mesos layer, protected from physical damage by the outer beta layer, is where the barrier lipids are localized (Fig. 3A, Inset). As stated above, the complete replacement of the barrier requires an ecdysis (periodic molt of the entire skin). However, if only a small part of the skin is damaged, as in tape stripping experiments (27), a hyperproliferation of the alpha cells seal off the damage, without generating the beta and mesos layers. This is comparable to an "epidermal scar," a temporary patchwork without differentiation of the beta and mesos layers; the latter is considered crucial for the barrier. Whether the TEWL in this localized area is different from the rest of the body has not been investigated. However, as these layers are formed only when the next pan-body molt occurs, it can be assumed that the organism can survive with a certain number of imperfections in its barrier; i.e., a barrier that suffices for survival. A surface area that is leaky could also be a pointer to a certain threshold of total body water loss that triggers the whole barrier renewal. The presence of MGBs (similar to those seen in aves) in the alpha layer (28) indicates that lipids can be secreted by the cells below the mesos layer, yet, whether bilayered structures form in the alpha layer (like in xerically stressed birds), or whether the lipid remains as a "sebum-like" coating, remains to be determined. Such increased lipid secretion from the viable cell layers subjacent to the SC may also underlie how the lizard, *Anolis carolinensis*, responds by decreased evaporative water loss during acclimation to a low humidity (29). This decreased TEWL persists even when they are put back in a high humidity environment, since the corneous layers, and hence the deposited lipids, are lost only in a subsequent molt (skin shedding), and not by continuous desquamation as in birds and mammals.

Sebum-like lipids are indeed the basis of facultative waterproofing in the waxing monkey tree frog, *Phyllomedusae sauvegii*, where a complex wiping behavior spreads the waxy secretions of skin glands over its dorsal skin (30), helping conserve precious body water when temperatures go up. However, if the ambient temperatures soar, and evaporative cooling is crucial, the melting point of the wax coatings assist: they melt away, restoring evaporative water loss and cooling, allowing survival.

Marine mammals, such as cetaceans (dolphins, whales) and amphibious mammals, like the hippopotamus, have entirely different challenges with regard to the permeability barrier. It is also challenging to study their barrier properties, as their TEWL cannot be assessed by the conventional means employed for terrestrial mammals. The highly thickened, parakeratotic cetacean epidermis shows an abundance of LBs, as well as free lipid droplets. Electron microscopy shows that the LBs are secreted, but the lipid droplets are retained in the corneocytes (stratum externum). The post-secretory processing of the LB contents is also limited in comparison to terrestrial mammals: much of the glycolipids are not processed to ceramides, and the intercorneocyte lamellae are not tightly packed as in terrestrial mammals (31). Conventional wisdom would suggest that such a morphology is predictive of a defective permeability barrier, but it is safe to assume that the barrier is good enough, or even perfect for the environmental challenges of the cetaceans, mammals evolved from terrestrial ancestors (32). The ceramide-enriched lipid bilayers of the terrestrial mammalian SC, known to be disrupted by hydration (33), would not work for an aquatic species. It is conceivable that a continuous release of the glycolipid-enriched skin lipids at the boundary layer water can reduce frictional drag, and therefore make swimming more efficient. Recently, Baum et al. (34) proposed that the "zymogel" of enzymes and lipids on whale skin prevents the settling of larvae of sessile organisms like barnacles, and hence provide a barrier against biofowling.

WHY DO LESSONS FROM COMPARATIVE BIOLOGY MATTER TO THE BARRIER RESEARCHERS?

Comparative and evolutionary perspectives of skin barrier provide rare insights into the relevance of many observations that we make in the course of our investigations, but relegate to being an epiphenomenon. An example would be the hydration damage to the barrier structures, where an hour of occlusion with water disrupts the barrier lipid structures (33). From the standpoint of transdermal delivery, or real-life situations (an olympic swimmer practicing for several hours), it is important to see how barrier homeostasis works: does adaptation to regular and prolonged periods of hydration involve changes in the epidermal lipogenesis/lipid metabolism or lipid processing, so as to provide more polar SC lipids akin to that of aquatic mammals? Comparative studies also provide opportunities for validating/testing new and often revolutionary hypothesis that are proposed to explain the formation of the barrier, such as the plastic crystalline theory of Norlen (35), who proposed that LBs are artifacts of preparation, parts of cubic lipid structures from the SG, which continuously flow out and attain a lamellar configuration on dehydration (in the SC). Prima facie, this may indeed seem to be the case with marine mammals, whose SC remains highly hydrated and lacking in multiple lamellar structures. If this were the case, the Norlen hypothesis would be restricted to the mammalian barrier, rather than being universally applicable to the vertebrate skin barrier. Nevertheless, the findings of defective lamellar structures in Gaucher's disease and its animal models (36) lacking a single enzyme that cleaves sugars off the pro-barrier lipids following secretion, as well as the isolation of LBs as discreet organelles (37) are in contrast to this hypothesis. Once again, the existence of MGBs in the avian epidermis (high TEWL values), their conversion into free lipid droplets in situ without being secreted at the SC–stratum transitivum junction under basal conditions, and the correlated lack of lamellar lipid structures (22) are worth recalling. MGBs are secreted under stress, which adds lamellar structures (rather than amorphous lipids) to the SC interstices, curtailing TEWL: a sequence of events that provides credence to the view that the unique lamellar organization of SC lipids is needed to curtail TEWL values (38). All of the above facts that are reviewed also argue against the view that cubic lipid structures flow out in a continuum from the granulocytes, and not as individual lamellar bodies, which provides the ability to fine tune the barrier as and when needed.

Another point of interest to investigators exploring the permeability barrier is to compare the barrier repair data from hairless mice and human experiments. Animal studies point to a repair over 24–36 hours. In contrast, human studies show a prolonged repair phase (48–70 hours). This difference may be due to the fact that a fast response is not crucial for the survival of humans compared with animals, since we have evolved to such a degree as to modify our microenvironments (temperature and humidity control, clothing, etc.). On the other hand, the differences may merely reflect the comparatively small and negligible percentage of the skin surface affected in the human experiments; i.e., it is possible that there exists a threshold of total evaporative water loss that triggers a barrier repair response. It is interesting to speculate if human barrier repair will be faster following delipidization of the whole arm rather than just a few centimeters of the volar forearm. If there is indeed a threshold, a small area where the barrier is disrupted and which remains as an open window for longer duration, can further be modified by occlusion or metabolic intervention approaches (39), a sound rationale for transdermal drug delivery.

Yet another factor that affects the human permeability barrier homeostasis is stress, be it physical, hormonal, or psychological. Although it has been in the focus of the barrier researchers only recently (40–42), there is enough evidence that the permeability barrier repair is retarded by stress. Although the details of how stress impacts the barrier are not fully understood, observations such as a decrease in the circulating white blood cells, resulting from its mobilization to the skin (41), the presence of corticotropin-releasing hormone in the sebaceous gland (43), etc. point to an intimate association of the permeability barrier with innate immunity. I speculate that a small dysfunction in the permeability barrier is involved in the proper priming of the immune responses, crucial to the survival of the individual. Possibly, an efficient barrier repair may blunt the mounting of a full immune response, as does an extremely high hygiene and sterile microenvironment, which weakens the immune system.

In summary, it could be argued that TEWL may be a good index of the skin permeability barrier, but a tighter water barrier does not always indicate the "best" for any given species. As an interactive boundary layer, the skin senses and responds with appropriate adjustments in its defenses against whatever environmental aggressors (heat, cold, damaging UV radiation, etc.) that are most crucial. This could also vary according to the seasons, geographic locations (in migrating organisms), or the stage in the life history of the organism. "When the barrier is good enough" depends on what provides the individual with the best survival strategy.

REFERENCES

1. Menon GK, Elias PM. The epidermal barrier and strategies for surmounting it. In: Hegge UR, Volc-Platzer B, eds. The Skin and Gene Therapy. Berlin: Springer-Verlag, 2001:3–26, 301.
2. Schaefer H, Redelmeier TE. Skin Barrier. Basel: Karger, 1996:310.
3. Elias PM, Friend D. Permeability barrier of mammalian epidermis. J Cell Biol 1975; 65:180–191.
4. Holleran WM, Takagi Y, Feingold KR, Menon GK, Legler G, Elias PM. Processing of epidermal glucosylceramides is required for optimal mammalian permeability barrier function. J Clin Invest 1993; 91:1656–1664.
5. Menon GK, Feingold KR, Elias PM. The lamellar body secretory response to barrier disruption. J Invest Dermatol 1992; 98:279–289.
6. Newnham RE, Ruschau GR. Smart electroceramics. Am Ceram Soc Bull 1996; 75:51–61.
7. Menon GK, Brandsma J, Schwartz P. Gene gun and the human skin: ultrastructural study of the distribution of gold particles in the epidermis [abstr]. J Invest Dermatol 1997; 110:637.
8. Downing DT. Lipids: their role in epidermal structure and function. Cosmet Toilet 1991; 106:63–69.
9. Elias PM. Epidermal lipids, barrier function and desquamation. J Invest Dermatol 1983; 80:44–49.
10. Forslind B, Lindberg M, eds. Skin, Hair, and Nails. New York, Basel: Marcel Dekker Inc., 2004.

11. Elias PM, Cullander C, Mauro T, Rssner U, Komuves L, Brown B, Menon GK. The secretory granular cell: the outermost granular cell as a specialized secretory cell. J invest Dermatol Symp Proc 1998; 3:87–100.

12. Holbrook K. Ultrastructure of the epidermis. In: Leigh IM, Lane BE, Watts FM, eds. The Keratinocyte Handbook. Oxford: Cambridge University Press, 1994:3–39.

13. Elias PM, Brown BE. The mammalian cutaneous permeability barrier: defective barrier function in essential fatty acid deficiency correlates with abnormal intercellular lipid deposition. Lab Invest 1978; 39:574–583.

14. Menon GK, Ghadially R. Morphology of lipid alterations in the epidermis: a review. Microsc Res Tech 1997; 37:180–192.

15. Flynn GL. Mechanisms of percutaneous absorption from physiochemical evidence. In: Branaugh RL, Maibach HI, eds. Percutaneous absorption. New York: Marcel Dekker, 1989:27–51.

16. Menon GK, Elias PM. Morphological basis for a pore-pathway in mammalian stratum corneum. Skin Pharmacol 1997; 10:235–246.

17. Lucas AM, Stettenheim PR. Avian Anatomy: Integument. Agriculture Handbook 362, US Department of Agriculture, Washington DC, 1972.

18. Lucas AM. Avian functional anatomical problems. Fed Proc 1970; 29:1641–1648.

19. Menon GK, Aggarwal SK, Lucas AM. Evidence for the holocrine nature of lipoid secretion by avian epidermal cells: a histochemical and ultrastructural study of rictus and the uropygial gland. J Morphol 1981; 167:185–199.

20. Menon GK, Menon JG. Avian epidermal lipids: functional considerations and relationship to feathering. Am Zool 2000; 40:540–552.

21. Menon GK. When is the barrier good enough? Comparative biology provides an overview. J Skin Barrier Res 2003; 5:19–26.

22. Menon GK, Hou SYE, Elias PM. Avian permeability barrier function reflects mode of sequestration and organization of stratum corneum lipids: reevaluation using ruthenium tetroxide staining and lipase cytochemistry. Tissue Cell 1991; 23:445–456.

23. Menon GK, Baptista LF, Brown BE, Elias PM. Avian epidermal differentiation II. Adaptive response of permeability barrier to water deprivation and replenishment. Tissue Cell 1989; 21:83–92.

24. Menon GK, Maderson PFA, Drewes RC, Baptista LF, Price LF, Elias PM. Ultrastructural organization of avian stratum corneum lipids as the basis of facultative waterproofing. J Morphol 1996; 227:1–13.

25. Peltonen L, Arieli Y, Pyomila A, Marder J. Adaptive changes in epidermal structure of the heat-acclimated pigeon (Columba livia): a comparative electron microscopic study. J Morphol 1996; 235:17–29.

26. Maderson PFA. The squammate epidermis: new light has been shed. Symp Zool Soc Lond 1984; 52:111–126.

27. Maderson PFA, Zucker AH, Roth SI. Epidermal regeneration and percutaneous water loss following cellophane stripping of reptile epidermis. J Exp Zool 1978; 204:11–32s.

28. Tu MC, Lillywhite HB, Menon JG, Menon GK. Postnatal ecdysis establishes the permeability barrier in snakeskin: new insights into barrier lipid structures. J Exp Biol 2002; 205:3019–3030.

29. Kattan GH, Lillywhite HB. Humidity acclimation and skin permeability in the lizard, Anolis carolinensis. Physiol Zool 1989; 62:593 606.

30. McClanahan LL, Stinner JN, Shoemaker VH. Skin lipids, water loss and energy metabolism in a South American Tree frog (*Phyllomedusa sauvaegei*). Physiol Zool 1978; 51: 179–187.

31. Elias PM, Menon GK, Greyson S, Brown BE, Rehfield SJ. Avian sebokeratinocytes and marine mammal lipokeratinocytes: structural, lipid biochemical and functional considerations. Am J Anat 1987; 180:161–177.

32. Pffiffer CJ. Molecular and Cell Biology of Marine Mammals. Malabar, FL: Krieger Publishing, 2002:429.

33. Warner RR, Boissy YL, Lilly NA, McKillop K, Marshall JA, Stone KJ. Water disrupts stratum corneum lipid lamellae: damage is similar to surfactants. J Invest Dermatol 1999; 113:960–966.

34. Baum C, Meyer W, Roessner D, Siebers D, Fleischer LG. A zymogel enhances the self-cleaning abilities of the skin of the pilot whale (Globicephala melas). Comp Biochem Physiol 2001; 130:835–847.

35. Norlen L. Barrier structure and function: the single gel phase model. J Invest Dermatol 2001; 117:830–836.

36. Holleran WM, Sidransky E, Menon GK, Fartasch M, Grundmann JU, Ginns EI, Elias PM. Consequences of B-glucocerebrosidase deficiency in epidermis: ultrastructure and permeability barrier alterations in Gaucher's disease. J Clin Invest 1994; 93:1756–1764.

37. Greyson S, Johnson-Winegar AG, Wintraub BU, Epstein EH Jr, Elias PM. Lamellar body-enriched fractions from neonatal mice: preparative techniques and partial characterization. J Invest Dermatol 1985; 85:289–295.

38. Friberg SE, Kayali I, Beckerman W, Rhein L, Simion A. Water permeation of reaggregated stratum corneum with model lipids. J Invest Dermatol 1990; 94:377–380.

39. Elias PM, Feingold KR, Tsai J, Thornfeldt C, Menon GK. Metabolic approach to transdermal drug delivery. In: Guy RH, Hadgraft J, eds. Transdermal Drug Delivery. 2nd ed. New York, Basel: Marcel Dekker Inc., 2003:285–304, 383.

40. Denda M, Tsuchiya T, Elias PM, Feingold KR. Stress alters cutaneous permeability barrier homeostasis. Am J Physiol Regul Integr Comp Physiol 2000; 278:R367–R372.

41. Dhabhar FS, Miller AH, McEwen BS, Spencer RL. Effects of stress on immune cell distribution. Dynamics and hormonal mechanisms. J Immunol 1995; 154:5511–5527.

42. Garg A, Chren MM, Sands LP, Matsui MS, Maraenus KD, Feingold KR, Elias PM. Psychological stress perturbs epidermal permeability barrier homeostasis. Implications for the pathogenesis of stress-associated skin disorders. Arch Dermatol 2001; 137:53–59.

43. Zouboulis CC, Seltmann H, Hiroi N, Chen W, Young Y, Oeff M, Scherbaum WA, Orfanos CE, McCann SM, Bornstein SR. Corticotropin-releasing hormone: an autocrine hormone that promotes lipogenesis in human sebocytes. Proc Natl Acad Sci USA 2002; 99:7148–7153.

14

SC pH: Measurement, Origins, and Functions

Theodora M. Mauro

Department of Dermatology, University of California, San Francisco, California, U.S.A.

INTRODUCTION

Stratum corneum (SC) acidity, or the "acid mantle," has been recognized since the 1920s (1,2). The pace of discoveries concerning SC acidity has accelerated during the last decade, partly due to the development of new technology for assessing SC pH, and partly due to the development of new animal models. In addition, SC acidity now is acknowledged to be essential not only in establishing the epidermal permeability barrier, but also in producing the epidermal antimicrobial barrier and in controlling SC integrity and cohesion. SC acidification has been studied in two discrete clinical presentations: establishment during perinatal life and re-establishment after epidermal permeability barrier insult. Current research indicates that these two processes parallel each other, and employ many of the same components.

SC pH: MEASUREMENT

Traditionally, SC pH has been assessed using a flat pH electrode, measuring surface pH only (3), or accessing progressively lower layers of the SC by removal of sequential SC layers with tape-stripping (4). Flat electrode measurements remain the most common method of assessing SC pH as this method is quick, simple to perform, and yields reproducible pH measurements. However, flat electrode measurements can only assess mean pH across a wide area. Thus, this method can neither distinguish between intracellular and extracellular pH nor identify localized areas of acidity ("microdomains") within the SC. Moreover, measuring the SC pH gradient with sequential tape-stripping is inherently disruptive to the SC. pH-sensitive fluorescent dyes also have been used as a less invasive technique. Unfortunately, assessing SC pH with these dyes is difficult, as non-uniform dye concentration and photobleaching artifacts prevent accurate measurements (5). To address these concerns, fluorescence life-time imaging (FLIM) was developed recently (6). FLIM can both localize SC acidity to the upper or lower SC, and differentiate with great precision between acidities in the intracellular and extracellular compartments. Unlike tape-stripping,

FLIM does not disrupt the SC to measure pH in the lower SC layers. Moreover, FLIM measurements eliminate other artifacts usually inherent in fluorescent dye measurements, as they do not result in photobleaching and are independent of pH-sensing dye concentration. Although cumbersome and expensive, FLIM therefore provides novel insights into the generation and spatial distribution of acidic microdomains (7).

SC pH: ORIGIN

Using progressive tape-stripping to remove sequential layers of the SC, Ohman and Vahlquist demonstrated that SC pH was inhomogeneous, distributed with a progressively neutral pH as one proceeds from the apex to the base of the stratum corneum (4). Subsequently, this gradient was found to be composed of heterogeneous discrete areas (microdomains) of acidity embedded in larger areas of neutral pH (7). SC acidity begins in extracellular microdomains at the base of the SC both in establishing the perinatal SC pH gradient and in re-establishing the adult pH gradient after barrier abrogation (7,8). The increasing acidity of the upper SC layers derives from an increasing number of uniformly acidic microdomains, rather than from increasing acidity of a fixed number of individual microdomains (7,8). While exogenous sources, such as microbial metabolism or lactate from sweat, seem to make only minor contributions, recent research demonstrates that three endogenous processes contribute to SC acidity: $trans$-urocanic acid (tUCA) production, free fatty acid (FFA) production via secretory phospholipase A (sPLA$_2$), and H$^+$ secretion by the keratinocyte plasma membrane Na$^+$/H$^+$ antiporter (NHE1) (Fig. 1) (7,9,10).

tUCA is produced through the deimination of filaggrin-derived histidine, catalyzed by the enzyme histidase. It is produced through the catabolism of filaggrin in the SC, thereby increasing in concentration in the upper SC, in parallel with measured SC acidity (9). Acidity generated through this pathway thus may be more

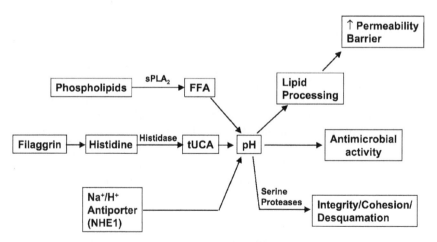

Figure 1 Origins and functions of SC acidity. The SC acidity is generated by the combined effects of at least three endogenous processes: FFA production via sPLA$_2$; tUCA generation from histidine, catalyzed by the enzyme histadase; H$^+$ secretion by the Na$^+$/H$^+$ antiporter NHE1. In turn, SC acidity enhances three essential aspects of epidermal physiology: the permeability barrier, antimicrobial activity, and optimum regulation of SC integrity, cohesion, and desquamation.

important in controlling processes such as desquamation from the SC surface, rather than processes such as lipid processing or the initial proteolytic attack on corneodesmosomes (see Functions, below). tUCA may also act as a humectant (9), and its UV-induced cis-isomer is a suspected, endogenous immunosuppressive agent (11,12), linked to UV-induced skin cancers (13).

Although SC acidity increases progressively toward the outer SC surface, essential lipid processing (see Functions, below) occurs at the SC/stratum granulosum (SG) interface, or in the innermost layers of the SC (14–16), suggesting that pathways other than tUCA generation may predominate in enhancing lipid processing. A second endogenous pathway is produced by the breakdown of secreted phospholipids, catalyzed by one or more of the co-secreted secretory phospholipases ($sPLA_2$) (17–19). $sPLA_2$ enzyme activity, localized to lamellar bodies (20,21), is liberated into the SC when the lamellar bodies empty their lipid contents at the SG/SC interface (20–23). $sPLA_2$ hydrolyzes membrane phospholipids to form FFAs, thereby contributing H^+ to the extracellular spaces of the SC. Since $sPLA_2$ has a neutral pH optimum (18), it might be expected to operate either in the lower SC or in areas outside the previously identified acidic microdomains.

NHE1 is the major NHE isoform present in epidermis (24). Since Na^+/H^+ antiporters require an Na^+ concentration gradient for activity, NHE1-mediated acidification would most likely be active at the SC/SG interface, and therefore may be the initial SC acidifying mechanism (8). The NHE1 establishes localized extracellular acidic microdomains, commencing immediately above the SG/SC interface (7,8). NHE antiporters do not consume energy, and require only an intact Na^+ extracellular versus intracellular gradient to operate. NHE activity is upregulated by increasing intracellular H^+ and/or Ca^{2+}, both conditions that might be found as viable SG keratinocytes transition into non-viable corneocytes (25,26).

Studies using pharmacologic or molecular strategies to block a single endogenous pathway reveal that no single pathway predominates in establishing the SC pH gradient. Histademic humans (27) do not display clinical alterations or altered barrier function. Pharmacologic inhibition of NHE1 or $sPLA_2$, or NHE1-deficient mice each suffer partial, but not complete impairment of SC pH and barrier function (7,19,28). Thus, it is likely that not only these three, but also additional pathways act in an additive or a redundant manner to form, maintain, or restore the SC pH gradient.

SC pH: FUNCTIONS IMPACTED

Recent research has demonstrated that SC acidity is essential in several epidermal functions: epidermal permeability barrier, epidermal antimicrobial barrier, epidermal inflammation, and SC integrity and cohesion (Fig. 2).

Epidermal Permeability Barrier

The epidermal permeability barrier is established by lipid bilayer formation between corneocytes of the SC. Lipid is secreted from lamellar bodies in the SG keratinocytes. Secreted lipid does not form an effective permeability barrier until it is processed into lipid bilayers. While Ca^{2+} and K^+ control lipid secretion (29), H^+ controls lipid processing (30). Acidification is essential for the epidermal permeability barrier, as shown by the observation that barrier recovery proceeds normally at an acidic pH, but is delayed at a neutral pH (i.e., pH 7–7.4) as a result of impaired

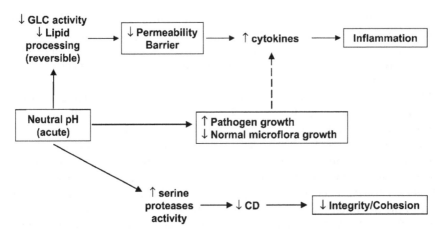

Figure 2 Pathological consequences of neutral SC pH. An abnormally neutral SC pH impairs formation of the epidermal permeability barrier through down-regulation of the pH-sensitive enzyme β-glucocerebrosidase (GLC). Further, integrity/cohesion of corneodesmosomes (CD) are decreased by neutral SC pH, mediated by serine proteases. Finally, neutral SC pH enhances pathogenic bacterial growth. Decreased permeability barrier functions and pathogenic bacteria combine to enhance inflammation.

postsecretory processing of secreted, extracellular lipids in the lower SC, while lipid secretion remains normal (30). Finally, neutral pH also may disrupt normal SC lipid packing (31).

Elegant studies by Holleran et al. (14) demonstrated that H^+ acts by activating pH-sensitive enzymes that process secreted lipid to functional bilayers. Chief among these enzymes are β-glucocerebrosidase (GLC), as well as acid sphingomyelinase (ACM) (14,15,32). Inhibiting GLC, experimentally or in human disease, reproduces the impaired lipid processing and incomplete establishment of the epidermal permeability barrier seen by neutralizing SC pH (14,33). Blocking NHE1 or sPLA$_2$ decreases GLC activity (8,10). Thus, SC acidity, regardless of the source, seems to act through the same process of GLC activation, processing secreted SC lipids into functional lipid bilayers.

Antimicrobial Activity and Inflammation

SC acidity also is integral to epidermal antimicrobial barrier function (34,35), supporting growth of normal microflora and inhibiting skin pathogen growth. For example, micrococci, a normal flora, grow best at an acidic pH (36), while *Staphylococcus* and *Candida* grow best at pH 7.5 but are suppressed at pH 5 to 6 (36).

Since a break in epidermal permeability barrier releases inflammatory cytokines (37,38), leading to an inflammatory cascade, the inflammatory and antimicrobial processes are closely linked. Diapered neonatal skin displays a more neutral pH than uncovered skin (39), worsened by urine and feces (40). This neutral skin pH enhances contact dermatitis (40). In addition, pathogens that grow at neutral pH worsen diaper dermatitis (41), setting up a vicious cycle where neutral pH, pathogen growth, and inflammatory cytokine release combine to produce an inflamed, colonized skin with impaired permeability and antimicrobial barriers.

Integrity/Cohesion

A third function, controlling corneosome integrity and cohesion, has been identified recently in SC pH (10,42,43). Neutral SC pH, via exposure to neutral pH buffers, pharmacologic sPLA₂ inhibition, or application of "superbases" to the skin, produces SC that is more easily removed by tape-stripping (decreased integrity). In addition, more SC proteins are removed with each individual tape-stripping (decreased cohesion) (19,43). Since neonates are born with neutral SC pH (39), the decreased integrity/cohesion seen with neutral SC pH may serve a physiologic function of allowing SC desquamation soon after birth.

In contrast to the epidermal permeability barrier, a single pathway, catalyzed by the serine proteases, seems to predominate in controlling SC integrity/cohesion. The chymotryptic and tryptic serine proteases are active in neutral pH (44,45), and enhance corneodesmosome degradation, especially the essential corneodesmosome protein desmoglein 1 (43). Serine protease activity is upregulated in neonates, and decreases as the SC is acidified (10).

CONCLUSION

SC pH regulates several essential SC barrier functions: the epidermal permeability barrier, the epidermal antimicrobial barrier, and SC desquamation. SC acidity is not formed passively, but instead is produced by at least three coordinated, regulated processes. Finally, SC H^+ concentration enhances or inhibits specific pH-sensitive enzymes to establish or maintain the SC permeability barrier and SC integrity/cohesion.

REFERENCES

1. Schade H. Zur physikalischen chemie der hautoberflache. Arch Dermatol Syphilis 1928; 154:690–716.
2. Marchionini A, Hausknecht W. Sauremantel der haut and bakterienabwehr. Klin Wochenschr 1938; 17:663–666.
3. Blank IH. Measurement of pH of the skin surface. II. pH of the exposed surfaces of adults with no apparent skin lesions. J Invest Dermatol 1939; 2:75–79.
4. Ohman H, Vahlquist A. In vivo studies concerning a pH gradient in human stratum corneum and upper epidermis. Acta Derm Venereol 1994; 74:375–379.
5. Turner NG, Cullander C, Guy RH. Determination of the pH gradient across the stratum corneum. J Invest Dermatol Symp Proc 1998; 3:110–113.
6. Hanson KM, Behne MJ, Barry NP, Mauro TM, Gratton E, Clegg RM. Two-photon fluorescence lifetime imaging of the skin stratum corneum pH gradient. Biophys J 2002; 83:1682–1690.
7. Behne MJ, Meyer JW, Hanson KM, Barry NP, Murata S, Crumrine D, Clegg RW, Gratton E, Holleran WM, Elias PM, Mauro TM. NHE1 regulates the stratum corneum permeability barrier homeostasis. Microenvironment acidification assessed with fluorescence lifetime imaging. J Biol Chem 2002; 277:47399–47406.
8. Behne MJ, Barry NP, Hanson KM, Aronchik I, Clegg RW, Gratton E, Feingold K, Holleran WM, Elias PM, Mauro TM. Neonatal development of the stratum corneum pH gradient: localization and mechanisms leading to emergence of optimal barrier function. J Invest Dermatol 2003; 120:998–1006.
9. Krien P, Kermici M. Evidence for the existence of a self-regulated enzymatic process within human stratum corneum—an unexpected role for urocanic acid. J Invest Dermatol 2000; 115:414–420.

10. Fluhr J, Behne M, Brown BE, Moskowitz DG, Selden C, Mauro T, Elias PM, Feingold K. Stratum corneum acidification in neonatal skin: I. Secretory phospholipase A2 and the NHE1 antiporter acidify neonatal rat stratum corneum. J Invest Dermatol 2004 Feb; 122(2):320–329.

11. Ross JA, Howie SE, Norval M, Maingay J, Simpson TJ. Ultraviolet-irradiated urocanic acid suppresses delayed-type hypersensitivity to herpes simplex virus in mice. J Invest Dermatol 1986; 87:630–633.

12. Beissert S, Ruhlemann D, Mohammad T, Grabbe S, El-Ghorr A, Norval M, Morrison H, Granstein RD, Schwarz T. IL-12 prevents the inhibitory effects of cis-urocanic acid on tumor antigen presentation by Langerhans cells: implications for photocarcinogenesis. J Immunol 2001; 167:6232–6238.

13. Reeve VE, Greenoak GE, Canfield PJ, Boehm-Wilcox C, Gallagher CH. Topical urocanic acid enhances UV-induced tumour yield and malignancy in the hairless mouse. Photochem Photobiol 1989; 49:459–464.

14. Holleran WM, Takagi Y, Imokawa G, Jackson S, Lee JM, Elias PM. Beta-glucocerebrosidase activity in murine epidermis: characterization and localization in relation to differentiation. J Lipid Res 1992; 33:1201–1209.

15. Takagi Y, Kriehuber E, Imokawa G, Elias PM, Holleran WM. Beta-glucocerebrosidase activity in mammalian stratum corneum. J Lipid Res 1999; 40:861–869.

16. Jensen JM, Schutze S, Forl M, Kronke M, Proksch E. Roles for tumor necrosis factor receptor p55 and sphingomyelinase in repairing the cutaneous permeability barrier. J Clin Invest 1999; 104:1761–1770.

17. Mazereeuw-Hautier J, Redoules D, Tarroux R, Charveron M, Salles JP, Simon MF, Cerutti I, Assalit MF, Gall Y, Bonafe JL, Chap H. Identification of pancreatic type U secreted phospholipase A2 in human epidermis and its determination by tape stripping. Br J Dermatol 2000; 142:424–431.

18. Schadow A, Scholz-Pedretti K, Lambeau G, Gelb MH, Furstenberger G, Pfeilschifter J, Kaszkin M. Characterization of group X phospholipase A(2) as the major enzyme secreted by human keratinocytes and its regulation by the phorbol ester TPA. J Invest Dermatol 2001; 116:31–36.

19. Fluhr JW, Kao J, Jain M, Ahn SK, Feingold KR, Elias PM. Generation of free fatty acids from phospolipids regulates stratum corneum acidification and integrity. J Invest Dermatol 2001; 117:44–51.

20. Elias PM, Nau P, Hanley K, Cullander C, Crumrine D, Bench G, Sideras-Haddad E, Mauro T, Williams ML, Feingold KR. Formation of the epidermal calcium gradient coincides with key milestones of barrier ontogenesis in the rodent. J Invest Dermatol 1998; 110:399–404.

21. Elias PM, Cullander C, Mauro T, Rassner U, Komuves L, Brown BE, Menon GK. The secretory granuler cell the outermost granular cell as a specialized secretory cell. J Invest Dermatol Symp Proc 1998; 3:87–100.

22. Graysonb S, Johnson-Winegar AG, Wintroub BU, Isseroff RR, Epstein EH Jr, Elias PM. Lamellar body-enriched fractions from neonatal mice: preparation techniques and partial characterization. J Invest Dermatol 1985; 85:289–294.

23. Freinkel RK, Traczyk TN. Acid hydrolases of the epidermis: subcellular localization and relationship to cornification. J Invest Dermatol 1983; 80:441–446.

24. Sarangarajan R, Shumaker H, Soleimani M, Le Poole C, Boissy RE. Molecular and functional characterization of sodium–hydrogen exchanger in skin as well as cultured keratinocytes and melanocytes. Biochim Biophys Acta 2001; 1511:181–192.

25. Haworth RS, McCann C, Snabaitis AK, Roberts NA, Avkiran M. Stimulation of the plasma membrane Na^+/H^+ exchanger NHE1 by sustained intracellular acidosis. Evidence for a novel mechanism mediated by the ERK pathway. J Biol Chem 2003; 278:31676–31684.

26. Maly K, Strese K, Kampfer S, Ueberall F, Baier G, Ghaffari–Tabrizi N, Grunicke HH, Leitges M. Critical role of protein kinase C alpha and calcium in growth factor induced activation of the Na(+)/H(+) exchanger NHE1. FEBS Lett 2002; 521:205–210.

27. Taylor RG, Levy IIL, McInnes RR. Histidase and histidinemia. Clinical and molecular considerations. Mol Biol Med 1991; 8:101–116.

28. Mao-Qiang M, Jain M, Feingold KR, Elias PM. Secretory phospholipase A2 activity is required for permeability barrier homeostasis. J Invest Dermatol 1996; 106:57–63.

29. Lee SH, Elias PM, Feingold KR, Mauro T. A role for ions in barrier recovery after acute perturbation. J Invest Dermatol 1994; 102:976–979.

30. Mauro T, Holleran WM, Grayson S, Gao WN, Man MQ, Kriehuber E, Behne M, Feingold KR, Elias PM. Barrier recovery is impeded at neutral pH, independent of ionic effects: implications for extracellular lipid processing. Arch Dermatol Res 1998; 290:215–222.

31. Bouwsta JA, Gooris GS, Dubbelaar FE, Ponec M. Phase behavior of skin barrier model membranes at pH 7.4. Cell Mol Biol (Noisy-le-grand) 2000; 46:979–992.

32. Schmuth M, Man MQ, Weber F, Gao W, Feingold KR, Fritsch P, Elias PM, Holleran WM. Permeability barrier disorder in Niemann-Pick disease: sphingomyelin-ceramide processing required for normal barrier homeostasis. J Invest Dermatol 2000; 115:459–466.

33. Holleran WM, Ginns EI, Menon GK, Grundmann JU, Fartasch M, McKinney CE, Elias PM, Sidransky E. Consequences of beta-glucocerebrosidase deficiency in epidermis. Ultrastructure and permeability barrier cohesion. J Invest Dermatol 2003; 121:345–353.

34. Aly R, Shirley C, Cunico B, Maibach HI. Effect of prolonged occlusion on the microbial flora, pH, carbon dioxide, and transepidermal water loss on human skin. J Invest Dermatol 1978; 71:378–381.

35. Puhvel SM, Reisner RM, Amirian DA. Quantification of bacteria in isolated pilosebaceous follicles in normal skin. J Invest Dermatol 1975; 65:525–531.

36. Korting HC, Hubner K, Greiner K, Hamm G, Braun-Falco O. Differences in the skin surface pH and bacterial microflora due to the long-term application of synthetic detergent preparations of pH 5.5 and pH 7.0. Results of a crossover trial in healthy volunteers. Acta Derm Venereal 1990; 70:429–431.

37. Wood LC, Stalder AK, Liou A, Campbell IL, Grunfeld C, Elias PM, Feingold KR. Barrier disruption increase gene expression of cytokines and the 55 kDa TNF receptor in murine skin. Exp Dermatol 1997; 6:98–104.

38. Nickoloff BJ, Naidu Y. Perturbation of epidermal barrier function correlates with initiation of cytokine cascade in human skin. J Am Acad Dermatol 1994; 30:535–546.

39. Visscher MO, Chatterjee R, Munson KA, Pickens WL, Hoath SB. Changes in diapered and non-diapered infant skin over the first month of life. Pediatr dermatol 2000; 17: 45–51.

40. Berg RW, Milligan MC, Sarbaugh FC. Association of skin wetness and pH with diaper dermatitis. Pediatr Dermatol 1994; 11:18–20.

41. Ferrazzini G, Kaiser RR, Hirsig Cheng SK, Wehrli M, Della Casa V, Pohlig G, Gonser S, Graf F, Jorg W. Microbiological aspects of diaper dermatitis. Dermatology 2003; 206:136–141.

42. Ohman S, Vahlquist A. The pH gradient over the stratum corneum differs in x-linked recessive and autosomal dominant ichthyosis: a clue to the molecular origin of the "acid skin mantle"? J Invest Dermatol 1998; 111:674–677.

43. Hachem JP, Crumrine D, Fluhr J, Brown BE, Feingold KR, Elias PM. pH directly regulates epidermal permeability barrier homeostasis and stratum corneum integrity/cohesion. J Invest Dermatol 2003; 121:345–353.

44. Ekholm IE, Brattsand M, Egelrud T. Stratum corneum tryptic enzyme in normal epidermis: a missing link in the desquamation process? J Invest Dermatol 2000; 114:56–63.

45. Lundstrom A, Egelrud T. Stratum corneum chymotryptic enzyme: a proteinase which may be generally present in the stratum corneum and with a possible involvement in desquamation. Acta Derm Venereol 1991; 71:471–474.

15

Stratum Corneum Lipid Processing: The Final Steps in Barrier Formation

Walter M. Holleran
Departments of Dermatology and Pharmaceutical Chemistry, Schools of Medicine and Pharmacy, University of California San Francisco and Department of Veterans Affairs Medical Center, San Francisco, California, U.S.A.

Yutaka Takagi
Biological Science Laboratories, Kao Corporation, Haga-gun, Tochigi, Japan

INTRODUCTION

The importance of extracellular lipids for mammalian epidermal barrier function is well established. The specific roles in epidermal function for the predominant lipid species by weight, ceramides (Cer), have been revealed in studies in both normal and diseased humans, as well as in animal models and in model membranes in vitro. Specifically, contents of these lipids are altered in patients with both atopic dermatitis (AD) (1,2) and psoriasis (3,4). Likewise, cholesterol (Chol), as well as essential and non-essential free fatty acids (FFAs) play separate, critical roles in barrier homeostasis. As all three of the major stratum corneum lipid classes, Chol, Cer, and FFAs derive from their respective precursor lipids, the enzymatic pathways responsible for producing these lipid end-products have garnered much recent attention. This chapter will review these critical enzymatic steps in the generation of epidermal barrier lipids, including details regarding their regulation, as well as their association with cutaneous disease states. Given that the human stratum corneum (SC) contains at least nine major Cer fractions, many of which are unique to the epidermis, including omega(ω)-hydroxylated and ω-acylated forms, as well as covalently attached Cer species, special emphasis is accorded herein to this unique class of lipids. Finally, where appropriate, the role of these lipids and/or their precursors in epidermal proliferation, differentiation, and/or apoptosis, will also be discussed.

LAMELLAR MEMBRANE STRUCTURES IN MAMMALIAN STRATUM CORNEUM

Mammalian SC contains extensive quantities of lipids, localized in the extracellular domains (interstices), corresponding to nearly 11% of the total weight of this tissue (see P. Wertz, Chap. 5 of this monograph). These intercellular lipids comprise nearly equimolar quantities of Cer, Chol, and FFAs, a ratio that is imperative for normal lamellar membrane organization and epidermal barrier homeostasis (5,6). Cer constitute approximately half of the total intercellular lipid content by weight, and are critical for the lamellar membrane structures (7–9) that constitute the epidermal permeability barrier (reviewed in Ref. 10). Given the structural complexity of these Cer (i.e., nine major Cer species to date—see below), it is intriguing that the epidermis forms these and other barrier lipids as *precursor* species, storing them with other lipid precursors in membrane-limited organelles called lamellar bodies (LBs) (see scheme in Fig. 1). It is only following the fusion of LBs with the apical plasma membrane of the outer stratum granulosum (SG) cells that secretion of their combined lipid and protein contents occurs (11,12). Hydrolysis of Cer, Chol, and FFA precursors comprises the final "processing" step that facilitates effective permeability barrier formation.

Only recently have studies begun to reveal one possible purpose for this apparently inefficient cycle of lipid precursor formation and subsequent hydrolysis during extracellular lipid processing; i.e., there is evidence that it protects the epidermis from adverse intracellular events that could stem from an excessive accumulation of bioactive lipids within the differentiating epidermal cell compartments. For example, various Cer species and metabolites now have recognized roles in signaling different cell fates, such as proliferation, differentiation, and/or apoptosis (reviewed in Refs. 13,14). Inappropriate accumulation of Cer species leads to cell death in keratinocytes (15–19), as in other cell types (reviewed in Ref. 20). Given

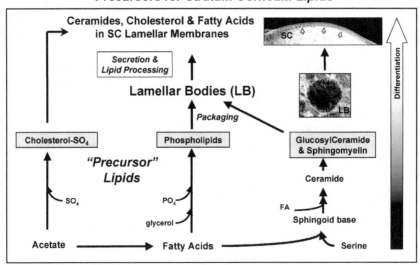

Figure 1   The three major lipid classes in mammalian SC (i.e., cholesterol, free fatty acids, and ceramides) are generated from their respective precursor lipids (cholesterol-sulfate, phospholipids, and glucosylceramide/sphingomyelin). These precursor lipids are first synthesized, packaged into lamellar bodies (LB), and then released into the extracellular domains following fusion of the LB with the apical plasma membrane of granular cells during the normal process of epidermal differentiation. Subsequent lipid processing yields the mature SC lipids, a process critical for the formation of normal lamellar membrane structures in the SC.

that specific phospholipid (PL) metabolites, including lysophospholipids, can also participate in signaling and cell fate pathways, a similar argument can be proposed for the sequestration of PLs, as precursors for SC free fatty acids, within the LB. Thus, the sequential formation of Cer precursor lipids, which are then sequestrated within the LB secretory system, followed by post-secretion extracellular hydrolysis to regenerate free Cer species, allows for the orderly accumulation of Cer required for the barrier, while at the same time minimizing risks from adverse Cer signaling events.

Given the location of the epidermis at the interface with the environs, it is not surprising that this tissue has developed mechanisms that protect it against the potential deleterious effects of Cer accumulation. An excellent example is the keratinocyte response to ultraviolet light, in which elevated Cer synthesis is progressively attenuated by an increased diversion of Cer into glucosylCer (GlcCer) (19,21), and by increased Cer hydrolysis (Uchida and Holleran, submitted). However, this requirement for high Cer levels to subserve epidermal functions in the face of their proapoptotic potential, poses a unique challenge to the differentiating keratinocyte. The epidermis appears to have developed multiple mechanisms to address this conundrum, with extracellular lipid processing being a major contributor. It is therefore important to understand the enzymatic steps that are critical for barrier lipid processing in the outer epidermis. Although significant progress has been made toward elucidating these metabolic pathways and their specific role(s) in cutaneous structure, function, and disease, it will become readily evident in this review that the study of lipid processing and epidermal "lipidomics" is still in its infancy.

GLUCOSYLCERAMIDES AS A MAJOR SOURCE OF STRATUM CORNEUM CERAMIDES

The pathway for epidermal sphingolipid synthesis begins with the enzyme serine palmitoyltransferase (SPT), the first committed and rate-limiting step that generates the distinct sphingoid base structures unique to this class of lipids (22–24). Subsequently, the amino group of sphinganine is N-acylated by Cer synthase to form dihydroCer (25), followed by C4-5 trans-desaturation (26) to generate Cer. Given that each Cer by definition contains the sphingoid base structure, this class of lipids is collectively referred to as "sphingolipids."

The synthesis of Cer species, although occurring throughout the epidermis (27), increases with epidermal differentiation, consistent with elevated sphingolipid generation and content in the more-differentiated epidermal layers (28–30). The importance of sphingolipid production for mammalian barrier function was first demonstrated in a series of studies performed on hairless mice. Specifically, acute disruption of the permeability barrier causes an upregulation of sphingolipid synthesis that is dependent upon increased SPT activity (31). Likewise, upregulation of SPT mRNA occurs in murine and human epidermis during barrier repair following acute disruption (32,33), showing the link between sphingolipid generation and mammalian permeability barrier homeostasis. The delay in permeability barrier recovery that results from the inhibition of SPT activity (and sphingolipid generation) (34) further demonstrates the importance of ongoing sphingolipid production both for barrier recovery and for maintenance of baseline function.

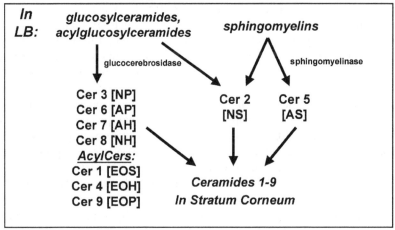

Figure 2 The nine major stratum corneum (SC) ceramide species (Cer 1-9) are derived from both glucosylceramide and sphingomyelin precursors, with all nine species available through glucocerebrosidase activity, while only two species (Cer 2 and Cer 5) are generated through sphingomyelin hydrolysis via sphingomyelinase. *Abbreviations*: N, non-hydroxy-FA; A, alpha-hydroxy-FA; O, omega-hydroxy FA; E, esterified (omega)-FA; S, sphingosine base; P, phytosphingosine base; H, 6-hydroxy-sphingosine base. *Source*: From Ref. 3.

In the epidermis, the varied Cer species destined for the SC are further modified at the 1-hydroxy position either to GlcCer species by GlcCer synthase (i.e., UDP-glucose:ceramide glucosyltransferase or GlcT1; EC 2.4.1.80) (35,36), or to sphingomyelin (SM) species by choline-phosphorylation (37,38). Although the majority of Cer species contained within LBs are glucosylated (39–43), PL including SM species (i.e., Cer containing a phosphoryl-choline group rather than glucose at the 1-OH position) are also present in substantial quantities (40,41). Consistent with this, GlcCer synthase activity increases during epidermal differentiation both in vitro (44,45) and in vivo (46), and as the permeability barrier forms in utero (47). Moreover, inhibitor studies have shown that GlcCer synthase is required for normal barrier homeostasis (46).

Human SC Cer are comprised of at least nine distinct molecular species (designated Cer 1–9), including three unique ω-hydroxylated Cer (48–51) (refer to Fig. 2; see also Chap. 6 by Y. Uchida and S. Hamanaka, this monograph for detailed review of epidermal Cer structures and nomenclature). The precursor–product relationship for each of the SC Cer species has been delineated recently (52,53). Analysis of epidermal SM species using gas chromatography–mass spectrometry, fast atom bombardment–mass spectrometry, and nuclear magnetic resonance for Cer characterization, revealed three major subfractions with distinctive amide-linked (*N*-acyl) fatty acid (FA) composition; i.e., containing either long-chain FA (SM-1; C22–C26), shorter-chain FA (SM-2; primarily C16), or short-chain alpha-hydroxy FA (SM-3; C16–C18). In addition, these three major epidermal SM species contain either sphingosine or sphinganine, but they lack phytosphingosine as the sphingoid base backbone. Thus, only two of the nine SC Cer species, Cer 2 (NS)[a] and Cer 5 (AS), derive from SM precursors (52).

A comparable analysis of epidermal GlcCer indicates conversely that distinctive epidermal GlcCer correspond to all Cer species in epidermis and SC (52,53). Thus, all nine Cer species, including the omega(ω)-hydroxy fatty-acid-containing Cer species; i.e., Cer 1 (EOS), Cer 4 (EOP), and the most-recently described Cer 9 (EOH) (51), derive from GlcCer, while only two Cer species [Cer 2 (NS) and Cer 5 (AS)], also derive in part from corresponding SM precursors (Fig. 3). These results provide further details about sphingolipid processing, and suggest potential divergent roles for GlcCer- vs. SM-derived Cer species in epidermal structure and function.

Localization of GlcCer'ase in Mammalian Epidermis

Biochemical studies have revealed that the increase in Cer levels that occur during the final stages of mammalian epidermal differentiation, corresponds with a decrease in GlcCer and SM levels, following a peak of these latter sphingolipids in the SG (28–30,54). These marked shifts in sphingolipid content can also be visualized in normal human epidermis by immunoelectron microscopy, using antibodies to both GlcCer and Cer (55). A precipitous decline in phospholipids (PL) with a more gradual hydrolysis of cholesterol-sulfate (CholSO$_4$), accompanied by concomitant increases in free FA and Chol, respectively, also accompanies terminal differentiation (see below).

Although at least two enzymes can catalyze the hydrolysis of β-linked glucose-moieties, only glucocerebrosidase (β-GlcCer'ase; EC 3.2.1.45) specifically hydrolyzes GlcCer-to-Cer (Fig. 3); therefore, this enzyme appears to be responsible for this key lipid processing step in the epidermis. A number of early reports described a β-glucosidase activity in whole skin as well as isolated epidermis (56,63). This β-glucosidase activity in porcine epidermis was both active at acidic pH (62), and the activity in epidermis and palatal epithelium exceeded that in non-keratinized buccal epithelium (63). The relative inactivity of β-glucosidase in non-keratinized epithelium not only is consistent with the persistence of GlcCer species to the epithelial surface (64,65), but also less stringent barrier in non-keratinized oral epithelium (66). Subsequent studies revealed that the specificity of this activity toward GlcCer substrate(s) was a consequence of β-GlcCer'ase activity. Interestingly, the epidermis also was found to contain at least a 10-fold higher β-GlcCer'ase activity than other mammalian tissue, including brain, liver, and spleen, when enzyme activity is expressed per amount of protein (67). Consistent with this, β-GlcCer'ase mRNA expression in murine epidermis exceeds the levels encountered in these extracutaneous tissues (67), suggesting that this specific enzyme is responsible for the observed epidermal activity. Moreover, this specific β-GlcCer'ase activity is even higher in the outer, more differentiated epidermal cell layers, extending into the enucleate SC (67,68), with elevated β-glycosidase activity being evident in serial frozen sections at the region corresponding to the SG–SC transition (69). Immunohistochemical staining for β-GlcCer'ase protein later revealed an enhanced fluorescent signal in the outer nucleated layers of the human epidermis, concentrated at the apex and margins of SG cells, as well as within membrane domains of the lower SC (55).

---

[a] Abbreviations for Cer species to delineate structures (as per Motta S., et al., 2003 [Citation #3]), containing as follows: N, non-hyroxy-FA; A, alpha-hydroxy-FA; O, omega-hydroxy FA; E, esterified (omega) FA; S, sphingosine base; P, phytosphingosine base; H, 6-hydroxy-sphingosine base.

ß-Glucocerebrosidase
(ß-GlcCer'ase)

Glucosylceramide ⟶ Ceramide + Glucose
(GlcCer)   (Cer)

Figure 3 The conversin of glucosylceramide (GlcCer) species to ceramide (Cer) and glucose is catalyzed by the enzyme β-glucocerebrosidase (β-GlcCer'ase) (EC 3.2.1.45). This enzyme releases glucose specifically from beta-linked GlcCer substrates, a process in mammalian epidermis that occurs in the extracellular domains of the SC as a requirement for normal lamellar membrane formation and permeability barrier function.

Moreover, in extracts from individual epidermal layers, β-GlcCer'ase activity is present throughout murine epidermis, with the highest activity in the SC, peaking in the lower-to-mid SC (67,68). Membrane couplets, consisting of segments of cornified envelopes (CEs) with intact lipid membrane domains prepared from isolated SC sheets, also demonstrate significant GlcCer'ase activity, with 2- to 8-fold higher activity than that of other acid hydrolases (68).

Yet, despite findings about enzymatic *protein*, whether or not this enzyme retains its *activity* within the hydrophobic, extracellular domains of the SC required further resolution. Using a novel in situ zymographic technique for both whole skin and tissue sections, highest levels of GlcCer'ase activity are found to be present in the upper SG and the lower SC (68,70,71). Thus, the activity profile of GlcCer'ase parallels the protein gradient of this enzyme in epidermis. Together, these data strongly suggest that the processing of GlcCer-to-Cer within the outer epidermis is attributable to the retention of specific enzymatic activity within SC extracellular domains.

GLUCOSYLCERAMIDE PROCESSING IS REQUIRED FOR EPIDERMAL BARRIER FUNCTION

The link between GlcCer-to-Cer conversion and normal permeability barrier homeostasis became evident when it was shown that both mRNA and enzyme activity levels for GlcCer'ase were increased during barrier recovery, following an acute abrogation in murine epidermis (72). However, the importance of enzymatic processing for the maintenance of epidermal permeability barrier function in mammalian SC was first demonstrated with a pharmacologic (i.e., inhibitor-based) approach in murine epidermis. In vivo inhibition of GlcCer'ase using a single topical application of bromoconduritol B-epoxide (BrCBE), a potent and specific inhibitor of this enzyme (73), reduced epidermal GlcCer'ase activity by > 90%, and significantly delayed the recovery of barrier function in this murine model (72,74). This functional delay was due to the replacement of normal, highly ordered, SC lamellar membrane arrays by disordered linear arrays of incompletely processed, immature-appearing membrane structures (74). Furthermore, repeated, daily applications of the same inhibitor to intact murine skin not only increased SC GlcCer levels, but also diminished barrier function, with similar alterations of SC membrane lipid domains (75) to those noted in the acute barrier repair model described above.

These inhibitor studies were subsequently extended to a null-allele GlcCer'ase-deficient mouse (76,77), which retains less than 1% residual enzyme activity, a model that was originally developed as a murine analog for Gaucher disease (78). The homozygous GlcCer'ase-deficient animals displayed nearly identical SC ultrastructural abnormalities to those present in the inhibitor-based model described above; i.e., linear, yet highly disordered and "immature" membrane arrays (75). A severely compromised barrier was also evident in the homozygous GlcCer'ase-deficient animals, with the profile of SC and epidermal lipid contents revealing both increased GlcCer levels, and diminished Cer, consistent with a deficiency of this enzyme. The epidermis of heterozygous animals, which retains approximately 50% of the normal GlcCer'ase activity, did not reveal the lipid biochemical, ultrastructural, or the functional abnormalities that were evident in the more-severely deficient animals (75). This knockout approach convincingly demonstrated not only the importance of GlcCer-to-Cer conversion for barrier homeostasis, but also that a single GlcCer'ase gene product solely accounts for this activity in mammalian epidermis.

Subsequent studies with skin samples from human Gaucher patients with severe GlcCer'ase-deficiency, i.e., neonatal Type 2 disease, demonstrated similar SC structural abnormalities (75,79). Interestingly, Gaucher patients with less severe disease do not display significant abnormalities in the SC ultrastructure (79), consistent with the findings in the mice heterozygous for GlcCer'ase deficiency described above. Together, these results suggest that an excess of this enzyme is available in the normal epidermis under basal conditions, and conversely that a minimal threshold of epidermal enzyme activity, which can no longer support the normal SC lamellar membrane formation and barrier integrity, exists in severe Gaucher disease.

Additional murine models that more closely mirror the molecular mutations in human Gaucher disease have since revealed similar findings. Specifically, while animals homozygous for GlcCer'ase point mutations equivalent to the common mutations found in human Gaucher disease (e.g., L444P) revealed no neurologic pathology, severe ichthyotic and histologic abnormalities were evident in the epidermis (80). These animals do not survive beyond the initial 24 hrs postpartum, presumably because of an abnormally high water loss resulting from the epidermal lipid processing defect (80). Examination of the SC ultrastructure (using ruthenium tetroxide post-fixed samples) from these animals revealed marked structural abnormalities in the SC membrane lipid domains, including incompletely processed LB contents throughout the SC interstices (Holleran et al., unpublished), as in β-GlcCer'ase deficiency of genetic or inhibitor-based origin.

These studies on β-GlcCer'ase were the first to demonstrate a critical requirement of enzymatic hydrolysis of lipid precursors (GlcCer) to specific products (Cer) for permeability barrier homeostasis. Interestingly, in moist keratinizing epithelia, such as oral mucosa and marine cetacean epidermis, both of which have less stringent barrier requirements, SC GlcCer content remains elevated (65,81,82), corresponding with lower endogenous β-glucosidase activity(ies) (63,69) (see also Chap. 13).

REGULATION OF GlcCer'ase ACTIVITY IN THE EPIDERMIS AND SC

Role of pH

The post-secretory processing of GlcCer precursors into Cer within the SC interstices is catalyzed by β-GlcCer'ase, a lysosomal, acidic-pH optimum enzyme. The activity of epidermal β-GlcCer'ase has been shown to possess an acidic pH optimum, with peak in vitro activity at pH 5.2, and absent or significantly reduced activity at neutral pH (7.4) (62,67,68). The fact that barrier homeostasis is perturbed when the normally acidic SC is neutralized (70,83), strongly suggests a role for SC acidification in epidermal function(s), including lipid processing events. Specifically, permeability barrier recovery proceeds normally when barrier-disrupted murine skin is exposed externally to solutions buffered to an acidic pH (70). In contrast, the initiation of barrier recovery slows when the barrier-disrupted skin is exposed to a neutral pH, independent of buffer composition. Interestingly, both the formation and secretion of LB proceed comparably when skin is exposed either to an acidic (pH 5.5) or to neutral (pH 7.4) conditions. However, exposure to a pH of 7.4 (but not pH 5.5) results in the persistence of immature, extracellular lamellar membrane structures accompanied by a marked decrease in the in situ activity of GlcCer'ase (70). Indeed, despite an increased pH toward neutrality in the lower SC, the extracellular "microdomains" remain acidic (84), strongly suggesting that β-GlcCer'ase could be activated by localized changes in SC pH. Consistent with the membrane localization of an acidic pH in the lower SC, increased β-GlcCer'ase activity is evident with increasing depth of tape stripping of mammalian skin (68,85).

The importance of SC acidification for permeability barrier homeostasis via regulation of lipid processing enzymes was further revealed in studies with mouse epidermis in vivo. It should be noted that while short-term changes in pH reversibly activate/inactivate β-GlcCer'ase (83), more prolonged elevations in pH ultimately result in an irreversible loss of enzyme content/activity due to a serine protease–mediated degradation of β-GlcCer'ase (86). Thus, extracellular pH in the SC has an important role in regulating GlcCer-to-Cer processing through an enzyme-dependent hydrolysis.

Role of Saposins

Additional mechanisms are likely to modulate the post-translational changes in GlcCer'ase activity. In extracutaneous tissues, β-GlcCer'ase is activated by small molecular weight glycoproteins called saposins (SAPs) (reviewed in Ref. 87). In particular, SAP-A and SAP-C can upregulate GlcCer'ase activity in reconstituted, in vitro enzyme systems (88,89). Four of the SAP proteins, i.e., SAP-A–SAP-D, each of which is expressed in human epidermis (Holleran et al., unpublished results), are derived by proteolytic processing of a common precursor protein, prosaposin (90). Given the importance of GlcCer'ase activity in mammalian epidermis, it is not surprising therefore that prosaposin-deficient mice display GlcCer accumulation, sub-normal levels of Cer, and immature SC lamellar membranes (91), as in Gaucher disease (see above). Furthermore, the decreased levels of epidermal prosaposin protein (92), may also explain, in part, the apparent decrease in sphingomyelinase (SM'ase) activities in patients with AD (93), contributing to the diminished SC Cer content of these patients (see below). Finally, the striking abnormality in SC membrane domains in prosaposin-deficient mice was further accompanied by an accumulation of GlcCer species that are covalently attached to CE proteins (91), showing that deglucosylation of ω-OH–GlcCer occurs after attachment to the CE (see below). Together, these results suggest that extracellular SAP activation of β-GlcCer'ase activity is important for normal SC lipid processing.

LIPID PROCESSING OF THE CORNEOCYTE LIPID ENVELOPE

Mammalian SC contains a lipid layer that is covalently attached to the external surface of CE proteins of fully differentiated corneocytes. This so-called "corneocyte lipid envelope" (CLE) consists of ω-OH Cer covalently attached to CE proteins (94–96). The ω-OH group on the Cer is required for CLE formation (97,98), as this moiety represents the attachment point between the Cer and specific amino acids of CE proteins, including involucrin (99) (see Fig. 4). Although purified transglutaminase 1 (TG-1) has been shown to perform this "ceramidation" reaction in vitro (100) (Fig. 4, Step 1), whether this enzyme is solely responsible for this reaction remains unresolved, because TG-1 deficient epidermis from a patient reveals the presence of sporadic normal CLE structures (101), as well as near-normal quantities of covalently-attached Cer (102).

Similar to the formation of membrane bilayer structures in the SC described above, lipid processing is also required to generate the mature CLE structure. A number of findings support this contention. First, in epidermis lacking GlcCer'ase activity, the CLE contains only ω-OH GlcCer species (91,103). Second, CLE structures are also evident in Gaucher mouse SC by ultrastructural analysis (Uchida and Holleran, submitted), despite the parallel accumulation of covalently attached ω-OH GlcCer and an absence of the corresponding covalently bound ω-OH Cer species in β-GlcCer'ase–deficient epidermis (91,103). Thus, deglucosylation, though clearly required for lamellar membrane formation/organization (72,74,75), *is not required* for initial CLE formation. However, since the covalent attachment of Cer to the

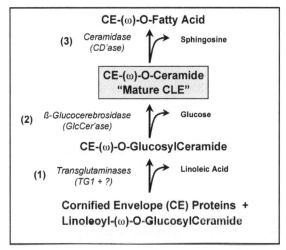

Figure 4 Formation of the mature corneocyte lipid envelope (CLE) requires a step-wise process, including: (1) covalent-attachment of omega (ω)-glucosylceramide (via the ω-hydroxy position) to cornified envelope (CE) proteins by transglutaminase(s) or other as yet-unidentified processes; (2) the release of glucose from the covalently-attached (ω)-O-glucosylceramide by β-glucocerebrosidase; and finally, (3) the hudrolysis of a portion of the covalently-attached (ω)-O-Cer to generate CE-(ω)-O-Cer to generate CE-(ω)-O-fatty acids and free sphingosine base species.

CE involves the ω-OH groups (98), the (bulky) hydrophilic glucose residue, facing toward the extracellular domains, could further interfere with the organization of the compact lamellar membranes required for competent barrier function. Together, these findings reveal that mature CLE formation occurs in a sequential manner; i.e., attachment of ω-OH GlcCer followed by subsequent enzymatic deglucosylation by GlcCer'ase (Fig. 4, Steps 1 & 2).

In recent studies with essential fatty acid–deficient (EFAD) mice, reduced content of both acylGlcCer and its downstream SC metabolite, ω-OH Cer, have been noted (Uchida and Holleran, submitted). The previously reported decrease in covalently attached ω-OH Cer species in EFAD epidermis (104) was also confirmed (Uchida and Holleran, submitted). Given that EFAD skin is also characterized by epidermal hyperplasia and altered differentiation (105), decreased CE "acceptor" proteins for ω-OH Cer might account, at least in part, for the observed decrease in CLE content. However, this interpretation seems unlikely since CLE–ω-OH Cer levels are normal-to-increased in another cutaneous disease, lamellar ichthyosis (101,102), which displays defective CE due to abnormal-to-deficient (TG-1) activity (106,107). Instead, it appears more likely that the ω-esterified linoleate moiety of acylGlcCer could play a critical role in the formation of the mature CLE structure (Fig. 4, Step 1). Thus, linoleic acid is not only important for acylCer/acylGlcCer formation, but also appears to be the preferred ω-O-esterified FA moiety that facilitates the covalent attachment of ω-OH GlcCer to CE proteins.

SPHINGOMYELINASE ACTIVITY IN THE GENERATION OF SC BARRIER LIPIDS

A number of studies have revealed that the enzymatic processing of SM to Cer by SM'ase; (EC 3.1.4.12) is also critical for SC structure and epidermal barrier homeostasis (Fig. 5). At least two isoenzymes in human skin can hydrolyze SM to Cer, including a lysosomal-type acid-pH optimum SM'ase (a-SM'ase) and a non-lysosomal, magnesium-dependent neutral-pH optimum SM'ase (n-SM'ase). The epidermal a-SM'ase has optimal activity at pH 4.5–5.0, and is activated by Triton X-100 (0.1% w/v) in vitro (108,109).

Although both the acidic- and neutral-SM'ase enzymes are involved in the recovery of permeability barrier function following an acute challenge (110), a number of findings reveal that at an acidic pH, the lysosomal enzyme appears to be primarily responsible for the extracellular hydrolysis of SM-to-Cer in the SC. For example, a-SM'ase activity in SC localizes primarily to intercellular membrane domains (11,111), making it ideally situated to catalyze this critical lipid processing

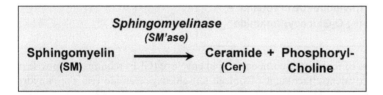

Figure 5 The conversion of sphingomyelin species to ceramide (Cer) and phosphorylcholine is catalyzed by the enzyme sphingomyelinase (SM'ase) (EC 3.1.4.12). This activity in the extracellular domains of the SC also facilitates lamellar membrane formation, and permeability barrier homeostasis.

step. In addition, a-SM'ase activity increases in parallel with the accumulation of lipids within LBs, during the maturation of these critical epidermal organelles (11). Moreover, in both normal hairy ($hr^{+/+}$) and hairless ($hr^{-/-}$) mice, a-SM'ase activity increased two hours following an acute barrier abrogation, an effect not observed in tumor necrosis factor-receptor (TNF-R)–deficient ($hr^{1/+}$) mouse epidermis (110). More importantly, inhibition of this increase in a-SM'ase activity by two independent approaches, a structural analog, PDHS, or intracellular inhibitors at the level of the lamellar body [i.e., either imipramine (110) or desipramine (109)], significantly delayed barrier recovery. This functional delay was accompanied by an increase in SM content, as well as a reduction of normal extracellular lamellar membrane structures in the SC (109). Electron microscopy of ruthenium tetroxide post-fixed skin samples reveals that inhibition of a-SM'ase activity interferes with the final stages of lamellar membrane maturation in the extracellular domains of the SC. Moreover, patients with Niemann–Pick (type A) disease, characterized by a deficiency of lysosomal a-SM'ase, demonstrate an abnormal permeability barrier homeostasis, including delayed recovery kinetics following an acute barrier disruption (109). Given that the inhibitor-induced delays in barrier recovery discussed above can be overridden by topical co-application of Cer (109), alteration of the Cer-to-SM ratio, rather than SM accumulation itself, appears to be responsible for the alteration in epidermal barrier function. Interestingly, this last finding contrasts with the consequences of absent β-GlcCer'ase (see Section "Regulation of GlcCer'ase Activity in the Epidermis and SC") or steroid sulfatase (SSase) (see Section "Processing of Cholesterol Sulfate by Steroid Sulfatase"), where accumulation of enzyme *substrates* (GlcCer or cholesterol-sulfate species, respectively) in SC, rather than reduction of enzyme *products* is responsible for the resultant membrane alterations and diminished barrier function; i.e., neither Cer nor Chol significantly override these abnormal parameters (74,112,113).

The contribution of specific SM precursors to SC Cer species was further addressed by a structural analysis of human epidermal SM species (see above) (52). Given that only two of the nine known human SC Cer species, i.e., Cer 2 (NS) and Cer 5 (AS), are generated in part by SM hydrolysis, and that all nine major SC Cer species are derived from GlcCer precursors (52,53) (for a more detailed analysis, refer to Chap. 6 by Y. Uchida and S. Hamanaka, this monograph), the GlcCer-to-Cer pathway appears to have a more critical role for generating the full spectrum of unique Cer species that comprise the epidermal barrier. Consistent with this interpretation is the more-significant epidermal barrier dysfunction that is evident with GlcCer'ase deficiency (i.e., in either severe Gaucher disease or GlcCer'ase knockout mice) (75,79) than that so-far has been observed with a-SM'ase deficiency (i.e., Niemann–Pick disease) (109,110).

Finally, the role of n-SM'ase in epidermal structure and function is less-well resolved. As noted above, a-SM'ase activity appears primarily responsible for the majority of SM-to-Cer hydrolysis that occurs in the extracellular domains of the SC. However, n-SM'ase activity also appears to be important for epidermal homeostasis. Studies by Jensen, Proksch, and colleagues have revealed a delayed barrier recovery following an acute challenge in FAN-deficient skin, suggesting a role for n-SM'ase activity in epidermal barrier homeostasis (114). In addition, delayed barrier recovery and *unchanged* a- and n-SM'ase activities were noted in TNF-R55–deficient mouse skin (110). Although these latter studies do not distinguish between a- and n-SM'ase-dependent events, they are consistent with the importance of the SM-to-Cer conversion being critical for epidermal barrier homeostasis.

The results summarized above represent strong evidence for the dynamic events occurring during the final stage of epidermal/barrier differentiation and development. As such, it should now be readily apparent that extracellular lipid processing of both SM and GlcCer precursors is critical for mammalian epidermal structure and function. Interestingly, the importance of the gradual decline in epidermal SM'ase activity (115) for the decline in barrier function in aging (116) has yet to be fully explored (see also Summary). Finally, given that SM-to-Cer turnover (and recycling) has been implicated in myriad cellular processes (13,20), and that active sphingolipid remodeling is ongoing within proliferating and more differentiated keratinocytes (Uchida & Holleran; unpublished observations), it is highly likely that additional important roles will be revealed for both SM and GlcCer in cutaneous function and disease.

PROCESSING OF GLYCEROPHOSPHOLIPIDS BY SECRETORY PHOSPHOLIPASES

FFAs represent one of the three key lipid components of the SC membrane bilayer system, and appear to be derived in large part by the hydrolytic processing of secreted PL. Specifically, inhibition of secretory phospholipase A2 (sPLA$_2$) activity by the topical application of either BPB or MJ33, irreversible and reversible sPLA$_2$ inhibitors, respectively, following acute disruption of the permeability barrier, results in a delay in barrier recovery (117). This delayed recovery is accompanied by the persistence of "immature" and disordered lamellar membrane arrays within the SC interstices (117,118). These changes in function and membrane structure can be reversed when the inhibitor-treated SC is co-treated in vitro with palmitic or stearic acids, but less efficiently following co-treatment with unsaturated FA species or with the lyso-phospholipid, lyso-lecithin, which lacks one FA moiety. These results indicate first, that the barrier perturbation induced by the phospholipase inhibition is due to a failure to generate FFAs rather than to an accumulation of PL, and therefore, that extracellular processing of PL to FA is required for normal barrier homeostasis. Second, these results suggest that sPLA2 generates a pool of non-essential FA, required as structural barrier ingredients, independent of the well-known requirement for linoleate as the ω-acylated FA in acylCer (see above).

Although the inhibitor-based studies discussed above strongly suggest that secretory PLA$_2$ activity is primarily responsible for the extracellular processing of PLs to the FFAs within the SC, the specific PLA$_2$ isozyme(s) involved has/have yet to be identified (Fig. 6). For example, several subtypes of type 2 sPLA$_2$ have recently been reported in both normal and psoriatic human skin. Immunofluorescence revealed the expression of sPLA$_2$-IB, -IIF, and -X predominately within the suprabasal

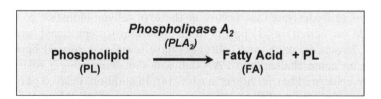

Figure 6 The release of fatty acids (FA) species from phospholipid precursors is largely catalyzed by a phospholipase A2 enzyme activity, a process that occurs primarily in the extracellular domains of mammalian stratum corneum for barrier homeostasis.

epidermal layers, while sPLA$_2$-V and -IID were detected in both basal and spinous layers (119). Additional isoforms are either weakly expressed (e.g., PLA$_2$-IIA), or are not detected (sPLA$_2$-IIE and -XIIA) by immunofluorescence of normal epidermis. Given the evidence that sPLA$_2$ activity and the generation of FFAs within the SC are critical for mammalian permeability barrier homeostasis (117,118,120), as well as the possible alterations in phospholipid hydrolysis in inflammatory dermatoses such as psoriasis (see below), much additional work will be required to delineate the role of individual sPLA$_2$ isoforms in PL processing, as well as in epidermal structure, function, and disease.

CERAMIDASES IN EPIDERMAL LIPID PROCESSING AND FUNCTION

Ceramidase (CD'ase) enzymes (EC 3.5.1.23) catalyze the hydrolysis of Cer to sphingosine and FFA (Fig. 7). Similar to Cer, sphingosine and its phosphorylated analog, sphingosine-1-phosphate (S1P), represent important cell-signaling molecules (reviewed in Refs. 21,22). The discovery of receptors with specificity for S1P binding in various tissues, including epidermis and keratinocytes (123,124), has unleashed a wave of interest in the mechanisms that regulate the levels of this key biomediary lipid. Given that sphingosine, and by analogy S1P, are formed exclusively via CD'ase-dependent Cer hydrolysis, the role of this enzymatic sequence in cellular functions is of particular interest. Five distinct mammalian CD'ase enzymes have been reported to date, including neutral (n-CD'ase) (125–127), acid (a-CD'ase) (128,129), phytoalkaline (phyto-CD'ase) (130), as well as an alkaline isoform (alk-CD'ase) that is highly expressed in mammalian skin (131). A fifth human CD'ase isozyme has been recently described as an additional alkaline isoform (C. Mao, personal communication). Acid-CD'ase is a lysosomal enzyme (128,129), whose deficiency results in the lysosomal storage disorder, Farber disease, which is associated with significant Cer accumulation in brain and other neuronal tissues (128,132,133). Interestingly, while the skin of the patients with Farber disease appears normal by light microscopy (134), an a-CD'ase–deficient mouse model displays abnormal skin findings: whereas the complete knockout (−/−) mouse was early-embryonic lethal (135), heterozygous (+/−) animals show skin abnormalities (R. Kolesnick, personal communication) that have not yet been fully characterized. Neutral-CD'ase is a type II integral membrane protein that localizes to the plasma membrane (136,137), which appears to play a key role in the metabolism of SM,

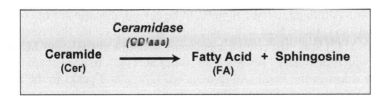

Figure 7 Ceramide hydrolysis to free fatty acid (FA) and sphingoid base is catalyzed by a family of ceramidase enzymes (EC 3.5.1.23). A number of ceramidase enzymes are present in mammalian epidermis, with specific roles for each of these enzymes in epidermal function yet to be resolved.

and which has a detoxifying role against inadvertent Cer accumulation in response to a variety of extracellular factors (138).

Whether CD'ase is involved with normal SC lipid processing remains unresolved. Earlier studies demonstrated both the presence of CD'ase within SC isolates (139), as well as free sphingosine in human and porcine SC (140,141), suggesting that CD'ase is active in this epidermal compartment. Furthermore, the presence of ω-OH FFA in CLE preparations (91,94,96,103) implies that a percentage of the covalently attached ω-OH Cer species are hydrolyzed by CD'ase(s) subsequent to their covalent attachment to the CE. Although no gross difference in Cer levels between outer and inner SC has been observed (142,143), limited and localized hydrolysis of SC Cer species still appears plausible.

A number of earlier studies revealed that the mammalian epidermis contains an alkaline CD'ase activity associated with a plasma membrane fraction that has maximal activities between pH 7.5 and 8.5 (139,144). Human skin was confirmed to have a high alkaline CD'ase activity as well (131). Recently, expression of all four CD'ase enzymes has been confirmed in the epidermis (145). Given also that diminished Cer and sphingosine levels have been reported in patients with AD, as well as an apparent association between diminished sphingosine levels and increased bacterial colonization in AD skin (see Section "Altered Lipid Processing in Psoriasis"), the function(s) of CD'ase activity(ies) within the epidermis is an issue of great potential clinical importance.

Finally, similar to findings in a related transgenic model, i.e., the prosaposin-deficient mouse (91), a virtual absence of covalently bound free ω-OH FA has been noted in β-GlcCer'ase–deficient (Gaucher) mouse SC (Uchida & Holleran, unpublished results). Thus, as anticipated, glucosylated ω-OH Cer species appear to be poor substrates for subsequent CD'ase activity. Moreover, the progressive hydrolysis of covalently bound ω-OH Cer to generate covalently attached ω-OH FA might accompany normal maturation of the CLE, facilitating later SC desquamation, perhaps by reducing the interaction between CLE and unbound acylCer in the SC.

PROCESSING OF CHOLESTEROL SULFATE BY STEROID SULFATASE

The content of cholesterol sulfate ($CholSO_4$) increases during normal epidermal differentiation, with the peak levels (i.e., approximately 5.2% of the total lipid content) evident in SG, and lesser amounts in subjacent nucleated layers (i.e., 3.4% of total lipids in the combined stratum basale and spinosum) (146). The SC also contains lower $CholSO_4$ levels (2.6% of total SC lipid content), with further decreases in the outer SC (142) being consistent with elevated steroid sulfatase (SSase) activity in outer epidermal layers (146). Although initially thought to be devoid of SSase activity (40) (Fig. 8), biochemical and cytochemical techniques have recently revealed the presence of SSase within LBs (147) and extracellular membrane domains in the lower SC of normal epidermis, with little residual activity in the outer SC (147). In normal epidermis, SS'ase activity is low in the basal and spinous cell layers, and peaks in the SG (146). High activity persists in the SC, particularly in membrane domains (146).

The critical role of SSase for epidermal homeostasis is readily evident from the cutaneous abnormalities that characterize patients with recessive X-linked ichthyosis (RXLI) who lack this enzyme (148–150) (Elias, et al.; Chap. 28 of this monograph). Genetic deficiency of SS'ase leads to diminished processing of $CholSO_4$ to Chol with

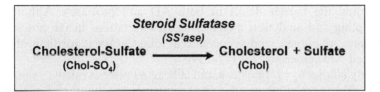

Figure 8 The conversion of cholesterol-sulfate to cholesterol is catalyzed by steroid sufatase (SS'ase). The lack of steroid sulfatase leads to accumulation of cholesterol sulfate and severe alterations in SC membrance domains characteristic of recessive X-linked ichthyosis (RXLI).

subsequent accumulation of this precursor lipid within SC (146,151). In normal epidermis, CholSO$_4$ accounts for approximately 5% of the total SG lipids, and it decreases to about 1% of lipids in the outer SC. Conversely, in RXLI, the SC contains about 10-fold elevated levels of CholSO$_4$, a lipid alteration associated with significant structural and functional epidermal abnormalities. Specifically, elevated SC CholSO$_4$ does not alter membrane structure, but instead it induces lamellar–non–lamellar phase separations within membrane domains (113). In model membrane bilayers, CholSO$_4$ not only segregates into distinct lamellar domains (152), but excess CholSO$_4$ also induces the asymmetric distribution of Chol within individual lamellar membrane domains, revealing large, asymmetric density increases (153). The limited ability of topical Chol to improve either the desquamation abnormality or barrier function in CholSO$_4$-treated mice (112), further suggests that it is retention of the sulfated lipid, rather than a lack of Chol, which accounts for the barrier abnormality in RXLI (113). Thus, retention of the hydrophilic sulfate group disrupts the normal organization of extracellular lipids within the SC interstices.

Given that the hyperkeratosis in RXLI is attributed to delayed desquamation, rather than excessive epidermal proliferation (154), elevated SC CholSO$_4$ likely has effects on the SC that extend beyond the above described changes in lamellar membrane domains. For example, the persistence of corneodesmosomes into the upper SC of these patients strongly suggests a role for CholSO$_4$ in regulating proteolytic processes in this tissue as well. The recent demonstration of diminished serine protease activity in RXLI SC by zymography is consistent with a direct role for these lipids in desquamation, perhaps through an inhibitory effect on serine protease activity (147). Interestingly, hair and nail retain approximately 5% CholSO$_4$, further suggesting a possible role for this sulfated lipid in corneocyte cohesion. Finally, CholSO$_4$ is a transcriptional regulator of corneocyte protein expression (155), as well as an activator of the gamma-isoform of protein kinase C (PKC-γ) (156), suggesting that the excess SC in RXLI could represent a form of "hyperdifferentiation." Thus, the enzymatic processing of CholSO$_4$ to Chol represents an important lipid hydrolytic step for the normal epidermal differentiation and function.

LIPID PROCESSING ALTERATIONS IN ATOPIC DERMATITIS

The contribution of SC lipid abnormalities to the pathogenesis of certain cutaneous disorders continues to be an active area of research. For example, there have been numerous studies attempting to link the distinctive barrier abnormality in patients with AD to altered SC lipid content, most notably, diminished Cer levels (1,2,157) (see also Chap. 26 of this monograph by H. Tagami an K. Kikochi) for more information regarding the barrier defect in both AD and psoriasis). Although differences in sampling and analytical methods lead to variations in the absolute levels of these changes, all of these studies concur that total Cer levels are diminished in the SC of affected AD epidermis (1,2,157–159).

However, early studies by G. Imokawa and colleagues also revealed no significant differences in either GlcCer'ase or alk-CD'ase activities in tape strippings from patients with AD (160). Subsequent studies by these same investigators revealed not only the high activity of a novel enzyme with properties of a sphingomyelin deacylase (161,162), but also an elevated content of the unique end-product of this enzymatic activity, sphingosyl–phosphorylcholine (SPC or lyso-sphingomyelin) (163) (Fig. 9). Additional studies later demonstrated a similar GlcCer deacylase activity (164). Since the responsible enzyme(s) has/have neither been cloned nor further identified, due in part, to the apparent low baseline expression in normal epidermis, it remains unclear whether this latter activity either represents a novel enzyme (164), a single enzyme with combined GlcCer and SM deacylase activities (165), or is possibly of bacterial origin. Despite this limitation, elevation of one or both of these novel enzyme activity(ies) could explain both the diminished Cer and sphingosine levels in the SC of AD patients (166) (Fig. 9, Step 2), and thus, contribute to the barrier abnormality, as well as other aspects of the disease. Indeed, SPC, coupled with decreased sphingosine could contribute to the increased proliferation, altered keratinization, inflammation, and even an increased tendency for secondary bacterial infections in patients with AD (166–168).

Interestingly, atopic SC was shown to be deficient not only in free Cer species (1,2,157–159), but also in covalently bound ω-OH Cer (corneocyte-bound lipid envelope) (169). In both lesional and non-lesional skin, covalently attached ω-OH Cer species were significantly reduced, i.e., 10–25 and 23–28 weight percent (wt.%), respectively, from the normal 46–53 wt.% of total protein-bound lipid content (169). Significant decreases in de novo synthesis of ω-esterified Cer 4 (EOH), and Cer 3 (NP) were also noted in keratinocytes from lesional skin (169) (Fig. 9, Step 1).

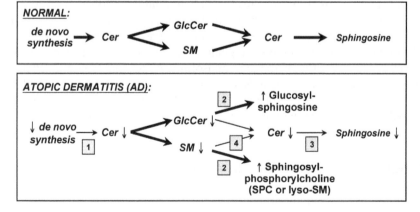

Figure 9 A number of possible mechanisms may account for the decreased ceramide content noted in the SC of atopic dermatitis patients, including: (1) a decrease in de novo ceramide synthesis, (2) lyase activity to generate glucosyl-sphingosine and/or sphingosyl-phosphorylcholine, (3) increased ceramidase activity, and (4) decreased sphingomyelinase activity.

Thus, lesional epidermis in patients with AD contains significant deficiencies of key barrier Cer species that may contribute to the alterations in not only the permeability barrier function, but also other functional defects (e.g., antimicrobial).

At least four CD'ase activities are present in mammalian epidermis (145) (see above), with high alk-CD'ase activity reported in SC (139). Although no alteration in alk-CD'ase activity was noted in atopic skin samples versus age-matched controls (160,166), a reduction of a-CD'ase activity is evident (166). Thus, the decreased sphingosine levels in involved AD skin (166) suggest that, in addition to elevations in the novel GlcCer/SM lyase activities (Fig. 9, Step 2; see also above), reduced CD'ase activitiy(ies) could also underlie this abnormality (Fig. 9, Step 3). In addition, speculation continues regarding possible contributions of bacterial CD'ase both to normal epidermal function and to atopic progression (170–172). Although elevated bacterial colonization correlates with the severity of atopic skin lesions, an effect attributed to diminished content of the natural anti-bacterial sphingosine (166,173), the extent to which these changes in endogenous and/or exogenous CD'ase activity(ies) contribute to the pathogenesis of AD has yet to be resolved.

Finally, contrary to the earlier studies that reported either no significant alterations in SM'ase activity in AD skin (161) or increases in SM'ase protein levels by quantitative immunoblot analysis (174), Proksch and colleagues have recently demonstrated reductions of both a-SM'ase and n-SM'ase activities in lesional AD skin (93) (Fig. 9, Step 4, see also Chapter by Proksch, this volume). In addition, the levels of prosaposin, the precursor for sphingolipid activator proteins, and/or saposin D itself, also appear to be diminished in psoriatic epidermis (92), representing yet another potential contributing factor to altered lipid processing in the epidermis of these patients. Despite these contrasting findings regarding enzyme activities that likely represent differences in sampling and/or assay techniques, a better understanding of the relative contributions of each of the above-mentioned alterations in lipid processing enzymes to the reduction in epidermal Cer content, and the associated permeability barrier abnormality in AD (175,176), could reveal the most appropriate therapeutic (non–immune-based) approaches to this debilitating dermatitis (177).

ALTERED LIPID PROCESSING IN PSORIASIS

Not surprisingly, the severity of barrier defect in psoriatic skin is proportional to the disease phenotype (see Chap. 26, this volume). Although a number of studies suggest a role for altered lipid processing in psoriasis, whether these alterations are involved in the pathogenesis, or simply represent a consequence of this complex cutaneous disorder, remain unresolved. A number of reports cite altered Cer distribution and/or content in psoriatic epidermis. For example, Motta and colleagues reported a decreased content of specific Cer species in psoriatic scale versus normal SC, i.e., Cer 1 (EOS), as well as phytosphingosine-containing Cer species, Cer 3 (NP) and Cer 6 (AP), with simultaneous increases in other Cer species, such that the total Cer content remained unchanged (4,178). The contribution of altered lipid processing to these changes in lipid content has been explored, yielding contrasting results. An early report compared the in vitro activities of 14 distinct acid hydrolases in epidermal keratome samples from eight psoriatic versus 36 normal (non-diseased) patients (179,180). Significant *elevations* in total β-glucosidase activity (i.e., 11-fold over mean control values) were noted, with further elevations in arylsulfatase-A and -B activities (179). Conversely, Alessandrini and colleagues recently reported *diminished* β-GlcCer'ase mRNA in whole skin punch biopsies from lesional sites in five patients with psoriasis vulgaris, when compared with skin from healthy, non-affected controls (181). Immunohistochemical localization using an antibody produced against a GST fusion protein containing β-GlcCer'ase (cloned from human skin) also revealed a corresponding decrease in β-GlcCer'ase protein in lesional psoriatic epidermis (181). Interestingly, non-lesional skin also showed a significant decrease in epidermal mRNA level and immunostaining for β-GlcCer'ase versus normal control skin, with both of these parameters lower than that in lesional skin. Decreased immunostaining for a-SM'ase in SC from lesional versus non-lesional psoriatic skin has also been reported (182). These results are consistent with additional findings from this group, wherein they demonstrated a decrease in prosaposin mRNA and protein levels in psoriatic skin (182). Immunohistochemical analysis revealed a significant decrease in prosaposin protein levels in lesional skin from both active- and chronic-type plaque, compared with non-lesional and normal skin (182). Given that individual SAP proteins are co-activator proteins for both GlcCer'ase and SM'ase enzymes (87,183–186), as well as for a-Cer'ase activity (187), and that prosaposin-deficient animals retain GlcCer species in the SC associated with diminished permeability barrier function (91), altered GlcCer (and SM) lipid processing could contribute to disease expression in psoriasis.

Alterations in PL processing in psoriatic skin have also been described. For example, a 46% decrease in FA content in psoriatic scale versus normal SC has been reported (3). Given that PLs represent a major precursor for FAs generated in the SC (117,120), this result is consistent with diminished PL processing in psoriatic epidermis. Furthermore, although sPLA$_2$-X is normally expressed in the suprabasal epidermal layers (see Section "Cermidases in Epidermal Lipid Processing and Functions"), its expression is markedly diminished in psoriatic epidermis, while it is simultaneously in evidence in psoriatic dermis, in conjunction with sPLA$_2$-Iia, -IID, and IB isoforms (119). Given the well-established, dual roles for PLA$_2$ enzymes first in the generation of FFAs for the barrier, and second in the generation of pro-inflammatory eicosanoids through the release of arachidonic acid, these intriguing findings suggest potential roles for sPLA$_2$ isozymes in the pathogenesis of psoriasis. In summary, abnormal expression and/or activity of enzymes important for SC lipid processing may have additional roles/functions in cutaneous disease processes such as psoriasis.

ALTERED LIPID PROCESSING WITH AGING

Although baseline barrier function in aging skin appears normal or possibly improved over younger skin, repair of the permeability barrier is delayed following an acute disruption (116,188). Consistent with this reduction in barrier function, each of the three major lipid species, i.e., Chol, FA, and Cer, were all significantly decreased in aged human SC (> 80 versus 23–30 years) (116), with more profound decreases reported for Chol or Cer species (189). Selective changes in specific SC Cer species (i.e., Cer 2 [NS]), with concurrent increases in Cer 3 (NP) relative to total Cer content, have also been noted in aged epidermis (190). Similarly, decreases in total SC lipid content have also been reported in aged murine skin, with little change in the distribution of Cer to other SC lipids (116).

Although an earlier study that revealed diminished epidermal lipid synthesis appears to account for the delayed barrier repair in aged mice (188), a role for altered lipid processing in epidermal aging has also been proposed. Specifically, Tezuka and colleagues reported *reduced* a-SM'ase activity in aged whole human epidermis (i.e., eighth decade) versus young adults (second decade) (115). Although this enzyme activity was not specifically localized to the SC, overall results of this work suggest an altered turnover of SM in aged epidermis. Interestingly, in liver cells from aged rats (191), as well as in a human fibroblast cell line (192), both Cer content and SM'ase activity are elevated, suggesting instead an *increased* SM turnover with aging, at least in these tissues/cell types. As noted above (see Sections "Glucosylceramides as a Major Source of Stratum Corneum Ceramides" and "Ceramidases in Epidermal Lipid Processing and Function"), SM'ase that generates long (C24) and short (C16) chain-containing Cer species is critical for epidermal barrier function (109,110). These data again reveal the likely importance of the SM-to-Cer conversion in the epidermis, a lipid turnover process that could be compromised in aged skin.

Interestingly, elevated CD'ase activity was reported in aged atopic human SC (tape strips), which may also contribute to the decreased Cer content of aged atopic skin (160). Given that mammalian epidermis contains five distinct CD'ase enzymes, two of which are elevated in the more-differentiated keratinocytes and epidermis (145), including an alkaline isoform that is selectively expressed in the skin (131), with an additional human alkaline isoform recently revealed (C. Mao, personal communication), the extent to which individual CDase isoform activities are altered with aging remains unresolved.

SUMMARY

Studies into the metabolic activities localized within the SC are driving a continued re-evaluation of the concept that this epidermal compartment is an inert accumulation of dead (enucleate) cells surrounded by static lipid-enriched domains. We now appreciate that the early bricks and mortar representation of the SC does not do full justice to the myriad biochemical and structural alterations required to subserve its numerous critical functions. The studies reviewed above reveal some of the biochemical complexities required for the normal formation and maturation of these protective lipid domains. However, the role that these key lipid changes play not only in orchestrating the normal corneocyte transition between the lower and outer layers, but also in disease pathogenesis and/or progression, remain highly fertile areas for future study. Thus, the study of epidermal lipidomics will likely drive a continuing transformation of our concepts of the SC as a dynamic lipid and protein environ.

REFERENCES

1. Imokawa G, Abe A, Jin K, Higaki Y, Kawashima M, Hidano A. Decreased level of ceremides in stratum corneum of atopic dermatitis: an etiologic factor in atopic dry skin? J Invest Dermatol 1991; 96:523–526.
2. Melnik B, Hollmann J, Plewig G. Decreased stratum corneum ceramides in atopic individuals—a pathobiochemical factor in xerosis? [letter]. Br J Dermatol 1988; 119:547–549.
3. Motta S, Sesana S, Ghidoni R, Monti M. Content of the different lipid classes in psoriatic scale. Arch Dermatol Res 1995; 287:691–694.

4. Motta S, Monti M, Sesana S, Caputo R, Carelli S, Ghidoni R. Ceramide composition of the psoriatic scale. Biochim Biophys Acta 1993; 1182:147–151.

5. Man MM, Feingold KR, Thornfeldt CR, Elias PM. Optimization of physiological lipid mixtures for barrier repair. J Invest Dermatol 1996; 106:1096–1101.

6. Man MQ, Feingold KR, Elias PM. Exogenous lipids influence permeability barrier recovery in acetone-treated murine skin. Arch Dermatol 1993; 129:728–738.

7. Swartzendruber DC, Wertz PW, Kitko DJ, Madison KC, Downing DT. Molecular models of the intercellular lipid lamellae in mammalian stratum corneum. J Invest Dermatol 1989; 92:251–257.

8. Bouwstra JA, Cheng K, Gooris GS, Weerheim A, Ponec M. The role of ceramides 1 and 2 in the stratum corneum lipid organisation. Biochim Biophys Acta 1996; 1300:177–186.

9. Bouwstra JA, Gooris GS, Weerheim A, Kempenaar J, Ponec M. Characterization of stratum corneum structure in reconstructed epidermis by X-ray diffraction. J Lipid Res 1995; 36:496–504.

10. Elias PM, Menon GK. Structural and lipid biochemical correlates of the epidermal permeability barrier. Adv Lipid Res 1991; 24:1–26.

11. Rassner U, Feingold KR, Crumrine DA, Elias PM. Coordinate assembly of lipids and enzyme proteins into epidermal lamellar bodies. Tissue Cell 1999; 31:489–498.

12. Elias PM, Friend DS, McNutt NS. Epidermal permeability barrier: transformation of lamellar granule-disks into intercellular sheets by a membrane fusion process [letter]. J Invest Dermatol 1987; 88:459–460.

13. Futerman AH, Hannun YA. The complex life of simple sphingolipids. EMBO Rep 2004; 5:777–782.

14. Smith WL, Merrill AH Jr. Sphingolipid metabolism and signalling minireview series. J Biol Chem 2002; 277:25841–25842.

15. Wakita H, Tokura Y, Yagi H, Nishimura K, Furukawa F, Takigawa M. Keratinocyte differentiation is induced by cell-permeant ceramides and its proliferation is promoted by sphingosine. Arch Dermatol Res 1994; 286:350–354.

16. Geilen CC, Wieder T, Orfanos CE. Ceramide signalling: regulatory role in cell proliferation, differentiation and apoptosis in human epidermis. Arch Dermatol Res 1997; 289: 559–566.

17. Bektas M, Dullin Y, Wieder T, Kolter T, Sandhoff K, Brossmer R, Ihrig P, Orfanos CE, Geilen CC. Induction of apoptosis by synthetic ceramide analogues in the human keratinocyte cell line HaCaT. Exp Dermatol 1998; 7:342–349.

18. Takami Y, Abe A, Matsuda T, Shayman JA, Radin NS, Walter RJ. Effect of an inhibitor of glucosylceramide synthesis on cultured human keratinocytes. J Dermatol 1998; 25:73–77.

19. Uchida Y, Murata S, Schmuth M, Behne MJ, Lee JD, Ichikawa S, Elias PM, Hirabayashi Y, Holleran WM. Glucosylceramide synthesis and synthase expression protect against ceramide-induced stress. J Lipid Res 2002; 43:1293–1302.

20. Pettus BJ, Chalfant CE, Hannun YA. Ceramide in apoptosis: an overview and current perspectives. Biochim Biophys Acta 2002; 1585:114–125.

21. Uchida Y, Nardo AD, Collins V, Elias PM, Holleran WM. De novo ceramide synthesis participates in the ultraviolet B irradiation-induced apoptosis in undifferentiated cultured human keratinocytes. J Invest Dermatol 2003; 120:662–669.

22. Braun PE, Morell P, Radin NS. Synthesis of C18-dihydrosphingosines and C20-dihydrosphingosines, ketodihydrosphingosines, and ceramides by microsomal preparations from mouse brain. J Biol Chem 1970; 245:335–341.

23. Williams RD, Wang E, Merrill AH Jr. Enzymology of long-chain base synthesis by liver: characterization of serine palmitoyltransferase in rat liver microsomes. Arch Biochem Biophys 1984; 228:282–291.

24. Holleran WM, Williams ML, Gao WN, Elias PM. Serine-palmitoyl transferase activity in cultured human keratinocytes. J Lipid Res 1990; 31:1655–1661.

25. Merrill AH Jr, Wang E. Biosynthesis of long-chain (sphingoid) bases from serine by LM cells. Evidence for introduction of the 4-trans-double bond after de novo biosynthesis of N-acylsphinganine(s). J Biol Chem 1986; 261:3764–3769.

26. Michel C, van Echten-Deckert G, Rother J, Sandhoff K, Wang E, Merrill AH Jr. Characterization of ceramide synthesis. A dihydroceramide desaturase introduces the 4,5-trans-double bond of sphingosine at the level of dihydroceramide. J Biol Chem 1997; 272:22432 22437.

27. Holleran WM, Gao WN, Feingold KR, Elias PM. Localization of epidermal sphingo-lipid synthesis and serine palmitoyl transferase activity: alterations imposed by perme-ability barrier requirements. Arch Dermatol Res 1995; 287:254–258.

28. Gray GM, Yardley HJ. Different populations of pig epidermal cells: isolation and lipid composition. J Lipid Res 1975; 16:441–447.

29. Elias PM, Brown BE, Fritsch P, Goerke J, Gray GM, White RJ. Localization and com-position of lipids in neonatal mouse stratum granulosum and stratum corneum. J Invest Dermatol 1979; 73:339–348.

30. Lampe MA, Williams ML, Elias PM. Human epidermal lipids: characterization and modulations during differentiation. J Lipid Res 1983; 24:131–140.

31. Holleran WM, Feingold KR, Man MQ, Gao WN, Lee JM, Elias PM. Regulation of epidermal sphingolipid synthesis by permeability barrier function. J Lipid Res 1991; 32:1151–1158.

32. Harris IR, Farrell AM, Grunfeld C, Holleran WM, Elias PM, Feingold KR. Perme-ability barrier disruption coordinately regulates mRNA levels for key enzymes of cholesterol, fatty acid, and ceramide synthesis in the epidermis. J Invest Dermatol 1997; 109:783–787.

33. Stachowitz S, Alessandrini F, Abeck D, Ring J, Behrendt H. Permeability barrier disruption increases the level of serine palmitoyltransferase in human epidermis. J Invest Dermatol 2002; 119:1048–1052.

34. Holleran WM, Man MQ, Gao WN, Menon GK, Elias PM, Feingold KR. Sphingolipids are required for mammalian epidermal barrier function. Inhibition of sphingolipid synthesis delays barrier recovery after acute perturbation. J Clin Invest 1991; 88:1338–1345.

35. Basu S, Kaufman B, Roseman S. Enzymatic synthesis of ceramide-glucose and ceramide-lactose by glycosyltransferases from embryonic chicken brain. J Biol Chem 1968; 243:5802–5804.

36. Ichikawa S, Sakiyama H, Suzuki G, Hidari KI, Hirabayashi Y. Expression cloning of a cDNA for human ceramide glucosyltransferase that catalyzes the first glycosylation step of glycosphingolipid synthesis. Proc Natl Acad Sci USA 1996; 93:12654.

37. Yamaoka S, Miyaji M, Kitano T, Umehara H, Okazaki T. Expression cloning of a human cDNA restoring sphingomyelin synthesis and cell growth in sphingomyelin synthase-defective lymphoid cells. J Biol Chem 2004; 279:18688–18693.

38. Huitema K, van den Dikkenberg J, Brouwers JF, Holthuis JC. Identification of a family of animal sphingomyelin synthases. EMBO J 2004; 23:33–44.

39. Wertz PW, Downing DT, Freinkel RK, Traczyk TN. Sphingolipids of the stratum corneum and lamellar granules of fetal rat epidermis. J Invest Dermatol 1984; 83: 193–195.

40. Grayson S, Johnson-Winegar AG, Wintroub BU, Isseroff RR, Epstein EH Jr, Elias PM. Lamellar body-enriched fractions from neonatal mice: preparative techniques and partial characterization. J Invest Dermatol 1985; 85:289–294.

41. Freinkel RK, Traczyk TN. Lipid composition and acid hydrolase content of lamellar granules of fetal rat epidermis. J Invest Dermatol 1985; 85:295–298.

42. Hamanaka S, Nakazawa S, Yamanaka M, Uchida Y, Otsuka F. Glucosylceramide accumulates preferentially in lamellar bodies in differentiated keratinocytes. Br J Dermatol 2005; 152:426–434.

43. Madison KC, Sando GN, Howard EJ, True CA, Gilbert D, Swartzendruber DC, Wertz PW. Lamellar granule biogenesis: a role for ceramide glucosyltransferase, lysosomal enzyme tansport, and the golgi. J Invest Dermatol Symp Proc 1998; 3:80–86.

44. Sando GN, Howard EJ, Madison KC. Induction of ceramide glucosyltransferase activity in cultured human keratinocytes. Correlation with culture differentiation. J Biol Chem 1996; 271:22044–22051.

45. Watanabe R, Wu K, Paul P, Marks DL, Kobayashi T, Pittelkow MR, Pagano RE. Up-regulation of glucosylceramide synthase expression and activity during human keratinocyte differentiation. J Biol Chem 1998; 273:9651–9655.

46. Chujor CS, Feingold KR, Elias PM, Holleran WM. Glucosylceramide synthase activity in murine epidermis: quantitation, localization, regulation, and requirement for barrier homeostasis. J Lipid Res 1998; 39:277–285.

47. Hanley K, Jiang Y, Holleran WM, Elias PM, Williams ML, Feingold KR. Glucosylceramide metabolism is regulated during normal and hormonally stimulated epidermal barrier development in the rat. J Lipid Res 1997; 38:576–584.

48. Wertz PW, Downing DT. Ceramides of pig epidermis: structure determination. J Lipid Res 1983; 24:759–765.

49. Robson KJ, Stewart ME, Michelsen S, Lazo ND, Downing DT. 6-Hydroxy-4-sphingenine in human epidermal ceramides. J Lipid Res 1994; 35:2060–2068.

50. Stewart ME, Downing DT. A new 6-hydroxy-4-sphingenine-containing ceramide in human skin. J Lipid Res 1999; 40:1434–1439.

51. Ponec M, Weerheim A, Lankhorst P, Wertz P. New acylceramide in native and reconstructed epidermis. J Invest Dermatol 2003; 120:581–588.

52. Uchida Y, Hara M, Nishio H, Sidransky E, Inoue S, Otsuka F, Suzuki A, Elias PM, Holleran WM, Hamanaka S. Epidermal sphingomyelins are precursors for selected stratum corneum ceramides. J Lipid Res 2000; 41:2071–2082.

53. Hamanaka S, Hara M, Nishio H, Otsuka F, Suzuki A, Uchida Y. Human epidermal glucosylceramides are major precursors of stratum corneum ceramides. J Invest Dermatol 2002; 119:416–423.

54. Cox P, Squier CA. Variations in lipids in different layers of porcine epidermis. J Invest Dermatol 1986; 87:741–744.

55. Vielhaber G, Pfeiffer S, Brade L, Lindner B, Goldmann T, Vollmer E, Hintze U, Wittern KP, Wepf R. Localization of ceramide and glucosylceramide in human epidermis by immunogold electron microscopy. J Invest Dermatol 2001; 117:1126–1136.

56. Ockerman PA. Acid hydrolases in human skin. Acta Derm Venereol 1969; 49:139–141.

57. Goldberg MF, Cotlier E, Fichenscher LG, Kenyon K, Enat R, Borowsky SA. Macular cherry-red spot, corneal clouding, and -galactosidase deficiency. Clinical, biochemical, and electron microscopic study of a new autosomal recessive storage disease. Arch Intern Med 1971; 128:387–398.

58. Ohkawara A, Halprin K, Taylor J, Levine V. Acid hydrolases in the human epidermis. Br J Dermatol 1972; 83450–83459:450–459.

59. Mier PD, van den Hurk JJ. Lysosomal hydrolases of the epidermis. I. Glycosidases. Br J Dermatol 1975; 93:1–10.

60. Wolff K, Schreiner E. Epidermal lysosomes. Electron microscopic-cytochemical studies. Arch Dermatol 1970; 101:276–286.

61. Nemanic MK, Whitehead JS, Elias PM. Alterations in membrane sugars during epidermal differentiation: visualization with lectins and role of glycosidases. J Histochem Cytochem 1983; 31:887–897.

62. Wertz PW, Downing DT. Beta-glucosidase activity in porcine epidermis. Biochim Biophys Acta 1989; 1001:115–119.

63. Chang F, Wertz PW, Squier CA. Comparison of glycosidase activities in epidermis, palatal epithelium and buccal epithelium. Comp Biochem Physiol B 1991; 100:137–139.

64. Squier CA, Cox P, Wertz PW. Lipid content and water permeability of skin and oral mucosa. J Invest Dermatol 1991; 96:123–126.

65. Squier CA, Wertz PW, Cox P. Thin-layer chromatographic analyses of lipids in different layers of porcine epidermis and oral epithelium. Arch Oral Biol 1991; 36:647–653.
66. Lesch CA, Squier CA, Cruchley A, Williams DM, Speight P. The permeability of human oral mucosa and skin to water. J Dent Res 1989; 68:1345–1349.
67. Holleran WM, Takagi Y, Imokawa G, Jackson S, Lee JM, Elias PM. Beta Glucocerebrosidase activity in murine epidermis: characterization and localization in relation to differentiation. J Lipid Res 1992; 33:1201–1209.
68. Takagi Y, Kriehuber E, Imokawa G, Elias PM, Holleran WM. Beta-glucocerebrosidase activity in mammalian stratum corneum. J Lipid Res 1999; 40:861–869.
69. Chang F, Wertz PW, Squier CA. Localization of beta-glucosidase activity within keratinizing epithelia. Comp Biochem Physiol Comp Physiol 1993; 105:251–253.
70. Mauro T, Holleran WM, Grayson S, Gao WN, Man MQ, Kriehuber E, Behne M, Feingold KR, Elias PM. Barrier recovery is impeded at neutral pH, independent of ionic effects: implications for extracellular lipid processing. Arch Dermatol Res 1998; 290:215–222.
71. Fluhr JW, Mao-Qiang M, Brown BE, Hachem JP, Moskowitz DG, Demerjian M, Haftek M, Serre G, Crumrine D, Mauro TM, Elias PM, Feingold KR. Functional consequences of a neutral pH in neonatal rat stratum corneum. J Invest Dermatol 2004; 123:140–151.
72. Holleran WM, Takagi Y, Menon GK, Jackson SM, Lee JM, Feingold KR, Elias PM. Permeability barrier requirements regulate epidermal beta-glucocerebrosidase. J Lipid Res 1994; 35:905–912.
73. Legler G, Bieberich E. Active site directed inhibition of a cytosolic beta-glucosidase from calf liver by bromoconduritol B epoxide and bromoconduritol F. Arch Biochem Biophys 1988; 260:437–442.
74. Holleran WM, Takagi Y, Menon GK, Legler G, Feingold KR, Elias PM. Processing of epidermal glucosylceramides is required for optimal mammalian cutaneous permeability barrier function. J Clin Invest 1993; 91:1656–1664.
75. Holleran WM, Ginns EI, Menon GK, Grundmann JU, Fartasch M, McKinney CE, Elias PM, Sidransky E. Consequences of beta-glucocerebrosidase deficiency in epidermis. Ultrastructure and permeability barrier alterations in Gaucher disease. J Clin Invest 1994; 93:1756–1764.
76. Tybulewicz VL, Tremblay ML, LaMarca ME, Willemsen R, Stubblefield BK, Winfield S, Zablocka B, Sidransky E, Martin BM, Huang SP, et al. Animal model of Gaucher's disease from targeted disruption of the mouse glucocerebrosidase gene. Nature 1992; 357:407–410.
77. Sidransky E, Sherer DM, Ginns EI. Gaucher disease in the neonate: a distinct Gaucher phenotype is analogous to a mouse model created by targeted disruption of the glucocerebrosidase gene. Pediatr Res 1992; 32:494–498.
78. Barranger JA, Ginns EI, Glucosylceramide lipidoses: Gaucher disease. In: Scriver CR, et al. eds. Metabolic Basis of Inherited Disease. New York: McGraw-Hill, 1989: 1677–1698.
79. Sidransky E, Fartasch M, Lee RE, Metlay LA, Abella S, Zimran A, Gao W, Elias PM, Ginns EI, Holleran WM. Epidermal abnormalities may distinguish type 2 from type 1 and type 3 of Gaucher disease. Pediatr Res 1996; 39:134–141.
80. Liu Y, Suzuki K, Reed JD, Grinberg A, Westphal H, Hoffmann A, Doring T, Sandhoff K, Proia RL. Mice with types 2 and 3 Gaucher disease point mutations generated by a single insertion mutagenesis procedure. Proc Natl Acad Sci USA 1998; 95:2503–2508.
81. Wertz PW, Cox PS, Squier CA, Downing DT. Lipids of epidermis and keratinized and non-keratinized oral epithelia. Comp Biochem Physiol B 1986; 83:529–531.
82. Elias PM, Menon GK, Grayson S, Brown BE, Rehfeld SJ. Avian sebokeratocytes and marine mammal lipokeratinocytes: structural, lipid biochemical, and functional considerations. Am J Anat 1987; 180:161–177.

83. Hachem JP, Crumrine D, Fluhr J, Brown BE, Feingold KR, Elias PM. pH directly regulates epidermal permeability barrier homeostasis stratum corneum integrity/cohesion. J Invest Dermatol 2003; 121:345–353.

84. Behne MJ, Meyer J, Hanson KM, Barry NP, Murata S, Crumrine D, Clegg RR, Gratton E, Holleran WM, Elias PM, Mauro TM. NHE1 regulates the stratum corneum permeability barrier homeostasis: microenvironment acidifcation assessed with FLIM. J Biol Chem 2002; 277:47399–406.

85. Redoules D, Tarroux R, Assalit MF, Peri JJ. Characterisation and assay of five enzymatic activities in the stratum corneum using tape-strippings. Skin Pharmacol Appl Skin Physiol 1999; 12:182–192.

86. Hachem JP, Man MQ, Crumrine D, Uchida Y, Brown BE, Rogiers V, Roseeuw D, Feingold KR, Elias PM. Sustained serine protease activity by prolonged increase in pH leads to degradation of lipid processing enzymes and profound alterations of barrier function and stratum corneum integrity. J Invest Dermatol. 2005. In press.

87. O'Brien JS, Kishimoto Y. Saposin proteins: structure, function, and role in human lysosomal storage disorders. FASEB J 1991; 5:301–308.

88. Morimoto S, Martin BM, Yamamoto Y, Kretz KA, O'Brien JS, Kishimoto Y. Saposin A: second cerebrosidase activator protein. Proc Natl Acad Sci USA 1989; 86:3389–3393.

89. Morimoto S, Kishimoto Y, Tomich J, Weiler S, Ohashi T, Barranger JA, Kretz KA, O'Brien JS. Interaction of saposins, acidic lipids, and glucosylceramidase. J Biol Chem 1990; 265:1933–1937.

90. Hiraiwa M, O'Brien JS, Kishimoto Y, Galdzicka M, Fluharty AL, Ginns EI, Martin BM. Isolation, characterization, and proteolysis of human prosaposin, the precursor of saposins (sphingolipid activator proteins). Arch Biochem Biophys 1993; 304:110–116.

91. Doering T, Holleran WM, Potratz A, Vielhaber G, Elias PM, Suzuki K, Sandhoff K. Sphingolipid activator proteins are required for epidermal permeability barrier formation. J Biol Chem 1999; 274:11038–11045.

92. Cui CY, Kusuda S, Seguchi T, Takahashi M, Aisu K, Tezuka T. Decreased level of prosaposin in atopic skin. J Invest Dermatol 1997; 109:319–323.

93. Jensen JM, Folster-Holst R, Baranowsky A, Schunck M, Winoto-Morbach S, Neumann C, Schutze S, Proksch E. Impaired sphingomyelinase activity and epidermal differentiation in atopic dermatitis. J Invest Dermatol 2004; 122:1423–1431.

94. Wertz PW, Downing DT. Covalent attachment of omega-hydroxyacid derivatives to epidermal macromolecules: a preliminary characterization. Biochem Biophys Res Commun 1986; 137:992–997.

95. Wertz PW, Downing DT. Covalently bound omega-hydroxyacylsphingosine in the stratum corneum. Biochim Biophys Acta 1987; 917:108–111.

96. Wertz PW, Madison KC, Downing DT. Covalently bound lipids of human stratum corneum. J Invest Dermatol 1989; 92:109–111.

97. Behne M, Uchida Y, Seki T, de Montellano PO, Elias PM, Holleran WM. Omega-hydroxyceramides are required for corneocyte lipid envelope (CLE) formation and normal epidermal permeability barrier function. J Invest Dermatol 2000; 114:185–192.

98. Stewart ME, Downing DT. The omega-hydroxyceramides of pig epidermis are attached to corneocytes solely through omega-hydroxyl groups. J Lipid Res 2001; 42:1105–1110.

99. Marekov LN, Steinert PM. Ceramides are bound to structural proteins of the human foreskin epidermal cornified cell envelope. J Biol Chem 1998; 273:17763–17770.

100. Nemes Z, Marekov LN, Fésüs L, Steinert PM. A novel function for transglutaminase 1: attachment of long-chain omega-hydroxyceramides to involucrin by ester bond formation. Proc Natl Acad Sci USA 1999; 96:8402–8407.

101. Elias PM, Schmuth M, Uchida Y, Rice RH, Behne M, Crumrine D, Feingold KR, Holleran WM, Pharm D. Basis for the permeability barrier abnormality in lamellar ichthyosis. Exp Dermatol 2002; 11:248–256.

102. Paige DG, Morse-Fisher N, Harper JI. Quantification of stratum corneum ceramides and lipid envelope ceramides in the hereditary ichthyoses. Br J Dermatol 1994; 131:23–27.

103. Doering T, Proia RL, Sandhoff K. Accumulation of protein-bound epidermal glucosyl-ceramides in beta-glucocerebrosidase deficient type-2 Gaucher mice. FEBS Lett 1999; 447:167–170.
104. Meguro S, Arai Y, Masukawa Y, Uie K, Tokimitsu I. Relationship between covalently bound ceramides and transepidermal water loss (TEWL). Arch Dermatol Res 2000; 292:463–468.
105. Hou SY, Mitra AK, White SH, Menon GK, Ghadially R, Elias PM. Membrane structures in normal and essential fatty acid-deficient stratum corneum: characterization by ruthenium tetroxide staining and x-ray diffraction. J Invest Dermatol 1991; 96:215–223.
106. Russell LJ, DiGiovanna JJ, Rogers GR, Steinert PM, Hashem N, Compton JG, Bale SJ. Mutations in the gene for transglutaminase 1 in autosomal recessive lamellar ichthyosis. Nat Genet 1995; 9:279–283.
107. Huber M, Rettler I, Bernasconi K, Frenk E, Lavrijsen SP, Ponec M, Bon A, Lautenschlager S, Schorderet DF, Hohl D. Mutations of keratinocyte transglutaminase in lamellar ichthyosis [see comments]. Science 1995; 267:525–528.
108. Bowser PA, Gray GM. Sphingomyelinase in pig and human epidermis. J Invest Dermatol 1978; 70:331–335.
109. Schmuth M, Man MQ, Weber F, Gao W, Feingold KR, Fritsch P, Elias PM, Holleran WM. Permeability barrier disorder in Niemann–Pick disease: sphingomyelin-ceramide processing required for normal barrier homeostasis. J Invest Dermatol 2000; 115:459–466.
110. Jensen JM, Schütze S, Förl M, Krönke M, Proksch E. Roles for tumor necrosis factor receptor p55 and sphingomyelinase in repairing the cutaneous permeability barrier. J Clin Invest 1999; 104:1761–1770.
111. Menon GK, Grayson S, Elias PM. Cytochemical and biochemical localization of lipase and sphingomyelinase activity in mammalian epidermis. J Invest Dermatol 1986; 86:591–597.
112. Maloney ME, Williams ML, Epstein EH Jr, Law MY, Fritsch PO, Elias PM. Lipids in the pathogenesis of ichthyosis: topical cholesterol sulfate-induced scaling in hairless mice. J Invest Dermatol 1984; 83:252–256.
113. Zettersten E, Man MQ, Sato J, Denda M, Farrell A, Ghadially R, Williams ML, Feingold KR, Elias PM. Recessive x-linked ichthyosis: role of cholesterol-sulfate accumulation in the barrier abnormality. J Invest Dermatol 1998; 111:784–790.
114. Kreder D, Krut O, Adam-Klages S, Wiegmann K, Scherer G, Plitz T, Jensen JM, Proksch E, Steinmann J, Pfeffer K, Krönke M. Impaired neutral sphingomyelinase activation and cutaneous barrier repair in FAN-deficient mice. EMBO J 1999; 18:2472–2479.
115. Yamamura T, Tezuka T. Change in sphingomyelinase activity in human epidermis during aging. J Dermatol Sci 1990; 1:79–83.
116. Ghadially R, Brown BE, Sequeira-Martin SM, Feingold KR, Elias PM. The aged epidermal permeability barrier. Structural, functional, and lipid biochemical abnormalities in humans and a senescent murine model. J Clin Invest 1995; 95:2281–2290.
117. Mao-Qiang M, Feingold KR, Jain M, Elias PM. Extracellular processing of phospholipids is required for permeability barrier homeostasis. J Lipid Res 1995; 36:1925–1935.
118. Mao-Qiang M, Jain M, Feingold KR, Elias PM. Secretory phospholipase A2 activity is required for permeability barrier homeostasis. J Invest Dermatol 1996; 106:57–63.
119. Haas U, Podda M, Behne M, Gurrieri S, Alonso A, Furstenberger G, Pfeilschifter J, Lambeau G, Gelb MH, Kaszkin M. Characterization and differentiation dependent regulation of secreted phospholipases A in human keratinocytes and in healthy and psoriatic human skin. J Invest Dermatol 2005; 124:204–211.
120. Fluhr JW, Kao J, Jain M, Ahn SK, Feingold KR, Elias PM. Generation of free fatty acids from phospholipids regulates stratum corneum acidification and integrity. J Invest Dermatol 2001; 117:44–51.
121. Cuvillier O, Pirianov G, Kleuser B, Vanek PG, Coso OA, Gutkind S, Spiegel S. Suppression of ceramide-mediated programmed cell death by sphingosine-1-phosphate. Nature 1996; 381:800–803.

122. Cuvillier O, Rosenthal DS, Smulson ME, Spiegel S. Sphingosine 1-phosphate inhibits activation of caspases that cleave poly(ADP-ribose) polymerase and lamins during Fas-mediated and ceramide-mediated apoptosis in Jurkat T lymphocytes. J Biol Chem 1998; 273:2910–2916.

123. Vogler R, Sauer B, Kim DS, Schafer-Korting M, Kleuser B. Sphingosine-1-phosphate and its potentially paradoxical effects on critical parameters of cutaneous wound healing. J Invest Dermatol 2003; 120:693–700.

124. Sauer B, Vogler R, von Wenckstern H, Fujii M, Anzano MB, Glick AB, Schafer-Korting M, Roberts AB, Kleuser B. Involvement of Smad signalling in sphingosine 1-phosphate-mediated biological responses of keratinocytes. J Biol Chem 2004; 279: 38471–38479.

125. El Bawab S, Roddy P, Qian T, Bielawska A, Lemasters JJ, Hannun YA. Molecular cloning and characterization of a human mitochondrial ceramidase. J Biol Chem 2000; 275:21508–21513.

126. El Bawab S, Bielawska A, Hannun YA. Purification and characterization of a membrane-bound nonlysosomal ceramidase from rat brain. J Biol Chem 1999; 274:27948–27955.

127. Mitsutake S, Tani M, Okino N, Mori K, Ichinose S, Omori A, Iida H, Nakamura T, Ito M. Purification, characterization, molecular cloning, and subcellular distribution of neutral ceramidase of rat kidney. J Biol Chem 2001; 276:26249–26259.

128. Koch J, Gärtner S, Li CM, Quintern LE, Bernardo K, Levran O, Schnabel D, Desnick RJ, Schuchman EH, Sandhoff K. Molecular cloning and characterization of a full-length complementary DNA encoding human acid ceramidase. Identification of the first molecular lesion causing Farber disease. J Biol Chem 1996; 271:33110–33115.

129. Bernardo K, Hurwitz R, Zenk T, Desnick RJ, Ferlinz K, Schuchman EH, Sandhoff K. Purification, characterization, and biosynthesis of human acid ceramidase. J Biol Chem 1995; 270:11098–11102.

130. Mao C, Xu R, Szulc ZM, Bielawska A, Galadari SH, Obeid LM. Cloning and characterization of a novel human alkaline ceramidase. A mammalian enzyme that hydrolyzes phytoceramide. J Biol Chem 2001; 276:26577–26588.

131. Mao C, Xu R, Szulc ZM, Bielawski J, Becker KP, Bielawska A, Galadari SH, Hu W, Obeid LM. Cloning and characterization of a mouse endoplasmic reticulum alkaline ceramidase: an enzyme that preferentially regulates metabolism of very long chain ceramides. J Biol Chem 2003; 278:31184–31191.

132. Dulaney J, Moser HW, Sidbury J, Milunsky A. The biochemical defect in Farber's disease. Adv Exp Med Biol 1976; 68:403–411.

133. Dulaney JT, Milunsky A, Sidbury JB, Hobolth N, Moser HW. Diagnosis of lipogranulomatosis (Farber disease) by use of cultured fibroblasts. J Pediatr 1976; 89:59–61.

134. Abenoza P, Sibley RK. Farber's disease: a fine structural study. Ultrastruct Pathol 1987; 11:397–403.

135. Li CM, Park JH, Simonaro CM, He X, Gordon RE, Friedman AH, Ehleiter D, Paris F, Manova K, Hepbildikler S, Fuks Z, Sandhoff K, Kolesnick R, Schuchman EH. Insertional mutagenesis of the mouse acid ceramidase gene leads to early embryonic lethality in homozygotes and progressive lipid storage disease in heterozygotes. Genomics 2002; 79:218–224.

136. Tani M, Okino N, Sueyoshi N, Ito M. Conserved amino acid residues in the COOH-terminal tail are indispensable for the correct folding and localization and enzyme activity of neutral ceramidase. J Biol Chem 2004; 279:29351–29358.

137. Tani M, Iida H, Ito M. O-glycosylation of mucin-like domain retains the neutral ceramidase on the plasma membranes as a type II integral membrane protein. J Biol Chem 2003; 278:10523–10530.

138. Choi MS, Anderson MA, Zhang Z, Zimonjic DB, Popescu N, Mukherjee AB. Neutral ceramidase gene: role in regulating ceramide-induced apoptosis. Gene 2003; 315: 113–122.

139. Wertz PW, Downing DT. Ceramidase activity in porcine epidermis. FEBS Lett 1990; 268:110–112.
140. Wertz PW, Downing DT. Free sphingosine in human epidermis. J Invest Dermatol 1990; 94:159–161.
141. Wertz PW, Downing DT. Free sphingosines in porcine epidermis. Biochim Biophys Acta 1989; 1002:213–217.
142. Long SA, Wertz PW, Strauss JS, Downing DT. Human stratum corneum polar lipids and desquamation. Arch Dermatol Res 1985; 277:284–287.
143. Weerheim A, Ponec M. Determination of stratum corneum lipid profile by tape stripping in combination with high-performance thin-layer chromatography. Arch Dermatol Res 2001; 293:191–199.
144. Yada Y, Higuchi K, Imokawa G. Purification and biochemical characterization of membrane-bound epidermal ceramidases from guinea pig skin. J Biol Chem 1995; 270:12677–12684.
145. Houben E, Uchida Y, Mao C, Obeid LM, Elias PM, Holleran WM. Differentiation-dependent expression of ceramidase isoforms in human keratinocytes and epidermis. J Invest Dermatol 2004; 122:76a.
146. Elias PM, Williams ML, Maloney ME, Bonifas JA, Brown BE, Grayson S, Epstein EH Jr. Stratum corneum lipids in disorders of cornification. Steroid sulfatase and cholesterol sulfate in normal desquamation and the pathogenesis of recessive X-linked ichthyosis. J Clin Invest 1984; 74:1414–1421.
147. Elias PM, Crumrine D, Rassner U, Hachem JP, Menon GK, Man W, Choy MH, Leypoldt L, Feingold KR, Williams ML. Basis for abnormal desquamation and permeability barrier dysfunction in RXLI. J Invest Dermatol 2004; 122:314–319.
148. Marinkovic-Ilsen A, Koppe JG, Jobsis AC, de Groot WP. Enzymatic basis of typical X-linked ichthyosis. Lancet 1978; 2:1097.
149. Koppe G, Marinkovic-Ilsen A, Rijken Y, De Groot WP, Jobsis AC. X-linked icthyosis. A sulphatase deficiency. Arch Dis Child 1978; 53:803–806.
150. Webster D, France JT, Shapiro LJ, Weiss R. X-linked ichthyosis due to steroid-sulphatase deficiency. Lancet 1978; 1:70–72.
151. Williams ML, Elias PM. Stratum corneum lipids in disorders of cornification: increased cholesterol sulfate content of stratum corneum in recessive x-linked ichthyosis. J Clin Invest 1981; 68:1404–1410.
152. Rehfeld SJ, Williams ML, Elias PM. Interactions of cholesterol and cholesterol sulfate with free fatty acids: possible relevance for the pathogenesis of recessive X-linked ichthyosis. Arch Dermatol Res 1986; 278:259–263.
153. McIntosh TJ. Organization of skin stratum corneum extracellular lamellae: diffraction evidence for asymmetric distribution of cholesterol. Biophys J 2003; 85:1675–1681.
154. Williams ML. Lipids in normal and pathological desquamation. Adv Lipid Res 1991; 24:211–262.
155. Hanley K, Wood L, Ng DC, He SS, Lau P, Moser A, Elias PM, Bikle DD, Williams ML, Feingold KR. Cholesterol sulfate stimulates involucrin transcription in keratinocytes by increasing Fra-1, Fra-2, and Jun D. J Lipid Res 2001; 42:390–398.
156. Denning MF, Kazanietz MG, Blumberg PM, Yuspa SH. Cholesterol sulfate activates multiple protein kinase C isoenzymes and induces granular cell differentiation in cultured murine keratinocytes. Cell Growth Differ 1995; 6:1619–1626.
157. Di Nardo A, Wertz P, Giannetti A, Seidenari S. Ceramide and cholesterol composition of the skin of patients with atopic dermatitis. Acta Derm Venereol 1998; 78:27–30.
158. Melnik B, Hollmann J, Hofmann U, Yuh MS, Plewig G. Lipid composition of outer stratum corneum and nails in atopic and control subjects. Arch Dermatol Res 1990; 282:549–551.
159. Yamamoto A, Serizawa S, Ito M, Sato Y. Stratum corneum lipid abnormalities in atopic dermatitis. Arch Dermatol Res 1991; 283:219–223.

160. Jin K, Higaki Y, Takagi Y, Higuchi K, Yada Y, Kawashima M, Imokawa G. Analysis of beta-glucocerebrosidase and ceramidase activities in atopic and aged dry skin. Acta Derm Venereol 1994; 74:337–340.

161. Murata Y, Ogata J, Higaki Y, Kawashima M, Yada Y, Higuchi K, Tsuchiya T, Kawainami S, Imokawa G. Abnormal expression of sphingomyelin acylase in atopic dermatitis: an etiologic factor for ceramide deficiency? J Invest Dermatol 1996; 106: 1242–1249.

162. Hara J, Higuchi K, Okamoto R, Kawashima M, Imokawa G. High-expression of sphingomyelin deacylase is an important determinant of ceramide deficiency leading to barrier disruption in atopic dermatitis. J Invest Dermatol 2000; 115:406–413.

163. Okamoto R, Arikawa J, Ishibashi M, Kawashima M, Takagi Y, Imokawa G. Sphingosylphosphorylcholine is upregulated in the stratum corneum of patients with atopic dermatitis. J Lipid Res 2003; 44:93–102.

164. Ishibashi M, Arikawa J, Okamoto R, Kawashima M, Takagi Y, Ohguchi K, Imokawa G. Abnormal expression of the novel epidermal enzyme, glucosylceramide deacylase, and the accumulation of its enzymatic reaction product, glucosylsphingosine, in the skin of patients with atopic dermatitis. Lab Invest 2003; 83:397–408.

165. Higuchi K, Hara J, Okamoto R, Kawashima M, Imokawa G. The skin of atopic dermatitis patients contains a novel enzyme, glucosylceramide sphingomyelin deacylase, which cleaves the N-acyl linkage of sphingomyelin and glucosylceramide. Biochem J 2000; 350(Pt 3):747–756.

166. Arikawa J, Ishibashi M, Kawashima M, Takagi Y, Ichikawa Y, Imokawa G. Decreased levels of sphingosine, a natural antimicrobial agent, may be associated with vulnerability of the stratum corneum from patients with atopic dermatitis to colonization by Staphylococcus aureus. J Invest Dermatol 2002; 119:433–439.

167. Imokawa G, Takagi Y, Higuchi K, Kondo H, Yada Y. Sphingosylphosphorylcholine is a potent inducer of intercellular adhesion molecule-1 expression in human keratinocytes. J Invest Dermatol 1999; 112:91–96.

168. Higuchi K, Kawashima M, Takagi Y, Kondo H, Yada Y, Ichikawa Y, Imokawa G. Sphingosylphosphorylcholine is an activator of transglutaminase activity in human keratinocytes. J Lipid Res 2001; 42:1562–1570.

169. Macheleidt O, Kaiser HW, Sandhoff K. Deficiency of epidermal protein-bound omega-hydroxyceramides in atopic dermatitis. J Invest Dermatol 2002; 119:166–173.

170. Okino N, Ichinose S, Omori A, Imayama S, Nakamura T, Ito M. Molecular cloning, sequencing, and expression of the gene encoding alkaline ceramidase from Pseudomonas aeruginosa. Cloning of a ceramidase homologue from Mycobacterium tuberculosis. J Biol Chem 1999; 274:36616–36622.

171. Ohnishi Y, Okino N, Ito M, Imayama S. Ceramidase activity in bacterial skin flora as a possible cause of ceramide deficiency in atopic dermatitis. Clin Diagn Lab Immunol 1999; 6:101–104.

172. Okino N, Tani M, Imayama S, Ito M. Purification and characterization of a novel ceramidase from Pseudomonas aeruginosa. J Biol Chem 1998; 273:14368–14373.

173. Miller SJ, Aly R, Shinefeld HR, Elias PM. In vitro and in vivo antistaphylococcal activity of human stratum corneum lipids. Arch Dermatol 1988; 124:209–215.

174. Kusuda S, Cui CY, Takahashi M, Tezuka T. Localization of sphingomyelinase in lesional skin of atopic dermatitis patients. J Invest Dermatol 1998; 111:733–738.

175. Fartasch M, Diepgen TL. The barrier function in atopic dry skin. Disturbance of membrane-coating granule exocytosis and formation of epidermal lipids? Acta Derm Venereol Suppl 1992; 176:26–31.

176. Fartasch M. Epidermal barrier in disorders of the skin. Microsc Res Tech 1997; 38: 361–372.

177. Proksch E, Jensen JM, Elias PM. Skin lipids and epidermal differentiation in atopic dermatitis. Clin Dermatol 2003; 21:134–144.

178. Motta S, Monti M, Sesana S, Mellesi L, Ghidoni R, Caputo R. Abnormality of water barrier function in psoriasis. Role of ceramide fractions. Arch Dermatol 1994; 130: 452–456.

179. Mier PD, van den Hurk JJ. Acid hydrolases in psoriatic epidermis. Br J Dermatol 1976; 94:219–220.

180. Mier PD, van den Hurk JJ. Lysosomal hydrolases of the epidermis. 6. Changes in disease. Br J Dermatol 1976; 95:271–274.

181. Alessandrini F, Pfister S, Kremmer E, Gerber JK, Ring J, Behrendt H. Alterations of glucosylceramide-beta-glucosidase levels in the skin of patients with psoriasis vulgaris. J Invest Dermatol 2004; 123:1030–1036.

182. Alessandrini F, Stachowitz S, Ring J, Behrendt H. The level of prosaposin is decreased in the skin of patients with psoriasis vulgaris. J Invest Dermatol 2001; 116:394–400.

183. Ho MW, O'Brien JS. Gaucher's disease: deficiency of 'acid'-glucosidase and reconstitution of enzyme activity in vitro. Proc Natl Acad Sci USA 1971; 68:2810–2813.

184. Wilkening G, Linke T, Sandhoff K. Lysosomal degradation on vesicular membrane surfaces. Enhanced glucosylceramide degradation by lysosomal anionic lipids and activators. J Biol Chem 1998; 273:30271–30278.

185. Morimoto S, Martin BM, Kishimoto Y, O'Brien JS. Saposin D: a sphingomyelinase activator. Biochem Biophys Res Commun 1988; 156:403–410.

186. Tayama M, Soeda S, Kishimoto Y, Martin BM, Callahan JW, Hiraiwa M, O'Brien JS. Effect of saposins on acid sphingomyelinase. Biochem J 1993; 290(Pt 2):401–404.

187. Linke T, Wilkening G, Sadeghlar F, Mozcall H, Bernardo K, Schuchman E, Sandhoff K. Interfacial regulation of acid ceramidase activity. Stimulation of ceramide degradation by lysosomal lipids and sphingolipid activator proteins. J Biol Chem 2001; 276: 5760–5768.

188. Ghadially R, Brown BE, Hanley K, Reed JT, Feingold KR, Elias PM. Decreased epidermal lipid synthesis accounts for altered barrier function in aged mice. J Invest Dermatol 1996; 106:1064–1069.

189. Rogers J, Harding C, Mayo A, Banks J, Rawlings A. Stratum corneum lipids: the effect of ageing and the seasons. Arch Dermatol Res 1996; 288:765–770.

190. Denda M, Koyama J, Hori J, Horii I, Takahashi M, Hara M, Tagami H. Age-dependent and sex-dependent change in stratum corneum sphingolipids. Arch Dermatol Res 1993; 285:415–417.

191. Lightle SA, Oakley JI, Nikolova-Karakashian MN. Activation of sphingolipid turnover and chronic generation of ceramide and sphingosine in liver during aging. Mech Ageing Dev 2000; 120:111–125.

192. Venable ME, Lee JY, Smyth MJ, Bielawska A, Obeid LM. Role of ceramide in cellular senescence. J Biol Chem 1995; 270:30701–30708.

16

The Epidermal Lamellar Body as a Multifunctional Secretory Organelle

Peter M. Elias
Dermatology Service, VA Medical Center, and Department of Dermatology, University of California, San Francisco, California, U.S.A.

Kenneth R. Feingold
Department of Medicine and Dermatology, University of California, San Francisco, California, U.S.A.

Manigé Fartasch
Department of Dermatology, University of Erlanger, Federal Republic of Germany

LAMELLAR BODIES—SPECIES AND TISSUE DISTRIBUTION AS AN INDICATOR OF PERMEABILITY BARRIER FUNCTION

The epidermal lamellar body (LB) is an ovoid, $1/3 \times 1/4 \mu m$ membrane bilayer–encircled, secretory organelle that is unique to mammalian epidermis (Fig. 1), and some other keratinizing epithelia, including those of the hard palate, the esophagus, and the vagina (reviewed in Refs. 1,2). Their absence in certain other, specialized keratinizing epithelia (e.g., hair and nail), which minimally impede transcutaneous water loss (TEWL), underscores the central role of this organelle in permeability barrier homeostasis. Likewise, few or no LB are present in the severe disorder of cornification, Harlequin ichthyosis (3–6), with drastic consequences for permeability barrier homeostasis (7). Even when barrier requirements are minimal, as in marine cetaceans, pinnipeds, and oral/genital epithelia, abundant LBs continue to be present, though they display subtle differences in structure and composition that reflect requirements unique to a near-isotonic or fully hydrated environment [(7,8); see also Chap. 13]. Thus, based upon its species and tissue distribution alone, LB can be assumed to play a central role in permeability barrier homeostasis.

Functions Attributed to Lamellar Bodies

Early workers attributed a broad range of additional/alternative functions to this organelle, opinions that can now be either discarded or vindicated (Table 1). To some extent, these differing functions reflect the range of names attached to LB by their earlier students. Initial observers of LBs speculated that they were effete mitochondria,

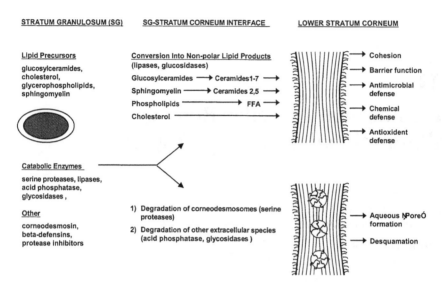

Figure 1 Lamellar body secretion delivers lipids, enzymes, antimicrobial peptides, and structural proteins that mediate multiple protective functions.

a view disputed initially by Odland (1), who suspected their physiologic importance (hence, LB are still often called Odland bodies in his honor). Because of their hydrolytic enzyme content, they also have been considered to be modified lysosomes—the term "keratinosome" reflects their putative role in hydrolytic events leading to desquamation (9,10). Yet, it is important to note that, despite possessing a selected array of hydrolytic enzymes (Table 2), LB lack certain classic lysosomal content markers, such as aryl sulfatase A/B and β-glucuronidase (11). Moreover, LB reportedly also lack classic lysosomal membrane markers, such as LAMP-1 (11,12). Instead, they appear to express markers of a secretory organelle, such as caveolin-1 (12).

Some early workers proposed that LB secrete materials, such as sugars, that coat the surface of corneocytes. Hence, the term "cementsome" has been applied to these organelles (13). Indeed, recent studies have shown that the ω-hydroxyceramides (Cer) that coat the external surface of corneocytes, forming the corneocyte lipid envelope (CLE), are initially glucosylated. Normally, these external-facing sugars are progressively removed within the lower SC by β-glucocerebrosidase, but when this enzyme is missing, as in Gaucher's disease, ω-OH-(and other extracellular) ceramides remain glucosylated at all levels of the SC (14).

Other early workers called these organelles "membrane coating granules," because of a putative relationship to the formation of the thickened cornified envelope (CE) (15). While this relationship does not match recent ultrastructural observations, it is interesting to note that LB secretes at least one CE protein precursor, the serine protease inhibitor, elafin (16).

Early workers focused neither on the potential roles of the LB in the permeability barrier, nor on its role as a pluri-functional organelle. Current preference for the term, "lamellar body," which does not attempt to restrict its functional attributes, is increasingly justified, because the number of functions linked to this organelle continue to increase (Table 2). Although the term "lamellar granule" is also occasionally used, it is less desirable, because LB are membrane-bound organelle, while intracellular "granules" typically are non-membrane-bound.

Table 1 Historical Overview of Terminology and Functional Attributes

Term	Attributed functions	Early evidence	Recent validation
Udland body	Udland refuted concept of LB as an effete mitochondrion	Distinctive internal structure	N/A
Cementsome	Cohesion	Saccharide staining of corneocyte surface	LB secrete corneodesmosin, a corneodesmosome structural protein that prevents premature desquamation
Keratinosome	Desquamation	Lysosomal enzyme contents	LB secrete lipases, proteases and glycosidases
Membrane coating granule	Cornification	Organelle contents lead to formation of cornified envelope (CE)	LB secrete SKALP (elafin), and cystatin M/E, CE precursor peptides, also important for desquamation
Lamellar body or "granule"	Barrier	Tracer blockade	Lipid contents destined for barrier function
	Hydration	Fusion of LB expands surface area: volume ratio	Fusion of LB generates CLE, which regulates water uptake into corneocyte
	Antimicrobial	FFA and GlcCer are antimicrobial	LB-derived sphingosine is also antimicrobial; secrete antimicrobial peptides (hBD2, LL-37)

Abbreviations: N/A, not applicable; CLE, corneocyte-bound lipid envelope; LB, lamellar body; FFA, free fatty acid.

The role of the LB in the permeability barrier was first suspected from ultrastructural studies, which demonstrated the blockade of outward percolation of tracers at the level of the outer stratum granulosum (17,18), at sites where secreted LB contents initially engorge the intercellular spaces (19). By freeze–fracture these lamellar body contents were then shown to transform into hydrophobic lipids, which re-deploy into a series of broad lamellar membrane structures within the interstices of the lower SC (3,19) (Fig. 1).

It is indeed fortunate that a generic, broadly encompassing term (i.e., lamellar body) is used for this organelle, because subsequent studies demonstrated that LB contain not only pro-barrier lipids and their respective lipid processing enzymes, but also an ever-expanding list of additional structural proteins, antimicrobial peptides, and proteases that participate in cohesion, desquamation, and antimicrobial

Table 2   Enzymatic Contents of Epidermal Lamellar Bodies[a]

Enzymes	Function
Lipid Hydrolases[a]	
β-Glucocerebrosidase[b]	Converts glucosylceramides into ceramides
Acidic sphingomyelinase	Converts sphingomyelin into ceramides
Secretory phospholipase A2 (Group I)[b]	Converts phospholipids into free fatty acids
Acidic neutral lipase activities	Deacylates ω-esterified ceramides
Proteases	
SC chymotryptic enzymes	Degrades corneodesmosomes; activates IL-1β
Cathepsins	Desquamation
Glycosidases	Desquamation
Acid Phosphatase	Substrate unknown
Protease inhibitors	
Serine protease inhibitors (e.g., SKALP)	Desquamation
Cysteine protease inhibitors (e.g., cytatin M/E)	Cytokine activation

[a]Recent studies suggest that an additional lipid hydrolase, steroid sulfatase, is also present.
[b]Mucosal epithelia and perhaps cetacean epidermis, display reduced β-glucocerebrosidase and secretory phospholipase activities.

function (Fig. 1). For example, LB secrete corneodesmosin (CNDS), an epidermis-unique protein that coats the external surface of corneodesmosomes, rendering them temporarily resistant to proteolysis (20). CNDS-mediated cohesion is an important contributor to SC integrity; i.e., its resistance to shearing forces, and it is only as CNDS and other CD proteins are hydrolyzed that desquamation can occur (Chap. 11).

At least one β-defensins, hBD2, has been shown to accumulate in LB (21), and there is preliminary evidence that the carboxy-terminal fragment of cathelicidin, LL-37, may also localize to LB. In the case of hBD2, a prior inflammatory signal, such as IL-1α stimulation, is required for translocation of pro-hBD2 to the LB in preparation for secretion (21). Accordingly, hBD2 has been further localized to membrane domains of the SC in inflammatory dermatoses where cytokine expression is enhanced (22).

Not only lipid hydrolases, but also certain other proteases, as well as protease inhibitors, important for both desquamation and cytokine activation, are delivered to the SC interstices by LB secretion (Table 2) (Fig. 1). Of these proteases,kallikrein (KIK) 7, the SC chymotryptic protease (SCCE) has been the most intensively studied (23). The secreted LB product, pro-SCCE, is activated by another serine protease, KIKS, the SC tryptic enzyme, and together, these serine proteases appear to initiate desquamation in the lower SC (24). The activities of SCCE and SCTE are opposed by a series of serine protease inhibitors (SPI), at least three of which, elafin (or SKALP), secretory leucocyte protease inhibitor (SLPS), and LEKTI, are also known LB products (16). Finally, desquamation almost certainly requires the activities of additional proteases that exhibit acidic pH optima (Chap. 11), and it is possible that one or both of the responsible aspartate and cyteine proteases, cathepsin D (25) and SC cysteine protease (SCCP) (26), respectively, could be LB products. Pertinently, the cysteine protease inhibitor, cystatin C/K, is also a known LB product (27), in whose genetic absence a severe scaling disorder results (the Harlequin mouse) (27). Finally, LB secretion is disturbed in several inflammatory and keratinizing disorders, such as atopic dermatitis (28) and the ichthyoses. Together, these results demonstrate the multiple roles of LB as delivery agents for several key SC protective functions (29).

REGULATION OF LAMELLAR BODY SECRETION

Kinetics of LB Secretion

In both rodents and humans, acute disruption of the permeability barrier by mechanical forces, solvents, or detergents increases TEWL, initiating a homeostatic repair response that results in the rapid recovery of permeability barrier function (Fig. 2). The first step in the repair response is rapid secretion (within minutes) of pre-formed LB contents from cells of the outer SG (Fig. 3), which leaves the cytosol of these cells largely devoid of LB (30,31). Newly secreted LB contents initially unfurl, in a hinge-like process (30,31). Then, the unfurled segments appear to line up in elongated, lamellar arrays between adjacent corneodesmosomes (32). The final transformation of these aligned lamellar arrays into the moisture-resistant, mature lamellar membrane structures that regulate barrier function, requires further enzymatic (lipid) processing of secreted LB contents (Chap. 15).

After the initial wave of secretion, newly formed LBs begin to reappear in SG cells by 30 to 60 minutes, and by 3 to 6 hours the number of LBs in SG cells has returned to normal (30,31). Because secretion and organellogenesis are accelerated at between 30 minutes and 6 hours, secreted LB contents progressively accumulate at the SG–SC interface. Yet, because lipid processing also accelerates, lipid-enriched lamellar bilayers rapidly re-appear in the lower SC; i.e., by 2 hours (30,31).

The lamellar membrane lipids in the SC derive primarily from the exocytosis of LB, which are enriched in cholesterol, glucosylceramide, phospholipids, and lipid

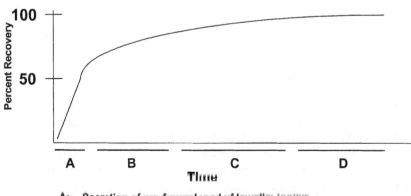

A: Osaration of pre-formed pool of lamellar bodies
B: Increased cholesterol/fatty acid synthesis
   Accelerated lamellar body formation/secretion
C: Increased ceramide synthesis
   Increased glucosylceramide processing
D: Increased DNA synthesis

Figure 2 Cutaneous stress test allows assessment of metabolic responses linked to barrier function.

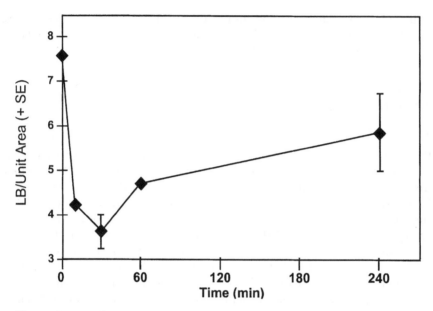

Figure 3 Lamellar body secretory response to acute barrier disruption. *Source*: Adapted from Ref. 31.

hydrolases enzymes (11) (Fig. 1). Thus, exocytosis of LB provides a pathway by which cells of the epidermis are able to deliver lipids and lipid-processing enzymes simultaneously to the extracellular spaces of the SC (33) (Chap. 15). Within the SC, the co-localized hydrolytic enzymes, including acid sphingomyelinase, β-glucocerebrosidase (β-GlcCer'ase), secretory phospholipase A_2 (sPLA$_2$), and steroid sulfatase (Chap. 28), catalyze the extracellular degradation of glucosylceramides and phospholipids (including sphingomyelin) to ceramides and FFA, respectively, thereby generating the key lipid products that form the mature lamellar membranes required for permeability barrier function (33). These morphological and biochemical changes, which are together termed "lipid processing," result in a parallel, progressive normalization of permeability barrier function (Fig. 2).

Regulation of LB Secretion

LB secretion is regulated by modulations in the epidermal Ca^{++} gradient. Under basal conditions, the high levels of extracellular Ca^{++} in the outer nucleated layers restrict LB secretion to low levels, still sufficient, however, to sustain basal barrier function (34,35). With acute barrier disruption, the Ca^{++} gradient is lost, and a wave of accelerated LB secretion occurs until the Ca^{++} gradient is restored (6–24 hour) (34). It has been shown that Ca^{++} levels, with an additional contribution of K^+, are the regulators of LB secretion, because exposure of acutely perturbed skin sites to a high Ca^{++}/K^+ solution inhibits LB secretion (36–38). Conversely, sonophoretic or iontophoretic displacement of Ca^{++} induces LB secretion, independent of changes in barrier function (35). Finally, LB secretion can also be blocked by pharmacologic blockade using inhibitors such as brefeldin A and monensin, further proof that exocytosis of these organelles is a regulated, secretory process (39,40).

The increase in SP activity that occurs after acute barrier disruption has adverse effects on permeability barrier homeostasis (55), which are reversible by

Table 3 Structural and Metabolic Adaptations of Secretory Granulocyte

Structural
Widely disbursed trans-Golgi network
Compound exocytosis of lamellar bodies
Apical invaginations of SG–SC interface
Metabolic
Accelerated synthesis of three key SC lipids
Accelerated formation and secretion of LB
Transient down-regulation of structural protein synthesis (metabolic conservation)
Synthesis of structural proteins is restricted to filaggrin, loricrin

topical application of SPI (55). Very recently, the negative effects of SP were shown to operate by down regulation of LB secretion.

Structural and Metabolic Adaptations that Facilitate LB Secretion

Structural Adaptations

LB secretion is largely restricted to the outermost SG cell under both basal (maintenance) conditions and after acute perturbations (10,31). Although these cells remain highly active, lipid-synthetic factories (Table 3), they also possess a highly keratinized cytosol and a partially formed cornified envelope (41). Certain structural features have evolved in these cells to facilitate the delivery of LB-derived lipid and enzyme contents to the SG–SC interface under basal conditions; these also allow amplified delivery of organelle contents after acute perturbations (31) (Table 3). These adaptations include: first, a widely disbursed, tubulo-reticular trans-Golgi network that extends throughout the apical cytosol (31), which generates nascent LB by "budding" and "consumption" of TGN mechanisms (Table 4). Second, these cells generate deep invaginations of the SG–SC interface, between adjacent corneodesmosomes (32), that form an extensive honeycomb/latticework, and are continuous with the intercellular domains (31).

Interestingly, Norlen (42,43) has interpreted these images of the invaginations and secreted LB contents quite differently. Norlen proposes that the invaginations reflect a non–energy-requiring, physico-chemical unfurling of lipids. The evidence against this model, however, is overwhelming: (i) high levels of extracellular Ca^{++} impede LB secretion (as mentioned above); (ii) metabolic inhibitors of LB formation block delivery of lipids to the SC (39,40); (iii) both LB formation and secretion are impaired at low temperatures (38,44); and (iv) chemical inhibitors of lipid synthesis block organellogenesis (45). Thus, the "unfolding" interpretation ignores a large body of evidence that has demonstrated that both LB assembly and secretion are regulated, energy-requiring processes.

Table 4 Characteristics of Lamellar Body (LB) Generation

LB are products of the trans-Golgi network (TGN)
LB form both by budding off and by consumption of TGN
LB accumulate enzyme proteins and lipids in parallel, but protein delivery is dependent on prior lipid deposition
Lipids (physiological only) can be delivered to LB from either endogenous or exogenous sources

The apical cytosol of the outermost SG cell is replete with columns of contiguous LB that undergo compound exocytosis (organelle-to-organelle, rather than solely organelle-to-plasma membrane fusion) following acute perturbations (31). In fact, following acute perturbations, the apical invaginations extend still deeper into the apical cytosol by the dual processes of accelerated fusion and compound exocytosis of LB. The apical invaginations form at the moment each subjacent SG cell moves into the outer SG; i.e., as the outermost SG cell begins to form a CE, thereby establishing portals to the intercellular space, potentially allowing initial CE formation to occur around the orifices of these invaginations (31) (Table 4). Finally, it is likely that the invaginations provide a potential starting point for endocytosis, allowing not only the uptake of topical lipids (39,40,46,47), but also the possibility of lipid recycling (Table 4).

Metabolic Adaptations

Whereas the epidermis is a highly active, lipid-synthetic capacity that is able to synthesize all three key classes of lipids (48), as described in chapter, SG cells can further up-regulate both lipid synthesis (49) and lamellar body secretion in response to barrier perturbation (30). More recently, we demonstrated an interesting anomaly—the SG cells retain the capacity to synthesize certain proteins in abundance (e.g., loricrin and filaggrin), but synthesis is transiently down-regulated in parallel with the loss of calcium that accompanies acute barrier disruption (50). Synthesis of these structural proteins is regulated by calcium at both a transcriptional and a post-transcriptional level (Chap. 18). The transient decline in protein synthesis may have an important teleological basis; i.e., it could allow temporary diversion of cellular energy towards lipid production (i.e., the response could be a form of metabolism conservation, as occurs, for example, in liver during the acute phase response) (50) (Table 3).

Together, these structural and metabolic modifications explain the ability of the outermost SG cell to function as a secretory cell, despite being both heavily keratinized and in possession of a partially developed CE (Tables 3 and 4). As a result of these observations, we have designated the outermost SG cell as the "secretory granulocyte" (31).

Table 5 Pathophysiology of the Lamellar Body Secretory System

Formation		Secretion		Post-secretory processing:
Increased	Decreased	Increased	Decreased	Decreased
Psoriasis	Harlequin ichthyosis	Psoriasis	Epidermolytic hyperkeratosis	Gaucher's disease
UV-B, x-irradiation	PAR-2 agonists	Barrier disruption	Atopic dermatitis	Niemann-Pick disease
Retinoid Rx	Glucocorticoid Rx	PAR-2 antagonists	Congenital ichthyosiform erythroderma	Netherton's syndrome
Barrier disruption	Aging	Netherton's syndrome		Psoriasis
Netherton's syndrome				Retinoid Rx

PATHOPHYSIOLOGY OF LAMELLAR BODY SECRETION

LB secretion can either increase or decrease in disease states, serving as an indicator of either an impending barrier recovery or a sustained defect, respectively (Table 5). Since LB secretion is amplified, as part of the barrier-repair response, it is not surprising that these organelles are produced in large numbers in skin disorders, where barrier function is impaired, as in psoriasis (51). High-dose UV-B and X-irradiation provoke an initial wave of apoptosis, which produces a transient barrier abnormality, as secretion-incompetent, apoptotic cells pass through the SG layers (52,53). Then, a hyperplastic response in the lower nucleated layers delivers an excess number of LB to the SG, guaranteeing that the barrier abnormality will be short-lived. In Nethertons syndrome, despite accelerated formation and secretion of LB contents, barrier function never normalizes, presumably reflecting accelerated degradation of organelle contacts (54) Yet, the accelerated secretion may be life-saving in NS, by providing a partial barrier within the nucleated layers of the epidermis (57).

Conversely, due to a variety of unrelated mechanisms, LB production may be inappropriately decreased (Table 5). In Harlequin ichthyosis decreased ABCA12 expression results not only in reduced lipid delivery to LB, but also in abnormal delivery of enzymes to the SC extracellular spaces. The result is two-fold, i.e., both an often profound barrier abnormality and a delay in desquamation; manifesting as excess scale (Chap. 27). Harlequin ichthyosis is the most devastating example of this dual outcome (8). Finally, there are other diseases where LB secretion is impeded. Impaired secretion in the face of normal lamellar body formation can be assessed by the extent to which lamellar body proteins are delivered to the SC interstices (29). For example, the cytoskeletal abnormality in epidermolytic hyperkeratosis interferes with LB secretion. Moreover, the global deficiency in SC lipids in atopic dermatitis may also be due to a failure of lamellar body extrusion (28), although the structural/enzymatic basis for impaired secretion in AD is not known.

REFERENCES

1. Odland G, Reed T. Epidermis. In: Zelickson A, ed. Ultrastructure of Normal and Abnormal Skin. Philadelphia: Lea & Febiger, 1967:54–75.
2. Odland GF, Holbrook K. The lamellar granules of epidermis. Curr Probl Dermatol 1981; 9:29–49.
3. Elias PM, Goerke J, Friend DS. Mammalian epidermal barrier layer lipids: composition and influence on structure. J Invest Dermatol 1977; 69:535–546.
4. Elias PM, Fritsch P, Epstein EH. Staphylococcal scalded skin syndrome. Clinical features, pathogenesis, and recent microbiological and biochemical developments. Arch Dermatol 1977; 113:207–219
5. Dale BA, Holbrook KA, Fleckman P, Kimball JR, Brumbaugh S, Sybert VP. Heterogeneity in harlequin ichthyosis, an inborn error of epidermal keratinization: variable morphology and structural protein expression and a defect in lamellar granules. J Invest Dermatol 1990; 94:6–18.
6. Milner ME, O'Guin WM, Holbrook KA, Dale BA. Abnormal lamellar granules in harlequin ichthyosis. J Invest Dermatol 1992; 99:824–829.
7. Moskowitz DG, Fowler AJ, Heyman MB, Cohen SP, Crumrine D, Elias PMML, Williams . Pathophysiological basis for growth failure in children with ichthyosis: an evalua-

tion of cutaneous ultrastructure, epidermal permeability barrier function, and energy expenditure. J Pediatr 2004; 145:82–92.

8. Elias PM, Fartasch M, Crumrine D, Behne M, Uchida Y, Holleran WM. Origin of the corneocyte lipid envelope (CLE): observations in harlequin ichthyosis and cultured human keratinocytes. J Invest Dermatol 2000; 115:765–769.

9. Wolff K, Holubar K. Keratinosomes as epidermal lysosomes. Arch Klin Exp Dermatol 1967; 231:1–19.

10. Weinstock M, Wilgram GF. Fine-structural observations on the formation and enzymatic activity of keratinosomes in mouse tongue filiform papillae. J Ultrastruct Res 1970; 30:262–274.

11. Grayson S, Johnson-Winegar AG, Wintroub BU, Isseroff RR, Epstein EH Jr, Elias PM. Lamellar body-enriched fractions from neonatal mice: preparative techniques and partial characterization. J Invest Dermatol 1985; 85:289–294.

12. Madison KC. Barrier function of the skin: "la raison d'etre" of the epidermis. J Invest Dermatol 2003; 121:231–241.

13. Hashimoto K. Intercellular spaces of the human epidermis as demonstrated with lanthanum. J Invest Dermatol 1971; 57:17–31.

14. Doering T, Holleran WM, Potratz A, Vielhaber G, Elias PM, Suzuki K, Sandhoff K. Sphingolipid activator proteins are required for epidermal permeability barrier formation. J Biol Chem 1999; 274:11038–11045.

15. Matoltsy AF, Papakkal P. Keratinization. In: Zelickson AS, ed. Ultrastructure of Normal and Abnormal Skin. Philadelphia: Lea & Febiger, 1967:76–104.

16. Nakane H, Ishida-Yamamoto A, Takahashi H, Iizuka H. Elafin, a secretory protein, is cross-linked into the cornified cell envelopes from the inside of psoriatic keratinocytes. J Invest Dermatol 2002; 119:50–55.

17. Schreiner E, Wolff K. The permeability of the intercellular space of the epidermis for low molecular weight protein. Electron microscopic cytochemical studies with peroxidase as a tracer substance. Arch Klin Exp Dermatol 1969; 235:78–88.

18. Squier CA. The permeability of keratinized and nonkeratinized oral epithelium to horseradish peroxidase. J Ultrastruct Res 1973; 43:160–177.

19. Elias PM, Friend DS. The permeability barrier in mammalian epidermis. J Cell Biol 1975; 65:180–191.

20. Serre G, Mils V, Haftek M, Vincent C, Croute F, Reano A, Ouhayoun JP, Bettinger S, Soleilhavoup JP. Identification of late differentiation antigens of human cornified epithelia, expressed in re-organized desmosomes and bound to cross-linked envelope. J Invest Dermatol 1991; 97:1061–1072.

21. Oren A, Ganz T, Liu L, Meerloo T. In human epidermis, beta-defensin 2 is packaged in lamellar bodies. Exp Mol Pathol 2003; 74:180–182.

22. Huh WK, Oono T, Shirafuji Y, Akiyama H, Arata J, Sakaguchi M, Huh NH, Iwatsuki K. Dynamic alteration of human beta-defensin 2 localization from cytoplasm to intercellular space in psoriatic skin. J Mol Med 2002; 80:678–684.

23. Lundstrom A, Egelrud T. Stratum corneum chymotryptic enzyme: a proteinase which may be generally present in the stratum corneum and with a possible involvement in desquamation. Acta Derm Venereol 1991; 71:471–474.

24. Ekholm IE, Brattsand M, Egelrud T. Stratum corneum tryptic enzyme in normal epidermis: a missing link in the desquamation process? J Invest Dermatol 2000; 114:56–63.

25. Horikoshi T, Igarashi S, Uchiwa H, Brysk H, Brysk MM. Role of endogenous cathepsin D-like and chymotrypsin-like proteolysis in human epidermal desquamation. Br J Dermatol 1999; 141:453–459.

26. Bernard D, Mehul B, Thomas-Collignon A, Simonetti L, Remy V, Bernard MA, Schmidt R. Analysis of proteins with caseinolytic activity in a human stratum corneum extract revealed a yet unidentified cysteine protease and identified the so-called "stratum corneum thiol protease" as cathepsin l2. J Invest Dermatol 2003; 120:592–600.

27. Zeeuwen PL, Dale BA, de Jongh GJ, van Vlijmen-Willems IM, Fleckman P, Kimball JR, Stephens K, Schalkwijk J. The human cystatin M/E gene (CST6): exclusion candidate gene for harlequin ichthyosis. J Invest Dermatol 2003; 121:65–68.

28. Fartasch M, Bassukas ID, Diepgen TL. Disturbed extruding mechanism of lamellar bodies in dry non-eczematous skin of atopics. Br J Dermatol 1992; 127:221 227.

29. Menon GK, Ghadially R, Williams ML, Elias PM. Lamellar bodies as delivery systems of hydrolytic enzymes: implications for normal and abnormal desquamation. Br J Dermatol 1992; 126:337–345.

30. Menon GK, Feingold KR, Elias PM. Lamellar body secretory response to barrier disruption. J Invest Dermatol 1992; 98:279–289.

31. Elias PM, Cullander C, Mauro T, Rassner U, Komuves L, Brown BE, Menon GK. The secretory granular cell: the outermost granular cell as a specialized secretory cell. J Invest Dermatol Symp Proc 1998; 3:87–100.

32. Fartasch M, Bassukas ID, Diepgen TL. Structural relationship between epidermal lipid lamellae, lamellar bodies and desmosomes in human epidermis: an ultrastructural study. Br J Dermatol 1993; 128:1–9.

33. Elias PM, Menon GK. Structural and lipid biochemical correlates of the epidermal permeability barrier. Adv Lipid Res 1991; 24:1–26.

34. Menon GK, Elias PM, Lee SH, Feingold KR. Localization of calcium in murine epidermis following disruption and repair of the permeability barrier. Cell Tissue Res 1992; 270:503–512.

35. Menon GK, Elias PM, Feingold KR. Integrity of the permeability barrier is crucial for maintenance of the epidermal calcium gradient. Br J Dermatol 1994; 130:139–147.

36. Lee SH, Elias PM, Proksch E, Menon GK, Mao-Quiang M, Feingold KR. Calcium and potassium are important regulators of barrier homeostasis in murine epidermis. J Clin Invest 1992; 89:530–538.

37. Lee SH, Elias PM, Feingold KR, Mauro T. A role for ions in barrier recovery after acute perturbation. J Invest Dermatol 1994; 102:976–979.

38. Elias P, Ahn S, Brown B, Crumrine D, Feingold KR. Origin of the epidermal calcium gradient: regulation by barrier status and role of active vs. passive mechanisms. J Invest Dermatol 2002; 119:1269–1274.

39. Mao-Qiang M, Feingold KR, Jain M, Elias PM. Extracellular processing of phospholipids is required for permeability barrier homeostasis. J Lipid Res 1995; 36: 1925–1935.

40. Mao-Qiang M, Brown Be, Wu-Pong S, Feingold KR, Elias PM. Exogenous nonphysiologic vs. physiologic lipids. Diverfent mechanisms for correction of permeability barrier dysfunction. Arch Dermatol 1995; 131:809–816.

41. Steinert PM, Marekov LN. Direct evidence that involuerin is a major early isopeptide cross-linked component of the keratinocyte cornified envelope. J Biol Chem 1997; 17: 2021–2030.

42. Norlen L. Skin barrier formation: the single gel phase model. J Invest Dermatol 2001; 117:830–836.

43. Norlen L. Skin barrier formation: the membrane folding model. J Invest Dermatol 2001; 117:823–829.

44. Halkier-Sorensen L, Menon GK, Elias PM, Thestrup-Pedersen K, Feingold KR. Cutaneous barrier function after cold exposure in hairless mice: a model to demonstrate how cold interferes with barrier homeostasis among workers in the fish-processing industry. Br J Dermatol 1995; 132:391–401.

45. Feingold KR. The regulation and role of epidermal lipid synthesis. Adv Lipid Res 1991; 24:57–82.

46. Mao-Qiang M, Feingold KR, Elias PM. Inhibition of cholesterol and sphingolipid synthesis causes paradoxical effects on permeability barrier homeostasis. J Invest Dermatol 1993; 101:185–190.

47. Mao-Qiang M, Elias PM, Feingold KR. Fatty acids are required for epidermal permeability barrier function. J Clin Invest 1993; 92:791–798.
48. Monger DJ, Williams ML, Feingold KR, Brown BE, Elias PM. Localization of sites of lipid biosynthesis in mammalian epidermis. J Lipid Res 1988; 29:603–612.
49. Proksch E, Elias PM, Feingold KR. Localization and regulation of epidermal 3-hydroxy-3-methylglutaryl-coenzyme A reductase activity by barrier requirements. Biochim Biophys Acta 1991; 1083:71–79.
50. Elias PM, Ahn SK, Denda M, Brown BE, Crumrine D, Kimutai LK, Komuves L, Lee SH, Feingold KR. Modulations in epidermal calcium regulate the expression of differentiation-specific markers. J Invest Dermatol 2002; 119:1128–1136.
51. Ghadially R, Reed JT, Elias PM. Stratum corneum structure and function correlates with phenotype in psoriasis. J Invest Dermatol 1996; 107:558–564.
52. Holleran WM, Uchida Y, Halkier-Sorensen L, Haratake A, Hara M, Epstein JH, Elias PM. Structural and biochemical basis for the UVB-induced alterations in epidermal barrier function. Photodermatol Photoimmunol Photomed 1997; 13:117–128.
53. Schmuth M, Sztankay A, Weinlich G, Linder DM, Wimmer MA, Fritsch PO, Fritsch E. Barrier function in skin exposed to ionizing radiation. Arch Dermatol 2001; 137: 1019–1023.
54. Fartasch M, Williams ML, Elias PM. Altered lamellar body secretion and stratum corneum membrane structure in Netherton syndrome: differentiation from other infantile erythrodermas and pathogenic implications. Arch Dermatol 1999; 135:823–832.

17

Skin Structural Development

Mathew J. Hardman
School of Biological Sciences, University of Manchester, Manchester, U.K.

Carolyn Byrne
Queen Mary School of Medicine and Dentistry, University of London, London, U.K.

INTRODUCTION

The structural development of human skin has been intensely studied and documented, first at the light microscopy level, then at the electron microscopy level (reviewed). These early observations have now been correlated with molecular localization data, primarily using immunohistochemical techniques. The outcome has been an extremely well-defined analysis of the structural development of the human skin, which underpins the analysis of cutaneous disease. This structural framework can be used to incorporate the flood of new data from genome projects, expression analyses using microarrays, and an abundance of functional data from animal models.

At present there is heavy reliance on the mouse model for the analysis of skin development, because it can be genetically manipulated and because of restrictions on access to human fetal material. Important goals in human skin development research are to identify new structural and molecular markers, and to use existing markers to compare precisely developing human and mouse skin (both temporally and regionally) so that murine data can be evaluated in the human skin. Further development and authentication of human embryonic/fetal experimental culture models will serve the unique needs of the human structural developmental biologists, both experimentally and as a source of material for an analysis of the human skin cells' transcriptome and proteome.

The aims of this chapter are to (i) summarize the very large body of data on human skin structural development, (ii) compare these data to the structural development in the mouse, and (iii) highlight the areas of human skin development where questions are raised or which remain unexplored, usually in the light of data from animal experimental models.

DEVELOPMENT OF HUMAN SKIN

Development of the skin involves the juxtaposition of tissues from mainly mesodermal/neural crest (body dermis/head dermis) and ectodermal (epidermal) origin. Experimental work on animals and human culture model shows that an interaction between the two tissues is necessary for differentiation of the epidermis to form the protective barrier residing in the stratum corneum, and formation of the skin appendages—hair follicles, glands and nails. The structure of adult human skin is shown in Figure 1.

A single-layered epithelium covers the human embryo from gastrulation and a cuboidal ectoderm overlying an undifferentiated mesenchyme is recorded by 5 weeks of development (2). Subsequent skin development has been classified according to

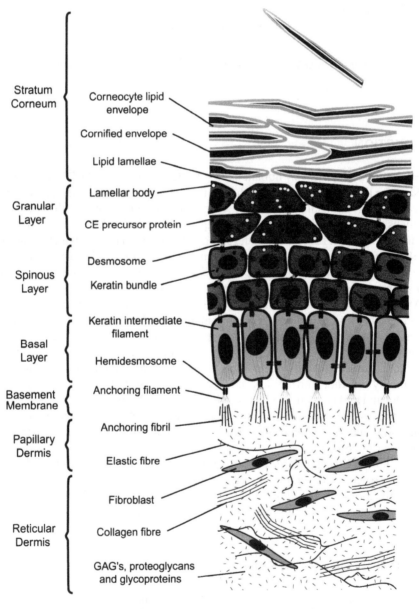

Figure 1   The structure of adult skin. Skin is composed of three separate layers, dermis, basement membrane, and epidermis. The epidermis can be subdivided into four further strata, each representing a specific stage during terminal differentiation.

embryonic/fetal developmental stages and these stages are extremely well defined and described (reviewed in Ref. 1) (Table 1; Fig. 2). These stages comprise:

    i.   the embryonic period (5 8 weeks),
    ii. the embryonic/fetal transition period (9–10 weeks),
    iii. the early fetal period (11–14 weeks),
    iv. the mid-fetal period (15–20 weeks), and
    v. the late fetal period (20 weeks to birth).

It is during the late fetal period that skin becomes functional—i.e., develops a protective barrier residing in the stratum corneum. Maturation of the stratum corneum is important for the health of the preterm infant and it is expected that, as morbidity and mortality rates of preterm infants fall due to improvements in the treatment for lung immaturity, the status of the preterm infant skin will become more of an issue in the treatment of the premature infant. A long-term goal in this field will be to develop an understanding of skin maturation sufficient to allow a pharmacologic manipulation of barrier function as currently now practiced for the augmentation of preterm lung function.

Several authors have globally assessed human skin development using parameters such as epidermal height (3) and proliferative activity (4,5). These data permit an interesting correlation of skin activity with fetal growth and environmental change. For example, a major increase in epidermal thickness is reported during weeks 5–13 (3), the period of organogenesis when rates of fetal size growth are slow (6). In contrast, epidermal height remains essentially unchanged during weeks 14–21 when there is a substantial increase in the size and skin surface area of the fetus, despite an increase in cell layers during this period (3). This period is marked by a decrease in the proliferative activity of epidermal cells (5). Foster and Holbrook (1988) propose that the increase in surface area is achieved substantially by a change in keratinocyte size and shape during this period.

The period of fetal growth deceleration (weeks 22–40) (6) correlates with a rigid stratum corneum formation (7,8). From this point, expansion of the skin is restricted due to reduced ability of the stratum corneum to expand horizontally. Subsequent horizontal growth must originate via a basal layer expansion and upward migration. It is possible that the requirement for rapid surface area increase precludes the stratum corneum formation during earlier development.

It is tempting to speculate as to why the barrier forms so early in the human skin, even though this inhibits subsequent epidermal expansion. During mouse, rat, and rabbit fetal development stratum corneum formation is delayed until several days before birth (9). One interesting theory is that the skin barrier activity is necessary during early human fetal development for protection from increasing levels of urine in amniotic fluid (10).

PERIDERM—THE EMBRYONIC SKIN LAYER OF UNKNOWN FUNCTION

The periderm is a transient epidermal layer that forms during the embryonic period (7,11) and is shed before birth, in conjunction with stratum corneum formation. The role of periderm is unknown since mutants lacking periderm have not been identified. However, periderm forms an interface between the embryo and amniotic fluid and during much of the gestational period, its morphology (surface microvilli and "bleb" -like protrusions which increase surface area; Table 1; Fig. 2) suggests an

Table 1 Stages of Human Skin Development with Mouse Comparisons

Stage	Human skin development		Mouse skin development	
	EGA (weeks)	Characteristics[a]	EGA (days)[b]	Characteristics[c]
Embryonic	5–8	Two-layered epidermis (basal layer and periderm)	8–11	Regional stratification to produce periderm
Embryonic/fetal transition	9–10	i) Formation of an epidermal intermediate laye xr	12–14	Hair germ formation, stratification to form intermediate layer
		ii) Induction of differentiation specific keratins (K1 andK10) in supra basal epidermal cells	14–15	Induction of differentiation-specific keratins (K1 and K10)
		iii) Dermal development		
Early fetal	11–14	Epidermal terminal differentiation, periderm forms surface "blebs"	15–16	Epidermal terminal differentiation
Mid fetal	15–20	Epidermal terminal differentiation, periderm regression		
Late fetal	20–40	Stratum corneum formation, barrier function, periderm disaggregation	16	Stratum corneum formation, barrier function
			17	Periderm disaggregation
	40	Birth	20	Birth

Abbreviations: EGA, estimated gestational age.

[a]From Refs. 11,13,25,39.

[b]Murine estimated gestational age or time since detection of the vaginal plug (day 0.5).

[c]From Refs. 20,35,76,77.

interactive role with amniotic fluid. This has led to speculation that periderm nourishes the underlying ectoderm prior to vascularization, or has an excretory role (11–13). Communication between the periderm and underlying keratinocytes is indicated by a clustering of connexins and gap junction proteins on borders between periderm and underlying cells (14). A role as an embryonic barrier is also probable and supported by the finding that the periderm cells are sealed by tight junctions (15,16).

During much of development the periderm cells express keratins normally associated with stressed or migratory epidermal cells (keratins 6/16/17) (17). In mice, migration and displacement of periderm cells is important in tissue fusions such as eyelid closure, thought to be analogous to the migration of keratin 6/16/17-positive epidermal cells during wound healing (18). The increased migratory/displacement capacity of the surface periderm cells may be important for major epidermal expansions and rearrangements during human development.

The periderm forms when the surface ectodermal cells are still single layered and undergoes a series of defined changes prior to regression and disaggregation (11,13) (Fig. 2). Initially, periderm cells proliferate, then later withdraw from the cell cycle, flatten, and increase in surface area. The cells are covered in microvilli, but, in addition, develop surface blebs or protusions, which later crenulate (13) (Fig. 2). These latter changes result in a further increase of surface area, fuelling speculation that the cells interact with the amniotic fluid (13). Finally, the periderm cells regress, a process involving nuclear degradation and subsequent disaggregation from the fetal surface, in conjunction with keratinization (13) (Fig. 2) (see below).

Embryonic Period (Post Gastrulation Embryo to 8 Weeks)

During the embryonic period the epidermis becomes two cell–layered, consisting of a proliferative basal layer and an outer surface of proliferative periderm cells. Epidermal keratinocytes express keratins characteristic of simple epithelia [keratins 8, 18, and 19 (19)]. Stratification could result due to a cell migration from the basal layer or basal cell division. However, stratification is difficult to observe and analyze in human embryos since it occurs early [embryos as early as 36 days EGA have already stratified to form the periderm layer (13)]. In contrast, periderm induction can easily be observed between 9 and 11 days in the mouse embryos (Table 1) where periderm formation is highly regional (20).

During the early embryonic period there is no appreciable dermis and no distinction between dermis and the underlying mesenchyme. The morphological development of human dermis has been thoroughly analyzed and reviewed by Smith et al. (1986) (21). These authors use morphological criteria to divide dermal development during the embryonic period into two stages. Initially, the subepidermal surface is cellular and devoid of detectable fibrous material. The second stage, beginning at two months, is associated with the definition of the dermal–subdermal boundary by vascular development (21).

During these early cellular stages of dermal development, deposition of protein at the basal lamina separating the epidermis and dermis, can be detected. Type IV collagen and laminin are present by 5 weeks (22,23) indicating the maturation of the basal lamina to a basement membrane. However, there are no hemidesmosomes i.e., the structures that anchor the keratinocytes to the basement membrane. The first traces of anchoring fibrils (type VII collagen fibrils which anchor the epidermis to the dermis) (Fig. 1) appear at 7–8 weeks (24).

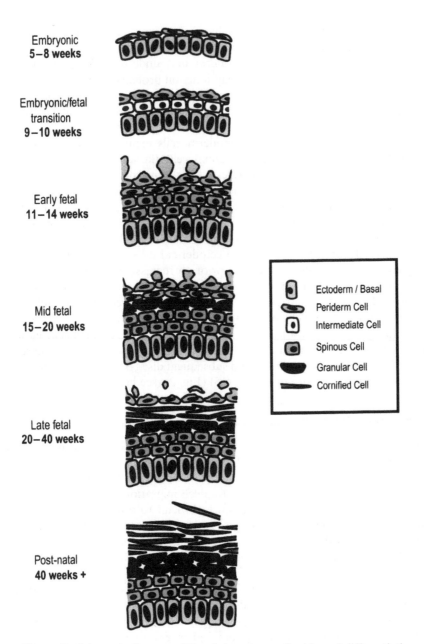

Figure 2 Schematic diagram of the six key stages of epidermal differentiation and periderm development. Epidermis develops from a single layer of undifferentiated ectoderm (5–8 weeks) to a multilayered stratified differentiated epithelia (40 weeks). Onset of terminal differentiation (the process where cells enter a defined programme of events culminating in formation of a functional stratum corneum) is triggered during the embryonic–fetal transition. In tandem, the periderm undergoes intense proliferation (11–14 weeks) and forms characteristic blebs and microvilli, thought to be functionally important. This is followed by regression and eventualy disaggregation (20–40 weeks). *Source*: Adapted from Ref. 44.

Embryonic Fetal Transition (9–10 Weeks, 60–70 Days)

The embryonic–fetal transition period in humans was first described on the basis of major morphological and biochemical change (25,26). This period is significant during the epidermal development in molecular terms, and signifies a switch in developmental programmes to enter terminal differentiation. Terminal differentiation initiated here will eventually result in the formation of the protective stratum corneum.

Embryonic ectoderm stratifies to form an intermediate layer at approximately 60 days EGA (25), followed by the induction of keratins associated with differentiating keratinocytes (keratin 1 and keratin 10) (26,27). The intermediate layer is initially proliferative (5) and fundamentally dissimilar to the adult suprabasal keratinoctyes.

During the embryonic–fetal transition period there is an associated maturation of the epidermal–dermal junction and an accelerated deposition of fibrous material and matrix in the dermis. (21,23,24). Anchoring filaments become more abundant (24) and hemidesmosomes are now detected (24,28) as well.

Hemidesmosomal integrin receptors, alpha 6 and beta 4 (Fig. 1), have been peri-cellularly expressed, but following stratification, are associated with hemidesmosomes at the basement membrane (28). Other epidermal adhesive structures, the desmosome and adherens junction, connect keratinocytes with each other and are located laterally and apically at sites of cell–cell contacts in the mature keratinocytes (Fig. 1). Before the embryonic–fetal transition, the protein components of desmosomes and adherens Junctions are also located peri-cellularly (29). Relocation of the proteins to cell–cell contacts on the lateral and apical membranes accompanies the embryonic–fetal transition, and it has been proposed that a polarization of basal keratinocytes into apical and basal compartments awaits the maturation of the basement membrane (29).

During the embryonic–fetal transition period non-keratinocyte epidermal cells are detected (24). Epidermal melanocytes are derived from the dorsal neural crest cells and migrate into the epidermis, and then later in to the hair follicles. Melanocytes are reported during the embryonic–fetal transition period (24) [though have been detected earlier (13)], as are the Langerhan cells (epidermal antigen–presenting/dendritic cells) that migrate to the skin from the fetal thymus and/or bone marrow.

An additional non-keratinocyte cell of the epidermis is the Merkel cell. Merkel cells are neurosecretory cells of the epidermal basal layer and the dermis. They function as mechanoreceptors, enclosing the endings of slowly adapting type 1 afferent fibres [reviewed (30)]. The origin of Merkel cells (epidermal or neural crest) was for many years the subject of debate, with the epidermal origin hypothesis being now generally accepted, due to the identification of keratins and desmosomes in Merkel cells [keratin 20 can distinguish epidermal Merkel cells from keratinocytes (31)] and developmental studies showing that Merkel cells appear first in the epidermis during development, and are then later detected in the dermis (31,32). Merkel cells have been detected as early as week eight of human development (33,34).

The murine equivalent of the human embryonic–fetal transition occurs over 2–3 developmental days (Table 1) with strong similarities to the transition that occurs in human development. Murine epidermis undergoes similar stratification to form a proliferative, intermediate layer that still expresses the basal cell–specific keratins at embryonic day 14, again indicating that this intermediate layer differs from a true spinous cell (20). Stratification in the mouse is achieved through cell division rather than migration (35). The expression of differentiation-specific keratins is delayed until embryonic day 15 (20,36) (Table 1). Stratification and keratin induction are highly regional in the mouse embryo, and a similar regional stratification has been reported in the human infant (11), complicating the comparison of data from different studies.

The human embryonic–fetal transition period may be modelled by the induction of keratinocyte terminal differentiation during the culture of isolated adult skin keratinocytes, either through calcium induction or serum withdrawal, with the caveat that the intrinsic differentiation properties of fetal keratinocytes can differ from those of the adult (37). Regulation of keratinocyte terminal differentiation is an area of very intense interest [reviewed (38,39)] and molecular signalling pathways identified in the adult keratinocyte culture models have been shown to be relevant to the early differentiation changes in the mouse (37), and are probably relevant to the embryonic–fetal transition in humans.

Early Fetal Period (11–14 Weeks, 70–100 Days)

During the early fetal period keratinocytes terminally differentiate, with the intermediate layer converting into a true spinous layer. The most conspicuous feature of the early fetal period in humans is the appearance of the germ cells of the hair at 12 weeks, reported to occur in a cephalocaudal direction (40,41).

The mouse does not provide an ideal model for either the early or the late fetal period, both of which are extended in the human and truncated in the mouse (Table 1). In addition, murine follicle development, which closely resembles human follicle development [reviewed (42)], occurs relatively earlier (Table 1), demonstrating that follicular development can be uncoupled from interfollicular development in mammals. However, the uncoupling has developmental consequences later (see below, stratum corneum formation).

Gap junction communication between the periderm cells and underlying keratinocytes is still indicated by connexion 26 clustering at cell–cell borders (14). Connexin 26 is usually associated with a hyperproliferative epidermis, or with cells undergoing a rapid growth. Intriguingly, the connexin 26 expression soon disappears from the skin, indicating the distinctive fetal nature of periderm and the underlying intermediate layer. Connexin 43, associated with the adult suprabasal keratinocyte gap junctions, now appears at the cell–cell borders of the intermediate cells (14), displaying an adoption of the characteristics of a true suprabasal layer.

At the epidermal-dermal junction.

There are abundant hemidesmosomes and anchoring fibrils (23). The density of cell–cell junctional complexes (desmosomes, adherens junctions and gap junctions) increases (29). This is a period of dermal maturation marked by an increasing fibrous and matrix deposition by the dermal cells (23), and at the end of this period (100 days) adipocytes are present in the dermis (43).

Mid Fetal Period (15–20 Weeks)

The mid-fetal period is marked by an increased epidermal stratification and a further maturation of hair follicles and additional appendages such as sweat glands and nails. Again, this period is truncated in the mouse. During the lengthy early and mid-fetal periods in humans, periderm morphological changes are one of the most noticeable changes occurring in the human skin (13), (Table 1; Fig. 2).

The epidermis has a true spinous layer rather than an embryonic intermediate layer and a granular layer (Fig. 2). At about 18 weeks the first sign of stratum corneum can be detected in the head region associated with the more mature hair follicles of the head (40,41). Stratum corneum formation is also accelerated over the nail bed, another type of epidermal appendage (44). Association of keratinization with hair follicle development does not occur in the mouse, except when hair follicle development is precocious, such as in the murine whisker pad and in association with nails (8). This presumably reflects the relatively late development of body hair in the mouse.

Late Fetal Period (20–40 Weeks)

Stratum Corneum Formation (Keratinization)

Human stratum corneum forms between 20 and 24 weeks (8,13,44). Stratum corneum formation is regional, being accelerated in the scalp, face, and plantar epidermis of the foot (sole region) (44). Association of keratinization with hair follicles in humans means that there is a regional acceleration of stratum corneum formation in association with the accelerated hair follicle formation of the head (40).

In the mouse (and additional mammals), stratum corneum formation is not linked with hair follicle formation, due to the relatively late development of follicles (8). A new type of regional stratum corneum development occurs, associated with skin initiation regions and apparent moving fronts of epidermal terminal differentiation (9). This type of regional stratum corneum formation is conserved in the human fetus (Fig. 2), although the pattern is complicated by follicle-associated keratinization.

A useful model of stratum corneum structure, the "bricks and mortar" model was proposed by Elias in 1983 [(45), reviewed 46]. The "bricks" represent flattened anucleate corneocytes (the results of keratinocyte terminal differentiation) with a 15 nm thick cornified envelope and an outer ceramide capsule or corneocyte lipid envelope [reviewed (47); Chap. 7], while the "mortar" consists of a heterogeneous mixture of predominantly non-polar lipids, arranged to form a complex lamellar bilayer structure [reviewed (48); Chap. 8]. The high degree of interdigitation and sheet-like non-polar intercellular lipid make the mature stratum corneum virtually impenetrable to water molecules and presumably confers much of the barrier qualities of the stratum corneum.

Stratum corneum is formed from multiple precursor proteins synthesized from week 18 onwards. In the mouse, key cornified envelope precursors are initially sequestered in keratohyalin granules (49), although these structures are far less prominent and significantly smaller in the human epidermis (50). In humans, most precursors are diffusely expressed throughout the cell (Fig. 1). Cornified envelope construction is initiated adjacent to the plasma membrane and involves sequential transglutaminase-mediated crosslinking of protein and lipid components. Transglutaminase activity is first detected in interfollicular non-periderm keratinocytes during the late fetal period (51).

The precise timing and sequence of envelope precursor incorporation has been the subject of intense study over recent years, mostly using murine and human keratinocyte culture models [reviewed in Ref. 52; Chap. 9]. The strong conservation between models suggests that the results are applicable to the fetal human. Briefly, as intercellular calcium levels rise, envelope scaffold proteins (envoplakin, periplakin and involucrin) move to the plasma membrane and are cross-linked via a membrane-bound transglutaminase 1 enzyme. These and other minor proteins form the initial envelope scaffold, a continuous cross-linked layer. In tandem with the initial scaffold formation, cross-bridging proteins (e.g., small proline-rich region proteins) in the cytoplasm become cross-linked by the cytoplasmically localized transglutaminase 3 enzyme to from small oligomers. These subsequently bind the cornified envelope precursor molecules (such as loricrin) and are incorporated into the envelope. Relatively late in envelope formation, the keratinocyte matrix protein, filaggrin, is proteolytically processed, binds keratin filaments internally, and attaches to the envelope surface (51) and further cross-linking proteins may bind and confer subtle changes to barrier properties (54).

In parallel with cornified envelope formation, extrusion of extracellular lipids and deposition of a lipid-bound envelope are key steps in stratum corneum formation. These lipids derive from abundant lamellar bodies synthesized in the early granular layer keratinocytes. The contents of lamellar bodies, non-polar lipids and lipid processing enzymes, are extruded into the extracellular space (55) and re-arranged into the lamellar sheets characteristic of mature stratum corneum. The lipid capsule forms around the extracellular (or inner) surface of the mature cornified envelope. Once again transglutaminase1 cross-links the lipid capsule, a key step in forming a water-tight barrier (56,57).

Skin Barrier Formation (20–34 Weeks)

An assumption, based on early tape-stripping experiments, which removed a part or all of the stratum corneum followed by barrier activity assessment, has been that barrier activity resides in the stratum corneum (reviewed 46). This view is bolstered by gene knockout mice where the knockout of transglutaminase 1 (58) or transcription factors that regulate cornified envelope proteins and lipids (59), (reviewed 60) results in the loss of barrier function leading to neonatal death. However, knockout of tight junction component claudin-1 in mouse shows that granular layer tight junctions are essential for barrier activity (61). In both fetal humans and mice, tight junctions appear in periderm cells, and then by the time of stratum corneum development and periderm disaggregation [22 weeks over most of the body (44)], they appear in the upper granular layers (15,16).

Other epidermal adhesive complexes, the desmosomes, may have a barrier function. Mice with altered desmosomal cadherins (the adhesive proteins of the desmosome can display barrier defects (62,63).

In situ permeability assays, which measure an extremely early stage in barrier formation, show that a barrier forms regionally in the human infant between 20 and 24 weeks gestation [(8); Fig. 3]. The barrier appears either at sites of hair follicle formation (in association with stratum corneum formation) or at initiation sites, which then propagates outward to cover the entire body. In the human infant, the barrier forms first around the head, face, and neck at 19–20 weeks, then several weeks later over the abdomen, followed by the back (8). Barrier formation correlates with an epidermal gradient of differentiation (Fig. 3).

Interestingly, lipid extrusion and cornified envelope (i.e., initiation of stratum corneum formation) actually precede barrier formation. Initial barrier formation correlates with several changes in the upper epidermal cell layer (8) (Fig. 3). These upper layer keratinocytes adopt a flattened electron-dense phenotype, forming a single stratum corneum precursor layer exactly at the site of barrier initiation. Formation of additional stratum corneum layers will contribute to further barrier acquisition.

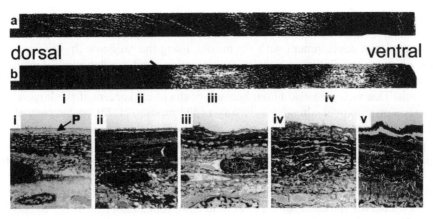

Figure 3 The epidermal permeability barrier is induced regionally in the human infant between 20 and 24 weeks. a) At 19 weeks a strip of skin from the torso of a preterm infant lacks barrier function (indicated by a dark result from a permeability assay), b) However, 2–3 weeks later, distinct barrier positive regions appear (white areas) and are propagated around the body as a ventral to dorsal wave (arrows). (i–iv) Specific ultrastructural changes accompany barrier induction. (i, ii) Immature epidermis, prior to barrier formation, retains periderm (P) attached to the outer epidermal surface. (iii, iv) Interfollicular epidermis from regions with barrier has prominent stratum cornuem (*bracket*) but has yet to achieve the thickness of that of the adult (v).

Subsequent barrier maturation can be monitored using an evaporimeter (64) to quantify trans-epidermal water loss (TEWL). Evaporimeter studies report a gradual maturation in skin barrier between 26 and 32 weeks (64–66). Barrier levels necessary for postnatal survival are reached several weeks before birth (68).

This feature of late gestational epidermis produces marked regional differences in the barrier function of preterm infant skin, which should be taken into account when managing treatment.

Periderm Disaggregation

Periderm undergoes terminal differentiation, including a type of "keratinization", in tandem with underlying embryonic epidermis prior to disaggregation (termed "regression"). The regressing cells form cornified envelopes and express other markers of terminal differentiation (52,69,70). If the role of the periderm was interactive or protective, then it will be redundant when underlying epidermis forms its protective barrier. Interestingly, periderm regression coincides with the formation of a functional barrier by the underlying epidermis at approximately 22–25 weeks (8,13). In mice, periderm dissociates in a similar pattern to that of the barrier formation over the surface of the animal (8), suggesting a link between stratum corneum maturation and periderm release, and supporting the idea that periderm had an interactive or protective role prior to epidermal barrier formation.

CONCLUSION

The wealth of detailed descriptive data on human development provides a resource for the exploitation of new gene expression and functional data arising from genome projects and animal models, provided that human development can be equated with animal or culture experimental models. In this review, emphasis has been placed on comparing human development with the mouse, using the rationale that the mouse, because of its susceptibility to genetic manipulation, and similar physiology and biochemistry to humans, is the most likely model for advancing human developmental research. This view was also taken because of the likely success of the large-scale mutagenesis programmes already underway in the mouse (71,72), and recent plans for an international effort for functional annotation of the mouse genome and to make publicly available knockout alleles for all mouse genes (73,74). It is highly probable that these efforts will yield mutant phenotypes relevant to the specific stages of skin development.

This comparison, however, shows that while the mouse will provide a good, accessible model for the embryonic period and embryonic–fetal transition, the acceleration of late gestational development in the mouse does not equate well temporally with the extended period of epidermal terminal differentiation in humans. Preterm mice cannot survive and provide a good model for barrier maturation in the preterm infant. In addition, we highlight in this review how the differences in synchronization of hair follicle formation and interfollicular terminal differentiation in humans and mice affect the nature of epidermal differentiation and barrier formation. Despite these difficulties mouse models provide a rich resource for understanding developmental change in humans.

The differences between the human and mouse models indicate that human culture models may provide part of the answer for researchers hoping to advance basic skin biology. Although acquisition of material is restricted by ethical considerations, particularly for the important late gestational period, there has been considerable advance in the generation of developmentally authentic organ cultures for human embryonic/fetal skin (27,28,75,76).

In this review, we highlight the regional nature of skin development in the human and the mouse. Regional development (e.g., hair follicle formation 40,41, onset of keratinization 11,77) was well established prior to discovery in the animals models (9). Regional modes of developmental change probably reflect a basic developmental process and are important in their own right, but regional change complicates the comparison of developmental status between laboratories and also between mutant or diseased individuals and healthy controls. We conclude that rather than relying simply on estimated gestational ages when making skin development comparison the way forward will be to compare samples for both morphological and biochemical markers, taking into account the anatomical regions from which the samples are derived. Human skin development research should now reap the benefits of many years of painstaking and meticulous morphological analysis.

REFERENCES

1. Holbrook KA. Skin structure and function of the developing human skin. In: Goldsmith LA, ed. Physiology, Biochemistry, and Molecular Biology of the Skin. 2nd ed. New York: Oxford University Press, 1991:63–110.
2. Verma KBL, Varma HC, Dayal SS. A histochemical study of human fetal skin. J Anat 1976; 121:185–191.
3. Foster CA, Bertram JF, Holbrook KA. Morphometric and statistical analyses describing the in utero growth of human epidermis. Anat Rec 1988; 222:201–206.

4. Stern IB. The uptake of tritiated thymidine by human fetal epidermis. J Invest Dermatol 1974; 63:268–272.
5. Bickenbach JR, Holbrook KA. Label-retaining cells in human embryonic and fetal epidermis. J Invest Dermatol 1987; 88:42–46.
6. Moore KL. The Developing Human (Clinically orientated embryology). Saunders Company, 1988:170–205.
7. Foster and Holbrook. 1988.
8. Holbrook KA, Odland GF. The fine structure of developing human epidermis: light, scanning and transmission electron microscopy of the periderm. J Invest Dermatol 1975; 65:16–38.
9. Hardman MJ, Moore L, Ferguson MWJ, Byrne C. Barrier formation in the human fetus is patterned. J Invest Dermatol 1999; 113:1106–1114.
10. Hardman MJ, Sisi P, Banbury DN, Byrne C. Patterned acquisition of barrier function during development. Development 1998; 128:1541–1552.
11. Parmley TH, Seeds AE. Fetal skin permeability to isotopic water (THO) in early pregnancy. Am J Obstet Gynecol 1970; 108:128–131.
12. Hoyes AD. Electron microscopy of the surface layer (periderm) of human foetal skin. J Anat 1968; 103:321–336.
13. Breathnach AS. The Herman Beerman lecture: embryology of human skin, a review of ultrastructural studies. J Invest Dermatol 1971; 57:133–143.
14. Holbrook KA, Odland GF. The fine structure of developing human epidermis: light, scanning, and transmission electron microscopy of the periderm. J Invest Dermatol 1975; 65:16–38.
15. Arita K, Akiyama M, Tsuji Y, McMillan JR, Eady RAJ, Shimizu H. Changes in gap junction distribution and connexion expression pattern during human fetal skin development. J Histochem Cytochem 2002; 50:1493–1500.
16. Morita K, Itoh M, Saitou M, Ando-Akatsuka Y, Furuse M, Yoneda K, Imamura S, Fujimoto K, Tsukita S. Subcellular distribution of tight junction-associated proteins (_ccluding, ZO-1, ZO-2) in rodent skin. J Invest Dermatol 1998; 110:862–866.
17. Pummi K, Malminen M, Aho H, Karvonen SL, Peltonen J, Peltonen S. Epidermal tight junctions: ZO-1 and _ccluding are expressed in mature, developing, and affected skin and in vitro differentiating keratinocytes. J Invest Dermatol 2001; 117:1050–1058.
18. Mazzalupo S, Coulombe PA. A reporter transgene based on a human keratin 6 gene promoter is specifically expressed in the periderm of mouse embryos. Mech Dev 2001; 100:65–69.
19. Paladini RD, Takahashi K, Bravo NS, Coulombe PA. Onset of re-epithelialization after skin injury correlates with a reorganization of keratin filaments in wound edge keratinocytes: defining a potential role for keratin 16. J Cell Biol 1996; 132:381–397.
20. Moll R, Moll I, Wiest W. Changes in the pattern of cytokeratin polypeptides in epidermis and hair follicles during skin development in human fetuses. Differentiation 1982; 23:170–178.
21. Byrne C, Tainsky M, Fuchs E. Programming gene expression in developing epidermis. Development 1994; 120:2369–2383.
22. Smith LT, Holbrook KA. Embryogenesis of the dermis in human skin. Pediatr Dermatol 1986; 3:271–280.
23. Fine JD, Smith LT, Holbrook KA, Katz SI. The appearance of four basement membrane zone antigens in developing human fetal skin. J Invest Dermatol 1984; 83:66–69.
24. Smith LT, Holbrook KA, Madri JA. Collagen types I, III, and V in human embryonic and fetal skin. Am J Anat 1986; 175:507–521.
25. Smith LT, Holbrook KA, Byers PH. Structure of the dermal matrix during development and in the adult. J Invest Dermatol 1982; 79:93s–104s.
26. Holbrook KA, Odland GF. Regional development of the human epidermis in the first trimester embryo and the second trimester fetus (ages related to the time of amniocentesis and fetal biopsy). J Invest Dermatol 1980; 74:161–168.

27. Dale BA, Holbrook KA, Kimball JR, Hoff M, Sun TT. Expression of epidermal keratins and filaggrin during human fetal skin development. J Cell Biol 1985; 101:1257–1269.

28. Fisher C, Holbrook KA. Cell surface and cytoskeletal changes associated with epidermal stratification and differentiation in organ cultures of embryonic human skin. Dev Biol 1987; 119:231–241.

29. Hertle MD, Adams JC, Watt FM. Integrin expression during human epidermal development in vivo and in vitro. Development 1991; 112:193–206.

30. Hentula M, Peltonen J, Peltonen S. Expression profiles of cell–cell and cell–matrix junction proteins in developing human epidermis. Arch Dermatol Res 2001; 293:259–267.

31. Johnson KO. The roles and functions of cutaneous mechanoreceptors. Curr Opin Neurobiol 2001; 11:455–461.

32. Moll I, Moll R, Franke WW. Formation of epidermal and dermal Merkel cells during human fetal skin development. J Invest Dermatol 1986; 87:779–787.

33. Moll R, Moll I, Franke WW. Identification of Merkel cells in human skin by specific cytokeratin antibodies: changes of cell density and distribution in fetal and adult plantar epidermis. Differentiation 1984; 28:136–154.

34. Moll I, Moll R. Early development of human Merkel cells. Exp Dermatol 1992; 1:180–184.

35. Kim DK, Holbrook KA. The appearance, density, and distribution of Merkel cells in human embryonic and fetal skin: their relation to sweat gland and hair follicle development. J Invest Dermatol 1995; 104:411–416.

36. Smart IH. Variation in plane of cell cleavage during the process of stratification in mouse epidermis. Br J Dermatol 1970; 82:276–282.

37. Bickenbach JR, Greer JM, Bundman JS, Roop DR. Loricrin expression is coordinated with other epidermal proteins and the appearance of the lipid lammelar granules in development. J Invest Dermatol 1995; 104:405–410.

38. Okuyama R, Nguyen BC, Talora C, Ogawa E, Tommasr di Vigano M, Chiorino G, Tagami H, Woo M, Dotto GP. High commitment of embryonic keratinocytes to terminal differentiation through a Notch1-caspase 3 regulatory mechanism. Dev Cell 2004; 6:551–562.

39. Dotto GP. Signal transduction pathways controlling the switch between keratinocyte growth and differentiation. Crit Rev Oral Med 1999; 10:442–447.

40. Lefort K, Paolo Dotto G. Notch signaling in the integrated control of keratinocyte growth/differentiation and tumor suppression. Semin Cancer Biol 2004; 14:374–386.

41. Holbrook KA, Odland GF. Structure of the human fetal hair canal and initial hair eruption. J Invest Dermatol 1978; 71:385–390.

42. Pinkus H. Embryology of hair. In: Montagna W, Ellis RA, eds. The Biology of Hair Growth. New York: Academic Press, 1958:1–32.

43. Paus R, Cotsarelis G. The biology of hair follicles. N Engl J Med 1999; 341:491–497.

44. Williams ML, Hincenbergs M, Holbrook KA. Skin lipid content during early fetal development. J Invest Dermatol 1988; 91:263–268.

45. Holbrook KA, Odland GF. Regional development of the human epidermis in the first trimester embryo and the second trimester fetus (ages related to the timing of amniocentesis and fetal biopsy). J Invest Dermatol 1980; 74:161–168.

46. Elias PM. Epidermal lipids, barrier function and desquamation. J Invest Dermatol 1983; 80:44–49.

47. Elias PM. The epidermal permeability barrier: from the early days at Harvard to emerging concepts. J Invest Dermatol 2004; 122:xxxvi–xxxix.

48. Nemes Z, Steinert PM. Bricks and mortar of the epidermal barrier. Exp Mol Med 1999; 31:5–19.

49. Wertz PW. Lipids and barrier function of the skin. Acta Derm Venereol Suppl (Stockh) 2000; 208:7–11.

50. Manabe M, O'Guin WM. Existence of trichohyalin–keratohyalin hybrid granules: co-localization of two major intermediate filament associated proteins in non-follicular epithelia. Differentiation 1994; 58:65–76.

51. Hashimoto K, Gross BG, Dibella RJ, Lever WF. The ultrastructure of the skin of human embryos: IV: the epidermis. J Invest Dermatol 1966; 106:317–335.

52. Akiyama M, Smith LT, Shimizu H. Expression of transglutaminase activity in developing human epidermis. Br J Dermatol 2000; 142:223–225.

53. Kalinin A, Kajava AV, Steinert PM. Epithelial barrier function: assembly and structural features of the cornified cell envelope. Bioessays 2002; 24:789–800.

54. Simon M, Haftek M, Sebbag M, Montezin M, Girbal-Neuhauser E, Shmftt D, Serre G. Evidence that filaggrin is a component of the cornified cell envelope in human planter epidermis. J Biochem 1996; 317:173–177.

55. Marshall D, Hardman MJ, Nield KM, Byrne C. Differentially expressed late constituents of the epidermal cornified envelope. Proc Natl Acad Sci USA 2001; 98:13031–13036.

56. Elias PM, Cullander C, Mauro T, Rassner U, Komuves L, Brown BE, Menon GK. The secretory granular cell: the outermost granular cell as a specialized secretory cell. J Invest Dermatol Symp Proc 1998; 3:87–100.

57. Behne M, Uchida Y, Seki T, De Montellano PO, Elias PM, Holleran WM. Omega-hydroxylceramides are required for comeocyte lipid envelope (CLE) formation and normal epidermal permeability barrier function. J Invest Dermatol 2000; 114:185–192.

58. Nemes Z, Marekov LN, Fésüs L, Steinert PM. A novel function for transglutaminase 1: attachment of long-chain omega-hydroxyceramides to involucrin by ester bond formation. Proc Natl Acad Sci USA 1999; 96:8402–8407.

59. Matsuki M, Yamashta F, Ishida-Yamamoto A, Yamada K, Kinoshita C, Fushiki S, Ueda E, Morishima Y, Tabata K, Yasuno H, Hashida M, Lizuki H, Ikawa M, Okabe M, Kondoh G, Kinoshita T, Takeda J, Yamanishi K. Defective stratum corneum and early neonatal death in mice lacking the gene for transglutaminase 1. Proc Natl Acad Sci USA 1998; 95:1044–1049.

60. Segre JA, Bauer C, Fuchs E. Klf4 is a transcription factor required for establishing the barrier function of the skin. Nat Genet 1999; 22:356–360.

61. Dai S, Segre JA. Transcriptional control of epidermal specification and differentiation. Curr Opin Genet Dev 2004; 14:485–491.

62. Furuse M, Hata M, Furuse K, Yoshida Y, Haratake A, Sugitani Y, Noda T, Kubo A, Tsukita S. Claudin-based tight junctions are crucial for the mammalian epidermal barrier: a lesson from claudin-1-deficient mice. J Cell Biol 2002; 156:1099–1111.

63. Elias PM, Matsuyoshi N, Wu H, Lin C, Wang ZH, Brown BE, Stanley JR. Desmoglein isoform distribution affects stratum corneum structure and function. J Cell Biol 2001; 153:243–249.

64. Chidgey M, Brakebusch C, Gustafsson E, Cruchley A, Hail C, Kirk S, Merritt A, North A, Tselepis C, Hewitt J, Byme C, Fassler R, Garrod D. Mice lacking desmocollin 1 show epidermal fragility accompanied by barrier defects and abnormal differentiation. J Cell Biol 2001; 155:821–832.

65. Nilsson GE. Measurement of water exchange through the skin. Med Biol Eng Comput 1977; 15:209–218.

66. Hammarlund K, Sedin G. Transepidenmal water loss in newborn infants: III. Relation to gestational age. Acta Paediatr Scand 1979; 68:795–801.

67. Wilson DR, Maibach HI. Transepidermal water loss in vivo: premature and term infants. Biol Neonate 1980; 37:180–185.

68. Harpin VA, Rutter N. Barrier properties of the newborn infant's skin. J Pediatr 1983; 102:419–425.

69. Kalia YN, Nonato LB, Lund CH, Guy RH. Development of skin barrier function in premature infants. J Invest Dermatol 1998; 111:320–326.

70. Akiyama M, Smith LT, Yoneda K, Holbrook KA, Hohl D, Shimizu H. Periderm cells form cornified cell envelope in their regression process during human epidermal development. J Invest Dermatol 1999; 112:903–909.

71. Lee SC, Lee JB, Kook JP, Seo JJ, Nam KI, Park SS, Kim YP. Expression of differentiation markers during fetal skin development in humans: immunohistochemical studies on

the precursor proteins forming the cornified cell envelope. J invest Dermatol 1999; 112:882–886.

72. Nolan PM, Peters J. A systematic, genome-wide, phenotype-driven rnutagenesis programme for gene function studies in the mouse. Nat Genet 2000; 25:440–443.

73. Stanford WL, Conn JB, Cordes SP. Gene-trap mutagenesis: past, present, and beyond. Nat Rev Genet 2001; 2:756–768.

74. Comprehensive Knockout Mouse Project Consortium. The knockout mouse project. Nat Genet 2004; 36:921–924.

75. The European Mouse Mutagenesis Consortium. The European dimension for the mouse genome mutagenesis program. Nat Genet 2004; 36:925–927.

76. Zeltinger J, Hoibrook KA. A model system for long-term serum-free suspension organ culture of human fetal tissues: experiments on digits and skin from multiple body regions. Cell Tissue Res 1997; 290:51–60.

77. Pinkus F. Development of the integument. In: Keibel F, Mall FP, eds. Manual of Embryology. J.B. Lippincott Co., 1910:243–291.

78. Sengel P. Morphogenesis of the Skin. Cambridge: Cambridge University Press, 1976.

79. Williams ML, Hanley K, Elias PM, Feingold KR. Ontogeny of the epidermal permeability barrier. J Invest Dermtol 1998; 3S:75–79.

18

Epidermal Calcium Gradient and the Permeability Barrier

Gopinathan K. Menon
Global Research and Development, Avon Products, Inc., Suffern, New York, U.S.A.

Seung Hun Lee
Department of Dermatology, Yonsei University College of Medicine, Seoul, Korea

INTRODUCTION

From a natural history perspective, the significance of calcium in the biology of the integument (the primary barrier of an organism) is readily apparent to the comparative biologists. The higher orders of invertebrates that preceded the vertebrates essentially possess a tough, calcium-enriched exoskeleton. Crustaceans, constrained by an inflexible exoskeleton, resort to periodic molt so that body growth can progress unrestricted for a period until the new exoskeleton gets calcified. Mollusks add new growth rings to their rather inflexible shell, while some of the highly mobile members of the phylum (cephalopods) internalize the shell as a skeletal support (cuttlebone). Many of the land snails have evolved shell-lessness. Shells are energetically expensive to produce, and require a large source of calcium in the environment, so it might have been advantageous to do away with shells, as long as they developed compensatory measures, such as living in non-xerotic microhabitats. Echinoderms have a unique endoskeleton, made of individual ossicles that are porous, having an internal latticework or labyrinth-like spaces filled with dermal cells and fibers. Developmentally, the skeleton begins as numerous, separate spicule-like elements, each behaving as a single calcite crystal. An epidermis covers this dermis, internalizing the exoskeleton. Vertebrates that developed a bony endoskeleton, which has the ability to grow and keep pace with the organism's growth dimensions, also evolved a flexible integument. The bones also provide a source of calcium that can be mobilized for the formation of eggshells (in oviparous forms) or the growing fetus. Although the vertebrate skin is not calcified in the literal sense, calcium continues to be critical for mammalian integumentary health and functions. In this chapter, we will examine some of the crucial functions of skin that are dependent on ionic calcium, and the skin dysfunctions that are correlated with altered calcium distribution and localization.

THE EPIDERMAL CALCIUM GRADIENT

The first significant finding that related calcium with murine keratinocyte proliferation and differentiation came from the in vitro studies of Yuspa and colleagues (1–3). In these landmark publications, they showed that (i) low calcium concentrations in media stimulated the keratinocyte proliferation, but, (ii) when switched to a high calcium medium, the cells undergo differentiation and stratification, and that (iii) calcium induces transglutaminase expression and the formation of glutaryl–lysine crosslinks in keratinocyte cornified envelopes. They also found that (iv) the expression of murine epidermal differentiation markers is tightly regulated by restricted extracellular calcium concentrations in vitro. These findings prompted us (4) to investigate the distribution pattern of ionic calcium in the mammalian epidermis that could correlate with the sequential events in epidermal stratification and differentiation, and formation of the permeability barrier.

We employed the technique of ion capture cytochemistry and electron microscopy (4) to visualize the ultrastructural localization of an exchangeable pool of calcium within the murine skin. As seen in Figure 1, calcium is localized both in the extracellular and cellular compartments of the epidermis. Extracellular calcium content is low in the basal and spinous layers, but increases gradually from the inner to the outer layers of stratum granulosum (SG), forming an extracellular reservoir of calcium within the SG—providing a means for rapid entry into the cytosol and triggering terminal differentiation. This extracellular calcium reservoir may be held in place by an apparent enrichment of calcium binding sites, demonstrated by staining with trivalent lanthanum (4). We postulated that the extracellular gradient of calcium in vivo, with negligible amounts surrounding the cells of stratum basale, promoted/favored cell proliferation, but the gradual increase in calcium concentration in the extracellular domains of SG provided a mechanism for their gradual differentiation. An influx of calcium ions into the uppermost SG cells (Fig. 2) was considered as a trigger for terminal differentiation [as well as an en mass secretion of lamellar bodies (LBs)]. We had also postulated that following such a calcium signal, and before the full formation of the cornified envelope, calcium is extruded from the cells, and the ions are recycled back to the extracellular reservoir. Whitfield (5) designated it as the "load and dump" hypothesis, and termed the terminal differentiation/programmed death of keratinocyte as "diffpoptosis." The cytochemically demonstrated calcium gradient was also validated by proton probe and X-ray microanalysis (6,7). Very recently, Behne et al. (8), employing Calcium Green-5N, achieved calcium-fluorescence lifetime imaging in ex vivo skin and showed increasing calcium concentrations from the basal to the granular layers, confirming the previous proton-induced X-ray emission analysis (PIXE) (9) and ultrastructural cytochemical demonstration of the epidermal calcium gradient.

The control of epidermal cell differentiation via calcium is not restricted to the mammalian epidermis, and exerts similar effects in the frog epidermal cells in vitro (9), suggesting that this regulatory mechanism may be highly conserved in the vertebrates. Although comparative cytochemical information on epidermal calcium distribution in vertebrates is not available, a clearly defined extracellular reservoir as seen in mice is not present in either the rat or the human epidermis (Fig. 3). Yet, a calcium gradient from the basal layer to the SG exists in both the instances, indicating that a high cytosolic calcium in the SG is tied to the process of terminal differentiation.

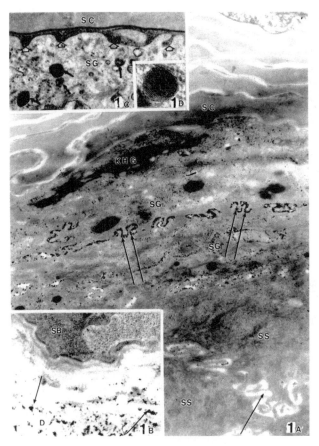

Figure 1 (A) Low magnification survey electron micrograph showing calcium localization in murine epidermis. Note the gradual accumulation of extracellular calcium (*arrows*) toward upper stratum granulosum (SG). In addition, uppermost cells of SG contain highest amounts of calcium precipitates. SS = stratum spinosum; KHG = keratohyalin granules; SC = stratum corneum. (B) Shows high calcium concentration in the dermis (D) and lack of precipitates above basement membrane. SB = stratum basale. (C) Electron micrograph of the SG–SC interface (*open arrows*), showing this domain is filled with secreted contents of lamellar bodies. Nascent Lamellar bodies (*arrows*) are present within the SG cytosol (OSO4 post-fixation). (D) High magnification electron micrograph of an individual Lamellar body showing the disk contents enveloped by the limiting membrane (RUO4 post-fixation). *Source*: Reprinted from Ref. 16, with kind permission of Springer-Verlag.

Several clues emerged from these empirical observations with respect to the roles of the calcium gradient in barrier formation. First, calcium was found to be associated with the nascent LBs in the cells of the SG, indicating its role in maintaining the LB structural integrity, or in the fusion of the LB membrane with the cell membrane leading to an exocytosis of the LB. Again, at the SG–SC interface, the secreted contents of the LBs also showed a cytochemical staining for calcium, but usually not above this level in the extracellular domains. Moreover, while some corneocytes show calcium precipitates within, most of the corneocytes do not— which raises an intriguing possibility of a heterogeneity in corneocytes, either regarding their calcium content, or the cellular permeability—points that are discussed later in this chapter.

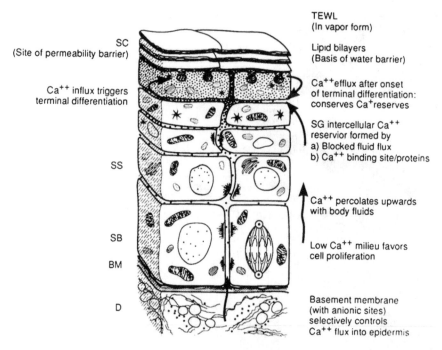

Figure 2 Diagrammatic representation of the epidermal calcium gradient formation, and how the "load and dump" hypothesis is correlated with terminal differentiation of keratinocytes and formation of permeability barrier. *Source*: Reprinted from Ref. 12 with permission of publishers, Blackwell Sciences Ltd., U.K.

ALTERED CALCIUM GRADIENT IN SKIN DYSFUNCTIONS

We have examined several skin dysfunctions involving altered cellular proliferation and differentiation, and found a loss of the epidermal calcium gradient in these instances, i.e., they have increased calcium content in all the layers of epidermis, and hence an obliteration of the ionic gradient that characterizes a healthy functioning epidermis. Animal models that display the loss of the gradient include mice that have a chronic barrier abnormality due to essential fatty acid deficiency (EFAD), and mice where repeated topical application of lovastatin results in an acute barrier disruption (10,11). Distinct differences from the normal murine epidermal calcium distribution are displayed by the EFAD mice (12), whose barrier abnormalities include epidermal hyperproliferation, hyperkeratosis, defective LB structure and lipid content, as well as an altered SC lipid lamellar structure that is reflected in high TEWL values. Instead of an increasing gradient of extracellular calcium toward the outer epidermis as in controls, abundant precipitates are found in all levels, including the basal and spinous layers. Keratinocytes in all suprabasal layers display variable, but relatively high levels of calcium precipitates in the cytosol, as well as in the extracellular spaces. Additionally, large clusters of calcium precipitates appear frequently within the extracellular domains of the SC (12).

In mice treated topically with lovastatin for 7 days, the epidermis shows hyperproliferation, accumulation of lipid droplets within keratinocytes, scaly SC, defective LBs, and elevated transepidermal water loss (TEWL) values. The epidermal calcium

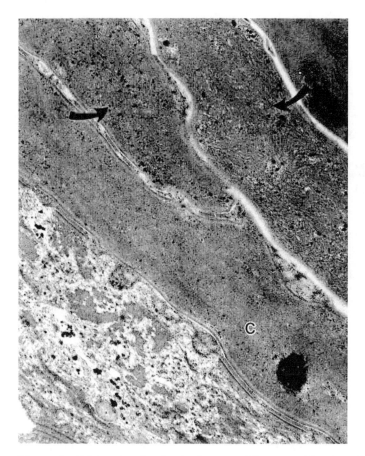

Figure 3 Calcium localization in the normal human epidermis. While the extracellular calcium reservoirs are absent, a calcium gradient is still present within the stratified epidermis. *Arrows* show calcium contents within some corneocytes. *Abbreviations*: C, corneocyte; D, desmosome; SG, stratum granulosum.

distribution in these mice resemble that seen in mice with EFAD, with the additional feature of large aggregates of calcium in association with the cytosolic lipid droplets. In the epidermis of the tail skin of mice, where normal epidermal differentiation is parakeratotic, the extracellular calcium reservoir (as seen in their orthokeratotic body epidermis) is absent (Fig. 4), indicating the inherent differences in calcium signaling for ortho- versus para keratotic terminal differentiation of keratinocytes.

Human diseases such as psoriasis (Fig. 5) and X-linked ichthyosis (RXLI) also display abnormalities of the epidermal calcium gradient (13,14). All these conditions share a basic feature of defective permeability barrier, resulting from a high rate of cell proliferation, defective LBs and altered differentiation that is reflected in dry, scaly skin conditions. In psoriasis, an increased calmodulin content of the epidermis has also been documented (15). In psoriatic patients, the uninvolved epidermis shows a calcium distribution, which generally resembles that of the normal human epidermis. However, several features distinguish the calcium localization pattern in the psoriatic lesions from the autologous uninvolved epidermis or epidermis from the non-psoriatics. These features are: (i) large quantities of calcium precipitates within the cytosol of all suprabasal cells; (ii) exceedingly small quantities of

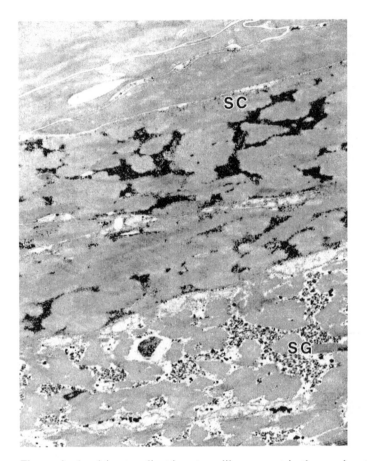

Figure 4 A calcium gradient is not readily apparent in the parakeratotic murine tail epidermis in contrast to body epidermis (orthokeratotic). Also note retention of nucleus in the SC. *Abbreviations*: LB, lamellar body; N, nucleus.

calcium precipitate in the extracellular domains of the basal layer; and (iii) nuclear localization of calcium in all the cell layers (as opposed to the basal layers in non-psoriatic/uninvolved epidermis). Additionally, an abnormally high amount of calcium is localized above the SG. While the extruded contents of LBs at the SG–SC interface display calcium precipitates (as in normal), in psoriatic lesions LB disks and calcium persist up to the higher levels of SC interstices, i.e., three to four cells above the granular layer. In these domains, wherever disk contents persist (instead of being processed into SC lamellar structures), they co-localize the calcium precipitates. As is the case with uninvolved skin and normal SC, small amounts of precipitates are seen in the cytosol of some individual corneocytes, while others do not show any deposits. The lipid droplets that accumulate within the corneocytes of psoriatic lesions are, by and large, free of calcium precipitates. The multiple abnormalities in the epidermal calcium distribution pattern in the plaque-type psoriasis suggest a drastically altered calcium gradient and microenvironment that are reflected in the defective epidermal differentiation and barrier formation. The maintenance of a normal calcium gradient in the epidermis may have a basis in the selective filtration of serum by the epidermal basement membrane, which in psoriatic lesions display defects such as basal cell hemiations or other functional alterations. The very low levels of extracellular calcium in the basal layers, and the reduced cell-to-cell contacts between adjacent basal and spinous cells of the involved epidermis, are consistent with the requirement of extracellular calcium for desmosomal assembly, and the lack of contact inhibition favoring an increased cell proliferation characteristic of psoriasis. The relatively high cytosolic and nuclear calcium in the basal and spinous layers may be related to the precocious expression of proteins such as involucrin in psoriatic lesions, as well as the activation of increased levels of calmodulin that are present in psoriatic epidermis (15). It is unlikely that an alteration in calcium metabolism is the primary defect in psoriasis, but it may be crucial to the clinical expression of the psoriatic lesion.

The epidermal calcium gradient is altered in the patients of RXLI as well. Specifically, all the cell layers in the SG show an elevated cytosolic calcium, which persist in the extracellular domains of the SC, particularly associated with the increased numbers of corneodesmosomes (14) that characterize this disorder of cornification. Elevated levels of cholesterol sulfate (CSO_4) which have been reported in SC lipids from patients with RXLI, and CSO_4 possibly inhibit the serine proteases responsible for desmosome degradation and normal desquamation of the corneocytes. Calcium, if present in sufficient quantities, could cross-link the highly anionic SO_4 group on adjacent lamellar bilayers, as well as stabilize the corneodesmosomes further, leading to an abnormally high corneocyte cohesion.

CALCIUM GRADIENT AND PERMEABILITY BARRIER: EXPERIMENTAL STUDIES

A logical extension of these morphologic studies was to evaluate the distribution of calcium in the epidermis following an acute barrier disruption, normal barrier recovery, post occlusion with water permeable versus impermeable membranes, and also with and without exposure to calcium ions (16,19). We found that barrier disruption caused an immediate depletion of both intracellular and extracellular calcium precipitates in the cells of the upper epidermal cell layers, resulting in the disappearance of the normal calcium distribution. However, the innermost SC, a site that was normally characterized by relatively few precipitates, displayed large clumps or precipitates in pools within the intercellular spaces. Between 1 and 2.5 hours after acetone treatment, calcium-containing precipitates gradually began to reappear in the cytosol of the upper SG cells, as well as in the extracellular domains. At the SG–SC interface, discrete calcium precipitates and larger aggregates occurred in association with the secreted LB contents. Thus, by 1 hour when the barrier has recovered by about 10%, a parallel restoration of epidermal calcium distribution begins.

By six hours of post-acetone treatment, when barrier function (indicated by TEWL) had recovered by about 60%, a further increase in calcium-containing precipitates was noted both within intra- and extracellular sites in the SG, resulting in the partial restoration of the apparent epidermal calcium gradient. Moreover, calcium precipitates were increased in the extracellular domains of the basal and spinous layers, suggesting that the epidermal calcium gradient re-forms from below. By 24 hours post-acetone treatment, during which time the barrier function recovered to near-normal levels, the intracellular calcium distribution became comparable with that of the normal epidermis, with the upper SG cells displaying abundant cytosolic calcium precipitates in comparison to the amounts in the lower epidermal cells. But, even by 24 hours, the extracellular calcium reservoir in the SG had not completely attained the fully replete normal profile, and larger accumulations of precipitates were still present in the intercellular spaces of the basal and spinous layers. These results suggest that the epidermal calcium gradient is largely restored by 24 hours. Cellophane tape stripping of the SC produced a barrier abrogation comparable to that seen with the acetone treatment (TEWL about $7.5\,mg/cm^2/h$). Just as seen with acetone treatment, a marked decrease both in intra- and extracellular calcium was evident in the upper epidermis, resulting in the loss of the normal epidermal calcium gradient.

Several lines of evidence suggested that the loss of extracellular calcium may signal the augmented synthesis and secretion of LBs, leading to barrier repair. First, barrier repair is inhibited when calcium ($\leq 0.01\,mM$) is added to an iso-osmolar sucrose solution in which the acetone-treated flank is immersed. In contrast, when the immersion solution lacks calcium, barrier recovery proceeds normally. However, the addition of calcium to the immersion bath normalizes the extracellular calcium around the SG cells, and an inhibition of the formation and secretion of LBs from the uppermost SG cells. In contrast, sites exposed to a calcium-free immersion bath demonstrated both decreased calcium in the upper, viable epidermis and a marked secretion of LBs by the SG cells. Again, as shown by several methods, water-permeable membranes allowed the restoration of the epidermal calcium levels, while vapor-impermeable membranes significantly delayed such a restoration.

Early studies on barrier recovery following an acute barrier disruption indicated that several metabolic responses, such as the synthesis of all three major classes of SC lipids, generation and secretion of LBs, and epidermal DNA synthesis may be regulated by the signal of increased TEWL (17). This theory was based on experiments that showed an artificial restoration of the barrier by occlusion with water vapor–impermeable, but not water-permeable wraps, wholly or partly blocked the various metabolic responses critical for the barrier repair. However, follow-up studies showed that the barrier recovered normally when perturbed skin sites were immersed in hypotonic, isotonic or hypertonic solutions, but when Ca and K ions were added to the solution, recovery is blocked (as in the case of occlusion), indicating that water loss is not the signal for initiating these metabolic responses (18). The inhibitory effects of added calcium could be reversed by co-treatment with inhibitors of either L-type calcium channels or calmodulin (18,19). These experimental studies reveal that the basal, high calcium content of the SG implies a "maintenance state" of the basal barrier function, allowing an increased comeocyte protein expression and a "housekeeping" level of LB secretion. On the other hand, the drastic loss of calcium following barrier disruption allows for a massive secretion of nascent LBs, as well as increased lipid synthesis, and assembly of new LBs and their secretion, all leading to barrier repair and restoration of the calcium gradient, which brings back the "maintenance state" of the basic barrier status (Fig. 1). Manipulating the epidermal Ca^{2+} gradient without extraction of the barrier lipids or removal of the SC could prove or disapprove this hypothesis.

Hence, to determine directly whether the LB secretion is regulated by alterations in extracellular calcium, we experimentally altered the extracellular calcium gradient without disrupting the barrier, using high-frequency sonophoresis (20). At appropriate frequencies, ultrasound enhances the transepidermal penetration of applied tracers without abrogating the permeability barrier. Because this process is accompanied by the bulk movement of extracellular fluids, we used it to manipulate the extracellular calcium reservoir, and examined the ultrastructural localization of calcium in the epidermis, as well as the LB secretory response, following sonophoresis of either water alone or iso-osmolar sucrose solutions with or without added calcium ions.

The most striking feature immediately following the sonophoresis of either distilled water or iso-osmolar sucrose was the absence of an extracellular calcium reservoir in the upper SG. Instead, large clumps of calcium precipitates appeared in the extracellular spaces of the lower nucleated layers, as well as within the superficial dermis, subjacent to the basement membrane. This reversal of the gradient, i.e., higher extracellular calcium within the lower cell layers, was noted in both distilled water and sucrose solution–permeated samples. This profile of epidermal calcium distribution persisted in the 3-hour posttreatment samples, but began to normalize again by 6-hour posttreatment. These results show that sonophoresis in the absence of exogenous calcium temporarily disrupts the epidermal calcium gradient, decreasing the calcium content of the upper epidermis by driving the extracellular calcium into the deeper nucleated layers (Fig. 5).

Immediately following the sonophoresis of sucrose solutions containing calcium ($\pm K^+$), the cytosol of all the nucleated layers of the epidermis showed increased calcium precipitates, thereby obliterating the calcium gradient. The high levels of cytosolic calcium effectively masked the extracellular calcium gradient, interfering with the comparison of the extracellular gradient under these conditions to either samples sonophoresed with calcium-free sucrose solutions or control samples. Moreover, calcium precipitates also appeared within corneocytes and at the SG–SC interface, sites that normally demonstrate only small amounts of precipitates. These results demonstrate that sonophoresis in the presence of exogenous calcium drives this ion both downward into the subjacent epidermal layers and into the cytosol. Moreover, this treatment results in an overall increase in the calcium content of the epidermis in all the epidermal cell layers.

Immediately following the sonophoresis of either distilled water or sucrose without calcium, increased LB contents appeared at the SG–SC interface, as well as between the cells of the SG. Moreover, deep invaginations of the apical plasma membrane of the uppermost granular cells appeared, which were filled with the secreted LB contents. Finally, the cytosol of the upper SG cells appeared, nearly devoid of nascent LBs. This finding was confirmed by stereologic measurements, which demonstrated that less than 2% of the cytosol of the outermost granular cells was occupied by LBs (20).

When the sonophoresed solution contained calcium ($\pm K^+$), which elevates the calcium content of the upper epidermis, LB secretion from the upper SG was inhibited. This was clearly evident from the presence of normal numbers of the LBs within the cytosol of the upper SG cells, a paucity of secreted LB contents at the SG–SC interface, and the virtual absence of secreted LB contents between the subjacent SG cell layers. These results show that the depletion of extracellular calcium at the level of the SG by sonophoresis leads to an accelerated LB secretion from the cells of the outer granular layers, a process that is inhibited when calcium is added to the sonophoresis solutions. The above-mentioned study provides direct evidence that the extracellular calcium content of the SG regulates the LB secretion. In addition, sonophoresis provides a potentially powerful investigative tool for the manipulation of epidermal extracellular ionic environments.

REGULATION OF THE CALCIUM GRADIENT

Based on these observations, a simplistic model of passive formation of the calcium gradient was proposed. In this schema, calcium ions from the dermis move into the

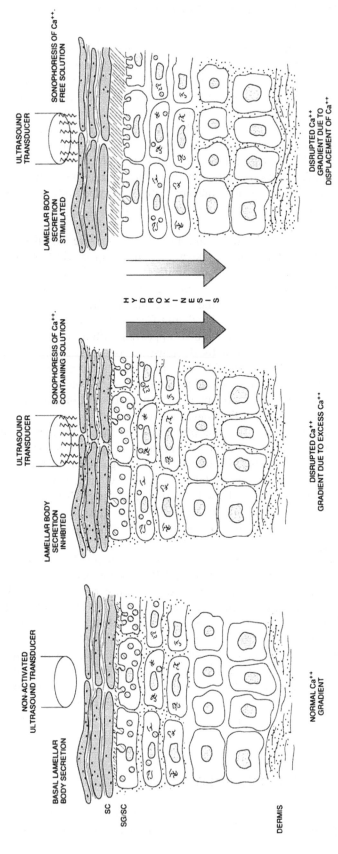

Figure 5   Diagrammatic representation of effects on the calcium gradient and lamellar body secretion in murine epidermis by sonophoresis of calcium solutions and non-calcium containing water. *Source:* Reprinted from Ref. 20 with permission of Blackwell Publishing, Inc.

epidermal compartment past the first barrier, i.e., the epidermal basement membrane, subsequently moving into the upper layers with the outward flux of water. At the SG–SC interface, the flux is blocked by the secreted LB contents, and only water in a vapor form crosses the SC. This results in a passive deposition of the calcium ions below the barrier lipids (the dam). An occlusive covering with water vapor–impermeable membrane (after barrier disruption) blocks the water movement through the epidermal layers and delays the restoration of the calcium content. This rather simplistic model gained experimental support from the following experiment done by the Elias group (21). Murine epidermal barrier was disrupted with tape stripping, and the barrier recovery and restoration of the calcium gradient were compared in skin sites covered with and without Gore-Tex, and exposed to cold (4°C) at 5 hours posttreatment. Previous studies had shown that exposure to cold blocks the barrier recovery after an acute perturbation due to metabolic slow-down, resulting in a deficient LB production (22). As expected, barrier-disrupted, unoccluded and cold-exposed sites did not show a barrier repair or a reappearance of the calcium gradient at 5 hours posttreatment, but similar sites covered with Gore-Tex showed a return of the calcium gradient, although with little barrier recovery. These results show that the barrier status (Gore-Tex occluding the surface providing a barrier, but being water vapor permeable, allowing for water movement across the epidermis) regulates the formation of the calcium gradient, and that a passive process alone can account for the formation of the calcium gradient. This does not take into account the active calcium pump mechanism in the epidermis, such as the Ca and Mg ATPase, with a distribution pattern that is opposite to that of the calcium gradient (23). The disappearance of Ca–Mg ATPase from the outermost granular cells correlates with the massive influx of calcium into these cells, triggering terminal differentiation and barrier formation. However, cold exposure can be expected to alter the epidermal calcium pump activity as well. The roles of such calcium pumps in the formation of the calcium gradient remain to be elucidated.

Another example wherein the formation of the calcium gradient coincides with barrier formation is the ontogeny of the permeability barrier during fetal development. Investigations of fetal rat and mouse skin using the ion capture cytochemistry, as well as PIXE analysis (24), have shown that a calcium gradient is not present at gestational days 16 to 18, prior to the permeability barrier formation, and that the formation of a calcium gradient coincides with the emergence of barrier competence (day 19 for the mice, and day 20 for the rats). While corroborating the role of calcium in key metabolic events leading to barrier formation, fetal barrier development does not offer any strong insights as to whether the gradient is formed actively or passively. A similar picture emerged from investigations on reconstituted skin equivalents. The reconstituted skin models, cultured in an air–water interface, are valuable as alternatives for animal testing, for toxicology assessments, and for human skin grafts. Yet, their use has been limited due to the inability to replicate the barrier competency of the in vivo integument. Vicanova et al. (25) made significant progress on this front by supplementing the cultures with vitamin C, wherein the organotypic cultures not only exhibited an improved morphology of the barrier lipids, but also displayed a calcium gradient.

An interesting set of experiments by Elias et al. (26) correlated the in vivo calcium content of the epidermis with keratinocyte differentiation in vivo at the post-transcriptional level, and completed the circle of the original cytochemical demonstration of calcium gradient, which was prompted by observations on the calcium effects on keratinocyte differentiation in vitro. As an acute barrier disruption reduces the calcium levels in the SG, they studied the regulation of murine epidermal differentiation after such calcium depletion and by exposure of such sites to low (0.03 M) and high (1.8 M) calcium. Three hours after barrier perturbation, coincidental with the loss of the extracellular calcium and accelerated LB secretion, both Northern blot and in situ hybridization techniques revealed a marked decrease in the mRNA levels of loricrin, profilaggrin and involucrin in the outer epidermis. Moreover, exposure of acutely barrier disrupted skin sites to low calcium solutions sustained the reduction in mRNA levels, whereas exposure to high calcium solutions restored normal mRNA levels. Such restoration was also blocked by the L-type calcium channel inhibitor, Nifedipine. These studies provided evidence that acute and sustained fluctuations in the epidermal calcium regulate the expression of differentiation-specific proteins in vivo, and that modulations in the epidermal calcium coordinately regulate events late in epidermal differentiation that together form the permeability barrier.

IMPLICATIONS OF EPIDERMAL CALCIUM GRADIENT FOR SKIN BIOLOGISTS

The presence of a calcium gradient in the mammalian epidermis is now a well-accepted fact, although there are differing views about the methodologies for imaging the calcium distribution. In spite of critiques of the ion capture cytochemistry (26), results obtained by this technique have been validated by other techniques, such as the PIXE and Proton probe techniques, as well as calcium dyes (8). Additionally, the demonstration of the gradient in several studies by different groups, its correlation with barrier formation in vivo (24) and in vitro (25), loss of the gradient with acute and chronic barrier disruption (12,19), as well as following experimental manipulations, such as sonophoresis (20) and iontophoresis (27), attest to the validity of the technique in experimental investigations.

Recent studies using molecular biology and transgenic mouse models have shed new light into how the epidermal cells sense the changes in extracellular calcium (29). The calcium-sensing receptor (CaSR), a G-protein coupled receptor (GPCR), which functions in sensing calcium and activating a calcium-signaling pathway in calcium-sensitive tissues like bone and parathyroid (30,31), appears to be functional in epidermal differentiation. Recently, Turksen and Troy (29) created transgenic mice overexpressing CaSR in the basal epidermal cells, thereby sensitizing these cells to calcium signaling, resulting in an accelerated terminal differentiation of keratinocytes, and an accelerated epidermal permeability barrier (compared to wild-type embryos at the same age), demonstrated by the dye exclusion method. It would be interesting to see if the calcium distribution pattern is altered within the epidermis of these transgenics.

There is much to be explored in how the epidermal calcium gradient influences the functioning of other resident cell types of the epidermal compartment, such as the Langerhans cells and the melanocytes. A possibility of inhibiting cutaneous contact hypersensitivity by the use of calcium transport inhibitors has been shown (32). There is evidence that the calcium gradient is altered after barrier disruption by UV irradiation (Fig. 6). As UVR also brings about immunosuppression and initiates an increased pigmentation, particularly in darker human phototypes, the role of calcium in modulating the activities of Langerhans cells and melanocytes are worth investigating. Calcium is known to trigger Beta Defensins 2 and 3 in the human keratinocytes (33). How the sentinel cells and Beta Defensin production are altered in

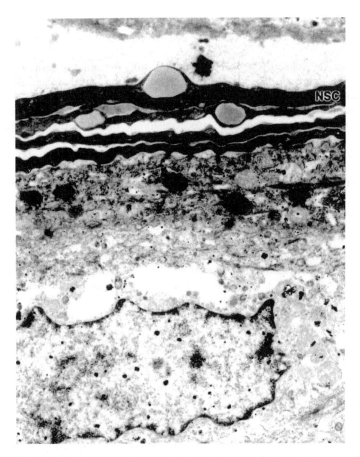

Figure 6 Electron micrograph showing loss of the calcium gradient in murine epidermis 72 hours post-UVB irradiation. Note the formation of a new SC (NSC) containing lipid droplets below the damaged epidermis (not in field). The new SG shows an abundance of LBs, and large precipitates of calcium (*arrows*). *Source*: Photograph by kind courtesy of Dr. Lars Halkier-Sorensen, from unpublished work (Halkier-Sorensen and Menon).

psoriatic lesions with their characteristically increased calcium concentrations, and whether these parameters can be modulated by manipulating the epidermal calcium by treatments including occlusive therapy (34) and/or influencing calcium binding proteins should be of considerable therapeutic interest.

ACKNOWLEDGMENTS

We acknowledge valuable editorial help from Sheri Lenc, and comments on an earlier draft by Ken Femgold. Dr. Halkier-Sorensen kindly provided an unpublished micrograph (Fig. 6), and permission to use it in this chapter.

REFERENCES

1. Hennings H, Michael D, Cheng C, Steinert P, Holbrook K, Yuspa SH. Calcium regulation of growth and differentiation of mouse epidermal cells in culture. Cell 1980; 19:245–254.

2. Hennings H, Holbrook K, Steinert P, Yuspa SH. Growth and differentiation of mouse epidermal cells in culture: effects of extracellular calcium. Curr Probl Dermatol 1980; 10:3–25.

3. Yuspa SH, Kilkenny AE, Steinert PM, Roop DR. Expression of murine epidermal differentiation markers is tightly regulated by restricted extracellular calcium concentration in vitro. J Cell Biol 1989; 109:1207–1217.

4. Menon GK, Grayson S, Elias PM. Ionic calcium reservoirs in mammalian epidermis: ultrastructural localization by ion-capture cytochemistry. J Invest Dermatol 1985; 84:509–512.

5. Whitfield JF. Calcium: Cell Cycle Driver, Differentiator and Killer. Austin, Texas: Landes Biosciences, 1997:164.

6. Forslind B. Quantitative X-ray microanalysis of skin. Acta Dermatol Venereol 1987; 134(suppl):1–8.

7. Malmquist KG, Carlsson LE, Forslind B, Roomans GM. Proton and electron microprobe analysis of human skin. Nuclear Inst Meth Phys Res 1984; 3:611–617.

8. Behne MJ, Barry N, Hanson K, Gratton E, Mauro T. Calcium fluorescence lifetime imaging in ex vivo skin II [abstr]. J Invest Dermatol 2004; 122:A81.

9. Mauro T, Bench C, Sidderas-Haddad E, Feingold K, Elias PM. Acute barrier perturbation abolishes the Ca^{2+} and K^+ gradients in murine epidermis: quantitative measurements using PIXIE. J Invest Dermatol 1998; 111:1198–1201.

10. Shimizu-Nishikawa K, Miller L. Calcium regulation of epidermal differentiation in the frog, Xenopus laevis. J Exp Zool 1991; 260:165–169.

11. Menon GK, Feingold KR, Man M-Q, Schaude M, Elias PM. Structural basis for the barrier abnormality following inhibition of HMG CoA reductase in murine epidermis. J Invest Dermatol 1992; 98:209–219.

12. Menon GK, Elias PM, Feingold KR. Integrity of the permeability barrier is crucial for maintenance of the epidermal calcium gradient. Br J Dermatol 1994; 130:139–147.

13. Menon GK, Elias PM. Ultrastructural localization of calcium in psoriatic and normal human epidermis. Arch Dermatol 1991; 127:57–63.

14. Elias PM, Crumrine D, Rassner U, Hachem J-P, Menon GK, Man W, Choy MHW, Leypoldt L, Feingold KR, Williams ML. Basis for abnormal desquamation and permeability barrier dysfunction in RXLI. J Invest Dermatol 2004; 122:314–319.

15. Fairley JA. Calcium metabolism and the pathogenesis of dermatologic diseases. Semin Dermatol 1991; 10:225–231.

16. Menon GK, Elias PM, Lee SH, Feingold KR. Localization of calcium in murine epidermis following disruption and repair of the permeability barrier. Cell Tissue Res 1992; 270:503–512.

17. Lee SH, Elias PM, Feingold KR, Mauro T. A role for ions in barrier recovery after acute perturbation. J Invest Dermatol 1994; 102:976–979.

18. Grubauer G, Elias PM, Feingold KR. Transdermal water loss: the signal for recovery of barrier structure and function. J Lipid Res 1989; 30:323–333.

19. Lee SH, Elias PM, Proksch E, Menon GK, Man M-Q, Feingold KR. Calcium and potassium are important regulators of barrier homeostasis in murine epidermis. J Clin Invest 1992; 89:530–538.

20. Menon GK, Price LF, Bommannan DB, Elias PM, Feingold KR. Selective obliteration of the epidermal calcium gradient leads to enhanced lamellar body secretion. J Invest Dermatol 1994; 102:789–795.

21. Elias PM, Ahn SK, Brown BE, Crumrine D, Feingold KR. Origin of the epidermal calcium gradient: regulation by barrier status and role of active vs. passive mechanisms. J Invest Dermatol 2002; 119:1269–1274.

22. Halkier-Sorensen L, Menon GK, Elias PM, Thestrup-Pederson K, Feingold KR. Cutaneous barrier function after cold exposure in hairless mice: a model to demonstrate how cold interferes with barrier homeostasis among workers in the fish-processing industry. Br J Dermatol 1995; 132:391–401.

23. Elias PM, Nau P, Hanley K, Cullander C, Crumrine D, Bench G, Sideras-Haddad E, Mauro T, Williams ML, Feingold KR. Formation of the epidermal calcium gradient coincides with key milestones of barrier ontogenesis in the rodent. J Invest Dermatol 1998; 110:399–404.
24. Vicanova J, Boelsma E, Mommaas AM, Kempenaar JA, Forslind B, Pallon J, Egelrud T, Koerten HK, Ponec M. Normalization of epidermal calcium distribution profile in reconstructed human epidermis is related to improvement of terminal differentiation and stratum corneum barrier formation. J Invest Dermatol 1998; 111:97–106.
25. Elias PM, Ahn SK, Denda M, Brown BE, Crumrine D, Kimutai LK, Komuves L, Lee SH, Feingold KR. Modulations in epidermal calcium regulate the expression of differentiation-specific markers. J Invest Dermatol 2002; 119:1128–1136.
26. Meldolesi J, Grohovaz F. Total calcium ultrastructure: advances in excitable cells. Cell Calcium 2001; 30:1–8.
27. Lee SH, Choi EH, Feingold KR, Jiang S, Ahn SK. Iontophoresis itself on hairless mouse skin induces the loss of epidermal calcium gradient without skin barrier impairment. J Invest Dermatol 1998; 111:39–43.
28. Turksen K, Troy T-C. Overexpression of the calcium sensing receptor accelerates epidermal differentiation and permeability barrier formation in vivo. Mech Dev 2003; 120: 733–744.
29. Brown EM. The extracellular calcium sensing receptor: central mediator of systemic calcium homeostasis. Ann Rev Nutr 2000; 20:507–533.
30. Brown EM, MacLeod RJ. Extracellular calcium sensing and extracellular calcium signaling. Physiol Rev 2001; 81:239–297.
31. Diezel W, Gruner S, Diaz LA, Anhalt GJ. Inhibition of cutaneous contact hypersensitivity by calcium transport inhibitors Lanthanum and Diltiazem. J Invest Dermatol 1989; 93: 322–326.
32. Pernet IM, Reymermier C, Guezennec A, Branks J-E, Guesnet J, Perrier E, Dezutter-Dambuyant C, Schmitt D, Viac J. Calcium triggers B-defensin (hBD-2 and hBD-3) and chemokine macrophage inflammatory protein-3 expression in monolayers of activated human keratinocytes. Exp Dermatol 2003; 12:755–760.
33. Hwang SM, Ann SK, Menon GK, Choi EH, Lee SH. Basis of occlusive therapy in psoriasis: correcting defects in permeability barrier and calcium gradient. Int Natl J Dermatol 2001; 40:223–231.

19

The Role of the Primary Cytokines, TNF, IL-1, and IL-6, in Permeability Barrier Homeostasis

Biao Lu, Peter M. Elias, and Kenneth R. Feingold
Department of Medicine and Dermatology, VA Medical Center, University of California, San Francisco, California, U.S.A.

INTRODUCTION

Over the last two decades studies have demonstrated that keratinocytes are capable of producing a wide array of cytokines. These cytokines play key roles in regulating epidermal function, and increase cytokines' participation in the pathogenesis of skin diseases. In this review we will focus on the role of the disruption of the cutaneous permeability barrier in increasing the secretion of TNF, IL-1, and IL-6, and the role of these cytokines in regulating permeability barrier homeostasis and inducing cutaneous inflammation.

INTERLEUKIN-1 FAMILY

General

IL-1 alpha and IL-1 beta are distinct gene products with 25% amino acid homology that interact with the same cellular receptors and have essentially identical biological properties (1). However, there are differences in the potency of IL-1 alpha and IL-1 beta in inducing certain effects. IL-1 is produced by a wide variety of cells including macrophages, endothelial cells, fibroblasts, lymphocytes, and keratinocytes (1–3). In most cell types, IL-1 beta is the predominant form of IL-1(1). However, in keratinocytes, IL-1 alpha predominates (3,4).

The synthesis of IL-1 is regulated at both transcriptional and translational steps that are under separate control (1). Other cytokines (TNF, GMCSF), and even IL-1 itself stimulate the production of IL-1, affecting both transcription and translation (1). Conversely, several cytokines (IL-4, IL-6, TGF beta) suppress IL-1 transcription (1). In most cells IL-1 genes are not constitutively expressed; however, in keratinocytes IL-1 alpha is constitutively produced at relatively high levels (3,4).

Both forms of IL-1 are initially synthesized as a pro–IL-1 31-kDa precursor without a defined signal peptide (1). Pro–IL-1 alpha is biologically active, whereas pro–IL-1 beta is inactive until it is cleaved to the mature 17-kDa form by a cysteine protease, interleukin-1 beta converting enzyme (ICE) (1). IL-1 alpha is processed to its mature form by a calcium-dependent protease, calpain. A significant portion of the pro–IL-I initially remains cell associated. The secretion of IL-1 is stimulated by endotoxin and cytokines (5). Cellular necrosis and apoptosis can also result in the release of IL-1 (6). In monocytes the ICE has been shown to cleave IL-1 beta to its active form (7,8). In addition, pro–IL-1 beta may also be cleaved to an active form by various proteases present in inflammatory tissues, such as plasmin, cathepsin G, collagenase, and serine proteases (1).

Both IL-1 alpha and IL-1 beta bind to the same cell-surface receptors (1,9). There are two major IL-1 receptors. The type I IL-1 receptor is an 80-kDa protein found in a variety of tissues including lymphocytes, endothelial cells, hepatocytes, and keratinocytes (1,9). The type II IL-1 receptor is a 60-kDa protein that is a member of the Ig superfamily and is present on B cells, neutrophils, and macrophages (1,9). There is 28% amino acid homology between the extracellular domains of the type I and II receptors, while the cytoplasmic domains are very different. The type I and II receptors contain 213 and 29 intracellular amino acids, respectively, making the type II receptor a "decoy" receptor that binds to IL-1 alpha and IL-1 beta, but elicits no biological response. In general, IL-1 alpha binds with higher affinity to the type I receptor, while IL-1 beta binds with higher affinity to the type II receptor.

The biological effects of IL-1 are pleiotropic, affecting the immune system and almost all other organ systems. The main systemic effects of IL-1 include fever, anorexia, malaise, and the production of the acute phase response (1,2). Of particular relevance to the epidermis, IL-1 has been shown to stimulate inflammation and to mediate the inflammatory response. In addition, IL-1 stimulates epidermal lipid synthesis, which may be important in permeability barrier homeostasis (10).

IL-1ra is an 18- to 25-kDa protein, which is a member of the IL-1 family (1,11). The size of IL-1ra depends on its degree of glycosylation, which does not affect its activity (2). IL-1ra has a 19% amino acid homology with IL-1 alpha and a 26% amino acid homology with IL-1 beta (1,11). IL-1ra binds to both the type I and II IL-1 receptors, but has no agonist activity, and has been shown to inhibit the ability of both IL-1 alpha and IL-1 beta to stimulate receptor activity (1,11). Because of the exquisite sensitivity of target tissues to small amounts of IL-1, excess quantities of IL-1ra must be present to effectively block IL-1 activity. The ratio of IL-1ra to IL-1 necessary to block 50% of the IL-1 response varies from 10 to 500 (1,11).

IL-1ra is produced in a variety of cells that also produce IL-1 alpha and IL-1 beta (for example monocytes and keratinocytes) (1,11). While IL-1ra is often produced at the same time as IL-1 alpha or IL-1 beta, a number of studies have demonstrated that the production of IL-1 and IL-1ra can be regulated independently (12).

IL-1 in the Epidermis

Primary keratinocyte cultures, transformed keratinocyte lines, and squamous cell cancer lines have all been shown to produce biologically active IL-1 (3). The mRNAs for both IL-1 alpha and beta are present in keratinocytes. However, while both IL-1 alpha and beta proteins are present in keratinocytes, only IL-1 alpha is present in a biologically active form (3). All of the immunoreactive IL-1 beta is in the pro–31-kDa form, which, as noted above, is not biologically active (13). Some IL-1 alpha is also present in the 31-kDa form, but in contrast, as discussed above, the 31-kDa form of IL-1 alpha displays biological activity (13). Although keratinocytes do not possess the protease ICE, which converts IL-1 beta into its active mature form, other extracellular proteases present in inflamed tissues and damaged stratum corneum could generate mature active IL-1 beta (13). Additionally, normal stratum corneum contains an enzyme, stratum corneum chymotryptic enzyme that has been shown to cleave IL-1 beta in an active molecule, although the cleavage sites differ from those attacked by ICE (14,15).

IL-1 production by keratinocytes increases in response to a variety of stimulants including mitogens (concanavalin A, phytohemagglutinin), tumor promoters (PMA), UV irradiation, and thermal energy (16–19). Additionally, cytokines such as TNF and GMCSF also increase IL-1 production in keratinocytes (20). Induction of keratinocyte differentiation with calcium treatment neither decreases nor markedly increases IL-1 levels suggesting that both differentiated and undifferentiated keratinocytes are capable of producing IL-1 (18).

Keratinocytes in culture also produce a variant form of IL-lra that contains seven additional amino acid residues at the N terminus (21,22). The first four amino acids are identical to the leader sequence of the monocyte form, while the remaining three amino acids are different. Because of the absence of the signal sequence, keratinocyte IL-lra is not secreted and remains intracellular (11,21). The role of intracellular IL-lra is unknown. The production of IL-1 alpha, beta, and IL-lra may be independently regulated. Keratinocyte differentiation stimulates IL-lra production without altering the IL-1 production (21).

In intact animals, IL-1 alpha and beta have been localized to the epidermis using assays of biological activity, ELISA's, Western blotting, or immunohistochemical localization at both the light and electron microscopic levels (23–29). Both diffuse cytosolic as well as membranous intercellular patterns of immunostaining for IL-1 alpha have been observed in the nucleated layers of the epidermis. Similar to cultured keratinocytes, in normal epidermis most of the IL-1 biological activity is accounted for by IL-1 alpha (25,27,28,30,31). In normal epidermis, IL-1 alpha mRNA is present indicating constituitive expression. In contrast, IL-1 beta mRNA is not abundantly expressed in normal epidermis (25,32). IL-1 alpha and beta proteins are present in all cell layers of the epidermis, but there is enrichment in the outer epidermis (stratum corneum and stratum granulosum) (4,18,23–27,33). Large quantities of IL-1 alpha are present in the stratum corneum (23,24,31). IL-lra is also present in large quantities in normal epidermis. Moreover, similar to IL-1 alpha and beta, IL-lra is concentrated in the outer epidermis.

IL-1 produces a wide variety of effects on keratinocytes. In some but not all studies, IL-1 has been shown to stimulate keratinocyte proliferation (20,34–36). In addition, IL-1 is a chemoattractant for keratinocytes (37). IL-1 also stimulates IL-6, IL-8, and GMCSF, as well as further IL-1 production by keratinocytes (38–40). This could result in a cascade effect with IL-1 having both direct effects and indirect effects mediated by other cytokines. In addition, by further stimulating IL-1 production the effects of IL-1 could be amplified.

Studies have suggested that the number of IL-1 receptors in normal epidermis is relatively small but increases with differentiation (18). Most of the IL-1 receptors in the epidermis are the type II 60-kDa "decoy" receptors, which would decrease the ability of IL-1 to activate keratinocytes (41). The number of IL-1 receptors, both full length and decoy, can increase markedly in disease states such as psoriasis.

The large quantities of pre-formed IL-1 in the epidermis provide a mechanism by which injuries could cause the rapid release of IL-1, which could then induce cellular responses, such as inflammation, enhanced cellular defense, wound repair, and so on, that would benefit the host. Underlying this hypothesis is the observation that most IL-1 remains cell associated, and under normal circumstances is not released but rather is harmlessly desquamated (42). Injuries to the stratum corneum result in the release of IL-1, in a non-energy-dependent manner, which could then either initiate and/or facilitate the response to the injury.

TNF FAMILY

General

TNF alpha and TNF beta (lymphotoxin), which are 30% homologous at the amino acid level, are the predominant members of a family of 10 proteins that comprise the TNF family (43). TNF alpha and beta bind to the same cellular receptors and have almost identical biological activity. TNF alpha is produced by many cells including monocytes/macrophages, neutrophils, lymphocytes, endothelial cells, and keratinocytes (43). TNF beta is produced by lymphocytes and has not been observed in keratinocytes or epidermis (43). TNF along with IL-1 are considered primary cytokines because they can initiate a cytokine cascade.

The production of TNF alpha in macrophages is stimulated by endotoxin both at the level of transcription and translation (43). TNF alpha is initially synthesized as a 26-kDa precursor protein that adheres to the plasma membrane (43). Evidence suggests that the active portion of the molecule is exposed on the outside of the cell enabling it to interact and activate adjacent cells. The mature 17-kDa form of TNF alpha is released from the plasma membrane after proteolytic cleavage, by a specific metalloprotease (43). Secreted TNF alpha is a soluble trimer of identical (17 kDa) subunits.

There are two distinct TNF receptors, 55 kDa and 75 kDa (43). The extracellular domains of both of these receptors are similar while the intracytoplasmic domains are unrelated. Most TNF responses, such as metabolic alterations, cytokine production, increased gene transcription, and apoptosis are mediated by the 55 kDa receptor. The 75 kDa receptor mediates T-cell development, the proliferation of cytotoxic T-lymphocytes, as well as cell death (44,45). Although most cell types express both receptors, the proportion of each receptor varies from tissue to tissue (43). As with IL-1 receptors, TNF receptors can be shed from cells and act as soluble inhibitors of TNF action. The mode of signal transduction induced by TNF appears to involve several pathways.

TNF has pleiotropic biological actions, which overlap considerably with those of IL-1 (46). TNF stimulates the production of a number of other cytokines including IL-1, IL-6, IL-8, and GMCSF (43,46). Additionally, TNF has been shown to alter lipid metabolism in liver, adipose tissue, and other sites (47,48).

TNF and the Epidermis

Multiple agents, such as endotoxin, UV light, and urushiol (the substance responsible for poison ivy/oak), can induce TNF alpha production in cultured keratinocytes (49). In intact animals, studies have demonstrated immunohistochemical staining for TNF alpha in the epidermis, predominantly in the stratum spinosum and granulosum (50). However, under normal basal conditions less TNF alpha is present in the epidermis. Similarly, in situ hybridization and Northern blotting studies have detected only small amounts of TNF alpha mRNA in normal epidermis (51). Importantly, following UV irradiation of intact skin or other injuries staining for TNF alpha increases and TNF is also seen in the basal layer (50).

Only the 55-kDa receptor is present on keratinocytes (52). TNF stimulates IL-1, IL-6, IL-8, and TGF production by keratinocytes (53). Thus, TNF, like IL-1, is capable of inducing a cascade of cytokines. In tissue culture, TNF alpha stimulates keratinocyte differentiation and inhibits proliferation (54). However, chronic TNF administration in vivo has been shown to stimulate epidermal proliferation (55).

INTERLEUKIN-6 FAMILY

General

Interleukin-6 (IL-6) belongs to a large family of cytokines, which include IL-6, IL-11, oncostatin M, leukemia inhibitory factor, ciliary neurotropic factor, cardiotropin 1, and novel neutrophin 1/B-lymphocyte–stimulating factor 3 (56–58). All members of this family have a molecular weight of 20 to 24 kDa in their non-glycosylated form (58). The homology among the members is very low and does not exceed 30%. However, they share a similar tertiary structure consisting of four antiparallel alpha-helices and exhibit high-affinity binding to their respective receptor complexes (58). In most cases, these cytokine–receptor complexes share a common signal transducing receptor component, the gpl30 molecule (56,58). Formation of these complexes triggers a cascade of intracellular events. Two pathways are usually activated, including the JAK/STAT and Ras/Raf-MAPK (59,60). An important characteristic of IL-6 family is overlapping biological activities (59). This functional redundancy may be explained by the shared usage of the signal transducer gpl30 in the multichain cytokine–receptor complexes (see below).

Human IL-6 is a variably glycosylated 22 to 27 kDa glycoprotein. The full-length cDNA of human IL-6 encodes a 212 amino acid molecule with a 28 amino acid signal peptide and an 184 amino acid mature protein (61–63). An alternative splice variant form of IL-6 (exon 2 deletion) has also been identified (64). This exon 2-deleted variant lacks a binding site for IL-6 transducing receptor gp130 and thus has no biological activity. Mouse and rat IL-6 have also been cloned and have approximately 40% amino acid identity to human IL-6 (65–67). Unlike human IL-6, mouse and rat IL-6 lack potential N-linked glycosylation sites. The presence or absence of glycosylation has no effect on activity. Many cells have been shown to produce IL-6, including monocytes/macrophages, neutrophiles, eosinophils, fibroblasts, endothelial cells, keratinocytes, mast cells, T cells, adipocytes, neurons, and many tumor cell lines (61,64,65,68 71). IL-6 production is generally correlated with cell activation, usually as a result of IL-1, TNF alpha, transforming growth factor beta, or lipopolysaccharide stimulation.

The receptors for IL-6 are complexes of two transmembrane glycoproteins: IL-6 receptor (IL-6R) and gpl30 (56,72,73). The interaction of IL-6 with its membrane receptors has revealed sequential events of receptor activation. First IL-6 binds to its membrane bound receptor IL-6R, and this IL-6/IL-6R complex then interacts with and recruits two 130-kDa signal-transducing molecules to form a functional signaling complex (56,73). Although most cell types express gpl30, the cytokine-specific IL-6R expression is much more limited (56). Therefore, the cellular response is largely determined by the regulated expression of cytokine-specific receptor and cytokine.

An intriguing feature of IL-6 receptor signaling pathway is the existence of soluble IL-6 receptors. IL-6R can shed from cellular surfaces by proteolysis. The soluble form of IL-6R retains IL-6–binding activity, and is able to associate with gpl30 on target cells. Thus, the IL-6 and soluble IL-6R complex may activate cells that express gpl30 but not IL-6R, a process that has been termed trans-signaling (74,75). Through trans-signaling, the potential IL-6 target cells may extend to cells devoid of IL-6R.

The biological effects of IL-6 are pleiotropic, affecting various aspects of host defense, immune response, and the growth or differentiation of numerous cell types (56). The major effects of IL-6 include regulating the immune response, stimulating the acute-phase reaction, and increasing IgA antibody production (76,77). In addition, IL-6 stimulates lipid synthesis in the liver (48,78–80).

IL-6 in Epidermis

Keratinocytes, which comprise 95% of the cells in the epidermis, have been shown to be the primary source of IL-6 in the epidermis, whereas macrophages, Langerhans cells, and fibroblasts in the dermis represent a minor source of this cytokine (81,82). In normal epidermis, IL-6 and IL-6 receptor immunoreactivities are preferentially localized in low amounts to keratinocytes in the basal, granular, and horny layers, but not in the spinous layer, suggesting cell-specific localization and a functional requirement (82). IL-6 mainly produces a mitogenic effect on keratinocytes (69,82,83).

IL-6 production by keratinocytes increases in response to a variety of agents including cytokines (IL-1 and TNF alpha), skin irritants, thermal injury, and UV light (53,69,83–86). In addition, increased levels of IL-6 are also present in several skin pathological conditions such as psoriasis and lupus erythematosus (69,87). In acute inflammatory settings, epidermal IL-6 production seems to be highly dependent upon the release of TNF alpha and preformed IL-1 alpha in keratinocytes; however, the exact mechanisms accounting for the increased IL-6 production in pathological conditions remains largely unknown (69,87).

EFFECT OF BARRIER DISRUPTION ON CYTOKINE HOMEOSTASIS IN THE EPIDERMIS

Acute barrier disruption by either acetone treatment or tape stripping, or chronic barrier disruption produced in essential fatty acid–deficient mice, increases epidermal mRNA levels of TNF alpha, IL-1 alpha, IL-1 beta, and IL-1ra (88–90). The time course of the increase in mRNAs differs with TNF reaching maximal levels one hour after acute disruption of the barrier while IL-1 alpha, IL-1 beta, and IL-lra mRNA levels peak at four hours (88). In each case the mRNA levels returned to control values by eight hours following acute barrier disruption. TNF alpha and IL-1 beta mRNA levels increased by 10 to 100 fold, while IL-1 alpha and IL-lra mRNA levels increased only two- to five-fold (88,89). This difference is probably due to the high levels of IL-1 alpha and IL-lra expressions in the epidermis under basal conditions as compared with the very low levels of TNF alpha and IL-1 beta mRNA.

Using a more sensitive multiprobe RNase protection assay it was observed that normal mouse epidermis expresses IL-6 in addition to TNF alpha and members of the IL-1 family (91). Following acute barrier disruption by tape stripping, TNF alpha, IL-1 alpha, IL-1 beta, and IL-6 mRNAs increase (91). In contrast, mRNAs encoding TNF beta, IL-2, IL-3, IL-4, and IL-5 were not detected in the epidermis either under basal conditions or following barrier disruption using RNase protection assays (91). Similarly, in a chronic model of barrier disruption, essential fatty acid deficiency, epidermal mRNA levels of TNF alpha, IL-1 alpha, IL-1 beta, and IL-6 were increased (88). In the dermis only IL-1 beta mRNA levels increased following barrier disruption.

With regards to cytokine receptors using RNase protection assays, the 80-kDa IL-1 receptor and the 75-kDa TNF receptor were not detectable in the epidermis (91). The 60-kDa IL-1 receptor (decoy receptor) and the IL-6 receptor were present in the epidermis, but their mRNA levels did not change following either acute or chronic barrier disruption (91). In contrast, the 55-kDa TNF receptor mRNA levels increased in the epidermis (91). Low levels of 55-kDa TNF receptors were present in the dermis, but were not increased following barrier disruption (91). The presence of receptors in the epidermis and dermis suggest that these tissues are capable of responding to cytokines in an autocrine or paracrine fashion. This suggests that epidermal cytokines produced after barrier disruption may initiate a cytokine cascade, which could regulate the epidermal response to barrier disruption and/or induce pathophysiologic abnormalities.

Further insights into the effect of barrier disruption on epidermal cytokine production were obtained by examining the effects of providing an artificial barrier by occlusion with a water-impermeable latex membrane. Occlusion of essential fatty acid–deficient mice for 24 to 48 hours lowered the epidermal mRNA levels of TNF alpha, IL-1 alpha, and IL-1ra to nearly control values, but had no effect on IL-1 beta mRNA levels (92). The absence of an effect of occlusion on IL-1 beta may reflect the origin of this cytokine in Langerhans cells, whereas the other cytokines studied are primarily produced by keratinocytes in the epidermis. In contrast to the results seen in animals with a chronic barrier disruption, occlusion did not inhibit the increase in TNF alpha, IL-1 alpha, IL-1 beta, or IL-1ra following acute barrier disruption by either acetone treatment or tape stripping (92). The increase in the 55-kDa TNF receptor in the epidermis that occurs with barrier disruption was also not blocked by occlusion (91). These results suggest that the acute increase in epidermal cytokine production may not be solely related to permeability barrier homeostasis, but also related to stratum corneum injury. Interestingly, while occlusion of normal mice with a water-impermeable membrane does not affect the mRNA levels of TNF alpha, IL-1 beta, or IL-1ra, occlusion dramatically decreases the mRNA levels of IL-1 alpha (92). Additionally, in mice with a chronic disruption of the barrier (EFAD) occlusion has been shown to decrease cytokine mRNA levels suggesting that both permeability barrier status and stratum corneum injury effect cytokine production (92).

The epidermis and, in particular, the stratum corneum contain large quantities of IL-1 alpha. It has been postulated that the epidermal pool of IL-1 alpha serves as a protective coating that is released upon injury to the outer layers of the skin. We used immunohistochemistry to determine the localization of IL-1 alpha following acute and chronic barrier disruptions in mice. In control mice, IL-1 alpha is present in the dermis and nucleated layers of the epidermis in a diffuse generalized pattern (4). In essential fatty acid–deficient mice (chronic barrier disruption) IL-1 alpha is present in all epidermal layers and the dermis with prominent stratum corneum staining (4). After acute barrier disruption with either acetone treatment or tape stripping, IL-1 alpha staining is increased throughout the epidermis and dermis within 10 minutes and remains elevated over controls for two to four hours but decreases to basal levels by 24 hours. Moreover, intense perinuclear basal cell staining is evident by 10 minutes after barrier disruption, which persists for four hours. Furthermore, prolonged occlusion of normal mice not only decreases epidermal mRNA levels, but also decreases basal immunostaining for IL-1 alpha, and blunts the expected increase in IL-1 alpha that usually is seen after acute barrier disruption (4).

The immediate increase in cutaneous IL-1 alpha following barrier disruption suggests that IL-1 alpha is released from a preformed pool in the epidermis. To address this hypothesis we showed that an increase in IL-1 alpha staining occurs after tape stripping even when the skin is maintained ex vivo at 4°C, conditions under which new protein synthesis would be markedly diminished (4). We observed that the intense perinuclear staining was not seen under these conditions, indicating that this intracellular staining, which is evident at 37°C, may represent newly synthesized IL-1 alpha (4). Furthermore, tape stripping stimulates the release of mature 17-kDa IL-1 alpha ex vivo, as measured by Western blotting and ELISA (4). Using these techniques, further studies demonstrated that a portion of this preformed pool of IL-1 alpha resides in the stratum corneum of normal mice. This suggests that acute barrier disruption increases cutaneous IL-1 alpha by triggering the release of IL-1 alpha from preformed pools and by stimulating IL-1 alpha production. The increased levels of IL-1 alpha in the epidermis may initiate the barrier repair process or signal an immune/inflammatory reaction.

With regards to TNF alpha, the increase in epidermal mRNA levels is accompanied by a simultaneous increase in the active 17-kDa form of TNF alpha as determined by Western-blot analysis (93). Furthermore, using immunohistochemistry it was found that (i) TNF alpha protein is present in normal mouse epidermis and is primarily localized to the upper nucleated layers where it displays a diffuse cytosolic pattern; (ii) acute barrier disruption results in TNF alpha staining that is more intense throughout all of the nucleated layers of the epidermis; (iii) the increase in TNF alpha staining occurs within two hours after barrier disruption, although, in some cases, staining was increased almost immediately after barrier disruption; and (iv) increased TNF alpha staining was present in the stratum corneum of essential fatty acid deficient mice (93). Thus, similar to IL-1 alpha, the increased levels of TNF alpha may play a role in barrier repair processes and/or signal an immune/inflammatory reaction.

With regards to IL-6, the increases in mRNA following barrier disruption were also accompanied by increased protein levels observed by both Western blotting and immunohistochemistry (82). The increase was observed in all nucleated layers of the epidermis (82). Additionally, IL-6 receptor protein levels also increased following barrier disruption (note mRNA levels of the receptor did not change) and was present in all nucleated layers. Notably, occlusion did not block the increase in either IL-6 or the IL-6 receptor.

ROLE IN BARRIER REPAIR

KO Mouse Studies

Studies in our laboratory demonstrated that in TNF type I (55 kDa) receptor knockout mice, barrier recovery following acute disruption of the barrier by acetone treatment, SDS treatment, or tape stripping was very similar to that in wild-type mice (94). In contrast, Jensen et al. (95) observed a delay in barrier repair following tape stripping in TNF type I receptor knockout mice but no change in TNF type II receptor knockout mice (95). The basis for this difference in results is not clear. In IL-1 type I (80 kDa) receptor knockout mice, we observed a delay in barrier recovery following acute barrier disruption with acetone treatment, SDS treatment, or tape stripping (94). Studies by Jensen et al. have also demonstrated a delay in barrier repair in IL-1 type I receptor deficient mice (96). Furthermore, recent studies have shown that barrier repair is delayed in IL-6 knockout mice (82). Additionally, studies have shown that the topical application and/or subcutaneous injection of TNF, IL-1, or IL-6 following barrier disruption accelerates barrier repair (82). Taken together, these results suggest that the increase in TNF, IL-1, and IL-6 following barrier disruption plays an important role in the barrier repair process that parallels the role of these cytokines in inducing inflammation.

Aged Mice

Previous studies have shown that the restoration of barrier function following acute barrier disruption is delayed in aged mice (97). Moreover, studies demonstrated that the expression of IL-1 alpha, but not TNF alpha, was reduced in aged mice both in the basal state and following barrier disruption (98). Moreover, treatment of aged mice with IL-1 improves barrier recovery following acute disruption (99). This IL-1–induced improvement in barrier recovery was associated with an increase in lamellar body secretion and the amount of organelle content at the stratum granulosum stratum corneum interface (99). In cultured keratinocytes, similar to what has been observed in other tissues such as the liver, IL-1 alpha increased fatty acid and cholesterol synthesis (99). One can speculate that this increase in lipid synthesis accounts for the increase in lamellar body formation and secretion, and the subsequent improvement in barrier homeostasis.

PATHOPHYSIOLOGIC CONSEQUENCES

As noted above, permeability barrier disruption and/or injuries to the stratum corneum result in a rapid and marked increase in the production and secretion of IL-1, TNF, and IL-6. These cytokines are well recognized to induce an inflammatory response both by their direct actions and by stimulating the production of other cytokines. In addition IL-1, TNF, and IL-6 stimulate epidermal cell proliferation. Thus, it is likely that the inflammation and epidermal hyperplasia that occurs following permeability barrier disruption and other injuries to the stratum corneum are mediated by increases in IL-1, TNF, and/or IL-6. Therefore disease states characterized by abnormalities in permeability barrier function are likely to be associated with increased cytokine expression, which could be either the primary process inducing the cutaneous abnormalities or in some circumstances could exacerbate or prolong skin diseases that lead to barrier abnormalities.

SUMMARY

Barrier disruption produces a rapid increase in the levels of TNF, IL-1, and IL-6 in the epidermis. It is likely that these increases are beneficial resulting in the restoration of barrier function. However, if barrier disruption is prolonged or frequent these increases in cytokine production could have harmful effects leading to inflammation and epidermal hyperproliferation.

REFERENCES

1. Dinarello CA. Interleukin-1 and interleukin-1 antagonism. Blood 1991; 77:1627–1652.
2. Dayer JM, Burger D. Interleukin-1, tumor necrosis factor and their specific inhibitors. Eur Cytokine Netw 1994; 5:563–571.
3. Kupper TS, Ballard DW, Chua AO, McGuire JS, Flood PM, Horowitz MC, Langdon R, Lightfoot L, Gubler U. Human keratinocytes contain mRNA indistinguishable from monocyte interleukin 1 alpha and beta mRNA. Keratinocyte epidermal cell-derived thymocyte-activating factor is identical to interleukin 1. J Exp Med 1986; 164:2095–2100.
4. Wood LC, Elias PM, Calhoun C, Tsai JC, Grunfeld C, Feingold KR. Barrier disruption stimulates interleukin-1 alpha expression and release from a pre-formed pool in murine epidermis. J Invest Dermatol 1996; 106:397–403.
5. Rubartelli A, Cozzolino F, Talio M, Sitia R. A novel secretory pathway for interleukin-1 beta, a protein lacking a signal sequence. EMBO J 1990; 9:1503–1510.
6. Hogquist KA, Nett MA, Unanue ER, Chaplin DD. Interleukin 1 is processed and released during apoptosis. Proc Natl Acad Sci USA 1991; 88:8485–8489.
7. Cerretti DP, Kozlosky CJ, Mosley B, Nelson N, Van Ness K, Greenstreet TA, March CJ, Kronheim SR, Druck T, Cannizzaro LA, et al. Molecular cloning of the interleukin-1 beta converting enzyme. Science 1992; 256:97–100.
8. Thornberry NA, Bull HG, Calaycay JR, Chapman KT, Howard AD, Kostura MJ, Miller DK, Molineaux SM, Weidner JR, Aunins J, et al. A novel heterodimeric cysteine protease is required for interleukin-1 beta processing in monocytes. Nature 1992; 356: 768–774.
9. Dower SK, Qwarnstrom EE, Page RC, Blanton RA, Kupper TS, Raines E, Ross R, Sims JE. Biology of the interleukin-1 receptor. J Invest Dermatol 1990; 94:68S–73S.
10. Feingold KR. The regulation and role of epidermal lipid synthesis. Adv Lipid Res 1991; 24:57–82.
11. Arend WP. Interleukin 1 receptor antagonist. A new member of the interleukin 1 family. J Clin Invest 1991; 88:1445–1451.
12. Arend WP, Smith MF Jr, Janson RW, Joslin FG. IL-1 receptor antagonist and IL-1 beta production in human monocytes are regulated differently. J Immunol 1991; 147:1530–1536.
13. Mizutani H, Black R, Kupper TS. Human keratinocytes produce but do not process pro-interleukin-1 (IL-1) beta. Different strategies of IL-1 production and processing in monocytes and keratinocytes. J Clin Invest 1991; 87:1066–1071.
14. Nylander-Lundqvist E, Egelrud T. Formation of active IL-1 beta from pro-IL-1 beta catalyzed by stratum corneum chymotryptic enzyme in vitro. Acta Derm Venereol 1997; 77:203–206.
15. Nylander-Lundqvist E, Back O, Egelrud T. IL-1 beta activation in human epidermis. J Immunol 1996; 157:1699–1704.
16. Ansel JC, Luger TA, Lowry D, Perry P, Roop DR, Mountz JD. The expression and modulation of IL-1 alpha in murine keratinocytes. J Immunol 1988; 140:2274–2278.
17. Kupper TS, Chua AO, Flood P, McGuire J, Gubler U. Interleukin 1 gene expression in cultured human keratinocytes is augmented by ultraviolet irradiation. J Clin Invest 1987; 80:430–436.
18. Blanton RA, Kupper TS, McDougall LK, Dower S. Regulation of interleukin 1 and its receptor in human keratinocytes. Proc Natl Acad Sci USA 1989; 86:1273–1277.
19. Nozaki S, Abrams JS, Pearce MK, Sauder DN. Augmentation of granulocyte/macrophage colony-stimulating factor expression by ultraviolet irradiation is mediated by interleukin 1 in Pam 212 keratinocytes. J Invest Dermatol 1991; 97:10–14.
20. Partridge M, Chantry D, Turner M, Feldmann M. Production of interleukin-1 and interleukin-6 by human keratinocytes and squamous cell carcinoma cell lines. J Invest Dermatol 1991; 96:771–776.
21. Bigler CF, Norris DA, Weston WL, Arend WP. Interleukin-1 receptor antagonist production by human keratinocytes. J Invest Dermatol 1992; 98:38–44.

22. Gruaz-Chatellard D, Baumberger C, Saurat JH, Dayer JM. Interleukin 1 receptor antagonist in human epidermis and cultured keratinocytes. FEBS Lett 1991; 294: 137–140.

23. Gahring LC, Buckley A, Daynes RA. Presence of epidermal-derived thymocyte activating factor/interleukin 1 in normal human stratum corneum. J Clin Invest 1985; 76:1585–1591.

24. Hauser C, Saurat JH, Schmitt A, Jaunin F, Dayer JM. Interleukin 1 is present in normal human epidermis. J Immunol 1986; 136:3317–3323.

25. Demezuk S. IL-1/ETAF activity and undetectable H-1 beta mRNA and minimal IL-1 alpha mRNA levels in normal adult heat separated epidermis. Biochem Biophys Res Commun 1988; 156:463–469.

26. Didierjean L, Salomon D, Merot Y, Siegenthaler G, Shaw A, Dayer JM, Saurat JH. Localization and characterization of the interleukin 1 immunoreactive pool (IL-1 alpha and beta forms) in normal human epidermis. J Invest Dermatol 1989; 92:809–816.

27. Romero LI, Ikejima T, Pincus SH. In situ localization of interleukin-1 in normal and psoriatic skin. J Invest Dermatol 1989; 93:518–522.

28. Camp R, Fincham N, Ross J, Bird C, Gearing A. Potent inflammatory properties in human skin of interleukin-1 alpha-like material isolated from normal skin. J Invest Dermatol 1990; 94:735–741.

29. Anttila HS, Reitamo S, Erkko P, Miettinen A, Didierjean L, Saurat JH. Membrane and cytosolic interleukin-1 alpha and beta in normal human epidermal cells: variability of epitope exposure in immunohistochemistry. J Invest Dermatol 1990; 95:31–38.

30. Gruaz D, Didierjean L, Grassi J, Frobert Y, Dayer JM, Saurat JH. Interleukin 1 alpha and beta in psoriatic skin: enzymoimmunoassay, immunoblot studies and effect of systemic retinoids. Dermatologica 1989; 179:202–206.

31. Cooper KD, Hammerberg C, Baadsgaard O, Elder JT, Chan LS, Sauder DN, Voorhees JJ, Fisher G. IL-1 activity is reduced in psoriatic skin. Decreased IL-1 alpha and increased nonfunctional IL-1 beta. J Immunol 1990; 144:4593–4603.

32. Takacs L, Kovacs EJ, Smith MR, Young HA, Durum SK. Detection of IL-1 alpha and IL-1 beta gene expression by in situ hybridization. Tissue localization of IL-1 mRNA in the normal C57BL/6 mouse. J Immunol 1988; 141:3081–3095.

33. Hirao T, Aoki H, Yoshida T, Sato Y, Kamoda H. Elevation of interleukin 1 receptor antagonist in the stratum corneum of sun-exposed and ultraviolet B-irradiated human skin. J Invest Dermatol 1996; 106:1102–1107.

34. Ristow HJ. A major factor contributing to epidermal proliferation in inflammatory skin diseases appears to be interleukin 1 or a related protein. Proc Natl Acad Sci USA 1987; 84:1940–1944.

35. Sauder DN. Biologic properties of epidermal cell thymocyte-activating factor (ETAF). J Invest Dermatol 1985; 85:176s–179s.

36. Hancock GE, Kaplan G, Cohn ZA. Keratinocyte growth regulation by the products of immune cells. J Exp Med 1988; 168:1395–1402.

37. Martinet N, Harne LA, Grotendorst GR. Identification and characterization of chemoattractants for epidermal cells. J Invest Dermatol 1988; 90:122–126.

38. Kupper TS, Lee F, Birchall N, Clark S, Dower S. Interleukin 1 binds to specific receptors on human keratinocytes and induces granulocyte macrophage colony-stimulating factor mRNA and protein. A potential autocrine role for interleukin 1 in epidermis. J Clin Invest 1988; 82:1787–1792.

39. Larson C, Oppenheim J, Matsushima K. Il-1 or TNF alpha stimulates the production of MAP/IL-8 by normal fibroblasts and keratinocytes. J Invest Dermatol 1989; 92:467–471.

40. Kirnbauer R, Kock A, Schwarz T, Urbanski A, Krutmann J, Borth W, Damm D, Shipley G, Ansel JC, Luger TA. IFN-beta 2, B cell differentiation factor 2, or hybridoma growth factor (IL-6) is expressed and released by human epidermal cells and epidermoid carcinoma cell lines. J Immunol 1989; 142:1922–1928.

41. Kupper TS, Groves RW. The interleukin-1 axis and cutaneous inflammation. J Invest Dermatol 1995; 105:62S–66S.

42. Kupper TS. Immune and inflammatory processes in cutaneous tissues. Mechanisms and speculations. J Clin Invest 1990; 86:1783–1789.
43. Vilcek J, Lee TH. Tumor necrosis factor. New insights into the molecular mechanisms of its multiple actions. J Biol Chem 1991; 266:7313–7316.
44. Tartaglia LA, Weber RF, Figari IS, Reynolds C, Palladino MA Jr, Goeddel DV. The two different receptors for tumor necrosis factor mediate distinct cellular responses. Proc Natl Acad Sci USA 1991; 88:9292–9296.
45. Heller RA, Song K, Fan N, Chang DJ. The p70 tumor necrosis factor receptor mediates cytotoxicity. Cell 1992; 70:47–56.
46. Grunfeld C, Palladino MA Jr. Tumor necrosis factor: immunologic, antitumor, metabolic, and cardiovascular activities. Adv Intern Med 1990; 35:45–71.
47. Grunfeld C, Soued M, Adi S, Moser AH, Dinarello CA, Feingold KR. Evidence for two classes of cytokines that stimulate hepatic lipogenesis: relationships among tumor necrosis factor, interleukin-1 and interferon-alpha. Endocrinology 1990; 127:46–54.
48. Feingold KR, Soued M, Serio MK, Moser AH, Dinarello CA, Grunfeld C. Multiple cytokines stimulate hepatic lipid synthesis in vivo. Endocrinology 1989; 125:267–274.
49. Kock A, Schwarz T, Kirnbauer R, Urbanski A, Perry P, Ansel JC, Luger TA. Human keratinocytes are a source for tumor necrosis factor alpha: evidence for synthesis and release upon stimulation with endotoxin or ultraviolet light. J Exp Med 1990; 172:1609–1614.
50. Oxholm A, Oxholm P, Staberg B, Bendtzen K. Immunohistological detection of interleukin 1-like molecules and tumor necrosis factor in human epidermis before and after UVB-irradiation in vivo. Br J Dermatol 1988; 118:369–376.
51. Majewski S, Hunzelmann N, Nischt R, Eckes B, Rudnicka L, Orth G, Krieg T, Jablonska S. TGF beta-1 and TNF alpha expression in the epidermis of patients with epidermodysplasia verruciformis. J Invest Dermatol 1991; 97:862–867.
52. Trefzer U, Brockhaus M, Loetscher H, Parlow F, Kapp A, Schopf E, Krutmann J. 55-kd tumor necrosis factor receptor is expressed by human keratinocytes and plays a pivotal role in regulation of human keratinocyte ICAM-1 expression. J Invest Dermatol 1991; 97:911–916.
53. Barker JN, Mitra RS, Griffiths CE, Dixit VM, Nickoloff BJ. Keratinocytes as initiators of inflammation. Lancet 1991; 337:211–214.
54. Pillai S, Bikle DD, Eessalu TE, Aggarwal BB, Elias PM. Binding and biological effects of tumor necrosis factor alpha on cultured human neonatal foreskin keratinocytes. J Clin Invest 1989; 83:816–821.
55. Piguet PF, Grau GE, Vassalli P. Subcutaneous perfusion of tumor necrosis factor induces local proliferation of fibroblasts, capillaries, and epidermal cells, or massive tissue necrosis. Am J Pathol 1990; 136:103–110.
56. Taga T, Kishimoto T. Gpl30 and the interleukin-6 family of cytokines. Annu Rev Immunol 1997; 15:797–819.
57. Miyajima A, Kinoshita T, Tanaka M, Kamiya A, Mukouyama Y, Hara T. Role of Oncostatin M in hematopoiesis and liver development. Cytokine Growth Factor Rev 2000; 11:177–183.
58. Bravo J, Heatti JK. Receptor recognition by gpl30 cytokines. EMBO J 2000; 19:2399–2411.
59. Taga T. Gpl30, a shared signal transducing receptor component for hematopoietic and neuropoietic cytokines. J Neurochem 1996; 67:1–10.
60. Hallek M, Neumann C, Schaffer M, Danhauser-Riedl S, von Bubnoff N, de Vos G, Druker B, Yasukawa K, Griffin J, Emmerich B. Signal transduction of interleukin-6 involves tyrosine phosphorylation of multiple cytosolic proteins and activation of Src-family kinases Fyn, Hck, and Lyn in multiple myeloma cell lines. Exp Hematol 1997; 25:1367–1377.
61. May LT, Helfgott DC, Sehgal PB. Anti-beta-interferon antibodies inhibit the increased expression of HLA-B7 mRNA in tumor necrosis factor-treated human fibroblasts: structural studies of the beta 2 interferon involved. Proc Natl Acad Sci USA 1986; 83: 8957–8961.

62. Hirano T, Yasukawa K, Harada H, Taga T, Watanabe Y, Matsuda T, Kashiwamura S, Nakajima K, Koyama K, Iwamatsu A, et al. Complementary DNA for a novel human interleukin (BSF-2) that induces B lymphocytes to produce immunoglobulin. Nature 1986; 324:73–76.

63. Zilberstein A, Ruggieri R, Korn JH, Revel M. Structure and expression of cDNA and genes for human interferon-beta-2, a distinct species inducible by growth-stimulatory cytokines. EMBO J 1986; 5:2529–2537.

64. Kestler DP, Agarwal S, Cobb I, Goldstein KM, Hall RE. Detection and analysis of an alternatively spliced isoform of interleukin-6 mRNA in peripheral blood mononuclear cells. Blood 1995; 86:4559–4567.

65. Chiu CP, Moulds C, Coffman RL, Rennick D, Lee F. Multiple biological activities are expressed by a mouse interleukin 6 cDNA clone isolated from bone marrow stromal cells. Proc Natl Acad Sci USA 1988; 85:7099–7103.

66. Van Snick J, Cayphas S, Szikora JP, Renauld JC, Van Roost E, Boon T, Simpson RJ. cDNA cloning of murine interleukin-HP1: homology with human interleukin 6. Eur J Immunol 1988; 18:193–197.

67. Northemann W, Braciak TA, Hattori M, Lee F, Fey GH. Structure of the rat interleukin 6 gene and its expression in macrophage-derived cells. J Biol Chem 1989; 264:16072–16082.

68. Xin X, Cai Y, Matsumoto K, Agui T. Endothelin-induced interleukin-6 production by rat aortic endothelial cells. Endocrinology 1995; 136:132–137.

69. Grossman RM, Krueger J, Yourish D, Granelli-Piperno A, Murphy DP, May LT, Kupper TS, Sehgal PB, Gottlieb AB. Interleukin 6 is expressed in high levels in psoriatic skin and stimulates proliferation of cultured human keratinocytes. Proc Natl Acad Sci USA 1989; 86:6367–6371.

70. Lacy P, Levi-Schaffer F, Mahmudi-Azer S, Bablitz B, Hagen SC, Velazquez J, Kay AB, Moqbel R. Intracellular localization of interleukin-6 in eosinophils from atopic asthmatics and effects of interferon gamma. Blood 1998; 91:2508–2516.

71. Melani C, Mattia GF, Silvani A, Care A, Rivoltini L, Parmiani G, Colombo MP. Interleukin-6 expression in human neutrophil and eosinophil peripheral blood granulocytes. Blood 1993; 81:2744–2749.

72. Yamasaki K, Taga T, Hirata Y, Yawata H, Kawanishi Y, Seed B, Taniguchi T, Hirano T, Kishimoto T. Cloning and expression of the human interleukin-6 (BSF-2/IFN beta 2) receptor. Science 1988; 241:825–828.

73. Hibi M, Murakami M, Saito M, Hirano T, Taga T, Kishimoto T. Molecular cloning and expression of an IL-6 signal transducer, gp130. Cell 1990; 63:1149–1157.

74. Mackiewicz A, Schooltink H, Heinrich PC, Rose-John S. Complex of soluble human IL-6-receptor/IL-6 up-regulates expression of acute-phase proteins. J Immunol 1992; 149:2021–2027.

75. Peters M, Muller AM, Rose-John S. Interleukin-6 and soluble interleukin-6 receptor: direct stimulation of gp130 and hematopoiesis. Blood 1998; 92:3495–3504.

76. Kopf M, Baumann H, Freer G, Freudenberg M, Lamers M, Kishimoto T, Zinkernagel R, Bluethmann H, Kohler G. Impaired immune and acute-phase responses in interleukin-6-deficient mice. Nature 1994; 368:339–342.

77. Ramsay AJ, Husband AJ, Ramshaw IA, Bao S, Matthaei KI, Koehler G, Kopf M. The role of interleukin 6 in mucosal IgA antibody responses in vivo. Science 1994; 264:561–563.

78. Metzger S, Hassin T, Barash V, Pappo O, Chajek-Shaul T. Reduced body fat and increased hepatic lipid synthesis in mice bearing interleukin-6-secreting tumor. Am J Physiol Endocrinol Metab 2001; 281:E957—E965.

79. Grunfeld C, Adi S, Soued M, Moser A, Fiers W, Feingold KR. Search for mediators of the lipogenic effects of tumor necrosis factor: potential role for interleukin 6. Cancer Res 1990; 50:4233–4238.

80. Nonogaki K, Fuller GM, Fuentes NL, Moser AH, Staprans I, Grunfeld C, Feingold KR. Interleukin-6 stimulates hepatic triglyceride secretion in rats. Endocrinology 1995; 136:2143–2149.

81. Castells-Rodellas A, CastelL JV, Ramirez-Bosca A, Nicolas JF, Valcuende-Cavero F, Thivolet J. Interleukin-6 in normal skin and psoriasis. Acta Derm Venereol 1992; 72: 165–168.

82. Wang XP, Schunck M, Kallen KJ, Neumann C, Trautwein C, Rose-John S, Proksch E. The interleukin-6 cytokine system regulates epidermal permeability barrier homeostasis. J Invest Dermatol 2004; 123:124–131.

83. Grellner W, Georg T, Wilske J. Quantitative analysis of proinflammatory cytokines (IL-lbeta, IL-6, TNF-alpha) in human skin wounds. Forensic Sci Int 2000; 113:251–264.

84. Kupper TS. Production of cytokines by epithelial tissues. A new model for cutaneous inflammation. Am J Dermatopathol 1989; 11:69–73.

85. Kupper TS, Min K, Sehgal P, Mizutani H, Birchall N, Ray A, May L. Production of IL-6 by keratinocytes. Implications for epidermal inflammation and immunity. Ann NY Acad Sci 1989; 557,454–464; discussion 464–465.

86. Urbanski A, Schwarz T, Neuner P, Krutmann L, Kirnbauer R, Kock A, Luger TA. Ultraviolet light induces increased circulating interleukin-6 in humans. J Invest Dermatol 1990; 94:808–811.

87. Nurnberg W, Haas N, Schadendorf D, Czarnetzki BM. Interleukin-6 expression in the skin of patients with lupus erythematosus. Exp Dermatol 1995; 4:52–57.

88. Wood LC, Jackson SM, Elias PM, Grunfeld C, Feingold KR. Cutaneous barrier perturbation stimulates cytokine production in the epidermis of mice. J Clin Invest 1992; 90: 482–487.

89. Wood LC, Feingold KR, Sequeira-Martin SM, Elias PM, Grunfeld C. Barrier function coordinately regulates epidermal IL-1 and IL-1 receptor antagonist mRNA levels. Exp Dermatol 1994; 3:56–60.

90. Nickoloff BJ, Naidu Y. Perturbation of epidermal barrier function correlates with initiation of cytokine cascade in human skin. J Am Acad Dermatol 1994; 30:535–546.

91. Wood LC, Stalder AK, Liou A, Campbell IL, Grunfeld C, Elias PM, Feingold KR. Barrier disruption increases gene expression of cytokines and the 55 kDa TNF receptor in murine skin. Exp Dermatol 1997; 6:98–104.

92. Wood LC, Elias PM, Sequeira-Martin SM, Grunfeld C, Feingold KR. Occlusion lowers cytokine mRNA levels in essential fatty acid-deficient and normal mouse epidermis, but not after acute barrier disruption. J Invest Dermatol 1994; 103:834–883.

93. Tsai JC, Feingold KR, Crumrine D, Wood LC, Grunfeld C, Elias PM. Permeability barrier disruption alters the localization and expression of TNF alpha/protein in the epidermis. Arch Dermatol Res 1994; 286:242–248.

94. Man MQ, Wood L, Elias PM, Feingold KR. Cutaneous barrier repair and pathophysiology following barrier disruption in IL-1 and TNF type I receptor deficient mice. Exp Dermatol 1999; 8:261–266.

95. Jensen JM, Schutze S, Forl M, Kronke M, Proksch E. Roles for tumor necrosis factor receptor p55 and sphingomyelinase in repairing the cutaneous permeability barrier. J Clin Invest 1999; 104:1761–1770.

96. Jensen JM, Kupper TS, Proksch E. IL-l/IL-1 receptor overexpression and knockout constructs in permeability barrier repair of transgenic mice. J Invest Dermatol 1988; 110499a(Abstract).

97. Ghadially R, Brown BE, Sequeira-Martin SM, Feingold KR, Elias PM. The aged epidermal permeability barrier. Structural, functional, and lipid biochemical abnormalities in humans and a senescent murine model. J Clin Invest 1995; 95:2281–2290.

98. Ye J, Garg A, Calhoun C, Feingold KR, Elias PM, Ghadially R. Alterations in cytokine regulation in aged epidermis: implications for permeability barrier homeostasis and inflammation. I. IL-1 gene family. Exp Dermatol 2002; 11:209–216.

99. Barland CO, Zettersten E, Brown BS, Ye J, Elias PM, Ghadially R. Imiquimod-induced interleukin-l alpha stimulation improves barrier homeostasis in aged murine epidermis. J Invest Dermatol 2004; 122:330–336.

20

Nuclear Hormone Receptors: Epidermal Liposensors

Matthias Schmuth
Department of Dermatology, Medical University Innsbruck, Innsbruck, Austria

Kenneth R. Feingold
Departments of Medicine and Dermatology, University of California, San Francisco, California, U.S.A.

THE NUCLEAR HORMONE RECEPTOR SUPER FAMILY

Nuclear hormone receptors are a large family of transcription factors. Currently, 48 nuclear hormone receptors have been identified in humans, making them one of the largest known families of transcription factors (1,2). The nuclear receptors can be divided into several classes. Class I receptors form homodimers and represent targets of the five classical steroid hormones (glucocorticoids, mineralocorticoids, androgen, estrogen, and progesterone). Class II receptors form heterodimers with retinoid X receptors (RXR). This class includes the thyroid receptor (TR), vitamin D receptor (VDR), retinoic acid receptor (RAR), peroxisome proliferator–activated receptors (PPAR), liver X receptor (LXR), farnesol X receptor (FXR), constitutive androstane receptor (CAR), and pregnane X receptor (PXR) (Fig. 1, Table 1). The role of this class of receptors in epidermal homeostasis and barrier function will be described in this chapter in more detail. Class III receptors lack identification of cognate ligands and are therefore called orphan receptors. Class IV receptors bind as monomers to a single hexameric core recognition motif flanked by additional sequences upstream of this motif. In this chapter, we will focus on recently described class II receptors (PPAR, LXR) that are powerful modulators of epidermal homeostasis and barrier function.

MECHANISM OF ACTION

Activation of nuclear hormone receptors occurs through the binding of an agonist with its cognate receptor initiating a complex cascade of events. The agonist receptor complex forms dimers, which regulate the expression of specific genes by interacting with specific enhancer elements in the promoters of their target genes

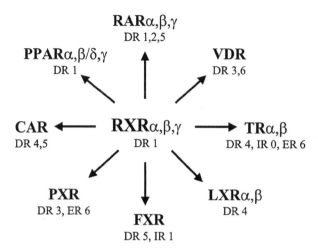

Figure 1 Class II nuclear hormone receptors heterodimerization partners of the retinoid X receptor.

(Figs. 2 and 3). The binding of receptor dimers to regulatory DNA elements results in the recruitment of a transcription initiation complex modulating the expression of a variety of genes. The transcription initiation complex comprises activating or suppressing co-regulators (3–5) that do not bind to the DNA directly, but modulate transcription by protein–protein interaction with the RNA polymerase machinery. Levels of co-regulators are crucial for nuclear receptor–mediated transcription and many co-regulators have been demonstrated to be targets for diverse intracellular signaling pathways and post-translational modifications. Ultimately, nuclear receptor binding results in the transcription of mRNA of downstream genes that subsequently are translated into the respective proteins to produce a physiological response (1,6).

Nuclear receptors are typically composed of three functional domains. The N-terminal domain harbors an activation domain. The central domain mediates

Table 1 Nuclear Hormone Receptors that Heterodimerize with the Retinoid X Receptor and their Activators

Receptor	Activators
RXR	9-cis retinoic acid, bexarotene
TR	Thyroid hormones
VDR	$1,25(OH)_2$ vitamin D, cholecalciferol, tacalcitol
RAR	All trans retinoic acid
PPAR-alpha	8-S-hydroxytetraenoic acid (8-S-HETE), leukotriene (LT) B4, fibrates, farnesol
PPAR-delta	Polyunsaturated Fatty acids, GW1514
PPAR-gamma	Prostaglandin J2, BLR49653, GI251929X, rosiglitazone, pioglitazone
LXR	Oxysterols, T0-901317, GW3965
FXR	Bile acids
PXR/CAR	Steroids, phenobarbital, antibiotics, antifungals, xenobiotics

Abbreviations: RXR, Retinoid X receptor; TR, thyroid receptor; VDR, vitamin D receptor; RAR, retinoic acid receptor; PPAR, peroxisome proliferator-activated receptors; LXR, liver X receptor; FXR, farnesoid X receptor; CAR, constitutive androstane receptor; PXR, pregnane X receptor.

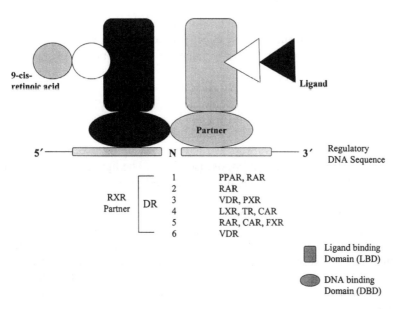

Figure 2 Nuclear hormone receptor binding to regulatory DNA sequences.

dimerization, nuclear localization, and DNA binding. It is composed of two four-cysteine zinc fingers mediating Zn^{2+} interaction. The C-terminal domain contains an activation domain for ligand binding, but also interacts with co-activators and molecular chaperones, and contains nuclear import and export sequences (1).

Regulatory elements within the promoter regions of target genes assure specificity as they contain highly conserved repeats of sequences related to AGGTCA, with the spacing between two motifs determining the choice of RXR partner (Figs. 2 and 3). Differentially spaced half-site DNA elements produce distinct transcriptional responses. Finally, the DNA-binding domain undergoes distinct conformational changes when binding to specific response elements, allowing the receptors to adopt different conformations at different binding sites. Because the binding to promoter regions in genes involves several additional regulatory systems: (i) the effect of promoter binding depends on the type of enhancer sequence, and (ii) the hormone–receptor complex interacts with other nuclear players, such as transcription factors, adapter proteins, co-regulators, and trans-acetylases, even different ligands, known as activators, of the same nuclear hormone

Direct Repeats (DR) A G G T C A - - - - -N- - - - - A G G T C A

Everse Repeats (ER) A C T G G A - - - - -N- - - - - A G G T C A

Inverse Repeats (IR) A G G T C A - - - - -N- - - - - A C T G G A

Figure 3 DNA-binding motifs.

receptor can exert differential effects on cellular physiology. Moreover, it has recently been shown that in addition to the genomic effects, certain effects of nuclear hormone receptor ligands occur by mechanisms independent of DNA-binding, i.e., protein-protein interactions (7).

LIGANDS

Several class II nuclear hormone receptors are activated by lipids, and by their metabolites, and have therefore been called "liposensors" (1). The ligands are chemically diverse and include hormones, vitamins, drugs, and lipid products of cellular metabolic pathways that may be produced within the cell (Table 1). The epidermis is a very active site of lipid synthesis (8). Numerous lipid species that are synthesized de novo in the epidermis, including fatty acids, various cholesterol species, and 1,25-dihydroxyvitamin D_3, have been shown to activate nuclear hormone receptors. Among the more recently discovered class II nuclear hormone receptors, PPAR and LXR are activated by such lipid metabolites and thus are good candidates for playing a regulatory role in stratum corneum (SC) formation and homeostasis. Thus, we here summarize recent results on the effects of this novel subgroup of nuclear hormone receptors on epidermal development, proliferation, cell death, differentiation, inflammation, and barrier function.

PEROXISOME PROLIFERATOR–ACTIVATED RECEPTORS (PPAR)

Of the PPARs, three isotypes have been described: PPAR-alpha (NR1C1), beta/delta (NR1C2), and gamma (NR1C3) (6,9). All three isotypes are expressed in the skin (10–12). They have been shown to be physiologically expressed during fetal rat skin development and to subsequently be down-regulated during postnatal life (12,13). Surprisingly, none of the mouse models with a deficiency of any of the three isotypes has revealed gross skin abnormalities (14–17), indicating redundancy of the isotypes.

PPAR-ALPHA

PPAR-alpha is expressed in liver, heart, kidney, muscle, and brown fat (11). PPAR-alpha activation stimulates the oxidation of fatty acids. In addition, PPAR-alpha activation increases serum HDL and decreases serum triglyceride levels (9). Clofibrate, gemfibrozil, and fenofibrate are drugs that activate PPAR-alpha and are widely used to treat dyslipidemias (9).

Epidermal Consequences of PPAR-alpha Deficiency

PPAR-alpha is expressed in keratinocytes and the epidermis, and mRNA levels increase during keratinocyte differentiation (10). Morphological analysis of adult PPAR-alpha $-/-$ knock out (KO) epidermis revealed a thinned stratum granulosum (SG) with fewer keratohyalin granules, focal parakeratosis, slightly decreased profilaggrin and loricrin mRNA, and protein expression (18). Electron microscopy revealed normal numbers of lamellar bodies and the quantity and structure of the lamellar membranes in the SC were not altered. Functional studies revealed that in PPAR-alpha KO mice, basal transepidermal water loss and permeability barrier repair after acute barrier disruption were normal as were SC water holding capacity, SC integrity and cohesion, and surface pH. However, a recent study has demonstrated that lack of PPAR-alpha impairs wound healing (13). Furthermore, in fetal PPAR-alpha KO mice, we observed that the formation of the SC is delayed (19) However, PPAR-alpha KO mice ultimately form a normal SC (a modest decrease in the expression of involucrin, loricrin, and filaggrin persists in PPAR-alpha KO adults).

In Vivo Effects of PPAR-Alpha Activation

In vivo, in adult mice, it was reported that topical treatment with PPAR-alpha activators, i.e., clofibrate and farnesol, decreased epidermal thickness, while expression of structural proteins of the upper spinous/granular layers (involucrin, profilaggrin/filaggrin, and loricrin) increased (both protein levels measured by immunohistochemistry and mRNA levels measured by in situ hybridization). Furthermore, topically applied PPAR-alpha activators also increased apoptosis and decreased cell proliferation. Experiments with PPAR-alpha KO mice showed that these effects are specifically mediated via PPAR-alpha. Topical clofibrate treatment did not cause any morphological changes or increase the expression of involucrin, loricrin, or profilaggrin in PPAR-alpha KO mice. Thus, in adult mice, activation of PPAR-alpha stimulates keratinocyte/epidermal differentiation and inhibits proliferation. Importantly, while no changes in TEWL occur under basal conditions, PPAR-alpha activation accelerated permeability barrier repair following abrogation of the permeability barrier by either tape stripping or detergent (10% SDS) treatment. Thus, topical PPAR-alpha activation accelerates barrier repair following acute abrogation in adult mice.

In hyperproliferative epidermis in hairless mice, induced either by repeated barrier abrogation (sub-acute model) or by essential fatty acid deficiency (chronic model) (20), topical treatment with PPAR-alpha activators substantially decreased epidermal hyperplasia in both the sub-acute and the chronic models of hyper-proliferation. Following topical treatment, anti-proliferating cell nuclear antigen (PCNA)-expressing cells were restricted to the basal layer, similar to that of normal epidermis. In hyperproliferative epidermis there was decreased expression of involu-crin, profilaggrin–filaggrin, and loricrin. Following topical treatment with PPAR-alpha activators, staining for these mRNAs and proteins increased toward normal levels. Finally, topically applied clofibrate also increased apoptosis in hyperprolifera-tive epidermis. These results demonstrate that treatment with PPAR-alpha activators normalizes cell proliferation and promotes epidermal differentiation, correcting the cutaneous pathology. Lastly, PPAR-alpha activators have been shown to reduce tumor formation in mice (21).

In Vitro Effects of PPAR-Alpha in Cultured Human Keratinocytes

In cultured human keratinocytes, Rivier et al. have shown that PPAR-alpha activators stimulate lipid synthesis, particularly ceramide and cholesterol synthesis (10). Further-more, we recently reported that the rate of cornified envelope formation was increased 3-fold, and involucrin and transglutaminase-1 were increased at both the mRNA level (2- to 7-fold) and the protein level (4- to 12-fold) by PPAR-alpha activators. Whereas the effect of PPAR-alpha activators was independent of calcium, it was additive to the effects of calcium on differentiation. Transfection of the involucrin promoter and the transglutaminase-1 promoter linked to luciferase revealed that clofibrate increased luciferase activity indicating that PPAR-alpha activators increase the expression of both involucrin and transglutaminase-1. Using deletions and mutations we further showed that the increase in involucrin expression requires an intact AP-1 response element at −2117 bp to −2111 bp (22). Finally, PPAR-alpha activators inhibited DNA synthesis (23). This demonstrates that PPAR-alpha activators induce differentiation and inhibit proliferation in human keratinocytes.

Role in Epidermal Development

In a series of in vitro and in vivo studies, we have shown that PPAR-alpha activators stimulate fetal epidermal development (24–26). Skin explants from rats on gestational day 17 (term is 22 days) are unstratified and lack a SC. After incubation in hormone-free media for three to four days, a multilayered SC replete with mature lamellar membranes in the interstices and a functionally competent barrier appears. PPAR-alpha stimulates both the formation of the extracellular lipid lamellar membranes and the expression of proteins required for epidermal differentiation (filaggrin, loricrin, and involucrin). Thus, PPAR-alpha activation accelerates epidermal development, resulting in mature lamellar membranes, a multilayered SC, and a competent barrier.

Anti-inflammatory Effects

PPAR-alpha agonists not only inhibit cytokine expression in macrophages (27) but also have anti-inflammatory effects on skin. In mouse models of irritant (experimentally induced by topical application of the phorbolester TPA) and allergic (oxazolone) contact dermatitis, topical treatment with PPAR-alpha activators reduces ear swelling, the magnitude of the inflammatory infiltrate, and epidermal cytokine expression, i.e., tumor necrosis factor (TNF)-alpha and interleukin (IL)-1 alpha (Table 2). Moreover, using KO mice we demonstrated that these effects are receptor mediated (28). In lesional skin from psoriasis patients, epidermal PPAR-alpha RNA expression is reduced (10) (similar to RAR, RXR, and TR). Furthermore, after UV exposure PPAR-alpha RNA expression is reduced in both cultured human keratinocytes and human skin in vivo. Conversely, topical application of PPAR-alpha agonists reduces the UV-induced erythema in human skin (29).

Table 2 Differential Effects of Class II Nuclear Hormone Receptor Activation in Cutaneous Homeostasis In Vivo

Receptor	Epidermal thickness	Differentiation	Barrier function	Inflammation	Expression in psoriasis
LXR	↓	↑	↑	↓	n.d.
PPARα	↓	↑	↑	↓	↓
PPARγ	n.c.	↑	↑	↓	↓
PPARβ/δ	n.c.	↑	↑	↓	↑
RAR	↑	n.c.	↓	↓	↓
TR	n.d.	n.d.	n.d.	n.d.	↓
VDR	↑	↑	↓	↓	n.c.

Abbreviations: n.d., not determined; n.c., no change.

PPAR-DELTA

PPAR-delta is expressed ubiquitously (11,12) and is activated by fatty acids (30). Drugs that activate PPAR-delta have been shown to markedly increase serum HDL levels while lowering serum triglyceride levels in obese rhesus monkeys (31). The increase in serum HDL is thought to be due to the increased expression of ABCA1, a transporter that is key in the efflux of cholesterol from cells to circulating HDL (31). Furthermore, studies have suggested a role for PPAR-delta in regulating the differentiation of adipocytes and oxidative metabolism in both adipose tissue and muscle (32–34).

Epidermal Consequences of PPAR-Delta Deficiency

In keratinocytes and in the epidermis, PPAR-delta is expressed at high levels, and its expression is not altered by differentiation (10,35). Homozygous PPAR-deficient mice have a high intrauterine mortality, and surviving animals have residual PPAR-beta/delta RNA transcripts (10,15,36). Nevertheless, despite partial expression, these animals display an increased susceptibility to phorbol ester-induced epidermal hyperplasia (15), while epidermal differentiation and hair cycling are normal (13). In addition homozygous, PPAR-delta deficient mice (PPAR-delta $+/-$) have been examined and wound healing has been reported to be impaired (13).

In Vivo Effects of PPAR-Delta Activation

In vivo effects show that PPAR-delta is increased by phorbol ester exposure, after hair plunking, wounding, and epidermal inflammation (13,15). After topical application of GW1514, a synthetic, selective PPAR-delta activator, an increased expression of filaggrin and loricrin was observed in mouse skin. Similar to what was observed in wild type animals, the increased expression of epidermal differentiation markers occurred in the epidermis of PPAR-alpha KO animals. This demonstrates that the GW1514 stimulation of keratinocyte differentiation is not mediated by activation of PPAR-alpha. In contrast, in RXR-alpha deficient mice, GW1514 did not stimulate either filaggrin or loricrin expression. This indicates that GW1514 requires RXR to stimulate differentiation and suggests that it is activating a receptor that heterodimerizes with RXR. These results strongly suggest, but do not definitively prove, that the pro-differentiating effects of GW1514 are mediated by PPAR-delta. Studies in PPAR-delta deficient mice are required to definitively demonstrate a role for PPAR-delta. However, mice with systemic deficiency in PPAR-delta are not viable and tissue (epidermis) specific KO mice have not been available for testing yet.

After topical treatment of mouse skin with GW1514, no significant decrease in epidermal thickness was detectable, in contrast to the effects of PPAR-alpha activators, which cause thinning of the epidermis. Conversely, the pool of proliferating cells was transiently increased at three days and unchanged after six days of treatment, while epidermal cell death detected by TUNEL staining was unchanged. In contrast, PPAR-alpha activators decreased keratinocyte proliferation and increased apoptosis, demonstrating that the effects of activation of epidermal liposensors can result in different effects on epidermal biology (Table 2). Again, in contrast to PPAR-alpha activators there was no effect on epidermal proliferation in a model of chronic epidermal hyperproliferation (38). Thus, similar to normal mouse skin, activation of PPAR-delta stimulates differentiation without affecting proliferation in this model.

The restoration of barrier homeostasis after acute barrier perturbation, either by mechanical methods (tape stripping), by solvent extraction (repeated topical acetone), or by detergent treatment (repeated topical sodium dodecyl sulfate), was accelerated in skin pre-treated with GW1514 regardless of the method of barrier perturbation, indicating a beneficial effect on barrier repair kinetics (Table 2). Moreover, in our model of repeated disruption of the permeability barrier of hairless mice by topical acetone application over three days inducing epidermal hyperplasia, topical treatment with GW1514 stimulated an increase in the expression of the differentiation markers, loricrin and filaggrin, returning expression levels toward normal in these mice (38).

In Vitro Effects of PPAR-Delta in Cultured Human Keratinocytes

In vitro, PPAR-delta protects from cell death by modulating Akt1, also known as protein kinase B-alpha (PKB-alpha). Akt1 is a major downstream effector of the phosphatidylinositol-3-kinase (PI3K). Akt1 signaling, in turn, occurs via phosphorylation of threonine 308 (T308) by the 3-phosphoinositide-dependent kinase-1 (PDK1) and of serine 473 (S473) by the integrin-linked kinase (ILK) (35,37). Westergaard et al. have shown that a non-selective PPAR-delta activator stimulates keratinocyte differentiation (35,37). Our laboratory has obtained similar results using the selective PPAR-delta activator GW1514. Conversely, others have reported that over-expression of PPAR-beta/delta stimulates differentiation in cultured keratinocytes (37) and that cytokine-induced keratinocyte differentiation requires the upregulation of PPAR-beta/delta via the stress-associated kinase cascade, that, in turn, targets an AP-1 site in the promoter (37).

Using microarray technology, we showed increases in multiple genes that are known to increase during keratinocyte differentiation by treatment with GW1514 (38). Specifically, we found that involucrin, SPRR 1B, SPRR 2C, SPRR 3, annexin A1, cystatin A, desmoplakin, and envoplakin were increased 24–48 hours after PPAR-beta/delta activation. It should be noted that this increase in the expression of these differentiation-related proteins was a late effect of PPAR-beta/delta activation. This suggests that the increased expression of these proteins is not a direct effect of PPAR-beta/delta on the promoter of these genes, but rather was due to PPAR-beta/delta activation stimulating other factors.

Furthermore, PPAR-beta/delta activation, aside from stimulating differentiation-related genes, additionally induced adipose differentiation-related protein (ADRP) and fasting-induced adipose factor (FIAF) mRNA in cultured keratinocytes, which was paralleled by increased oil red O staining indicative of lipid accumulation, the bulk of which were triglycerides (TG) (38). FIAF is expressed in adipocytes and its expression is increased during adipocyte differentiation, during fasting, and in mouse models of obesity and diabetes (6). The biological function of FIAF is unknown, but it is presumed to play a role in lipids metabolism. ADRP is a membrane-associated fatty acid binding protein that facilitates the transport of long chain fatty acids (39). Its expression is induced during adipocyte differentiation but it is also expressed in other tissues that are involved in triglyceride and fatty acids metabolism. Cells that either store or transport lipid express ADRP and it has been proposed that ADRP associates with lipid vacuoles. Recent studies have suggested that ADRP plays an important role in the uptake of surfactant lipids by alveolar type II epithelial cells (40). Studies have shown that there are nuclear hormone receptor response elements in the promoter of ADRP and that PPAR activation directly stimulates ADRP expression. That ADRP is a direct downstream target of PPAR-beta/delta is very compatible with the early increase in ADRP expression that we see with GW1514 treatment.

To follow up on these findings, indicating a novel link between keratinocyte differentiation and lipid metabolism, and also because studies by other investigators have shown that activation of PPAR-beta/delta stimulates adipocyte differentiation (31), we assessed if treatment of keratinocytes with PPAR-beta/delta activator was inducing an adipocyte phenotype in keratinocytes. Other genes that are expressed in adipocytes, adipsin, resistin, leptin, and aP2, and specific adipocyte markers were not expressed in either GW1514 treated or control keratinocytes (37). Keratinocytes also have the potential to become sebocytes, which store and secrete lipids. To determine if PPAR-beta/delta activation was stimulating the conversion of keratinocytes to sebocytes (41,42), we determined if the expression of sebocyte markers was increased in keratinocytes treated with GW1514. Keratin 7, keratin 19, and epithelial membrane antigen are sebocyte markers and the expression of these genes was not increased in keratinocytes by PPAR-beta/delta activator treatment (38). Thus, PPAR-beta/delta activation stimulates lipid accumulation in keratinocytes, but it is not clear at this time why this occurs or its functional significance.

Anti-inflammatory Effects

In addition to stimulating epidermal differentiation, there is also evidence that PPAR-beta/delta activation has anti-inflammatory effects. In a mouse model of irritant contact dermatitis (TPA treatment of ears), treatment with GW1514 decreased the degree of inflammation (38). This reduction in inflammation is similar to what is observed with topical glucocorticoid treatment, a standard anti-inflammatory therapy. Conversely, Peters et al. have reported that PPAR-beta/delta deficient mice have an increased inflammatory response to phorbol ester treatment, which suggests that PPAR-beta/delta plays a key role in down-regulating inflammation. Pertinently, in lesional psoriatic skin, the expression of PPAR-beta/delta is increased while the expression of PPAR-alpha and gamma is decreased (10). The increased expression of PPAR-beta/delta during cutaneous inflammation makes it an attractive therapeutic target for the treatment of diseases that are characterized by cutaneous inflammation (Table 2). However, in a recent clinical pilot trial, topical tetradecylthioacetic acid (TTA), a non-selective PPAR-delta agonist, did not improve lesional skin in psoriasis patients (43,44).

PPAR-GAMMA

PPAR gamma is predominantly expressed in adipocytes, colon, spleen, and adrenal tissues (11,12). Activation of PPAR-gamma stimulates free fatty acid uptake, lipogenesis, and differentiation. PPAR-gamma is the key transcription factor required for the differentiation of fibroblasts into adipocytes. Additionally it plays a key role in regulating insulin action. Drugs such as rosiglitazone and pioglitazone are being used to reduce insulin resistance in patients with Type 2 diabetes mellitus (45) (Table 1).

Epidermal Consequences of PPAR-Gamma Deficiency

PPAR-gamma is expressed in the epidermis (10–12,35). Keratinocyte differentiation results in an increase in PPAR-gamma mRNA levels. Nevertheless, the gross cutaneous appearance of mice deficient in PPAR-gamma in the epidermis is largely normal except for patchy hair loss in older animals (in young animals, <16 weeks of age, no abnormalities were observed) (46). Hematoxylin & Easin (H&E) stained sections of these animals revealed a modest increase in epidermal thickness in the PPAR-gamma deficient mice. In concordance with this increase in epidermal thickness, PCNA staining was slightly increased in the PPAR-gamma deficient mice, indicating increased keratinocyte proliferation. However, apoptosis, as measured by the TUNEL assay, was unchanged in the PPAR-gamma deficient mice. Similarly, the expression of differentiation markers was also not altered in PPAR-gamma deficient mice compared with wild type mice. Several key biophysical measurements yielded normal, non-pathological results i.e., SC pH, basal TEWL, and water-holding capacity of SC in PPAR-gamma deficient skin were all similar to wild type mice. Additionally, permeability barrier recovery following acute disruption by tape stripping was normal in PPAR-gamma deficient skin. PPAR-gamma deficient mice did not display any abnormalities in wound healing (13) and the cutaneous inflammatory response to TPA treatment was not different (45). Lastly, electron microscopy revealed that the number and the appearance of lamellar bodies and lamellar secretory system were similar in PPAR-gamma deficient and wild type mice. Thus, except for slight epidermal hyperplasia and patchy hair loss with aging, the structure and function of PPAR-gamma deficient murine skin appears normal.

In Vivo Effects of PPAR-Gamma Activation

However, in vivo, we have recently examined the effects of topical application of PPAR-gamma activators on epidermal structure and function. In these experiments, treatment with ciglitazone or troglitazone induced an increase in the expression of involucrin, loricrin, and filaggrin. In PPAR-gamma deficient mice, no pro-differentiating effect was observed indicating that the stimulation of differentiation by PPAR-gamma activators is mediated by PPAR-gamma. Interestingly, in contrast to observations with PPAR-alpha or -beta/delta activators, treatment with PPAR-gamma activators resulted in an increase in epidermal thickness. Accordingly, PCNA staining, a marker of cell proliferation, was slightly increased in ciglitazone treated mice. Additionally, topical treatment with PPAR-gamma activators accelerated barrier recovery following acute disruption by either tape stripping or acetone treatment, indicating an improvement in permeability barrier homeostasis (46).

In Vitro Effects of PPAR-Gamma in Cultured Human Keratinocytes

In recent experiments, we also demonstrated that ciglitazone treatment increased mRNA levels of both involucrin and transglutaminase-1 in keratinocytes grown in either low or high calcium. Of note, the increase in both involucrin and transglutaminase-1 mRNA levels induced by ciglitazone treatment was greater than that observed with high calcium, the standard method for stimulating keratinocyte differentiation (46). These results confirm the in vivo results from studies in mice, demonstrating that ciglitazone stimulates human keratinocyte differentiation.

Role in Epidermal Development

The PPAR-gamma ligands, prostaglandin J2 and troglitazone, were tested in our skin explants model from rats on gestational day 17 (term is 22 days) that display an unstratified epidermis and lack a SC. Neither prostaglandin J2 nor troglitazone modulated the development of barrier function or epidermal morphology as compared to vehicle control in this model (24).

Anti-inflammatory Effects

PPAR-gamma agonists have anti-inflammatory effects on macrophages, as well as in irritant and allergic contact dermatitis, which are accompanied by a reduction in inflammatory cytokines such as TNF-alpha and IL-1 alpha (46). Interestingly, however, PPAR-gamma activators inhibited inflammation in both PPAR-gamma deficient and wild type mouse skin, indicating that the inhibition of cutaneous inflammation by these PPAR-gamma activators does not require PPAR-gamma, an effect similar to that reported by others in macrophages. Similar to PPAR-alpha, and in contrast to PPAR-delta, PPAR-gamma RNA levels are reduced in lesional psoriatic skin and after UV exposure of normal human skin (10,29). Troglitazone, when used as an anti-diabetic compound, has been reported to have beneficial effects on skin lesions of diabetic patients with concurrent psoriasis (47). However, when applied topically to lesional skin, the PPAR-gamma agonist, rosiglitazone, did not improve psoriasis (43,44). Moreover, in a recent study, no association between polymorphisms in the PPAR-gamma gene and the clinical manifestation of psoriasis has been found (48).

LIVER X RECEPTOR (LXR)

Two genes encode LXR paralogues. LXR-alpha is expressed predominantly in the liver and to a lesser extent in kidneys, spleen, adrenal gland, and the small intestine, while LXR-beta is ubiquitously expressed (49). Activation of LXR increases the reverse cholesterol transport pathway (i.e., movement of cholesterol from peripheral cells to the liver for excretion into the bile) at several steps. Specifically, LXR activation (a) increases cholesterol efflux from cells by increasing the expression of the cholesterol transporter ABCA1 (50), (b) increases serum levels of cholesterol ester transport protein (CETP) which facilitates the movement of cholesterol to the liver (51), and (c) increases cholesterol 7-hydroxylase activity in the liver, which facilitates the synthesis of bile acids from cholesterol (52). In addition to regulating reverse cholesterol transport, LXR activation also inhibits cholesterol absorption in the small intestine by increasing the levels of ABC-G5 and -G8 in enterocytes (53). Lastly, LXR activation has been shown to increase the expression of the transcription factor SREBP-1c, which is an important regulator of fatty acids synthesis (this may provide a link between cholesterol levels and fatty acids metabolism) (53–55).

Epidermal Consequences of LXR Deficiency

Both LXR-alpha and -beta are present in human keratinocytes and fetal rat epidermis, while in mouse epidermis only LXR-beta is detectable. In LXR-alpha,

LXR-beta, and LXR-alpha, beta double KO mice, there were no gross cutaneous abnormalities (55). On examination by light microscopy, there was thinning of the epidermis. Immunohistochemical staining for loricrin, filaggrin, and involucrin revealed a modest decrease in the levels of these proteins in the outer epidermis. Electron microscopy revealed normal numbers of lamellar bodies, and the quantity and the structure of the lamellar membranes in the SC were not altered. Functional studies revealed that in both LXR-alpha and -beta KO mice that basal transepidermal water loss and permeability barrier repair after barrier disruption were normal as were SC water holding capacity, SC integrity and cohesion, and surface pH. Thus, there are reductions in the expression of differentiation-related proteins, but these changes do not result in either major functional or morphological abnormalities. Of note is a similar modest decrease in the expression of differentiation-related proteins in the absence of major functional and morphological abnormalities also occurs in VDR deficient mice (these mice have alopecia which is not seen in the PPAR-alpha or LXR KO mice) (57–58). The absence of a marked epidermal phenotype may indicate receptor redundancy, i.e., the absence of one receptor is compensated for by the presence of other receptors.

In Vivo Effects of LXR Activation

In vivo, topical treatment of normal hairless mice with 22(R)-hydroxycholesterol or 24(R)25-epoxycholesterol, LXR ligands, resulted in increased levels of involucrin, loricrin, and profilaggrin protein and mRNA in the epidermis, indicating that oxysterols stimulate epidermal differentiation. Topical oxysterol treatment induced differentiation in LXR-alpha KO mice, while in LXR-beta KO mice there was no increase in the expression of differentiation markers, indicating that these effects are receptor mediated. Additionally, topical oxysterol pretreatment decreased epidermal thickness and keratinocyte proliferation as determined by PCNA staining. These studies demonstrate that epidermal differentiation in mouse skin is regulated by LXR-beta and that oxysterols, acting via LXR-beta, can induce differentiation and inhibit proliferation in vivo.

Moreover, treatment of hyperproliferative epidermis with oxysterols restored epidermal homeostasis (i.e., decreased the hyperproliferation and stimulated differentiation). Importantly, we also examined the effects of topical LXR activation on barrier homeostasis. We did not observe any difference in basal TEWL following repeated oxysterol treatment; however, sites pretreated with 22(R)-hydroxycholesterol for three days demonstrated accelerated barrier repair kinetics compared with vehicle-treated sites after acute barrier disruption with either acetone or tape stripping (58). Thus, topical oxysterol treatment improves barrier homeostasis in adult mice.

In Vitro Effects of LXR in Cultured Human Keratinocytes

In cultured keratinocytes, mRNA and protein levels of involucrin and transglutaminase-1, increased 2- to 3-fold in normal human keratinocytes incubated in the presence of 25- or 22(R)-hydroxycholesterol in low calcium. In high calcium, which alone induces differentiation, mRNA levels were further increased by oxysterols (59,60). Rates of cornified envelope formation, an indicator of terminal differentiation, also increased 2-fold with oxysterol treatment. In contrast, the rate of DNA synthesis was inhibited by approximately 50% by oxysterols. Transactivation was assessed in keratinocytes transfected with either transglutaminase-1 or involucrin promoter-luciferase constructs. 22(R)-hydroxycholesterol increased transglutaminase-1 and involucrin promoter activity 2- to 3-fold. Either deletion of the −2452 bp to −1880 bp region of the involucrin promoter or mutation of the AP-1 site (−2117 bp to −2111 bp) within this region abolished oxysterol responsiveness. Treatment of keratinocytes transfected with an AP-1 response element luciferase construct with LXR activators demonstrated an increase in luciferase activity, indicating that LXR activators increase AP-1 activity. Moreover, increased AP-1 DNA binding was observed in oxysterol-treated keratinocytes by gel shift analyses, and among the constituent proteins of the AP-1 complex, Fra-1, c-Fos, and Jun-D were shown to be increased (60). These data indicate that LXR activators induce involucrin expression, an effect that requires an intact AP-1 response element and is mediated by an increase in AP-1 activity.

Role in Epidermal Development

To determine a potential role of LXR in epidermal development, 22(R)-hydroxycholesterol was injected into the amniotic fluid of fetal rats on gestational day 17. Fetal epidermal barrier function and morphology were assessed on day 19. Whereas vehicle-treated fetal rats displayed no measurable barrier (transepidermal water loss $>10 \, mg/cm^2/hour$), a measurable barrier was induced by the intra-amniotic administration of 22(R)-hydroxycholesterol (transepidermal water loss range 4.0–8.5 mg/ $cm^2/hour$). It was observed from light microscopy that control pups lacked a well-defined SC, whereas a distinct SC and a thickened stratum granulosum were present in treated pups (26). While using electron microscopy, the extracellular spaces of the SC in control pups revealed a paucity of mature lamellar unit structures, whereas these structures filled the SC interstices in treated pups. Additionally, protein and mRNA levels of loricrin and filaggrin, two structural proteins of SC, were increased in treated epidermis, as were the activities of two lipid catabolic enzymes critical to SC function, beta-glucocerebrosidase and steroid sulfatase (26).

Anti-inflammatory Effects

Following UV-B irradiation, LXR-alpha RNA levels were reduced while LXR-beta levels remained unchanged in cultured keratinocytes. Moreover, recent studies have demonstrated that LXR activators display potent anti-inflammatory activity in both irritant and allergic contact dermatitis animal models. Thus, we recently studied the anti-inflammatory effects of two oxysterols, 22(R)-hydroxycholesterol and 25-hydroxycholesterol, and a nonsterol activator of LXR, GW3965, in models of irritant and allergic contact dermatitis. Whereas TPA or oxazolone treatment alone induced an approximately 2-fold increase in ear weight and thickness, LXR activation markedly suppressed the increase (greater than 50% decrease), comparable to what was observed with 0.05% clobetasol treatment (61). Histology also revealed a marked decrease in cutaneous inflammation in oxysterol-treated animals. Immunohistochemistry demonstrated an inhibition in the production of the pro-inflammatory cytokines interleukin-1 alpha and tumor necrosis factor alpha in the oxysterol-treated sites from both TPA- and oxazolone-treated animals (61). As topical treatment with cholesterol did not reduce the TPA-induced inflammation, and the nonsterol LXR activator (GW3965) inhibited inflammation, the anti-inflammatory effects of oxysterols cannot be ascribed to a nonspecific sterol effect. In addition, 22(R)-hydroxycholesterol did not reduce inflammation in LXR-beta KO or LXR-alpha/beta double KO animals, indicating that LXR-beta is required for this anti-inflammatory effect. 22(R)-hydroxycholesterol also caused a partial reduction in ear thickness in LXR-alpha KO animals, however (approximately 50% of that observed in wild-type mice), suggesting that this receptor also mediates the anti-inflammatory effects of oxysterols. These studies demonstrate that activators of LXR display potent anti-inflammatory activity in both irritant and allergic contact models of dermatitis, requiring the participation of both LXR-alpha and LXR-beta.

CROSSTALK BETWEEN LIPIDS AND PROTEINS IN THE EPIDERMIS

A critical question is whether activation of these "liposensor" type nuclear hormone receptors, by epidermal lipids generated during the formation of lamellar bodies and/or by metabolic products of these lipids in the epidermis, could provide a mechanism that coordinately regulates the formation of the corneocytes ("bricks") and extracellular lipid membranes ("mortar") during epidermal differentiation. Epidermal lipids not only provide the structural building blocks for the SC but also serve as regulators of cellular functions. The protein versus lipid arms of keratinocyte differentiation and SC formation are traditionally viewed as concurrent, but independent processes. However, the ability of lipids, such as long chain fatty acids and oxysterols, to activate PPARs and LXR and the recent data, demonstrating that these transcription factors can stimulate keratinocyte proteins required for cornified envelope formation, suggest that there may be crosstalk between the two arms of keratinocyte differentiation (Fig. 4). One can speculate that as lipid precursors accumulate in stratum granulosum cells, these lipids or their metabolites could activate nuclear hormone receptors, which in turn stimulate other aspects of keratinocyte differentiation, such as increasing the expression of the structural proteins required to form the cornified envelope. This would allow for the coordinated formation of the SC (Fig. 4).

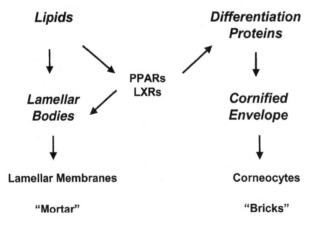

Figure 4 Coordinated regulation of lamellar body and cornified envelope components by class II nuclear hormone receptors in the epidermis.

REFERENCES

1. Mangelsdorf DJ, Evans RM. The RXR heterodimers and orphan receptors. Cell 1995; 83:841–850.
2. Chawla A, Repa JJ, Evans RM, Mangelsdorf DJ. Nuclear receptors and lipid physiology: opening the X-files. Science 2001; 294:1866–1870.
3. Yamamoto KR. Multilayered control of intracellular receptor function. Harvey Lect 1995; 91:1–19.
4. McKenna NJ, O'Malley BW. Combinatorial control of gene expression by nuclear receptors and coregulators. Cell 2002; 108:465–474.
5. Hermanson O, Glass CK, Rosenfeld MG. Nuclear receptor coregulators: multiple modes of modification. Trends Endocrinol Metab 2002; 13:55–60.
6. Kersten S, Desvergne B, Wahli W. Roles of PPARs in health and disease. Nature 2000; 405:421–424.
7. Reichardt HM, Kaestner KH, Tuckermann J, Kretz O, Wessely O, Bock R, Gass P, Schmid W, Herrlich P, Angel P, Schutz G. DNA binding of the glucocorticoid receptor is not essential for survival. Cell 1998; 93:531–541.
8. Feingold KR. The regulation and role of epidermal lipid synthesis. Adv Lipid Res 1991; 24:57–82.
9. Schoonjans K, Staels B, Auwerx J. The peroxisome proliferator activated receptors (PPARS) and their effects on lipid metabolism and adipocyte differentiation. Biochim Biophys Acta 1996; 1302:93–109.
10. Rivier M, Safonova I, Lebrun P, Griffiths CE, Ailhaud G, Michel S. Differential expression of peroxisome proliferator-activated receptor subtypes during the differentiation of human keratinocytes. J Invest Dermatol 1998; 111:1116–1121.
11. Braissant O, Foufelle F, Scotto C, Dauca M, Wahli W. Differential expression of peroxisome proliferator-activated receptors (PPARs): tissue distribution of PPAR-alpha, -beta, and -gamma in the adult rat. Endocrinology 1996; 137:354–366.
12. Braissant O, Wahli W. Differential expression of peroxisome proliferator-activated receptor-alpha, -beta, and -gamma during rat embryonic development. Endocrinology 1998; 139:2748–2754.
13. Michalik L, Desvergne B, Tan NS, Basu-Modak S, Escher P, Rieusset J, Peters JM, Kaya G, Gonzalez FJ, Zakany J, Metzger D, Chambon P, Duboule D, Wahli W. Impaired skin wound healing in peroxisome proliferator-activated receptor (PPAR) {alpha} and PPAR{beta} mutant mice. J Cell Biol 2001; 154:799–814.
14. Lee SS, Pineau T, Drago J, Lee EJ, Owens JW, Kroetz DL, Fernandez-Salguero PM, Westphal H, Gonzalez FJ. Targeted disruption of the alpha isoform of the peroxisome proliferator-activated receptor gene in mice results in abolishment of the pleiotropic effects of peroxisome proliferators. Mol Cell Biol 1995; 15:3012–3022.
15. Peters JM, Lee SS, Li W, Ward JM, Gavrilova O, Everett C, Reitman ML, Hudson LD, Gonzalez FJ. Growth, adipose, brain, and skin alterations resulting from targeted disruption of the mouse peroxisome proliferator-activated receptor beta(delta). Mol Cell Biol 2000; 20:5119–5128.
16. Barak Y, Nelson MC, Ong ES, Jones YZ, Ruiz-Lozano P, Chien KR, Koder A, Evans RM. PPAR gamma is required for placental, cardiac, and adipose tissue development. Mol Cell 1999, 4.585–595.
17. Kubota N, Terauchi Y, Miki H, Tamemoto H, Yamauchi T, Komeda K, Satoh S, Nakano R, Ishii C, Sugiyama T, Eto K, Tsubamoto Y, Okuno A, Murakami K, Sekihara H, Hasegawa G, Naito M, Toyoshima Y, Tanaka S, Shiota K, Kitamura T, Fujita T, Ezaki O, Aizawa S, Kadowaki T, et al.: PPAR gamma mediates high-fat diet-induced adipocyte hypertrophy and insulin resistance. Mol Cell 1999; 4:597–609..
18. Komuves LG, Hanley K, Lefebvre AM, Man MQ, Ng DC, Bikle DD, Williams ML, Elias PM, Auwerx J, Feingold KR. Stimulation of PPARalpha promotes epidermal keratinocyte differentiation in vivo. J Invest Dermatol 2000; 115:353–360.

19. Schmuth M, Schoonjans K, Yu QC, Fluhr JW, Crumrine D, Hachem JP, Lau P, Auwerx J, Elias PM, Feingold KR. Role of peroxisome proliferator-activated receptor alpha in epidermal development in utero. J Invest Dermatol 2002; 119:1298–1303.

20. Komuves LG, Hanley K, Man MQ, Elias PM, Williams ML, Feingold KR. Keratinocyte differentiation in hyperproliferative epidermis: topical application of PPARalpha activators restores tissue homeostasis. J Invest Dermatol 2000; 115:361–367.

21. Thuillier P, Brash AR, Kehrer JP, Stimmel JB, Leesnitzer LM, Yang P, Newman RA, Fischer SM. Inhibition of peroxisome proliferator-activated receptor (PPAR)-mediated keratinocyte differentiation by lipoxygenase inhibitors. Biochemical Journal 2002; 15:901–910.

22. Hanley K, Komuves LG, Ng DC, Schoonjans K, He SS, Lau P, Bikle DD, Williams ML, Elias PM, Auwerx J, Feingold KR. Farnesol stimulates differentiation in epidermal keratinocytes via PPARalpha. J Biol Chem 2000; 275:11484–11491.

23. Hanley K, Jiang Y, He SS, Friedman M, Elias PM, Bikle DD, Williams ML, Feingold KR. Keratinocyte differentiation is stimulated by activators of the nuclear hormone receptor PPARalpha. J Invest Dermatol 1998; 110:368–375.

24. Hanley K, Jiang Y, Crumrine D, Bass NM, Appel R, Elias PM, Williams ML, Feingold KR. Activators of the nuclear hormone receptors PPARalpha and FXR accelerate the development of the fetal epidermal permeability barrier. J Clin Invest 1997; 100:705–712.

25. Komuves LG, Hanley K, Jiang Y, Elias PM, Williams ML, Feingold KR. Ligands and activators of nuclear hormone receptors regulate epidermal differentiation during fetal rat skin development. J Invest Dermatol 1998; 111:429–433.

26. Hanley K, Komuves LG, Bass NM, He SS, Jiang Y, Crumrine D, Appel R, Friedman M, Bettencourt J, Min K, Elias PM, Williams ML, Feingold KR. Fetal epidermal differentiation and barrier development In vivo is accelerated by nuclear hormone receptor activators. J Invest Dermatol 1999; 113:788–795.

27. Chinetti G, Griglio S, Antonucci M, Torra IP, Delerive P, Majd Z, Fruchart JC, Chapman J, Najib J, Staels B. Activation of proliferator-activated receptors alpha and gamma induces apoptosis of human monocyte-derived macrophages. J Biol Chem 1998; 273:25573–25580.

28. Sheu MY, Fowler AJ, Kao J, Schmuth M, Schoonjans K, Auwerx J, Fluhr JW, Man MQ, Elias PM, Feingold KR. Topical peroxisome proliferator activated receptor-alpha activators reduce inflammation in irritant and allergic contact dermatitis models. J Invest Dermatol 2002; 118:94–101.

29. Kippenberger S, Loitsch SM, Grundmann-Kollmann M, Simon S, Dang TA, Hardt-Weinelt K, Kaufmann R, Bernd A. Activators of peroxisome proliferator-activated receptors protect human skin from ultraviolet-B-light-induced inflammation. J Invest Dermatol 2001; 117:1430–1436.

30. Willson TM, Brown PJ, Sternbach DD, Henke BR. The PPARs: from orphan receptors to drug discovery. J Med Chem 2000; 43:527–550.

31. Oliver WR, Shenk JL, Snaith MR, Russell CS, Kelli KD, Bodkin NL, Lewis MC, Winegar DA, Sznaidman ML, Lambert MH, Xu HE, Sternbach DD, Kliewer SA, Hansen BC, Willson TM. A selective peroxisome proliferator-activated receptor delta agonist promotes reverse cholesterol transport. Proc Natl Acad Sci U S A 2001; 98:5306–5311.

32. Bastie C, Luquet S, Holst D, Jehl-Pietri C, Grimaldi PA. Alterations of peroxisome proliferator-activated receptor delta activity affect fatty acid-controlled adipose differentiation. J Biol Chem 2000; 275:38768–38773.

33. Luquet S, Lopez-Soriano J, Holst D, Fredenrich A, Melki J, Rassoulzadegan M, Grimaldi PA. Peroxisome proliferator-activated receptor delta controls muscle development and oxidative capability. Faseb J 2003; 17:2299–2301.

34. Wang YX, Lee CH, Tiep S, Yu RT, Ham J, Kang H, Evans RM. Peroxisome-proliferator-activated receptor delta activates fat metabolism to prevent obesity. Cell 2003; 113:159–170.

35. Westergaard M, Henningsen J, Svendsen ML, Johansen C, Jensen UB, Schroder HD, Kratchmarova I, Berge RK, Iversen L, Bolund L, Kragballe K, Kristiansen K. Modulation of keratinocyte gene expression and differentiation by PPAR-selective ligands and tetradecylthioacetic acid. J Invest Dermatol 2001; 116:702–712.

36. Barak Y, Liao D, He W, Ong ES, Nelson MC, Olefsky JM, Boland R, Evans RM. Effects of peroxisome proliferator-activated receptor delta on placentation, adiposity, and colorectal cancer. Proc Natl Acad Sci U S A 2002; 99:303–308.

37. Tan NS, Michalik L, Noy N, Yasmin R, Pacot C, Heim M, Fluhmann B, Desvergne B, Wahli W. Critical roles of PPAR beta/delta in keratinocyte response to inflammation. Genes Dev 2001; 15:3263–3277.

38. Schmuth M, Haqq CM, Cairns WJ, Holder JC, Dorsam S, Chang S, Lau P, Fowler AJ, Chuang G, Moser AH, Brown BE, Mao-Qiang M, Uchida Y, Schoonjans K, Auwerx J, Chambon P, Willson TM, Elias PM, Feingold KR. Peroxisome proliferator-activated receptor (PPAR)-beta/delta stimulates differentiation and lipid accumulation in keratinocytes. J Invest Dermatol 2004; 122:971–983.

39. Gao J, Ye H, Serrero G. Stimulation of adipose differentiation related protein (ADRP) expression in adipocyte precursors by long-chain fatty acids. J Cell Physiol 2000; 182:297–302.

40. Schultz CJ, Torres E, Londos C, Torday JS. Role of adipocyte differentiation-related protein in surfactant phospholipid synthesis by type II cells. Am J Physiol Lung Cell Mol Physiol 2002; 283:L288–296.

41. Elias PM, Menon GK, Grayson S, Brown BE, Rehfeld SJ. Avian sebokeratocytes and marine mammal lipokeratinocytes: structural, lipid biochemical, and functional considerations. Am J Anat 1987; 180:161–177.

42. Ferraris C, Bernard BA, Dhouailly D. Adult epidermal keratinocytes are endowed with pilosebaceous forming abilities. Int J Dev Biol 1997; 41:491–498.

43. Kuenzli S, Saurat JH. Effect of topical PPARbeta/delta and PPARgamma agonists on plaque psoriasis. A pilot study.. Dermatology 2003; 206:252–256.

44. Kuenzli S, Saurat JH. Peroxisome proliferator-activated receptors in cutaneous biology. Br J Dermatol 2003; 149:229–236.

45. Spiegelman BM. PPAR-gamma: adipogenic regulator and thiazolidinedione receptor. Diabetes 1998; 47:507–514.

46. Mao-Qiang M, Fowler AJ, Schmuth M, Lau P, Chang S, Brown BE, Moser AH, Michalik L, Desvergne B, Wahli W, Li M, Metzger D, Chambon PH, Elias PM, Feingold KR. Peroxisome-proliferator-activated receptor (PPAR)-gamma activation stimulates keratinocyte differentiation. J Invest Dermatol 2004; 123(2):305–312.

47. Ellis CN, Varani J, Fisher GJ, Zeigler ME, Pershadsingh HA, Benson SC, Chi Y, Kurtz TW. Troglitazone improves psoriasis and normalizes models of proliferative skin disease: ligands for peroxisome proliferator-activated receptor-gamma inhibit keratinocyte proliferation. Arch Dermatol 2000; 136:609–616.

48. Mossner R, Kaiser R, Matern P, Kruger U, Westphal GA, Brockmoller J, Ziegler A, Neumann C, Konig IR, Reich K. Variations in the genes encoding the peroxisome proliferator-activated receptors alpha and gamma in psoriasis. Arch Dermatol Res 2004; 296:1–5.

49. Willy PJ, Umesono K, Ong ES, Evans RM, Heyman RA, Mangelsdorf DJ. LXR, a nuclear receptor that defines a distinct retinoid response pathway. Genes Dev 1995; 9:1033–1045.

50. Costet P, Luo Y, Wang N, Tall AR. Sterol-dependent transactivation of the ABC1 promoter by the liver X receptor/retinoid X receptor. J Biol Chem 2000; 275:28240–28245.

51. Luo Y, Tall AR. Sterol upregulation of human CETP expression in vitro and in transgenic mice by an LXR element. J Clin Invest 2000; 105:513–520.

52. Peet DJ, Turley SD, Ma W, Janowski BA, Lobaccaro JM, Hammer RE, Mangelsdorf DJ. Cholesterol and bile acid metabolism are impaired in mice lacking the nuclear oxysterol receptor LXR alpha. Cell 1998; 93:693–704.

53. Repa JJ, Turley SD, Lobaccaro JA, Medina J, Li L, Lustig K, Shan B, Heyman RA, Dietschy JM, Mangelsdorf DJ. Regulation of absorption and ABC1-mediated efflux of cholesterol by RXR heterodimers. Science 2000; 289:1524–1529.

54. Repa JJ, Mangelsdorf DJ. The role of orphan nuclear receptors in the regulation of cholesterol homeostasis. Annu Rev Cell Dev Biol 2000; 16:459–481.

55. Repa JJ, Liang G, Ou J, Bashmakov Y, Lobaccaro JM, Shimomura I, Shan B, Brown MS, Goldstein JL, Mangelsdorf DJ. Regulation of mouse sterol regulatory element-binding protein-1c gene (SREBP-1c) by oxysterol receptors, LXRalpha and LXRbeta. Genes Dev 2000; 14:2819–2830.

56. Komuves LG, Schmuth M, Fowler AJ, Elias PM, Hanley K, Man MQ, Moser AH, Lobaccaro JM, Williams ML, Mangelsdorf DJ, Feingold KR. Oxysterol stimulation of epidermal differentiation is mediated by liver X receptor-beta in murine epidermis. J Invest Dermatol 2002; 118:25–34.

57. Li YC, Pirro AE, Amling M, Delling G, Baron R, Bronson R, Demay MB. Targeted ablation of the vitamin D receptor: an animal model of vitamin D-dependent rickets type II with alopecia. Proc Natl Acad Sci U S A 1997; 94:9831–9835.

58. Xie Z, Komuves L, Yu QC, Elalieh H, Ng DC, Leary C, Chang S, Crumrine D, Yoshizawa T, Kato S, Bikle DD. Lack of the vitamin D receptor is associated with reduced epidermal differentiation and hair follicle growth. J Invest Dermatol 2002; 118:11–16.

59. Hanley K, Ng DC, He SS, Lau P, Min K, Elias PM, Bikle DD, Mangelsdorf DJ, Williams ML, Feingold KR. Oxysterols induce differentiation in human keratinocytes and increase Ap-1-dependent involucrin transcription. J Invest Dermatol 2000; 114:545–553.

60. Schmuth M, Elias PM, Hanley K, Lau P, Moser A, Willson TM, Bikle DD, Feingold KR. The effect of LXR activators on AP-1 proteins in keratinocytes. J Invest Dermatol 2004; 123:41–48.

61. Fowler AJ, Sheu MY, Schmuth M, Kao J, Fluhr JW, Rhein L, Collins JL, Willson TM, Mangelsdorf DJ, Elias PM, Feingold KR. Liver X receptor activators display anti-inflammatory activity in irritant and allergic contact dermatitis models: liver-X-receptor-specific inhibition of inflammation and primary cytokine production. J Invest Dermatol 2003; 120:246–255.

21

Permeability Barrier Homeostasis

Peter M. Elias
*Dermatology Service, VA Medical Center, and Department of Dermatology,
University of California, San Francisco, California, U.S.A.*

Kenneth R. Feingold
*Departments of Medicine and Dermatology, University of California,
San Francisco, California, U.S.A.*

STRUCTURAL AND BIOCHEMICAL BASIS FOR THE STRATUM CORNEUM BARRIER

Epidermal differentiation leads to the formation of the stratum corneum (SC), a heterogeneous tissue composed of lipid-depleted corneocytes embedded in a lipid-enriched extracellular matrix, which subserves the barrier (Fig. 1). These lipids derive from a highly active lipid-synthetic factory (1), operative in all of the nucleated cell layers of epidermis, which generates a unique lipid- and hydrolase-enriched secretory organelle, the epidermal lamellar body (LB) (2,3) (Chap. 16). LBs are $0.3–0.4 \times 0.25$ mm structures, which comprise about 10% of the cytosol of the stratum granulosum (SG) (2–4). Following secretion at the SG–SC interface, LB contents are processed from a polar lipid mixture into a hydrophobic mixture of ceramides, free fatty acids (FFAs), and cholesterol, and organized into the extracellular, lamellar membrane structures that form the hydrophobic matrix "mortar" within which corneocytes ("bricks") are embedded (Fig. 1) (4).

The Corneocyte

Whereas the importance of the extracellular lipid matrix for the permeability barrier is well known (see below), the role of the corneocyte in the permeability barrier is less well defined. Yet, the proteins of the corneocyte have been studied intensively as markers of epidermal differentiation (5,6) (Fig. 2), and they are well known to perform other critical epidermal functions [e.g., defense against external injury, UV filtration, and SC hydration (Chap. 24)] (7,8). One role of the corneocyte in the permeability barrier is to function as "spacers," i.e., they force water, microbes, and xenobiotics through the tortuous lipid-enriched extracellular pathway (9), and another role is their scaffold function for lamellar bilayer organization (see below).

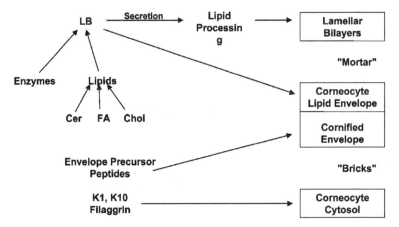

Figure 1 Major metabolic processes leading to formation of the two-compartment structure, the SC.

Proteins of the Cornified Envelope

The cornified envelope (CE) and its external ceramide-enriched, corneocyte lipid envelope (CLE) together provide a critical scaffold for the deposition and supramolecular organization of the extracellular lamellar membrane (see below). Moreover, CE-associated keratins and filaggrin contribute to the mechanical resistance of the SC by providing corneocyte rigidity (deformation). A distinctive feature of the CE is its stability to heating and to reducing or chaotropic agents, and its resistance to mechanical trauma. The CE is a 15-nm thick, peripheral product of terminal differentiation, which defines the formation of the SC (5,6). Yet, two types of CE occur in normal SC—a "fragile type" predominates in the lower SC and a rigid CE that becomes progressively more rigid, due to ongoing protein cross-linking, in the outer SC (10,11). In contrast,

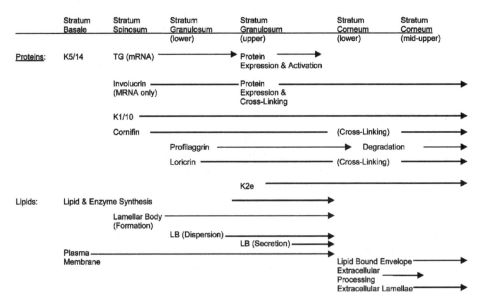

Figure 2 Parallel vertical differentiation pathways that generate the protein-enriched corneocyte and lipid-enriched extracellular matrix.

however, less "rigid" CE increases in proportion in hyperplastic and inflammatory skin conditions (10,11), consistent with increased rates of epidermal turn-over.

The CE consists of several highly cross-linked cytosolic proteins, including involucrin, loricrin, elafin, desmoplakin, envoplakin, cytostatin α, along with pancornulins/cornifins (small proline-rich proteins, SPRs) (12–14). Whereas involucrin predominates in the outer portion of the CE and accounts for 5–15% of the whole CE, loricrin accounts for up to 80% of CE protein mass, and the inner portion of the CE is also enriched with SPRs (12–14) (Table 1). Involucrin is a 68-kDa rod-shaped molecule, with a series of highly conserved 10 amino acid repeats, containing three glutamine residues, each serving as potential cross-linking sites (5,6,12). Expressed in the late spinous and SG layer, involucrin is the first envelope precursor that is cross-linked to nascent CEs by TG1, a process that begins in the outer SG (12). Loricrin is a cysteine (7%)-, serine (22%)-, and glycine (55%)-enriched 38-kDa highly insoluble peptide that comprises the principal component of L-type keratohyalin granules (12–14). Loricrin is expressed sequentially, late in differentiation, i.e., after K1/10 and involucrin are, and cross-linked to the CE immediately after LB secretion, coincident with cornification (15) (Fig. 2). A mutation resulting in elongation of the C-terminal domain of one loricrin allele occurs in some kindreds with Vohwinkle's disease (16). Patients with the loricrin defect display not only digital constrictions (pseudo-ainhum) and a dense honeycomb keratoderma, but also a mild generalized ichthyosis. Recent studies have shown that these patients also display a permeability barrier abnormality, which reflects an abnormal CE scaffold, as in lamellar ichthyosis (see below and Chap. 27).

Formation of the CE is catalyzed largely by the epidermal-specific, calcium-dependent enzyme, transglutaminase 1 (TG1), a 92-kDa protein, which catalyzes the formation of α-glutamyl-e-lysine isopeptide bonds between constituent precursor proteins (5,17). Although TG1 mRNA is expressed in the cytosol of both the spinous and granular layers, enzymatic activity is expressed primarily in the outermost granular cell (6). The activity distribution for TG1 coincides precisely with the peak in calcium (Ca) levels in the outer epidermis (18), consistent with the hypothesis that barrier-induced modulations in Ca regulate transcriptional expression of CE-associated proteins in vivo (Table 2). At least two other TG isoforms, TG2 (82 KDa) and TG3 (77 KDa), contribute variably to CE cross-linking. Yet, since the CEs from

Table 1 Protein Components of CE

	Characteristics
Outer portion	
Involucrin	Cross-linked earliest by TG1 (outer SG layer)
	Covalently attached to CLE
Inner portion	
Loricrin	Form bulk of inner portion of CE
Cornifin/SPRs, elafin	Also cross-linked after involucrin; cross-linking continues throughout SC
Filaggrin	Attached to CE by C-terminal region
Type II keratins (i.e., K1)	Attached to CE by V1 domain
Traverse CE	
Desmoglein, envoplakin	Attach to V1 domain of type II keratins

Abbreviations: CE, cornified envelope; TG, transglutaminase; CLE, cornified-bound lipid envelope; SG, stratum granulosum; SC, stratum corneum; SPR, small proline-rich proteins.

Table 2 Proposed Sequence of CE Formation and Associated Events

Layer	Ca++ gradient	Protein changes	Membrane changes
Outer SG layer	Peaks	Involucrin TG1 (+Ca++)	
Transitional cells	Declines	Involucrin-Involucrin TG1 (+Ca++) Loricrin, SPR's	Corneocyte lipid envelope SC extracellular lamellae
Above SG–SC interface	Disappears	Involucrin-Involucrin Loricrin, SPR's	Loss of plasma membrane Lamellar body secretion

Abbreviations: CE, cornified envelope; SG, stratum granulosum; SC, stratum corneum; TG, transglutaminase; SPR, small proline-rich protein.

the corneocytes of patients with lamellar ichthyosis are defective (19), residual TG2 and TG3 activities do not compensate completely for TG1 deficiency. TG1 is both the principal TG in the outer SG and the only isoform that is anchored to the plasma membrane (20), explaining the inability of lamellar ichthyosis keratinocytes to utilize their complement of TG2/TG3 to fully compensate for TG1 deficiency.

Whereas autosomal recessive forms of primary ichthyosis comprise a heterogeneous group, only patients with the severe classic lamellar ichthyosis phenotype display TG1 deficiency (21,22). A severe permeability barrier abnormality is present under basal conditions in lamellar ichthyosis skin (23–25). Yet, despite the attenuated CE in TG1-deficient patients (19), the increase in permeability occurs not across the defective CE, but rather through the SC interstices (24). Although the extracellular membranes in lamellar ichthyosis display minor abnormalities in interlamellar spacing (23,26), the basis for increased intercellular permeability is best explained by fragmentation of extracellular lamellae that occurs in these patients (24).

CE-associated proteins, while being necessary for the steady-state maintenance of normal barrier homeostasis, are transiently down-regulated following acute barrier perturbations, presumably as a form of metabolic conservation that conserves energy for lipid production (27). Thus, the lipid and protein pathways of epidermal differentiation do not operate as separate processes, but instead as parallel, interdependent, and co-regulated sequences (Table 2, Fig. 2). These two compartments, in turn, are linked firmly through the CE/CLE, together providing the scaffold necessary for the deposition of the extracellular matrix.

Structural Proteins of the Corneocyte Cytosol

Keratins are the most abundant structural proteins of the epidermis and its appendages, maintaining the mechanical properties of these epithelia, a role that is most vividly demonstrated in the epidermis (28,29) (Chap. 10). Keratins are of two types, type I or acidic (K9–20) and type II or basic (K1–8), which are co-expressed in pairs under a variety of conditions. All keratins display a similar secondary structure, with a central rod domain comprising four α helices, and distinctive, non-helical head and tail sequences. Whereas K5 and -14 are expressed in the basal layer, K1/2e/10 are expressed in suprabasal layers (29), eventually accounting for 80% of the mass of the corneocyte. Deletions of as few as 10 amino acids from the rod domain of either K1, 2e, or 10 result in keratin clumping, i.e., the defective allelic protein binds to its partner in a dominant-negative fashion, forming defective intermediate filaments, resulting in several forms of epidermolytic hyperkeratosis (EHK) (30,31) (Chap. 27). Patients in this group of autosomal dominant disorders display a variable phenotype, which shifts from a predominantly blistering disorder in neonates to predominant hyperkeratosis, after exposure to the xeric postnatal environment (32), while a milder phenotype with flexural accentuation and molting occurs with mutations of keratin 2e [ichthyosis bullosa of Siemens, IBS (33)]. The basis for the permeability barrier abnormality in EHK has been shown recently to result from the cytoskeleton abnormality, i.e., rather than being due to corneocyte fragility, the abnormal keratin pairs interfere with LB secretion, which results in decreased amounts of extracellular lipids (34).

Type II keratin filaments, with their partners, interact covalently with the CE via a single lysine residue in a highly conserved region of the VI subdomain of K1 (35) (Table 1). Accordingly, mutations in the Vl domain affecting a highly conserved lysine residue interfere with the insertion of type II keratins to desmoplakin in the

CE (35). These patients display a diffuse non-epidermolytic palmo-plantar kerato-derma with acral keratotic plaques (35,36). We have shown that this mutation results in detachment and retraction of keratin bundles from desmosomes in the SG and corneodesmosomes in the SC, resulting both in micro-vesiculation and deformation of the keratinocyte periphery (36) (i.e., corneocytes do not flatten properly). Whether this alteration impacts negatively on the barrier in non–palmar-plantar lesions of these patients, and how filament detachment leads to the putative barrier abnormality is not known.

Profilaggrin is a large histidine-rich, highly cationic phosphoprotein member of the S100 family of proteins (Chap. 9). It consists of numerous 37-kDa filaggrin repeats, connected by peptide segments enriched in hydrophobic amino acids (37). Profilaggrin is concentrated within keratohyalin granules, where it may sequester loricrin, which also localizes to keratohyalin. During terminal differentiation, profilaggrin is both dephosphorylated and proteolytically processed by a Ca^{++}-dependent protein convertase, furin, at the N-terminus to yield filaggrin (38), which ionically binds to K1/10, inducing the formation of macrofibrils in the corneocyte cytosol (39). Immunolocalization studies suggest that processed filaggrin peptides associate initially with the CE via their N-terminal domain in the lower SC (Table 1), but they later dissociate into precursors of hygroscopically active amino acids and deiminated products in the cytosol of the mid- to outer SC, in an external humidity-dependent fashion (40) (Chaps. 9 and 24).

Regulation of Corneocyte Protein Expression

Members of both the Class I and Class II families of nuclear hormone receptors (NHR) influence both epidermal permeability barrier homeostasis and development in utero (Tables 3 and 4). At least three ligands of the Class I family, which comprises receptors for the steroid hormones, such as glucocorticoids, estrogens, and androgens, have been shown to influence permeability barrier development in fetal skin, as well as barrier homeostasis in adult skin [reviewed in Ref. 41]. In fetal skin both exogenous glucocorticoids and estrogens, either administered in utero or added directly to fetal skin explants in organ culture, accelerate the development of a mature permeability barrier, while in contrast, administration of androgens retards barrier ontogenesis (Table 3). Although the impact of Class I ligands on barrier function in postnatal skin is less well understood, normal-to-supranormal levels of androgens provoke an analogous decline in permeability barrier homeostasis in adult murine and human skin (42). Yet in contrast, an increase in endogenous glucocorticoids, induced either by psychological stress (43) or by systemic administration of supraphysiologic levels

Table 3 NHR Activators Modulate Barrier Ontogenesis

Stimulate	No effect	Delay
Glucocorticoids	1,25(OH)$_2$D3	Androgens
Estrogens	9-*cis*-RA	
Thyroid hormone	Retinoids	
PPARα ligands	Growth factors (e.g., EGF)	
LXR ligands		

Abbreviations: NHR, nuclear hormone receptor; PPAR, peroxisome proliferator activator receptors; LXR, liver X receptor; EGF, epidermal growth factor.

Table 4 Cutaneous Effects of Liposensor vs. Classic Class II NHR Ligands

Receptor	Ligands/ activators	Fetal barrier development	Adult barrier homeostasis	Anti-inflammatory
Classic				
RAR	All-*trans*-retinoic acid	None	Worse	Improves
T₃R	Triiodothyronine (T3)	Accelerates	?	?
D₃R	1,25(OH)2 vitamin D3	None	Worse	Improves
Liposensor				
PPARα	Leukotriene B4, fatty acids, fibrates	Accelerates	Accelerates	Improves
PPARγ	Prostaglandin J₂, troglitazone	None	Accelerates	Improves
PPARβ/δ	Fatty acids, fibrates	?	Accelerates	Improves
LXR	Oxygenated sterols	Accelerates	Accelerates	Improves

Abbreviations: RAR, retinoic acid; T₃R thyroid hormone; D₃R, vitamin D₃; PPAR, peroxisome proliferator activator receptors; LXR Liver X receptors.

of exogenous steroids (44), alters both permeability barrier homeostasis and SC integrity/cohesion. Why the functional effects of some Class I ligands (e.g., effects of glucocorticoids) diverge in fetal versus postnatal skin is not yet known.

The Class II family of NHR includes not only receptors for well-known ligands, such as thyroid hormone (T₃R), retinoic acid (RAR), and 1,25(OH)2 vitamin D3 (D₃R), but also a number of other receptors ("liposensors") whose activators/ligands are endogenous lipids (45,46) (Table 4) (see also Chap. 20). The role of these receptors, which include that of the peroxisome proliferator activator receptors (PPARs) and liver X receptor (LXR), in epidermal function has been characterized recently (45,46) (Table 4). The activators for these liposensors, e.g., PPARα, PPARγ, PPARβ/γ, and LXRα/β, include lipid synthetic intermediates or their metabolites, including certain FFAs, leukotrienes, prostanoids, and oxygenated sterols (41). Over the last six years, activation of these liposensor receptors has been shown to both accelerate fetal skin development (47–49) and induce keratinocyte differentiation, both in vitro and in vivo (48,50–52). Both by regulating the transcription of key corneocyte proteins, e.g., involucrin, loricrin, and TG1 (50,53), and by stimulating both epidermal lipid synthesis and secretion (54), these liposensors can potentially influence both the "brick" and "mortar" compartments of the barrier (Fig. 3). Since increased quantities of sterol and FFA metabolites are generated during epidermal development (55) and also as co-products of the increased lipid synthesis that follows barrier disruption (see below), it becomes increasingly likely that processes leading to formation/restoration of the lipid matrix could concurrently promote corneocyte protein production (Fig. 3). Moreover, since these agents also reverse the barrier abnormalities, epidermal hyperplasia, and cutaneous inflammation in various animal models (50–58), they hold substantial promise as therapeutic agents in dermatology (59).

Extracellular Lipids of the SC

Whereas LB secretion delivers a large quantity of lipids to the SC interstices (≈10% of dry weight), it is the further processing of the secreted LB contents that generates a mixture of non-polar lipids, enriched in ceramides, cholesterol, and FFAs, in an

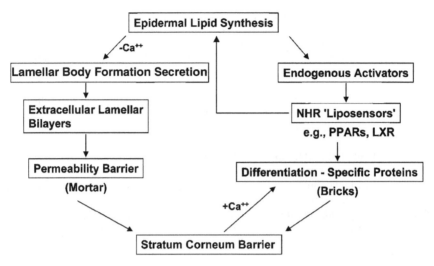

Figure 3 Co-ordinate regulation of epidermal differentiation and lamellar body secretion by calcium and nuclear hormone receptors.

approximately equimolar ratio (Table 5). Lesser and variable amounts of cholesterol esters, cholesterol sulfate, triglycerides, and diglycerides also persist, some of which may be of sebaceous gland origin (1,60,61) (Chap. 5). The FFAs comprise a mixture of essential (EFAs) and non-essential (NEFAs) FFAs, and both NEFAs and EFAs are required separately as critical structural ingredients of the barrier (60) (Table 5). NEFAs derive largely, if not entirely, from the hydrolysis of phospholipids, which are co-secreted with their respective secretory phospholipases at the SG–SC interface (62,63). These phospholipid-derived NEFAs are critical not only as structural ingredients of the barrier, but as described below, they also are key acidifiers of the SC interstices (64).

Exocytosis of LB contents delivers abundant cholesterol, which is secreted unchanged into the SC interstices. Additional, but lesser quantities of cholesterol derive also from the hydrolysis of cholesterol sulfate to cholesterol by the enzyme, steroid sulfatase (65). A variety of studies have shown that not only cholesterol, but also hydrolysis of cholesterol sulfate (i.e., elimination of excess substrate), is critical for permeability barrier function (66) (Chap. 28).

A third key lipid constituent of the mortar is a family of up to nine ceramide species (Fig. 4), which vary (67) according to their (i) sphingosine versus

Table 5 How Stratum Corneum Lipids Mediate Barrier Function

1. Extracellular localization (only intercellular lipids play role)
2. Amount of lipid (lipid wt%)
3. Elongated, tortuous pathway (increases diffusion path length)
4. Organization into lamellar membrane structures
5. Hydrophobic composition (absence of polar lipids and presence of very long chain saturated free fatty acids)
6. Correct molar ratio (approximately equimolar ratio of three key lipids: ceramides, cholesterol, and non-essential free fatty acids)
7. Unique, linoleic acid-bearing molecule structures (i.e., acylceramides)

Table 4 Cutaneous Effects of Liposensor vs. Classic Class II NHR Ligands

Receptor	Ligands/ activators	Fetal barrier development	Adult barrier homeostasis	Anti-inflammatory
Classic				
RAR	All-*trans*-retinoic acid	None	Worse	Improves
T₃R	Triiodothyronine (T3)	Accelerates	?	?
D₃R	1,25(OH)2 vitamin D3	None	Worse	Improves
Liposensor				
PPARα	Leukotriene B4, fatty acids, fibrates	Accelerates	Accelerates	Improves
PPARγ	Prostaglandin J₂, troglitazone	None	Accelerates	Improves
PPARβ/δ	Fatty acids, fibrates	?	Accelerates	Improves
LXR	Oxygenated sterols	Accelerates	Accelerates	Improves

Abbreviations: RAR, retinoic acid; T_3R thyroid hormone; D_3R, vitamin D_3; PPAR, peroxisome proliferator activator receptors; LXR Liver X receptors.

of exogenous steroids (44), alters both permeability barrier homeostasis and SC integrity/cohesion. Why the functional effects of some Class I ligands (e.g., effects of glucocorticoids) diverge in fetal versus postnatal skin is not yet known.

The Class II family of NHR includes not only receptors for well-known ligands, such as thyroid hormone (T_3R), retinoic acid (RAR), and 1,25(OH)2 vitamin D3 (D_3R), but also a number of other receptors ("liposensors") whose activators/ligands are endogenous lipids (45,46) (Table 4) (see also Chap. 20). The role of these receptors, which include that of the peroxisome proliferator activator receptors (PPARs) and liver X receptor (LXR), in epidermal function has been characterized recently (45,46) (Table 4). The activators for these liposensors, e.g., PPARα, PPARγ, PPARβ/γ, and LXRα/β, include lipid synthetic intermediates or their metabolites, including certain FFAs, leukotrienes, prostanoids, and oxygenated sterols (41). Over the last six years, activation of these liposensor receptors has been shown to both accelerate fetal skin development (47–49) and induce keratinocyte differentiation, both in vitro and in vivo (48,50–52). Both by regulating the transcription of key corneocyte proteins, e.g., involucrin, loricrin, and TG1 (50,53), and by stimulating both epidermal lipid synthesis and secretion (54), these liposensors can potentially influence both the "brick" and "mortar" compartments of the barrier (Fig. 3). Since increased quantities of sterol and FFA metabolites are generated during epidermal development (55) and also as co-products of the increased lipid synthesis that follows barrier disruption (see below), it becomes increasingly likely that processes leading to formation/restoration of the lipid matrix could concurrently promote corneocyte protein production (Fig. 3). Moreover, since these agents also reverse the barrier abnormalities, epidermal hyperplasia, and cutaneous inflammation in various animal models (56–50), they hold substantial promise as therapeutic agents in dermatology (59).

Extracellular Lipids of the SC

Whereas LB secretion delivers a large quantity of lipids to the SC interstices ($\approx 10\%$ of dry weight), it is the further processing of the secreted LB contents that generates a mixture of non-polar lipids, enriched in ceramides, cholesterol, and FFAs, in an

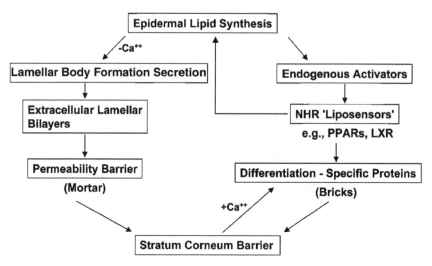

Figure 3 Co-ordinate regulation of epidermal differentiation and lamellar body secretion by calcium and nuclear hormone receptors.

approximately equimolar ratio (Table 5). Lesser and variable amounts of cholesterol esters, cholesterol sulfate, triglycerides, and diglycerides also persist, some of which may be of sebaceous gland origin (1,60,61) (Chap. 5). The FFAs comprise a mixture of essential (EFAs) and non-essential (NEFAs) FFAs, and both NEFAs and EFAs are required separately as critical structural ingredients of the barrier (60) (Table 5). NEFAs derive largely, if not entirely, from the hydrolysis of phospholipids, which are co-secreted with their respective secretory phospholipases at the SG–SC interface (62,63). These phospholipid-derived NEFAs are critical not only as structural ingredients of the barrier, but as described below, they also are key acidifiers of the SC interstices (64).

Exocytosis of LB contents delivers abundant cholesterol, which is secreted unchanged into the SC interstices. Additional, but lesser quantities of cholesterol derive also from the hydrolysis of cholesterol sulfate to cholesterol by the enzyme, steroid sulfatase (65). A variety of studies have shown that not only cholesterol, but also hydrolysis of cholesterol sulfate (i.e., elimination of excess substrate), is critical for permeability barrier function (66) (Chap. 28).

A third key lipid constituent of the mortar is a family of up to nine ceramide species (Fig. 4), which vary (67) according to their (i) sphingosine versus

Table 5 How Stratum Corneum Lipids Mediate Barrier Function

1. Extracellular localization (only intercellular lipids play role)
2. Amount of lipid (lipid wt%)
3. Elongated, tortuous pathway (increases diffusion path length)
4. Organization into lamellar membrane structures
5. Hydrophobic composition (absence of polar lipids and presence of very long chain saturated free fatty acids)
6. Correct molar ratio (approximately equimolar ratio of three key lipids: ceramides, cholesterol, and non-essential free fatty acids)
7. Unique, linoleic acid-bearing molecule structures (i.e., acylceramides)

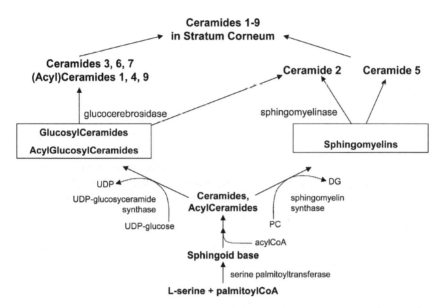

Figure 4 Ceramide fractions originate from either glucosylceramides and/or sphingomyelins.

phytosphingosine (extra-OH group) base, (ii) α- versus non–α-hydroxylated N-acyl fatty acids, which typically are >C30 in length, and (iii) the presence of an additional ω-esterified linoleic acid residue (Chap. 6). The latter (ceramides 1 and 4) are the principal repositories for linoleic acid, a critical structural ingredient in the barrier (Table 5). These epidermis-unique molecules appear to link adjacent bilayers through their highly elongated N-acyl chains (68) (Chap. 7). The importance of the esterified linoleate moiety for barrier function is shown by EFA deficiency, where the primary biochemical defect is a substitution of NEFA for linoleic acid, a biochemical alteration that results in a pronounced permeability barrier defect (60). Finally, it is important to note that sphingomyelin is a precursor for only two of the SC ceramides, while glucosylceramides can generate the full spectrum of SC ceramide (69).

Corneocyte Lipid Envelope

A 10-nm tightly apposed, electron-lucent, plasma membrane-like structure, now termed the corneocyte lipid envelope (CLE), replaces the plasma membrane on the external aspect of mammalian corneocytes (70,71). After aggressive solvent treatment (e.g., chloroform:methanol extraction), the CLE appears to comprise a single outer electron-dense leaflet, separated from the CE by an electron-lucent space (71). However, following the treatment with the polar solvent, pyridine, the CLE can be seen instead to comprise a trilaminar structure intimately related to the CE (72,73). Moreover, pyridine treatment also uniquely reveals images of the partially formed CE at the level of the SG (72), consistent with the evidence that involucrin cross-linking already occurs at this level of the epidermis (12). Indirect evidence supports the concept that involucrin cross-linking occurs early in epidermal differentiation (Table 2), forming a scaffold for CLE formation. The CLE comprises unique ω-hydroxyceramides (Cer) with very long chain N-acyl fatty acids (70,71,74), covalently bound to the CE. Involucrin-enriched CE fractions contain covalently bound lipid with a molecular mass and fatty acid composition that is comparable to ω-hydroxyceramides (12). Although it has been proposed that these ω-hydroxy-ceramides derive from the lipolytic hydrolysis of secreted acylceramides, it appears more likely that they result from the insertion of the ω-glucosyl hydroxyceramide–enriched limiting membrane of the LB into the apical plasma membrane of the outermost granular (SG) cells (74). Since the CLE forms in both cultured keratinocytes and Harlequin ichthyosis in the absence of LB with replete contents (73), it is likely that the CLE derives solely from the insertion of the limiting membrane of the LB into the plasma membrane. Bound glucosylated ω-hydroxy-ceramides are quickly deglucosylated (75). The CLE could serve (i) as a "molecular rivet" in SC cohesion (74), and/or (ii) as a scaffold for extracellular lamellar membrane organization (18,56) (Chap. 6 & 15). Despite its extreme hydrophobicity, the CLE's ability to restrict water movement is unclear, since solvent extraction of SC leaves the CLE intact, while the SC becomes completely porous to transcutaneous water loss (73). Yet, the CLE could still restrict transcutaneous water loss to extracellular domains, while minimizing both uptake of water into the corneocyte and egress of humectants out of the corneocyte cytosol.

METABOLIC REGULATION OF PERMEABILITY BARRIER HOMEOSTASIS

Although the SC has many functions, none is as important as its ability to serve as a protective barrier that prevents the loss of excess fluids and electrolytes (76). Hence, the mechanisms that maintain and restore permeability barrier function deserve special attention (1,7,8).

Dynamics of Barrier Recovery—The Cutaneous Stress Test

Acute barrier disruption, regardless of the method (organic solvent, detergent, tape stripping), depletes the SC of its complement of lipids, stimulating a series of lipid/DNA synthetic responses that leads to barrier recovery (61) (Fig. 5). Although the total time required for barrier recovery can vary, in all cases, there is an initial rapid recovery phase that leads to 50% to 60% recovery in normal murine epidermis by about six hours (1), followed by a prolonged recovery phase that requires about 35 hours for completion (77). In humans, the acute recovery phase is longer (about 12 hours), and the later recovery phase is prolonged to 72 hours (78). Restoration of barrier function is accompanied by re-accumulation of lipids within the SC interstices (77,78), visible with Nile red fluorescence, and by the re-appearance of membrane bilayers, as early as two hours after acute disruption.

Applications of the Cutaneous Stress Test

The kinetics of barrier recovery after acute perturbation have proved useful in assessing epidermal metabolic processes that contribute to permeability barrier homeostasis (Fig. 5). But this test has also been deployed as a physiologic challenge (i.e., stress test) to unearth abnormal function, even when basal parameters are normal. Thus, the "cutaneous stress" test is analogous to other types of clinical maneuvers that are deployed in the search for underlying clinical pathology (e.g., cardiac treadmill exam, overnight water deprivation for kidney function, etc.). Indeed, the cutaneous stress test reveals deficient function in both aged (78) and neonatal skin (79),

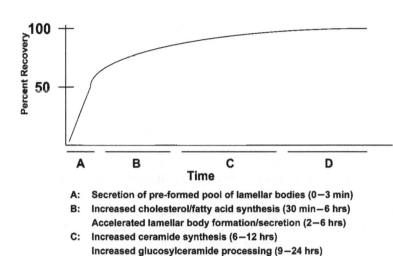

A: Secretion of pre-formed pool of lamellar bodies (0–3 min)
B: Increased cholesterol/fatty acid synthesis (30 min–6 hrs)
   Accelerated lamellar body formation/secretion (2–6 hrs)
C: Increased ceramide synthesis (6–12 hrs)
   Increased glucosylceramide processing (9–24 hrs)
D: Increased DNA synthesis (16–24 hrs)

Figure 5 The cutaneous stress test: acute barrier perturbations stimulate specific metabolic responses that normalize function.

as well as in the skin of individuals subjected to increased psychological stress (80) (Fig. 6). Further, it amplifies differences in barrier function among "normal" groups, e.g., in testosterone-replete versus deficient individuals (42), in subjects exposed to a humid environment (81), and in individuals with type 5–6 versus 1–2 pigmentation (82). Although clinicians have not yet fully exploited this tool, these results could explain the propensity for inflammatory dermatoses to be more severe in males than in females, for fair-skinned individuals to have "sensitive" (? atopic) skin, and for stress-induced flares of inflammatory skin disease. In Figure 6, we show how these additional factors could further aggravate skin disorders, which are already associated with abnormal barrier function, i.e., via amplification of the cytokine cascade (Chap. 2 & 19).

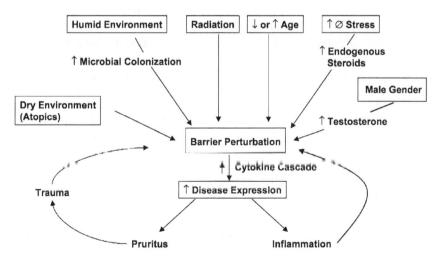

Figure 6 The cutaneous stress test reveals additional situations that can predispose to exacerbation or flares of dermatoses.

Lamellar Body (LB) Secretion and Post-Secretory Processing

In both rodents and humans, acute disruption of the permeability barrier by mechanical forces, solvents, or detergents increases transepidermal water loss, initiating a homeostatic repair response that results in the rapid recovery of permeability barrier function. The first step in the repair response that follows barrier disruption is the rapid secretion (within minutes) of a pool of performed LB contents from cells of the outer SG (Fig. 5), which leaves the cytosol of these cells largely devoid of LB (83) (Chap. 16). Abundant evidence supports the concept that LB secretion is signaled by the reduction of Ca^{++} that accompanies barrier disruptions (see below). Newly formed LB then begins to appear in SG cells by 30 to 60 minutes, and by three to six hours the number of LB in SG cells returns to normal (84). Because of accelerated secretion and organellogenesis between 30 minutes and six hours, the quantities of secreted LB contents increase at the SG–SC interface, and by two hours new, lipid-enriched lamellar bilayers re-appear in the lower SC (84).

The lamellar lipids in the SC interstices derive primarily from the exocytosis of LB chain, which are enriched in cholesterol, glucosylceramide, phospholipids, and co-secreted hydrolytic enzymes (85,86). Thus, exocytosis of LB provides a pathway by which the cells of the outer epidermis are able to deliver lipids and lipid-processing enzymes simultaneously to the extracellular spaces of the SC (Fig. 2) (Chap. 16). Within the SC, the co-localized hydrolytic enzymes, including acidic sphingomyelinase, β-glucocerebrosidase (β-GlcCer'ase), and secretory phospholipase A_2 (sPLA$_2$), catalyze the extracellular degradation of sphingomyelinase and glucosylceramides to ceramides, and phospholipids to FFA, respectively, thereby generating the key lipid products that form the mature lamellar membranes required for permeability barrier function (2,7,8). These morphological and biochemical changes are paralleled by a progressive normalization of permeability barrier function.

Regulation of Lipid Synthesis by Barrier Requirements

The rapid LB formation by the SG cells following barrier disruption requires the availability of the major lipid components of LB, namely cholesterol, glucosylceramides, and phospholipids. The epidermis is a very active site of lipid synthesis, and permeability barrier disruption results in a rapid, marked increase in the synthesis of cholesterol, ceramides, and fatty acids (87,88) (a major component of both phospholipids and ceramides) (Fig. 7). The increase in cholesterol synthesis is associated with an increase in the activity, protein levels, and mRNA levels of HMG CoA reductase (89), and in other key enzymes of the cholesterol synthetic pathway, i.e., HMG CoA synthase, farnesyl diphosphate synthase, and squalene synthase (Fig. 7) (90). Whereas, the increase in fatty acid synthesis is due to an increase in the activity and mRNA levels of both of the key enzymes of fatty acid synthesis, acetyl CoA carboxylase and fatty acid synthase (91). The increase in ceramide synthesis is due to an increase in the activity and mRNA levels of serine palmitoyl transferase (88) (Fig. 7), the enzyme that catalyzes the initial and first committed step in ceramide synthesis. Although the activity of glucosylceramide synthase, the enzyme which synthesizes glucosylceramides, does not increase following barrier disruption (92), glucosylceramide synthesis could still change depending upon the availability of ceramides and fatty acids. Thus, a specific, coordinate increase in the synthesis of the key lipid constituents of LB provides the pool of lipids that is required for the formation of new LB (Fig. 3).

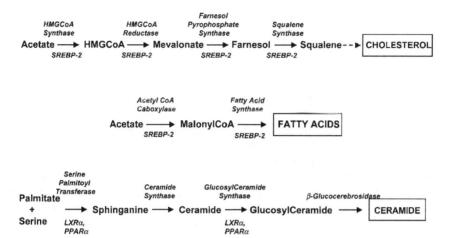

Figure 7 Metabolic pathways leading to synthesis of cholesterol, fatty acids, and ceramides.

Transcriptional Regulation of Epidermal Lipid Synthesis

Cholesterol and Fatty Acid Synthesis

Seminal studies by Brown and Goldstein in their laboratory have demonstrated that both cholesterol and fatty acid syntheses are feed-back regulated by a group of transcription factors, the sterol regulatory element–binding proteins (SREBPs) (93). Two SREBP genes (SREBP-1 and SREBP-2) encode three proteins, SREBP-1a, SREBP-1c, and SREBP-2 (94,95). These tripartite proteins, which are ≈1150 amino acids in length, with a ≈480 amino acid NH2-terminal segment facing the cytosol, are members of the basic helix–loop–helix leucine zipper family of transcription factors. This NH2-terminal segment is followed by a membrane attachment fragment of ≈80 amino acids, containing two membrane-spanning sequences separated by a ≈31 amino acid hydrophilic loop that projects into the lumen of the ER and nuclear envelope, and a COOH-terminal segment of ≈590 amino acids that projects into the cytosol. The cholesterol-sensing mechanism, which involves movement of pro-SREBP from the endoplasmic reticulum to the Golgi apparatus, is activated by sterol depletion (96,97). A two-step proteolytic process occurs that results in the release of the NH2-terminal segments, allowing them to enter the nucleus, where they bind as homodimers to cis-elements in the promoters of multiple SREBP-responsive genes stimulating various enzymes of cholesterol and fatty acid syntheses (93,95). In contrast, when excess cholesterol accumulates, proteolytic cleavage is inhibited and transcription of target genes declines (96,97). The two-step cleavage process that leads to the release of active SREBPs begins at site 1, between the Leu and Ser of the RSVLS sequence, in the middle of the hydrophilic loop (95). The site 1 protease (S1P) is a serine protease that splits the lumenal loop of SREBPs into two halves that remain attached by their membrane attachment domains. Because the S1P localizes to the Golgi apparatus, cleavage of SREBPs is initiated there. Transport of SREBPs from the endoplasmic reticulum to the Golgi apparatus is facilitated by SREBP cleavage-activating protein (SCAP), an elongated protein whose COOH terminus complexes with the COOH-terminus of SREBPs (97). The final release of the active NH2 fragment of SREBP requires a second proteolytic step at site 2, a Leu–Cys bond at the border of the cytosolic and membrane portion of the NH2 segment. Although the site 2 protease (S2P) is not regulated directly by changes in cholesterol levels, it can only act after prior site 1 cleavage has occurred. Together, this feedback system insures that cells obtain an uninterrupted supply of optimal levels of cholesterol and fatty acids, while also preventing their accumulation.

SREBP-1 and -2 activate the same family of genes, but in different proportions (93–95,98). In general, SREBP-2 is a more important regulator of cholesterol synthesis, e.g., cholesterol-depleted cells preferentially up-regulate SREBP-2, and SREBP-1 knockout animals up-regulate SREBP-2 and normalize cholesterol synthesis in response to decreased cellular sterols (94–97). SREBP-1a is as effective as SREBP-2 as a regulator of HMGCoA synthase and HMGCoA reductase (i.e., cholesterol synthesis), but it has a greater effect on fatty acid synthesis than does SREBP-2, while SREBP-1c primarily regulates fatty acid synthesis (94,95). Although both SREBP-1a and -1c are expressed in keratinocytes (99), SREBP-2 predominates in both murine epidermis and in cultured human keratinocytes (99). Moreover, SREBP-2 appears to coordinately regulate cholesterol and fatty acid syntheses in keratinocytes (Fig. 7), but its role in the transcriptional regulation of the lipid synthetic response to barrier disruption is not yet clear.

Ceramide Synthesis

Regulation of ceramide synthesis occurs predominantly by alterations in the activity of SPT and/or the availability of the FFA, palmitic acid, a substrate for SPT (88) (Figs. 3 and 7). Thus, alterations in FA synthesis, potentially regulated by SREBPs, could indirectly affect ceramide production (90). Yet, the expression of this enzyme is not regulated directly by SREBP, as SPT mRNA levels increase, rather than decrease, with oxysterol blockade of SREBP activation (99). In contrast, SPT expression increases in response to inflammatory stimuli, such as UV light, endotoxin, and cytokines (TNF and IL-1) (100). To what extent and how liposensor activators could regulate ceramide/glucosylceramides production is a subject of intense current study (98) (Fig. 3).

Barrier Homeostasis Requires Synthesis of Each of the Three Key Lipids

Using specific inhibitors of key synthetic enzymes, we demonstrated an individual requirement for cholesterol, fatty acids, ceramides, and glucosylceramides for barrier formation (1). For example, blockade of cholesterol synthesis with topical inhibitors of HMG CoA reductase (e.g., statins) delays barrier recovery, and selectively delays the return of cholesterol to the SC (101). These effects are due to a specific block in cholesterol synthesis, rather than to non-specific toxicity, because co-applications of either mevalonate (the immediate product of HMG CoA reductase) or cholesterol (the distal product) normalize barrier homeostasis. Likewise, topical 5-(tetradecyloxy)-2-furancarboxylic acid (TOFA), an inhibitor of acetyl CoA carboxylase, one of the two key enzymes of FA synthesis, inhibits epidermal fatty acid synthesis and delays barrier repair (102). TOFA-induced inhibition of barrier repair can also be overcome by topical co-applications of FFA, again demonstrating the specificity of the inhibitor effect. Beta-chloroalanine, a selective inhibitor of serine palmitoyl transferase, also delays barrier recovery after acute barrier disruption, and inhibition of barrier recovery can be overcome by co-applications of exogenous ceramides, again demonstrating specificity. Finally, PDMP, a selective inhibitor of glucosylceramide synthase, also inhibits barrier recovery after acute disruption (92). Inhibition of all of these enzymes results in a decrease in LB formation, contents, and secretion, as well as a decrease in extracellular lamellar bilayers. Thus, epidermal cholesterol, fatty acid, ceramide, and glucosylceramide syntheses are required individually for LB formation and barrier homeostasis (1,61).

The Three Key SC Lipids are Required in an Equimolar Distribution

Whereas the above-described studies clearly demonstrate the specific requirement for each of the three key lipids (cholesterol, fatty acids, and ceramides) for the permeability barrier, these lipids must be generated or supplied together in the proper proportions for normal barrier recovery (103). Topical applications of any one or two of the three key lipids to acutely perturbed skin actually result in a delay of barrier recovery. In contrast, when the three key lipids are applied in an equimolar mixture, recovery is normal (103). Both incomplete and complete mixtures of the three key lipids rapidly traverse the SC, internalize within the granular cell layer (103), bypassing the endoplasmic reticulum and proximal Golgi apparatus, while targeting distal sites (i.e., the trans-Golgi network), where LB are formed (104). Within the LB the exogenous and endogenous lipids mix, producing normal or abnormal LB contents and derived lamellar membrane structures depending on the molar distribution of the applied lipids. Further acceleration of barrier recovery can be achieved by increasing the proportion of any of the three key lipids to a 3:1:1 ratio (105). In contrast, non-physiologic lipids, like petrolatum, function like vapor-permeable membranes at the surface of the SC (106). Thus, physiologic mixtures of topical lipids affect barrier recovery, not by occluding the SC, but rather by contributing to the lipid pool within SG cells, thereby regulating the formation of LB. The contrasting features of non-physiologic and physiologic lipids dictate the clinical settings where each is uniquely useful (Table 6) (see also the Epilogue).

Table 6 Logical Barrier Repair Strategies–Clinical Indications

Repair strategy	Clinical indication
Dressings	
Vapor permeable	Healing wounds
Vapor impermeable	Keloids
NPL	
Petrolatum or lanolin	Radiation dermatitis or severe sunburn
	Premature infants (aged <34 weeks)
PL: optimal molar ratio	
Cholesterol-dominant	Aging or photoaging
Ceramide-dominant	Atopic dermatitis
Free fatty acid–dominant	Neonatal skin, including psoriasis, diaper dermatitis (with added NPL)
Cholesterol-, ceramide-, or free fatty acid–dominant	Irritant contact dermatitis (with added NPL)
	Glucocorticoid-treated
	Psychological stress

Abbreviations: NPL, non-physiologic lipids; PL, physiologic lipids.

Potential of Barrier Repair Therapy (See also the Epilogue)

Logically then, bolstering the skin's barrier status should increase the resistance to inflammation, and further decrease the susceptibility to those skin diseases which are triggered, sustained, or exacerbated by external perturbations, such as atopic dermatitis, contact dermatitis, and psoriasis. All of these diseases are characterized by a barrier abnormality, and the clinical severity is reflected by the extent of the barrier abnormality (107). Hence, the recent emergence of "barrier repair" strategies to decrease the susceptibility to these disorders. These repair approaches can be classified into three categories (108) (Table 6): (i) mixtures of all three *physiologic lipids* (ceramides, cholesterol, and FFAs) in appropriate molar ratios; (ii) one or more *non-physiologic* lipids (e.g., petrolatum, lanolin); and (iii) *dressings*, either vapor-permeable, which allow metabolic (repair) processes to continue in the underlying epidermis, or vapor-impermeable, which shut down metabolic responses in the underlying epidermis. But *caveat emptor*, the term "barrier repair" is frequently applied loosely to emollients, often based upon petrolatum alone, and often inappropriately to formulations that can do more harm than good, i.e., incomplete mixtures of physiologic lipids that impede rather than allow or facilitate normalization of barrier function. Nevertheless, we are now in an era of "choice of barrier" (108), and it now should be possible to select the most logical barrier repair strategy for a specific clinical indication, based upon the knowledge of disease pathogenesis.

Atopic dermatitis is characterized by a global decrease in SC lipids with a steep reduction in ceramides (109), attributable to increased sphingomyelin deacylase activity in affected epidermis (110). There is also a defect in LB secretion, which could contribute to the lipid deficiency (109). Hence, the logic and success of a recently deployed, ceramide-dominant mixture of physiologic lipids (111). In contrast, aged and photoaged epidermis exhibits a global reduction in SC lipids (78), with a further decrease in cholesterol synthesis (112). Hence, the success of a cholesterol-dominant mixture of physiological lipids in this setting (113). Yet, there are several clinical situations where physiologic lipids might not be effective, due to the absence of an intact LB secretory system. These include: radiation dermatitis [both UV-B and x-irradiation (114,115)], very premature infants (i.e., <33 weeks), and the initial stages of wound heading. In such situations non-physiologic lipids or dressing alone, with or without added physiologic lipids, become the most logical choice (108).

EXTRACELLULAR SIGNALS OF BARRIER HOMEOSTASIS

Calcium (Ca) and Other Ions

Signaling mechanisms can be inferred to be operative in the epidermis, based upon phenomenon such as the recovery response that follows acute barrier disruption, and the epidermal response to altered external humidities (see above). Even minor external perturbations stimulate sometimes profound, metabolic responses in the underlying, nucleated layers of the epidermis (116). A distinctive Ca^{++} gradient is present in epidermis (18), with the highest levels of Ca^{++} in the outer SG, tapering to very low levels in both the lower epidermis and SC (117). Recent studies have shown that this gradient is regulated passively by barrier integrity, i.e., changes in Ca^{++} distribution occur in response to an altered barrier (117,118) (Fig. 8). In the presence of high Ca^{++}, barrier recovery is inhibited, but recovery normalizes when Ca^{++} is co-applied with inhibitors of voltage-sensitive Ca^{++} channels (e.g., nifedipine, verapamil) (119).

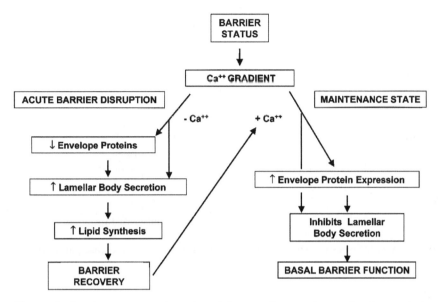

Figure 8 Barrier status regulates the calcium gradient, and opposite changes in intraepidermal calcium levels, in turn, regulate epidermal differentiation and lamellar body secretion.

Potassium exerts synergistic inhibitory effects with Ca^{++}, apparently through its ability to alter Ca influx via membrane depolarization (119,120).

Ca^{++} ion–induced regulation of barrier recovery targets LB secretion (27,121). Although Ca^{++} slows LB secretion, these low rates are nevertheless sufficient to meet basal barrier requirements (Fig. 8). In contrast, LB secretion rates accelerate quickly when Ca levels in surrounding granular cells decline in parallel with barrier disruption (27,117,121) (Fig. 8). While high Ca^{++} in the outer nucleated layers restricts LB secretion, these high levels of Ca^{++} conversely in the outer nucleated layers of the epidermis directly regulate epidermal differentiation (27). Thus, Ca^{++} coordinately regulates a critical subset of homeostatic responses in epidermis, i.e., those related to LB secretion and epidermal differentiation (Figs. 3 and 8).

Cytokines and Growth Factors

Production of several cytokines and growth factors increases following either acute or prolonged barrier disruption (122–124). Moreover, a portion of the large, pre-formal pool of IL-1α in the outer epidermis (125) is released in a non–energy-dependent fashion after acute barrier disruption (126). While the role of injury-provoked cytokine generation in epidermal pathophysiology is clear (Figs. 6 and 9), its importance as a regulatory signal for metabolic processes that lead to barrier recovery is still not well defined. The principal issue relates to the observation that occlusion, which artificially restores normal barrier function, fails to block the up-regulation of cytokine production that occurs after acute barrier disruption (127–129). Likewise, occlusion has little or no effect on the levels of receptors for these cytokines (130). Yet, occlusion does, in fact, down-regulate expression levels of primary cytokines in chronically perturbed skin (e.g., essential fatty acid deficiency) (128). Moreover, occlusion also blocks the up-regulation of certain growth factors, e.g., amphiregulin and nerve growth factor,

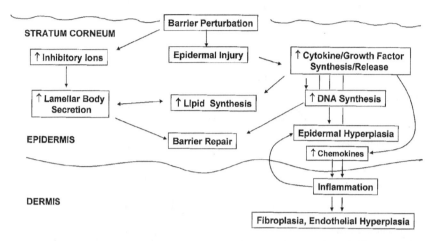

Figure 9 Divergent roles of cytokine cascade in barrier repair and disease pathogenesis.

whose expression also increases after acute barrier disruption (131). Finally, transgenic mice with double knockouts of both the functional IL-1 and/or TNF receptors display a delay in barrier recovery (132,133). Together, these results suggest that cytokines could be classic, "two-edged swords," serving simultaneously as pro-inflammatory mediators and as signals of the homeostatic repair response (Fig. 9).

Recent studies have shed light on how cytokines could serve as a regulator of barrier homeostasis. In extracutaneous tissues, primary cytokines, such as IL-1α, TNFα, and IL-6, are well known to stimulate lipid synthesis (134,135). Moreover, recent studies have shown that exogenous IL-1α stimulates keratinocyte lipid synthesis in vivo and in vitro (136). Moreover, IL-1 signaling selectively declines in aged epidermis (136), an abnormality that can be reversed by administration of either exogenous IL-1α (136) or a cytokine stimulator (i.e., imiquimod) (137). Together with the well-known capacity of both cytokines and growth factors to stimulate keratinocyte proliferation (125,138), it now appears likely that certain cytokines and growth factors regulate components of the repair response following barrier insults.

REFERENCES

1. Elias PM, Feingold KR. Lipids and the epidermal water barrier: metabolism, regulation, and pathophysiology. Semin Dermatol 1992; 11:176–182.
2. Odland GF, Holbrook K. The lamellar granules of epidermis. Curr Probl Dermatol 1981; 9:29–49.
3. Landmann L. The epidermal permeability barrier. Anat Embryol (Berl) 1988; 178:1–13.
4. Korting HC, Kober M, Mueller M, Braun-Falco O. Influence of repeated washings with soap and synthetic detergents on pH and resident flora of the skin of forehead and forearm. Results of a cross-over trial in health probationers. Acta Derm Venereol 1987; 67:41–47.
5. Eckert RL, Crish JF, Robinson NA. The epidermal keratinocyte as a model for the study of gene regulation and cell differentiation. Physiol Rev 1997; 77:397–424.
6. Hohl D. Cornified cell envelope. Dermatologica 1990; 180:201–211.
7. Elias PM, Feingold KR. Skin as an organ of protection. In: Freedberg I, et al, eds. Fitzpatrick's Dermatology in General Medicine. Philadelphia: McGraw-Hill, 1999: 164–174.

8. Elias PM, Williams ML, Feingold KR. In defense of skin defense: beyond the lymphocyte—the cutaneous interface. (Viewpoint 3 in What is the "true" function of skin? Chuong et al.) Exp Dermatol 2002; 11:159–187.

9. Potts RO, Francoeur ML. Lipid biophysics of water loss through the skin. Proc Natl Acad Sci USA 1990; 87:3871–3873.

10. Michel S, Schmidt R, Shroot B, Reichert U. Morphological and biochemical characterization of the cornified envelopes from human epidermal keratinocytes of different origin. J Invest Dermatol 1988; 91:11–15.

11. Harding C, Long S, Richardson J, Rogers J, Zhang Z, Bush A, Rawlings AV. The cornified cell envelope: an important marker of stratum corneum maturation in healthy and dry skin. Int J Cosm Sci 2003; 25:157–167.

12. Steinert PM, Marekov LN. Direct evidence that involucrin is a major early isopeptide crosslinked component of the keratinocyte cornified envelope. J Biol Chem 1997; 17:2021–2030.

13. Hohl D, Mehrel T, Lichti U, Turner ML, Roop DR, Steinert PM. Characterization of human loricrin. Structure and function of a new class of epidermal cell envelope proteins. J Biol Chem 1991; 266:6626–6636.

14. Ishida-Yamamoto A, Iizuka H. Structural organization of cornified cell envelopes and alterations in inherited skin disorders. Exp Dermatol 1998; 7:1–10.

15. Bickenbach JR, Greer JM, Bundman DS, Rothnagel JA, Roop DR. Loricrin expression is coordinated with other epidermal proteins and the appearance of lipid lamellar granules in development. J Invest Dermatol 1995; 104:405–410.

16. Maestrini E, Monaco AP, McGrath JA, Ishida-Yamamoto A, Camisa C, Hovnanian A, Weeks DE, Lathrop M, Uitto J, Christiano AM. A molecular defect in loricrin, the major component of the cornified cell envelope, underlies Vohwinkel's syndrome. Nat Genet 1996; 13:70–77.

17. Hennings H, Steinert P, Buxman MM. Calcium induction of transglutaminase and the formation of epsilon(gamma-glutamyl) lysine cross-links in cultured mouse epidermal cells. Biochem Biophys Res Commun 1981; 102:739–745.

18. Menon GK, Grayson S, Elias PM. Ionic calcium reservoirs in mammalian epidermis: ultrastructural localization by ion-capture cytochemistry. J Invest Dermatol 1985; 84:508–512.

19. Hohl D, Huber M, Frenk E. Analysis of the cornified cell envelope in lamellar ichthyosis. Arch Dermatol 1993; 129:618–624.

20. Chakravarty R, Rice RH. Acylation of keratinocyte transglutaminase by palmitic and myristic acids in the membrane anchorage region. J Biol Chem 1989; 264:625–629.

21. Russell LJ, DiGiovanna JJ, Rogers GR, Steinert PM, Hashem N, Compton JG, Bale SJ. Mutations in the gene for transglutaminase 1 in autosomal recessive lamellar ichthyosis. Nat Genet 1995; 9:279–283.

22. Huber M, Rettler I, Bernasconi K, Frenk E, Lavrijsen SP, Ponec M, Bon A, Lautenschlager S, Schorderet DF, Hohl D. Mutations of keratinocyte transglutaminase in lamellar ichthyosis. Science 1995; 267:525–528.

23. Lavrijsen AP, Bouwstra JA, Gooris GS, Weerheim A, Bodde HE, Ponec M. Reduced skin barrier function parallels abnormal stratum corneum lipid organization in patients with lamellar ichthyosis. J Invest Dermatol 1995; 105:619–624.

24. Elias PM, Schmuth M, Uchida Y, Rice RH, Behne M, Crumrine D, Feingold KR, Holleran WM, Pharm D. Basis for the permeability barrier abnormality in lamellar ichthyosis. Exp Dermatol 2002; 11:248–256.

25. Choate KA, Medalie DA, Morgan JR, Khavari PA. Corrective gene transfer in the human skin disorder lamellar ichthyosis. Nat Med 1996; 2:1263–1267.

26. Ghadially R, Williams ML, Hou SY, Elias PM. Membrane structural abnormalities in the stratum corneum of the autosomal recessive ichthyoses. J Invest Dermatol 1992; 99:755–763.

27. Elias PM, Ahn SK, Denda M, Brown BE, Crumrine D, Kimutai LK, Komuves L, Lee SH, Feingold KR. Modulations in epidermal calcium regulate the expression of differentiation-specific markers. J Invest Dermatol 2002; 119:1128–1136.

28. Fuchs E. Intermediate filaments and disease: mutations that cripple cell strength. J Cell Biol 1994; 125:511–516.
29. Fuchs E, Weber K. Intermediate filaments: structure, dynamics, function, and disease. Annu Rev Biochem 1994; 63:345–382.
30. Cheng J, Syder AJ, Yu QC, Letai A, Paller AS, Fuchs E. The genetic basis of epidermolytic hyperkeratosis: a disorder of differentiation-specific epidermal keratin genes. Cell 1992; 70:811–819.
31. Rothnagel JA, Dominey AM, Dempsey LD, Longley MA, Greenhalgh DA, Gagne TA, Huber M, Frenk E, Hohl D, Roop DR. Mutations in the rod domains of keratins 1 and 10 in epidermolytic hyperkeratosis. Science 1992; 257:1128–1130.
32. Williams ML, Elias PM. From basket weave to barrier. Unifying concepts for the pathogenesis of the disorders of cornification. Arch Dermatol 1993; 129:626–629.
33. Kremer H, Zeeuwen P, McLean WH, Mariman EC, Lane EB, van de Kerkhof CM, Ropers HH, Steijlen PM. Ichthyosis bullosa of Siemens is caused by mutations in the keratin 2e gene. J Invest Dermatol 1994; 103:286–289.
34. Schmuth M, Yosipovitch G, Williams ML, Weber F, Hintner H, Ortiz-Urda S, Rappersberger K, Crumrine D, Feingold KR, Elias PM. Pathogenesis of the permeability barrier abnormality in epidermolytic hyperkeratosis. J Invest Dermatol 2001; 117: 837–847.
35. Kimonis V, DiGiovanna JJ, Yang JM, Doyle SZ, Bale SJ, Compton JG. A mutation in the V1 end domain of keratin 1 in non-epidermolytic palmar-plantar keratoderma. J Invest Dermatol 1994; 103:764–769.
36. Candi E, Tarcsa E, Digiovanna JJ, Compton JG, Elias PM, Marekov LN, Steinert PM. A highly conserved lysine residue on the head domain of type II keratins is essential for the attachment of keratin intermediate filaments to the cornified cell envelope through isopeptide crosslinking by transglutaminases. Proc Natl Acad Sci USA 1998; 95:2067–2072.
37. Fleckman P, Dale BA, Holbrook KA. Profilaggrin, a high-molecular-weight precursor of filaggrin in human epidermis and cultured keratinocytes. J Invest Dermatol 1985; 85:507–512.
38. Resing KA, al-Alawi N, Blomquist C, Fleckman P, Dale BA. Independent regulation of two cytoplasmic processing stages of the intermediate filament-associated protein filaggrin and role of Ca^{2+} in the second stage. J Biol Chem 1993; 268:25139–25145.
39. Dale BA, Presland RB, Lewis SP, Underwood RA, Fleckman P. Transient expression of epidermal filaggrin in cultured cells causes collapse of intermediate filamenta networks with alteration of cell shape and nuclear integrity. J Invest Dermatol 1997; 108: 179–187.
40. Scott IR, Harding CR. Filaggrin breakdown to water binding compounds during development of the rat stratum corneum is controlled by the water activity of the environment. Dev Biol 1986; 115:84–92.
41. Williams ML, Hanley K, Elias PM, Feingold KR. Ontogeny of the epidermal permeability barrier. J Invest Dermatol Symp Proc 1998; 3:75–79.
42. Kao JS, Garg A, Mao-Qiang M, Crumrine D, Ghadially R, Feingold KR, Elias PM. Testosterone perturbs epidermal permeability barrier homeostasis. J Invest Dermatol 2001; 116:443–451.
43. Denda M, Tsuchiya T, Elias PM, Feingold KR. Stress alters cutaneous permeability barrier homeostasis. Am J Physiol Regul Integr Comp Physiol 2000; 278:R367–372.
44. Kao JS, Fluhr JW, Man MQ, Fowler AJ, Hachem JP, Crumrine D, Ahn SK, Brown BE, Elias PM, Feingold KR. Short-term glucocorticoid treatment compromises both permeability barrier homeostasis and stratum corneum integrity: inhibition of epidermal lipid synthesis accounts for functional abnormalities. J Invest Dermatol 2003; 120:456–464.
45. Duplus E, Forest C. Is there a single mechanism for fatty acid regulation of gene transcription? Biochem Pharmacol 2002; 64:893–901.

46. Fitzgerald ML, Moore KJ, Freeman MW. Nuclear hormone receptors and cholesterol trafficking: the orphans find a new home. J Mol Med 2002; 80:271–281.

47. Komuves LG, Hanley K, Jiang Y, Elias PM, Williams ML, Feingold KR. Ligands and activators of nuclear hormone receptors regulate epidermal differentiation during fetal rat skin development. J Invest Dermatol 1998; 111.429–433.

48. Hanley K, Komuves LG, Bass NM, He SS, Jiang Y, Crumrine D, Appel R, Friedman M, Bettencourt J, Min K, Elias PM, Williams ML, Feingold KR. Fetal epidermal differentiation and barrier development in vivo is accelerated by nuclear hormone receptor activators. J Invest Dermatol 1999; 113:788–795.

49. Gao J, Ye H, Serrero G. Stimulation of adipose differentiation related protein (ADRP) expression in adipocyte precursors by long-chain fatty acids. J Cell Physiol 2000; 182: 297–302.

50. Hanley K, Komuves LG, Ng DC, Schoonjans K, He SS, Lau P, Bikle DD, Williams ML, Elias PM, Auwerx J, Feingold KR. Farnesol stimulates differentiation in epidermal keratinocytes via PPARalpha. J Biol Chem 2000; 275:11484–11491.

51. Komuves LG, Hanley K, Lefebvre AM, Man MQ, Ng DC, Bikle DD, Williams ML, Elias PM, Auwerx J, Feingold KR. Stimulation of PPARalpha promotes epidermal keratinocyte differentiation in vivo. J Invest Dermatol 2000; 115:353–360.

52. Komuves LG, Schmuth M, Fowler AJ, Elias PM, Hanley K, Man MQ, Moser AH, Lobaccaro JM, Williams ML, Mangelsdorf DJ, Feingold KR. Oxysterol stimulation of epidermal differentiation is mediated by liver X receptor-beta in murine epidermis. J Invest Dermatol 2002; 118:25–34.

53. Hanley K, Ng DC, He SS, Lau P, Min K, Elias PM, Bikle DD, Mangelsdorf DJ, Williams ML, Feingold KR. Oxysterols induce differentiation in human keratinocytes and increase Ap-1-dependent involucrin transcription. J Invest Dermatol 2000; 114:545–553.

54. Rivier M, Castiel I, Safonova I, Ailhaud G, Michel S. Peroxisome proliferator-activated receptor-alpha enhances lipid metabolism in a skin equivalent model. J Invest Dermatol 2000; 114:681–687.

55. Hurt CM, Hanley K, Williams ML, Feingold KR. Cutaneous lipid synthesis during late fetal development in the rat. Arch Dermatol Res 1995; 287:754–760.

56. Fowler AJ, Sheu MY, Schmuth M, Kao J, Fluhr JW, Rhein L, Collins JL, Willson TM, Mangelsdorf DJ, Elias PM, Feingold KR. Liver X receptor activators display antiinflammatory activity in irritant and allergic contact dermatitis models: liver-X-receptor-specific inhibition of inflammation and primary cytokine production. J Invest Dermatol 2003; 120:246–255.

57. Sheu MY, Fowler AJ, Kao J, Schmuth M, Schoonjans K, Auwerx J, Fluhr JW, Man MQ, Elias PM, Feingold KR. Topical peroxisome proliferator activated receptor-alpha activators reduce inflammation in irritant and allergic contact dermatitis models. J Invest Dermatol 2002; 118:94–101.

58. Komuves LG, Hanley K, Man MQ, Elias PM, Williams ML, Feingold KR. Keratinocyte differentiation in hyperproliferative epidermis: topical application of PPARalpha activators restores tissue homeostasis. J Invest Dermatol 2000; 115:361–367.

59. Ellis CN, Varani J, Fisher GJ, Zeigler ME, Pershadsingh HA, Benson SC, Chi Y, Kurtz TW. Troglitazone improves psoriasis and normalizes models of proliferative skin disease: ligands for peroxisome proliferator-activated receptor-gamma inhibit keratinocyte proliferation. Arch Dermatol 2000; 136.609–616.

60. Schurer NY, Elias PM. The biochemistry and function of stratum corneum lipids. Adv Lipid Res 1991; 24:27–56.

61. Feingold KR. The regulation and role of epidermal lipid synthesis. Adv Lipid Res 1991; 24:57–82.

62. Mao-Qiang M, Feingold KR, Jain M, Elias PM. Extracellular processing of phospholipids is required for permeability barrier homeostasis. J Lipid Res 1995; 36:1925–1935.

63. Mao-Qiang M, Jain M, Feingold KR, Elias PM. Secretory phospholipase A2 activity is required for permeability barrier homeostasis. J Invest Dermatol 1996; 106:57–63.

64. Fluhr JW, Kao J, Jain M, Ahn SK, Feingold KR, Elias PM. Generation of free fatty acids from phospholipids regulates stratum corneum acidification and integrity. J Invest Dermatol 2001; 117:44–51.

65. Williams ML, Elias PM. Stratum corneum lipids in disorders of cornification: increased cholesterol sulfate content of stratum corneum in recessive x-linked ichthyosis. J Clin Invest 1981; 68:1404–1410.

66. Zettersten E, Man MQ, Sato J, Denda M, Farrell A, Ghadially R, Williams ML, Feingold KR, Elias PM. Recessive x-linked ichthyosis: role of cholesterol-sulfate accumulation in the barrier abnormality. J Invest Dermatol 1998; 111:784–790.

67. Wertz PW, Downing DT, Freinkel RK, Traczyk TN. Sphingolipids of the stratum corneum and lamellar granules of fetal rat epidermis. J Invest Dermatol 1984; 83:193–195.

68. Bos JD, Van Leent EJ, Sillevis Smitt JH. The millennium criteria for the diagnosis of atopic dermatitis. Exp Dermatol 1998; 7:132–138.

69. Uchida Y, Hara M, Nishio H, Sidransky E, Inoue S, Otsuka F, Suzuki A, Elias PM, Holleran WM, Hamanaka S. Epidermal sphingomyelins are precursors for selected stratum corneum ceramides. J Lipid Res 2000; 41:2071–2082.

70. Swartzendruber DC, Wertz PW, Madison KC, Downing DT. Evidence that the corneocyte has a chemically bound lipid envelope. J Invest Dermatol 1987; 88:709–713.

71. Marekov LN, Steinert PM. Ceramides are bound to structural proteins of the human foreskin epidermal cornified cell envelope. J Biol Chem 1998; 273:17763–17770.

72. Elias PM, Goerke J, Friend DS. Mammalian epidermal barrier layer lipids: composition and influence on structure. J Invest Dermatol 1977; 69:535–546.

73. Elias PM, Fartasch M, Crumrine D, Behne M, Uchida Y, Holleran WM. Origin of the corneocyte lipid envelope (CLE): observations in harlequin ichthyosis and cultured human keratinocytes. J Invest Dermatol 2000; 115:765–769.

74. Wertz PW, Swartzendruber DC, Kitko DJ, Madison KC, Downing DT. The role of the corneocyte lipid envelope in cohesion of the stratum corneum. J Invest Dermatol 1989; 93:169–172.

75. Doering T, Holleran WM, Potratz A, Vielhaber G, Elias PM, Suzuki K, Sandhoff K. Sphingolipid activator proteins are required for epidermal permeability barrier formation. J Biol Chem 1999; 274:11038–11045.

76. Scheuplein RJ, Blank IH. Permeability of the skin. Physiol Rev 1971; 51:702–747.

77. Grubauer G, Elias PM, Feingold KR. Transepidermal water loss: the signal for recovery of barrier structure and function. J Lipid Res 1989; 30:323–333.

78. Ghadially R, Brown BE, Sequeira-Martin SM, Feingold KR, Elias PM. The aged epidermal permeability barrier. Structural, functional, and lipid biochemical abnormalities in humans and a senescent murine model. J Clin Invest 1995; 95:2281–2290.

79. Behne MJ, Barry NP, Hanson KM, Aronchik I, Clegg RW, Gratton E, Feingold K, Holleran WM, Elias PM, Mauro TM. Neonatal development of the stratum corneum pH gradient: localization and mechanisms leading to emergence of optimal barrier function. J Invest Dermatol 2003; 120:998–1006.

80. Garg A, Chren MM, Sands LP, Matsui MS, Marenus KD, Feingold KR, Elias PM. Psychological stress perturbs epidermal permeability barrier homeostasis: implications for the pathogenesis of stress-associated skin disorders. Arch Dermatol 2001; 137:53–59.

81. Denda M, Sato J, Masuda Y, Tsuchiya T, Koyama J, Kuramoto M, Elias PM, Feingold KR. Exposure to a dry environment enhances epidermal permeability barrier function. J Invest Dermatol 1998; 111:858–863.

82. Reed JT, Ghadially R, Elias PM. Skin type, but neither race nor gender, influence epidermal permeability barrier function. Arch Dermatol 1995; 131:1134–1138.

83. Elias PM, Cullander C, Mauro T, Rassner U, Komuves L, Brown BE, Menon GK. The secretory granular cell: the outermost granular cell as a specialized secretory cell. J Invest Dermatol Symp Proc 1998; 3:87–100.

84. Menon GK, Feingold KR, Elias PM. Lamellar body secretory response to barrier disruption. J Invest Dermatol 1992; 98:279–289.

85. Grayson S, Johnson-Winegar AG, Wintroub BU, Isseroff RR, Epstein EH Jr, Elias PM. Lamellar body-enriched fractions from neonatal mice: preparative techniques and partial characterization. J Invest Dermatol 1985; 85:289–294.
86. Menon GK, Ghadially R, Williams ML, Elias PM. Lamellar bodies as delivery systems of hydrolytic enzymes: implications for normal and abnormal desquamation. Br J Dermatol 1992; 126:337–345.
87. Grubauer G, Feingold KR, Elias PM. Relationship of epidermal lipogenesis to cutaneous barrier function. J Lipid Res 1987; 28:746–752.
88. Holleran WM, Feingold KR, Man MQ, Gao WN, Lee JM, Elias PM. Regulation of epidermal sphingolipid synthesis by permeability barrier function. J Lipid Res 1991; 32:1151–1158.
89. Proksch E, Elias PM, Feingold KR. Regulation of 3-hydroxy-3-methylglutaryl-coenzyme A reductase activity in murine epidermis. Modulation of enzyme content and activation state by barrier requirements. J Clin Invest 1990; 85:874–882.
90. Harris IR, Farrell AM, Grunfeld C, Holleran WM, Elias PM, Feingold KR. Permeability barrier disruption coordinately regulates mRNA levels for key enzymes of cholesterol, fatty acid, and ceramide synthesis in the epidermis. J Invest Dermatol 1997; 109:783–787.
91. Ottey KA, Wood LC, Grunfeld C, Elias PM, Feingold KR. Cutaneous permeability barrier disruption increases fatty acid synthetic enzyme activity in the epidermis of hairless mice. J Invest Dermatol 1995; 104:401–404.
92. Corden LD, McLean WH. Human keratin diseases: hereditary fragility of specific epithelial tissues. Exp Dermatol 1996; 5:297–307.
93. Brown MS, Goldstein JL. Sterol regulatory element binding proteins (SREBPs): controllers of lipid synthesis and cellular uptake. Nutr Rev 1998; 56:S1–S3; Discussion S54–S75.
94. Smith JR, Osborne TF, Brown MS, Goldstein JL, Gil G. Multiple sterol regulatory elements in promoter for hamster 3-hydroxy-3-methylglutaryl-coenzyme A synthase. J Biol Chem 1988; 263:18480–18487.
95. Vallett SM, Sanchez HB, Rosenfeld JM, Osborne TF. A direct role for sterol regulatory element binding protein in activation of 3-hydroxy-3-methylglutaryl coenzyme A reductase gene. J Biol Chem 1996; 271:12247–12253.
96. Loewen CJ, Levine TP. Cholesterol homeostasis: not until the SCAP lady INSIGs. Curr Biol 2002; 12:R779–R781.
97. Rawson RB. The SREBP pathway—insights from Insigs and insects. Nat Rev Mol Cell Biol 2003; 4:631–640.
98. Narce M, Poisson JP. Lipid metabolism: regulation of lipid metabolism gene expression by peroxisome proliferator-activated receptor alpha and sterol regulatory element binding proteins. Curr Opin Lipidol 2002; 13:445–447.
99. Harris IR, Farrell AM, Holleran WM, Jackson S, Grunfeld C, Elias PM, Feingold KR. Parallel regulation of sterol regulatory element binding protein-2 and the enzymes of cholesterol and fatty acid synthesis but not ceramide synthesis in cultured human keratinocytes and murine epidermis. J Lipid Res 1998; 39:412–422.
100. Farrell AM, Uchida Y, Nagiec MM, Harris IR, Dickson RC, Elias PM, Holleran WM. UVB irradiation up-regulates serine palmitoyltransferase in cultured human keratinocytes. J Lipid Res 1998; 39:2031–2038.
101. Feingold KR, Man MQ, Menon GK, Cho SS, Brown BE, Elias PM. Cholesterol synthesis is required for cutaneous barrier function in mice. J Clin Invest 1990; 86:1738–1745.
102. Mao-Qiang M, Elias PM, Feingold KR. Fatty acids are required for epidermal permeability barrier function. J Clin Invest 1993; 92:791–798.
103. Man MQ, Feingold KR, Elias PM. Exogenous lipids influence permeability barrier recovery in acetone-treated murine skin. Arch Dermatol 1993; 129:728–738.

104. Mao-Qiang M, Brown BE, Wu-Pong S, Feingold KR, Elias PM. Exogenous nonphysiologic vs physiologic lipids. Divergent mechanisms for correction of permeability barrier dysfunction. Arch Dermatol 1995; 131:809–816.

105. Man MM, Feingold KR, Thornfeldt CR, Elias PM. Optimization of physiological lipid mixtures for barrier repair. J Invest Dermatol 1996; 106:1096–1101.

106. Ghadially R, Halkier-Sorensen L, Elias PM. Effects of petrolatum on stratum corneum structure and function. J Am Acad Dermatol 1992; 26:387–396.

107. Sugarman JL, Fluhr JW, Fowler AJ, Bruckner T, Diepgen TL, Williams ML. The objective severity assessment of atopic dermatitis score: an objective measure using permeability barrier function and stratum corneum hydration with computer-assisted estimates for extent of disease. Arch Dermatol 2003; 139:1417–1422.

108. Elias PM, Feingold KR. Does the tail wag the dog? Role of the barrier in the pathogenesis of inflammatory dermatoses and therapeutic implications. Arch Dermatol 2001; 137:1079–1081.

109. Fartasch M, Diepgen TL. The barrier function in atopic dry skin. Disturbance of membrane-coating granule exocytosis and formation of epidermal lipids? Acta Derm Venereol Suppl (Stockh) 1992; 176:26–31.

110. Hara J, Higuchi K, Okamoto R, Kawashima M, Imokawa G. High-expression of sphingomyelin deacylase is an important determinant of ceramide deficiency leading to barrier disruption in atopic dermatitis. J Invest Dermatol 2000; 115:406–413.

111. Chamlin SL, Kao J, Frieden IJ, Sheu MY, Fowler AJ, Fluhr JW, Williams ML, Elias PM. Ceramide-dominant barrier repair lipids alleviate childhood atopic dermatitis: changes in barrier function provide a sensitive indicator of disease activity. J Am Acad Dermatol 2002; 47:198–208.

112. Ghadially R, Brown BE, Hanley K, Reed JT, Feingold KR, Elias PM. Decreased epidermal lipid synthesis accounts for altered barrier function in aged mice. J Invest Dermatol 1996; 106:1064–1069.

113. Zettersten EM, Ghadially R, Feingold KR, Crumrine D, Elias PM. Optimal ratios of topical stratum corneum lipids improve barrier recovery in chronologically aged skin. J Am Acad Dermatol 1997; 37:403–408.

114. Haratake A, Uchida Y, Schmuth M, Tanno O, Yasuda R, Epstein JH, Elias PM, Holleran WM. UVB-induced alterations in permeability barrier function: roles for epidermal hyperproliferation and thymocyte-mediated response. J Invest Dermatol 1997; 108:769–775.

115. Schmuth M, Sztankay A, Weinlich G, Linder DM, Wimmer MA, Fritsch PO, Fritsch E. Permeability barrier function of skin exposed to ionizing radiation. Arch Dermatol 2001; 137:1019–1023.

116. Taljebini M, Warren R, Mao-Oiang M, Lane E, Elias PM, Feingold KR. Cutaneous permeability barrier repair following various types of insults: kinetics and effects of occlusion. Skin Pharmacol 1996; 9:111–119.

117. Menon GK, Elias PM, Feingold KR. Integrity of the permeability barrier is crucial for maintenance of the epidermal calcium gradient. Br J Dermatol 1994; 130:139–147.

118. Elias P, Ahn S, Brown B, Crumrine D, Feingold KR. Origin of the epidermal calcium gradient: regulation by barrier status and role of active vs. passive mechanisms. J Invest Dermatol 2002; 119:1269–1274.

119. Lee SH, Elias PM, Proksch E, Menon GK, Mao-Quiang M, Feingold KR. Calcium and potassium are important regulators of barrier homeostasis in murine epidermis. J Clin Invest 1992; 89:530–538.

120. Lee SH, Elias PM, Feingold KR, Mauro T. A role for ions in barrier recovery after acute perturbation. J Invest Dermatol 1994; 102:976–979.

121. Menon GK, Price LF, Bommannan B, Elias PM, Feingold KR. Selective obliteration of the epidermal calcium gradient leads to enhanced lamellar body secretion. J Invest Dermatol 1994; 102:789–795.

122. Elias PM, Wood LC, Feingold KR. Epidermal pathogenesis of inflammatory dermatoses. Am J Contact Dermat 1999; 10:119–126.
123. Elias PM, Ansel JC, Woods LD, Feingold KR. Signaling networks in barrier homeostasis. The mystery widens. Arch Dermatol 1996; 132:1505–1506.
124. Nickoloff BJ, Naidu Y. Perturbation of epidermal barrier function correlates with initiation of cytokine cascade in human skin. J Am Acad Dermatol 1994; 30:535–546.
125. Kupper TS. Immune and inflammatory processes in cutaneous tissues. Mechanisms and speculations. J Clin Invest 1990; 86:1783–1789.
126. Wood LC, Elias PM, Calhoun C, Tsai JC, Grunfeld C, Feingold KR. Barrier disruption stimulates interleukin-1 alpha expression and release from a pre-formed pool in murine epidermis. J Invest Dermatol 1996; 106:397–403.
127. Wood LC, Jackson SM, Elias PM, Grunfeld C, Feingold KR. Cutaneous barrier perturbation stimulates cytokine production in the epidermis of mice. J Clin Invest 1992; 90:482–487.
128. Wood LC, Elias PM, Sequeira-Martin SM, Grunfeld C, Feingold KR. Occlusion lowers cytokine mRNA levels in essential fatty acid-deficient and normal mouse epidermis, but not after acute barrier disruption. J Invest Dermatol 1994; 103:834–838.
129. Wood LC, Feingold KR, Sequeira-Martin SM, Elias PM, Grunfeld C. Barrier function coordinately regulates epidermal IL-1 and IL-1 receptor antagonist mRNA levels. Exp Dermatol 1994; 3:56–60.
130. Wood LC, Stalder AK, Liou A, Campbell IL, Grunfeld C, Elias PM, Feingold KR. Barrier disruption increases gene expression of cytokines and the 55 kDa TNF receptor in murine skin. Exp Dermatol 1997; 6:98–104.
131. Liou A, Elias PM, Grunfeld C, Feingold KR, Wood LC. Amphiregulin and nerve growth factor expression are regulated by barrier status in murine epidermis. J Invest Dermatol 1997; 108:73–77.
132. Jensen JM, Schutze S, Forl M, Kronke M, Proksch E. Roles for tumor necrosis factor receptor p55 and sphingomyelinase in repairing the cutaneous permeability barrier. J Clin Invest 1999; 104:1761–1770.
133. Kreder D, Krut O, Adam-Klages S, Wiegmann K, Scherer G, Plitz T, Jensen JM, Proksch E, Steinmann J, Pfeffer K, Kronke M. Impaired neutral sphingomyelinase activation and cutaneous barrier repair in FAN-deficient mice. EMBO J 1999; 18: 2472–2479.
134. Memon RA, Fuller J, Moser AH, Smith PJ, Feingold KR, Grunfeld C. In vivo regulation of acyl-CoA synthetase mRNA and activity by endotoxin and cytokines. Am J Physiol 1998; 275:E64–E72.
135. Memon RA, Holleran WM, Moser AH, Seki T, Uchida Y, Fuller J, Shigenaga JK, Grunfeld C, Feingold KR. Endotoxin and cytokines increase hepatic sphingolipid biosynthesis and produce lipoproteins enriched in ceramides and sphingomyelin. Arterioscler Thromb Vasc Biol 1998; 18:1257–1265.
136. Ye J, Garg A, Calhoun C, Feingold KR, Elias PM, Ghadially R. Alterations in cytokine regulation in aged epidermis: implications for permeability barrier homeostasis and inflammation. I. IL-1 gene family. Exp Dermatol 2002; 11:209–216.
137. Barland C, Zettersten E, Brown BS, YE J, Elias PM, Ghadially R. indirect other stimulation improves barrier homeostasis aged murine epidermis. J Invest Dermatol 2004; 122:330–336.
138. Sauder DN. The role of epidermal cytokines in inflammatory skin diseases. J Invest Dermatol 1990; 95:27S–28S.

22

Cutaneous Barriers in Defense Against Microbial Invasion

Anna Di Nardo and Richard L. Gallo
Department of Medicine-Dermatology Section, University of California,
San Diego, California, U.S.A.

INTRODUCTION

The skin is one of several epithelial systems positioned at an interface between internal organ sub-systems and the outside world. Uniquely, it has to combine multiple disparate functions into one organized system able to prevent excess water loss, limit percutaneous absorption, enable plasticity and elasticity, and provide protection against UV radiation. All these functions must also be integrated to provide a barrier against the natural tendency of microbes to establish and proliferate in the nutrient-rich environment established by the body. Microbes that are successful in exhibiting limited growth on the epithelial surface are defined as "nonpathogenic," and those that invade and have the potential for unrestrained growth are defined as "pathogenic." Ultimately, it is the immune barrier defense presented by the individual host that defines the pathogenic potential of any given microbe.

Recently, many substances have been discovered that are implicated in innate and acquired immune response of the skin. Many were discovered primarily for their antimicrobial properties; others like certain lipids, enzymes, chemokines, and neuropeptides have been known for quite some time, but have only recently been re-evaluated for their activity in fighting infection.

The skin is organized and differentiated into an organ that works like a transducer between two different environments, the dry and hostile outside world and the delicate inside environment. The most superficial layer, created by secretion and terminal differentiation of keratinocytes, must be able to recognize possible enemies, combating them if possible, and sending activation signals to the inner layers alerting them of possible invasion. Any modification of barrier homeostasis becomes a chemical signal for activating the inflammatory pathway.

The composition of the skin surface is optimized to prevent bacterial growth; it has a low content of carbohydrates and water, a pH of about 5.6, peptides with direct antibacterial, antifungal, and antiviral activities, and the degradation products of sebum-derived triglycerides. All of these factors appear to contribute to a barrier to microbial growth (Table 1).

Table 1 Antimicrobial Defense Structures of the Human Skin Barrier

Barrier	Components
Acidic pH	Sodium/hydrogen antiporter-1
	Urocanic acid
	Lactic acid
	Free fatty acids
Lipids	Free fatty acids
	Glycosphingolipids
	Phospholipids
	Sphingosines
Antimicrobial peptides	Defensins
	Cathelicidins
	Dermcidins
	Chemokines
	Enzymes
	Neuropeptides

SKIN SURFACE pH

Skin pH has a key role in fighting bacteria (1). It is known that at the skin's low pH (5.6–6.4) few species of bacteria can proliferate. Therefore, the development and maintenance of the correct surface pH is essential for skin defense. The skin surface pH is neutral at birth (2–5), and the absence of an acidic stratum corneum (SC) at birth has been associated with an increased risk of bacterial and yeast infections in neonates (6). In contrast, the acidic pH of both older neonates and adults is associated with decreased colonization by pathogenic bacteria (7,8) and with adhesion of nonpathogenic bacteria to the SC (9).

The development of an acidic pH is also important for permeability barrier recovery after acute insults (10), also accounting for an indirect antibacterial activity. The acidic pH is optimum for certain critical lipid-processing enzymes in the SC, those being β-glucocerebrosidase (11) and acidic sphingomyelinase (12,13), which generate a family of ceramides required for permeability barrier homeostasis (12,14).

Only recently has the formation of the acidic mantle been explained. It involves substances originating outside the skin such as microbial metabolites, free fatty acids (FFA) of sebaceous origin (8), and eccrine gland–derived lactic acid (15). Keratinocytes products are: urocanic acid (UCA) from histidine (16); FFA from phospholipid hydrolysis (17); and a sodium/proton antiporter, sodium/hydrogen antiporter-1 (NHE1) (18).

FFA antimicrobial activity is related to pH (19). Ushijima et al. found that the Minimum Inhibitory Concentration (MIC) of acetic and propionic acids for resident bacteria on normal human skin, such as *Pseudomonas acnes* and *Staphylococcus epidermidis*, was 25 mg/mL or more at pH higher than 5.5, while the MIC of the same acids for most of the transient bacteria was markedly decreased by lowering the pH (19). At those more acidic pH values the MIC was 6.25 mg/mL or less. The MIC of oleic acid for some strains of Gram-positive transient bacteria of *Streptococcus*, *Micrococcus*, or *Bacillus* was 100 µg/mL or less at all tested pH. *Staphylococcus aureus* was resistant to this acid at pH 6.8, but became as sensitive as *Streptococcus* when the pH was lowered. The growth of *P. acnes*, the most predominant resident bacterium, was enhanced markedly and reached a maximum level at MICs 6.25 mg/mL of propionic acid, 12.5 mg/mL of acetic acid, and 50 to 100 μg/mL of oleic acid.

THE SKIN LIPID BARRIER

The SC barrier consists of several layers of cornified keratinocytes embedded in a lipid matrix (20,21). Ceramides, cholesterol, and FFAs are the principal lipids of the SC. They form a continuous network in between corneocytes. The backbone of this network is represented by ceramides (22,23). They are covalently bound lipids consisting mainly of 30- through 34-carbon omega-hydroxyacids amide linked to sphingosine bases (24). Embedded in these main structural lipids are free sphingosine bases, free cholesterol, and FFAs. Free cholesterol, FFAs, and ceramides are keratinocyte-derived products. The surface of adult skin also contains the products of sebaceous gland, mainly consisting of squalene wax, wax esters, and triglycerides (25).

Some lipids have been known for quite some time for their antibacterial activities, and others have only recently been discovered. FFAs have been described to have antibacterial activity against *S. aureus*. To demonstrate skin barrier FFA activity, skin flora of hairless normal and essential fatty acid–deficient mice (EFAD) were examined, and the antimicrobial efficacy of lipids extracted from their SC compared (26). EFAD mice supported 100-fold more bacteria than normal mice did, and were the only group from which *S. aureus* were routinely isolated. Despite this greater carriage, in vitro experiments demonstrated that EFAD lipids are more lethal than normal lipids against *Streptococcus pyogenes*, *S. aureus*, *S. epidermidis*, and *Micrococcus* sp. Skin fungi were equally susceptible to both extracts. After thin layer chromatography, the most active fractions were found to be glycosphingolipids and phospholipids. EFAD extracts had 35% more FFAs and 75% more glycosphingolipids; normal extracts had more triglycerides and phospholipids. *S. aureus* strain 502A survived equally well on EFAD or normal mice. Normal lipids applied on EFAD mice had no additional effect, but EFAD lipids on normal mice brought about a 35% reduction of the inoculated bacteria.

Another free component of the lipid skin barrier is sphingosine. Sphingosine has been shown as a natural antibacterial agent, and the level of sphingosine in the upper SC is significantly reduced (by approximately 2.0-fold) in the uninvolved and involved skin of atopic dermatitis (AD) patients compared with healthy controls. This down-regulated production of sphingosine corresponds to increased colonization of the skin by *S. aureus* and other skin surface bacteria, which is significantly higher in AD compared with healthy controls. The reduced amounts of sphingosine and its relevance to the increased colonization of AD skin suggest that sphingosine plays the role of an innate defense mechanism against the proliferation of *S. aureus* in the SC of healthy control skin.

ANTIMICROBIAL PEPTIDES

The milieu that characterizes the skin surface contains specialized peptides and proteins that provide primary innate immune defense as a consequence of their ability to kill or inhibit the growth of microbes (Table 2). These antimicrobial peptides (AMPs) may exhibit a broad spectrum of activity or appear to function more as specialized agents targeted against specific classes of bacteria, viruses, or fungi.

Table 2 Peptides with Antimicrobial Activity in the Human Skin Barrier

Specialized antimicrobial peptides (discovered first based on antimicrobial function)	Other antimicrobials (discovered based on alternative functions)
Defensins	Chemokines: CXC3, Rantes, IP10/CXCL10, CXCL11, MIG/CXCL9
Cathelicidins	Neuropeptides: SP, NPY, PYY, alpha-MSH, proenkephalins, granulysin, adrenomedullin (AM)
Dermcidins	Enzymes: secretory leukocyte protease inhibitor (SLPI) elastase

Simply put, the AMPs are naturally occurring antibiotics that are encoded by genes, transcribed to mRNA, and assembled into proteins by a wide variety of cells. The manner in which they disrupt microbial growth is through disarrangement of the microbial membrane. Because it is difficult for a microbe to change the organization of its membrane without compromising essential characteristics of its growth, resistance to AMPs occurs at levels that are orders of magnitude lower than those observed for conventional antibiotics.

Defensins

The defensins are divided into two classes, (α) and (β), on the basis of the differences in their secondary structures. α-Defensins were first discovered in the granules of neutrophils, and later specialized forms were found in Paneth cells of the gut. The role of α-defensins in neutrophils is to kill bacteria by a non-oxidative pathway. Their function in the intestine is to control the number of growing bacteria. β-defensins are expressed by both circulating cells and a variety of epithelial cells. This AMP family has had four members most thoroughly investigated in humans [human β-defensin-1 (HBD-1) through -4] (27). HBD-1 is constitutively expressed by the epithelia, whereas the other three are induced by inflammation (28). Expression of HBD-2 appears to be localized to the upper Malpighian layer of the epidermidis of the SC, at the interface with the possible presence of pathogens.

Expression of HBD-2 peptide by human keratinocytes requires differentiation of the cells (either by increased calcium concentration or by growth and maturation in epidermal organotypic culture). They are effectively induced by interleukin-1 alpha and interleukin-1 beta. In interleukin-1 alpha–stimulated epidermal cultures, HBD-2 first appears in the cytoplasm in differentiated suprabasal layers of the skin, next in a more peripheral web-like distribution in the upper layers of the epidermis, and then over a few days migrates to the SC. By semi-quantitative Western blot analysis of epidermal lysates, the average concentration of HBD-2 in stimulated organotypic epidermal culture reached 15 to 70 µg per gram of tissue, i.e., 3.5 to 16 µM, well within the range required for antimicrobial activity (29).

Light microscopy shows HBD-2 is localized in the spinous and granular layers of the epidermis, and particularly around the periphery of keratinocytes. Immunogold staining and electron microscopy have shown HBD-2 to be localized with lamellar bodies (LB). Keratinocytes do not have a typical storage compartment, but they have LBs that transport lipids and hydrolytic enzymes to the surface where they release their contents and contribute to the barrier formation. These findings have relevance because they implicate that the AMPs are an integral part of the skin barrier system, and that they are released to the surface where they reach the maximum concentration in contact with bacteria. Moreover, AMP presence inside the LBs suggests that HBD-2 is following the skin barrier formation and repair roles (30).

Calcium is a regulator of keratinocyte differentiation and appears to be essential to control β-defensin expression in these cells. Modulating the extracellular calcium gradient is a method to induce keratinocyte maturation in vitro, and an increasing calcium gradient toward the surface is always present in normal skin. Moreover the presence of chronic inflammation or other factors that can alter the skin permeability barrier enables inducing an increase in calcium efflux. Thus, the induction of HBD-2 is coordinated with calcium to enable delivery at the appropriate epidermal layer and stage of maximal defense requirements (31).

During wound healing, a wide variety of growth factors are produced to stimulate repair and are needed to re-establish the physical epithelial barrier. Growth factors important in wound healing, such as insulin-like growth factor I and TGF-alpha, induce the expression of several AMPs/polypeptides including HBD-3, human cationic antimicrobial protein hCAP-18/LL-37, neutrophil gelatinase-associated lipocalin, and secretory leukocyte protease inhibitor (SLPI) in human keratinocytes (32).

The expression of HBD-2 can be induced consistently by *S. aureus*, *S. epidermidis*, *Escherichia coli*, and *Pseudomonas aeruginosa*, whereas strains of *S. pyogenes* were poor and variable inducers of HBD-2 (33). The sensitivity of skin pathogens to HBD-2 is inversely related to their ability to induce expression; *S. pyogenes* was significantly more sensitive to killing than *S. epidermidis* was. This ability to induce HBD-2 expression in combination with sensitivity to its antimicrobial effects may account for the gram negative bacteria ability to induce HBD-2 expression may account for the few Gram-negative bacterial infections in the skin, and the more frequent ability of *S. pyogenes* to cause skin disease. The combination of high induction of HBD-2 and the relative tolerance to it may enable *S. epidermidis* to survive on the skin surface and modulate HBD-2 expression when the SC barrier is disrupted (33).

Permeabilization of the bacterial membrane is essential to HBD activity. In experiments with artificial membranes, pore formation took place when a negative charge was applied to the side opposite the defensin-containing solvent. This experiment confirmed that the capacity of defensin to be inserted in membranes depends on electrical forces that act on the positively charged defensin and drive defensins into the membranes where they form pores (27).

HBDs are suspected to play a role in skin defense not only as direct killers of bacteria, but also as strong activators of cellular aspects of the immune system. Acting through the CCR6 receptor they are able to recruit and activate immature dendritic cells (34). HBD-2 can also promote histamine release from mast cells. These observations suggest the contribution of this family of AMPs to the barrier may be more complex than the simple function of defensins as natural antibiotics.

Cathelicidins

The term cathelicidins (Caths) applies to a variety of different peptides that are related by a similar precursor sequence termed the "cathelin domain." They are characterized by an amino terminal signal peptide of approximately 30 amino acids, a highly conserved pro-sequence of about 100 amino acids, and a cationic peptide at the C terminus that varies greatly in size and structure among individual cathelicidin genes.

To date, Caths have been found only in mammals. In human beings and rodents, Caths are represented by a single gene, while in other mammals, such as pigs, cows, and sheep, there are many. The cathelin domain is highly conserved between the members of the family, while the more variable domain, the anti-microbial peptide, is species specific. Cathelicidin is stored in an inactive precursor form that is enzymatically processed to cleave the cathelin from the C-terminal peptide. The C terminus is the most studied part of the molecule because of its potent antimicrobial activity.

So far only one Cath has been discovered in humans (hCAP18/LL-37), and only one in mice (mCRAMP) (35). Caths are mainly expressed by neutrophils, epithelial cells (36) and mast cells (37).

The biosynthesis and maturation process of Cath was first studied in myeloid cells. The precursor propeptide is stored in large granules of the neutrophil. At the moment of activation, elastase cleaves the active peptide. The presence of an elastase-specific inhibitor enables blocking this process in myelocytes. These experiments performed in bovine neutrophils suggested that the granules containing the propeptide are released, and then the cathelin domain is freed specifically by elastase-dependent proteolytic cleavage. However, in other situations other enzymes have been described with the ability to cleave and activate the Cath propeptide. For example, LL-37 can be cleaved from the propeptide hCAP18/LL-37 by proteinase 3, while in the vaginal epithelium the propeptide can be activated by gastricsin (pepsin C) when exposed to vaginal fluid with low pH (38).

Mature cathelicidin peptides exhibit a broad spectrum antimicrobial activity, against both Gram-positive and Gram-negative bacteria.

They are active against *S. aureus*, Group A streptococcus, *P. aeruginosa*, and even some types of *Candida*. Moreover they show activity against vaccinia viruses or parasites like *Cryptosporidium* (39,40).

To kill bacteria, Caths adhere to the bacterial membrane and assemble themselves to disrupt the membrane structure. However, other mechanisms are also probably involved for some members of this gene family. An example of another mechanism is porcine PR-39 that is also able to block the bacterial protein synthesis prior to membrane disruption (41).

The cathelin protein shares homology with the cystatin family of cysteine protease inhibitors. Cathelin protein once cleaved from the cathelicidin AMP can directly inhibit cysteine protease activity. Furthermore, cathelin was also tested for antimicrobial activity using solid-phase radial diffusion and liquid-phase killing assays. The cathelin prosequence, but not full-length hCAP18/LL-37, killed human pathogens including *E. coli* and methicillin-resistant *S. aureus* at concentrations ranging from 16 to 32 μM. Together these findings suggest that after proteolytic cleavage the cathelin domain can contribute to innate host defense through inhibition of bacterial growth and limitation of cysteine-proteinase–mediated tissue damage (42).

Cath, in the skin, is typically constitutively expressed only in specialized structures such as the hair and nail apparatus or in fetal and neonatal skin in the basal layer for eventual deposition in the SC (43). Immunohistochemistry and in situ hybridization demonstrated that abundant cathelicidin protein and mRNA are present in normal skin during the perinatal period 10- to 100-fold greater than in adult skin. The presence, in fetal and perinatal skin, of AMPs provides a safe barrier defense against bacteria in a period in which the acquired immune system is still deficient (43).

Cath is expressed also in sweat. In humans, LL-37 was localized to both the eccrine gland and sweat ductal epithelial cells; after secretion onto the skin surface, the CAMP gene product is processed by a serine protease–dependent mechanism into multiple AMPs distinct from the cathelicidin LL-37. These peptides show enhanced antimicrobial action, acquiring a stronger ability to kill skin pathogens such as *S. aureus* and *Candida albicans* (44).

Cath peptide expression differs in different diseases, and is possibly related to the level of bacterial colonization and infection associated with those diseases. In psoriasis, cathelicidin expression is elevated and secondary infections are rare, whereas in atopic dermatitis, in which cathelicidin level is low, infections are increased (45). Cath is produced by keratinocytes at high levels also during wound healing. The highest Cath levels are attained at 48 hours post-injury, declining to pre-injury levels upon wound closure. Cath is detected in the inflammatory infiltrate and in the epithelium migrating over the wound bed. On the contrary, in wounds that are chronically not healing, Cath expression is low or absent (46).

Cath processing in the skin is still under investigation. Very recent data have further elucidated the pathway of cathelin synthesis and release by keratinocytes. Using immunocytochemistry and confocal microscopy it has been possible to localize Cath origin in the Golgi apparatus and by electron microscopy (EM) inside the LB of fully differentiated keratinocytes.

Thus, like the defensins, cathelicidins are localized in the skin in such a way as to provide a coordinated defense with barrier lipids.

OTHER PROTEINS AND PEPTIDES WITH ANTIMICROBIAL PEPTIDE FUNCTIONS

Chemokines

After the discovery that defensins share some receptors with chemokines, interest in the antimicrobial activity of cytokines and chemokines has increased.

Chemokines are a large family of structurally related chemotactic factors that share the ability to stimulate leukocyte motility. They are conventionally divided into two subfamilies, CC and CXC (47). Resident cells in the skin that have been shown to produce chemokines include keratinocytes, fibroblasts, and epithelial cells. The CXC type is preferentially chemotactic for neutrophils. IL-8 belongs to this family as well as MGSA, GRO-alpha, gamma-IP-10, and MIP-2.

Members of the CC subfamily are primarily chemotactic for monocytes and T lymphocytes. Members of this family are MCP-1, MCP-2, MCP-3, MCP-4, RANTES, MIP-1alpha, and MIP-1beta.

Eleven chemokines were tested for antimicrobial activity against *E. coli* at pH 7.4, with representatives from the C, CC, CXC, and CX3C groups. The three ELR-CXC chemokines were antimicrobials. RANTES/CCL5 was not antimicrobial at pH 7.4 but it was in an acidic buffer (pH 5.5). When the antimicrobial activity against *E. coli* and *Listeria monocytogenes* was explored using an RDA in low (10 mM sodium phosphate, pH 7.4), medium (10 mM sodium phosphate, pH 7.4 + 50 mM NaCl), and high (10 mM sodium phosphate, pH 7.4 + 100 mM NaCl) ionic concentrations, the activity of IP-10/CXCL10, I-TAC/CXCL11, and MIG/CXCL9 were similar to that of an alpha-defensin (HNP-1) against *E. coli* and *L. monocytogenes*. The salt sensitivity of ELR-CXC chemokines was similar to defensins and many other AMPs (48).

Granulysin is a molecule expressed by human natural killer cells and activated T lymphocytes. It exhibits cytolytic activity against a variety of microbes and tumors. It is present within the skin only during inflammation and infections (49–51).

Neuropeptides

Neuropeptides are amphipathic molecules and they share this property with AMPs. Because of their biochemical properties, and known membrane activity, neuropeptides have been studied for antimicrobial activity. It is difficult to define when a neuropeptide has relevant antimicrobial activity because the physiological concentrations of these peptides are often difficult to determine. However, within systems like skin or the mucosa, neuropeptides have shown substantial importance. Substance P (SP) is present in sensory neurons within unmyelinated axons, the C-fibers for pain. In the skin, SP induces increased permeability, vasodilation, neutrophil and macrophage recruitment, mast cell degranulation, and keratinocyte proliferation. SP can thus be considered a pro-inflammatory molecule. SP has been shown in vitro to exhibit antimicrobial activity against *S. aureus*, *E. coli*, *E. faecalis*, *P. vulgaris*, and *C. albicans*.

Neuropeptide Y (NPY) is another example of a neuropeptide with antimicrobial activity. This substance is used as a mediator for several different neural processes and can affect behavior and metabolism within the brain.

These peptides also have antimicrobial properties. In vitro, NPY exhibits potent antifungal activity against *C. albicans*, *Cryptococcus neoformans*, and *Arthroderma simii* as well as activity against Gram-negative and Gram-positive microbes (52). Their contribution to skin defense may be due to expression in Langerhans cells (LC) and has been shown for NPY and PYY (53).

Alpha-MSH and Related Peptides

POMC peptides are neuro-hormones with anti-inflammatory activity in the skin. They were first described in the pituitary gland and later in the skin and other tissues. In the skin, keratinocytes, melanocytes, endothelial cells, mast cells, fibroblasts, and dendritic cells produce POMC peptides.

POMCs are post-translationally processed to alpha-MSH, beta-MSH, gamma-MSH, and beta-endorphin. Alpha-MSH is capable of suppressing both local and systemic immunological function in vivo (54). Recent studies have demonstrated that alpha-MSH has potent antimicrobial activity. Alpha-MSH and its carboxy-terminal tripeptide (11–13, KPV) have antimicrobial influences against two major and representative pathogens: *S. aureus* and *C. albicans*. Alpha-MSH peptides inhibit *S. aureus* colony formation and reversed the enhancing effect of urokinase on microbial growth. Antimicrobial effects occurred at physiological (picomolar) concentrations.

Proenkephalin A

Proenkephalin A is a precursor of the enkephalin opiod peptides, processed to yield several biologically active peptides (Met-enkephalin, Leu-enkephalin, Met-enkephalin-Arg-Phe, Met-enkephalin-Arg-Gly-Leu), enkelytin, and proenkephalin A–derived peptides (PEAP) like Peptide B. These peptides are mainly expressed in the brain and in the adrenal medulla, but they have recently been described in the skin (55).

PEA fragments have been evaluated for activity against several pathogens: vasostatin-I and chromofungin are potent inhibitors of fungi and yeast; enkelytin, a potent inhibitor of Gram-positive bacteria (including *M. luteus*, *B. megaterium* and the pathogenic strain *S. aureus*, in the 0.2–4.5 micromolar range); and Ub against Gram-positive bacteria and fungi. Vasostatin-I, enkelytin, and Ub correspond to highly conserved peptides, and their antimicrobial activities probably occurred early in evolution. Furthermore, they are widely distributed not only in endocrine, neuroendocrine, and nerve cells but also in immune cells. Therefore, in stress situations, these peptides might provide a highly beneficial strategy against pathogenic invasion (56).

Adrenomedullin

Adrenomedullin (AM) is a regulatory peptide that is synthesized and secreted by a wide number of cells and tissues. AM is a potent vasodilator, but also exerts other functions, such as regulating cell growth and antimicrobial defense. It acts through the binding with two receptors, L1 and calcitonin receptor-like receptor (CRLR), which are able to bind AM (57).

AM and its receptors are present in the suprabasal epidermis, in the melanocytes of the epidermis, and in sweat and sebaceous glands. AM protein is strongly expressed in the basal and suprabasal layers of the hair bulb and the proximal outer root sheath (58).

Keratinocytes do not store AM but secrete it constitutively. Cytokines interleukin-1-alpha and -1-beta, tumor necrosis factor-alpha and -beta, and the bacterial component lipopolysaccharide, all significantly stimulate adrenomedullin secretion from oral but not skin keratinocytes. Both transforming growth factor-beta1 and interferon-gamma are potent suppressors of adrenomedullin secretion from both cell types, as are forskolin, di-butyryl cyclic adenosine monophosphate, and adrenocorticotropin. The peptides thrombin and endothelin-1 increase adrenomedullin production, particularly from skin keratinocytes (57).

AM antimicrobial activity against the microflora of the human skin and oral mucosa has been demonstrated. Both pathogenic and commensal strains of bacteria are sensitive, Gram-positive and Gram-negative bacteria being equally susceptible. On the contrary, no activity against the yeast *C. albicans* was observed (59).

ENZYMES

Another class of molecules that possesses antimicrobial activity and may contribute to the antimicrobial properties of the skin barrier are enzymes or enzyme inhibitors such as SLPI. SLPI was originally described as a proteinase inhibitor produced by cells of mucosal surfaces. Chemically it consists of a tandemly repeated four disulfide core motifs, the second domain being structurally related to the C-terminal domain of members of the trappin gene family, which includes the proteinase inhibitor SKALP/elafin. SLPI is able to inhibit polymorphonuclear leukocyte elastase and cathepsin G (60), and mast cell chymase (61); moreover, it inhibits a chymotrypsin-like enzyme found in SC (62). In addition to its anti-proteinase activity, SLPI was shown to inhibit infection of T cells and monocytes by human immunodeficiency virus 1 (HIV-1) in vitro (63). The presence of SLPI in human saliva could explain the low HIV transmission rate by oral route. SLPI activity has been demonstrated in SC extracts, although the exact cellular source was not identified. SLPI acts as a multifunctional protein by protecting against excessive proteolysis and providing antimicrobial activity.

SLPI displays a marked antibacterial activity in vitro against *E. coli* and *S. aureus* (64).

The effect of SLPI on *P. aeruginosa* has been investigated, and it has been proven that SLPI is active against *P. aeruginosa* with potency similar to that of lysozyme. Recently, several other biologic properties of SLPI were discovered, such as antiviral, antibacterial, and LPS-modulating effects.

BARRIER IMPLICATIONS

The skin as a barrier must maintain water and electrolyte balance, but this function is correlated with a capacity to resist microbial invasion and subsequent infection. The balance of antimicrobial activity may influence the physical barrier properties. The specific combination of antimicrobial molecules at this site dictates the equilibrium between the resident flora and pathogens, contributing to the pH and the skin surface composition. Barrier modification accounts for lipid surface modification, calcium gradient modification, and pH modifications (Fig. 1).

Each of these parameters is able to induce a response intended to re-establish the normal skin barrier. Any alteration that triggers a change in surface ion composition provokes the release of a variety of inflammatory and antimicrobial mediators from the epithelial keratinocytes, thus eliciting an inflammatory response. Modification in the skin barrier is followed by a rapid release of new lipids, release of cytokines, and coincident activation of a cascade of transcription factors enabling appropriate new synthesis of molecules designed to repair and protect the defect (21). Pathogenic bacteria have a unique ability to exploit or induce barrier defects. It is known that many pathogens can easily grow on skin surface when the pH is impaired. *S. aureus* expresses sphingomyelinase and ceramidase (1) and can therefore

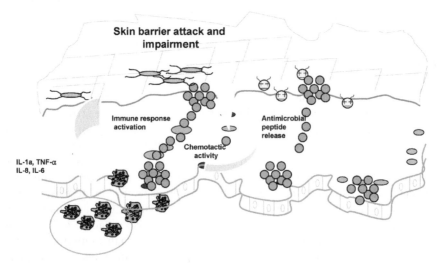

Figure 1   Skin barrier attack and impairment.

induce a modification in the skin barrier lipid composition, thus gaining access. Initiation of infection may depend on disruption of the corneal layer, allowing access of bacteria to differentiated upper spinous layer keratinocytes (65). Ready binding of bacteria to keratinocytes is consistent with the hypothesis that disruption of SC and adherence to keratinocytes is an important initiating step in the pathogenesis of skin infections. The bacterial disruption of SC and of the lipid barrier located at that level provokes a rapid reaction including rapid release of Oddland bodies with their lipid contents and AMP contents.

The second layer response to barrier impairment is related to keratinocyte response. Keratinocyte reactions include direct activation of the cell cycle, in part, due to Ca^{++}-activated events. Skin barrier invasion and bacterial adhesion to keratinocytes induce keratinocyte activation, and release of IL-1alpha (storage form), IL-8, and TNF-alpha (66,67). The "activated keratinocytes" and the pro-inflammatory cytokines connected to it induce activation of ceramide, sphingosine, cholesterol, and FFA syntheses aimed at re-establishing skin barrier permeability and pH (21).

With keratinocyte degranulation comes release of AMPs such as defensins and cathelicidins into the SC. The presence of activated LL-37 (the human neutrophil form of cathelicidins) on keratinocytes is strongly pro-inflammatory (68), and such activity is enhanced if the keratinocytes are in a low-calcium condition (basal layer) (unpublished personal data). In the presence of LL-37, keratinocytes release IL-8, IL-6, TNF-alpha, and IL-1. The chemotactic activity of LL-37 might further amplify the process by stimulating additional leukocytes recruitment through their interaction with formyl peptide receptor-like 1 and CCR-6, respectively (69).

CONCLUDING REMARKS

The inclusion of AMPs and AMP-related molecules into the complex mechanism with which the skin fights infections opens a new and wider window on the skin's capacity to preserve its integrity and function. Skin cells are able to produce a huge variety of biologically active substances from lipids and neuropeptides to enzymes. They also coordinate those disparate molecules by working together in the final aim of defending the skin from microbial invasion. Understanding these interactive mechanisms allows control of the anti-infective function of the skin, and allows the creation and manipulation of more sophisticated therapeutic approaches. This new pharmaceutical strategy will take into account not only the direct implications of delivering an antimicrobial, but also its ability to be stimulated by the peripheral nervous system, and in turn of stimulating the acquired immune response.

REFERENCES

1. Mempel M, Schmidt T, Weidinger S, Schnopp C, Foster T, Ring J, Abeck D. Role of Staphylococcus aureus surface-associated proteins in the attachment to cultured HaCaT keratinocytes in a new adhesion assay. J Invest Dermatol 1998; 111(3):452–456.
2. Behrendt H, Green M. Nature of the sweating deficit of prematurely born neonates. Observations on babies with the heroin withdrawal syndrome. N Engl J Med 1972; 286(26):1376–1379.
3. Hardman MJ, Sisi P, Banbury DN, Byrne C. Patterned acquisition of skin barrier function during development. Development 1998; 125(8):1541–1552.

4. Visscher MO, Chatterjee R, Munson KA, Pickens WL, Hoath SB. Changes in diapered and nondiapered infant skin over the first month of life. Pediatr Dermatol 2000; 17(1):45–51.
5. Yosipovitch G, Maayan-Metzger A, Merlob P, Sirota L. Skin barrier properties in different body areas in neonates. Pediatrics 2000; 106(1 Pt 1):105–108.
6. Leyden JJ, Kligman AM. The role of microorganisms in diaper dermatitis. Arch Dermatol 1978; 114(1):56–59.
7. Aly R, Maibach HI, Rahman R, Shinefield HR, Mandel AD. Correlation of human in vivo and in vitro cutaneous antimicrobial factors. J Infect Dis 1975; 131(5):579–583.
8. Puhvel SM, Reisner RM, Sakamoto M. Analysis of lipid composition of isolated human sebaceous gland homogenates after incubation with cutaneous bacteria. Thin-layer chromatography. J Invest Dermatol 1975; 64(6):406–411.
9. Bibel DJ, Aly R, Lahti L, Shinefield HR, Maibach HI. Microbial adherence to vulvar epithelial cells. J Med Microbiol 1987; 23(1):75–82.
10. Mauro T, Holleran WM, Grayson S, Gao WN, Man MQ, Kriehuber E, Behne M, Feingold KR, Elias PM. Barrier recovery is impeded at neutral pH, independent of ionic effects: implications for extracellular lipid processing. Arch Dermatol Res 1998; 290(4):215–222.
11. Takagi Y, Kriehuber E, Imokawa G, Elias PM, Holleran WM. Beta-glucocerebrosidase activity in mammalian stratum corneum. J Lipid Res 1999; 40(5):861–869.
12. Jensen JM, Schutze S, Neumann C, Proksch E. Impaired cutaneous permeability barrier function, skin hydration, and sphingomyelinase activity in keratin 10 deficient mice. J Invest Dermatol 2000; 115(4):708–713.
13. Schmuth M, Man MQ, Weber F, Gao W, Feingold KR, Fritsch P, Elias PM, Holleran WM. Permeability barrier disorder in Niemann-Pick disease: sphingomyelin-ceramide processing required for normal barrier homeostasis. J Invest Dermatol 2000; 115(3):459–466.
14. Holleran WM, Takagi Y, Menon GK, Legler G, Feingold KR, Elias PM. Processing of epidermal glucosylceramides is required for optimal mammalian cutaneous permeability barrier function. J Clin Invest 1993; 91(4):1656–1664.
15. Ament W, Huizenga JR, Mook GA, Gips CH, Verkerke GJ. Lactate and ammonia concentration in blood and sweat during incremental cycle ergometer exercise. Int J Sports Med 1997; 18(1):35–39.
16. Krien PM, Kermici M. Evidence for the existence of a self-regulated enzymatic process within the human stratum corneum -an unexpected role for urocanic acid. J Invest Dermatol 2000; 115(3):414–420.
17. Fluhr JW, Kao J, Jain M, Ahn SK, Feingold KR, Elias PM. Generation of free fatty acids from phospholipids regulates stratum corneum acidification and integrity. J Invest Dermatol 2001; 117(1):44–51.
18. Behne MJ, Meyer JW, Hanson KM, Barry NP, Murata S, Crumrine D, Clegg RW, Gratton E, Holleran WM, Elias PM, Mauro TM. NHE1 regulates the stratum corneum permeability barrier homeostasis. Microenvironment acidification assessed with fluorescence lifetime imaging. J Biol Chem 2002; 277(49):47399–47406.
19. Ushijima T, Takahashi M, Ozaki Y. Acetic, propionic, and oleic acid as the possible factors influencing the predominant residence of some species of Propionibacterium and coagulase-negative Staphylococcus on normal human skin. Can J Microbiol 1984; 30(5):647–652.
20. Elias PM, Brown BE, Ziboh VA. The permeability barrier in essential fatty acid deficiency: Evidence for a direct role for linoleic acid in barrier function. J Invest Dermatol 1984; 74:230–233.
21. Elias PM, Feingold KR. Coordinate regulation of epidermal differentiation and barrier homeostasis. Skin Pharmacol Appl Skin Physiol 2001; 14(Suppl 1):28–34.
22. Downing DT. Lipid and protein structures in the permeability barrier of mammalian epidermis. Journal of Lipid Research 1992; 33:301–313.

23. Wertz PW, Miethke MC, Long SA, Strauss JS, Downing DT. The composition of ceramides from human stratum corneum and from comedones. J Invest Dermatol 1985; 84:410–412.
24. Wertz PW, Downing DT. Acylglucosylceramides of pig epidermis: structure determination. J Lipid Res 1983; 24:753–758.
25. Yardley HJ, Summerly R. Lipid composition and metabolism in normal and diseased epidermis. Pharmacol Ther 1981; 13:357–381.
26. Bibel DJ, Miller SJ, Brown BE, Pandey BB, Elias PM, Shinefield HR, Aly R. Antimicrobial activity of stratum corneum lipids from normal and essential fatty acid-deficient mice. J Invest Dermatol 1989; 92(4):632–638.
27. Ganz T. Defensins: antimicrobial peptides of innate immunity. Nat Rev Immunol 2003; 3(9):710–720.
28. Fellermann K, Wehkamp J, Stange EF. Antimicrobial peptides in the skin. N Engl J Med 2003; 348(4):361–363.
29. Liu AY, Destoumieux D, Wong AV, Park CH, Valore EV, Liu L, Ganz T. Human beta-defensin-2 production in keratinocytes is regulated by interleukin-1, bacteria, and the state of differentiation. J Invest Dermatol 2002; 118(2):275–281.
30. Oren A, Ganz T, Liu L, Meerloo T. In human epidermis, beta-defensin 2 is packaged in lamellar bodies. Exp Mol Pathol 2003; 74(2):180–182.
31. Pernet I, Reymermier C, Guezennec A, Branka JE, Guesnet J, Perrier E, Dezutter-Dambuyant C, Schmitt D, Viac J. Calcium triggers beta-defensin (hBD-2 and hBD-3) and chemokine macrophage inflammatory protein-3 alpha (MIP-3alpha/CCL20) expression in monolayers of activated human keratinocytes. Exp Dermatol 2003; 12(6):755–760.
32. Sorensen OE, Cowland JB, Theilgaard-Monch K, Liu L, Ganz T, Borregaard N. Wound healing and expression of antimicrobial peptides/polypeptides in human keratinocytes, a consequence of common growth factors. J Immunol 2003; 170(11):5583–5589.
33. Dinulos JG, Mentele L, Fredericks LP, Dale BA, Darmstadt GL. Keratinocyte expression of human beta defensin 2 following bacterial infection: role in cutaneous host defense. Clin Diagn Lab Immunol 2003; 10(1):161–166.
34. Yang D, Chertov O, Oppenheim JJ. The role of mammalian antimicrobial peptides and proteins in awakening of innate host defenses and adaptive immunity. Cell Mol Life Sci 2001; 58(7):978–989.
35. Zanetti M. Cathelicidins, multifunctional peptides of the innate immunity. J Leukoc Biol 2004; 75(1):39–48.
36. Nizet V, Ohtake T, Lauth X, Trowbridge J, Rudisill J, Dorschner RA, Pestonjamasp V, Piraino J, Huttner K, Gallo RL. Innate antimicrobial peptide protects the skin from invasive bacterial infection. Nature 2001; 414(6862):454–457.
37. Di Nardo A, Vitiello A, Gallo RL. Cutting edge: mast cell antimicrobial activity is mediated by expression of cathelicidin antimicrobial peptide. J Immunol 2003; 170(5):2274–2278.
38. Sorensen OE, Gram L, Johnsen AH, Andersson E, Bangsboll S, Tjabringa GS, Hiemstra PS, Malm J, Egesten A, Borregaard N. Processing of seminal plasma hCAP-18 to ALL-38 by gastricsin: a novel mechanism of generating antimicrobial peptides in vagina. J Biol Chem 2003; 278(31):28540–28546.
39. Zanetti M, Gennaro R, Skerlavaj B, Tomasinsig L, Circo R. Cathelicidin peptides as candidates for a novel class of antimicrobials. Curr Pharm Des 2002; 8(9):779–793.
40. Howell MD, Jones JF, Kisich KO, Streib JE, Gallo RL, Leung DY. Selective killing of vaccinia virus by LL-37: implications for eczema vaccinatum. J Immunol 2004; 172(3):1763–1767.
41. Oren Z, Lerman JC, Gudmundsson GH, Agerberth B, Shai Y. Structure and organization of the human antimicrobial peptide LL-37 in phospholipid membranes: relevance to the molecular basis for its non-cell-selective activity. Biochem J 1999; 341(Pt 3):501–513.

42. Zaiou M, Nizet V, Gallo RL. Antimicrobial and protease inhibitory functions of the human cathelicidin (hCAP18/LL-37) prosequence. J Invest Dermatol 2003; 120(5):810–816.

43. Dorschner RA, Lin KH, Murakami M, Gallo RL. Neonatal skin in mice and humans expresses increased levels of antimicrobial peptides: innate immunity during development of the adaptive response. Pediatr Res 2003; 53(4):566–572.

44. Murakami M, Ohtake T, Dorschner RA, Schittek B, Garbe C, Gallo RL. Cathelicidin anti-microbial peptide expression in sweat, an innate defense system for the skin. J Invest Dermatol 2002; 119(5):1090–1095.

45. Ong PY, Ohtake T, Brandt C, Strickland I, Boguniewicz M, Ganz T, Gallo RL, Leung DY. Endogenous antimicrobial peptides and skin infections in atopic dermatitis. N Engl J Med 2002; 347(15):1151–1160.

46. Heilborn JD, Nilsson MF, Kratz G, Weber G, Sorensen O, Borregaard N, Stahle-Backdahl M. The cathelicidin anti-microbial peptide LL-37 is involved in re-epithelialization of human skin wounds and is lacking in chronic ulcer epithelium. J Invest Dermatol 2003; 120(3):379–389.

47. Rot A, Von Andrian UH. Chemokines in Innate and Adaptive Host Defense: Basic Chemokinese Grammar for Immune Cells. Annu Rev Immunol 2004; 22:891–928.

48. Cole AM, Ganz T, Liese AM, Burdick MD, Liu L, Strieter RM. Cutting edge: IFN-inducible ELR- CXC chemokines display defensin-like antimicrobial activity. J Immunol 2001; 167(2):623–627.

49. Modlin RL. Learning from leprosy: insights into contemporary immunology from an ancient disease. Skin Pharmacol Appl Skin Physiol 2002; 15(1):1–6.

50. Canaday DH, Wilkinson RJ, Li Q, Harding CV, Silver RF, Boom WH. CD4(+) and CD8(+) T cells kill intracellular Mycobacterium tuberculosis by a perforin and Fas/Fas ligand-independent mechanism. J Immunol 2001; 7(5):2734–2742.

51. Ochoa MT, Stenger S, Sieling PA, Thoma-Uszynski S, Sabet S, Cho S, Krensky AM, Rollinghoff M, Nunes Sarno E, Burdick AE, Rea TH, Modlin RL. T-cell release of granulysin contributes to host defense in leprosy. Nat Med 2001; 7(2):174–179.

52. Shimizu M, Shigeri Y, Tatsu Y, Yoshikawa S, Yumoto N. Enhancement of antimicrobial activity of neuropeptide Y by N-terminal truncation. Antimicrob Agents Chemother 1998; 42(10):2745–2746.

53. Lambert RW, Campton K, Ding W, Ozawa H, Granstein RD. Langerhans cell expression of neuropeptide Y and peptide YY. Neuropeptides 2002; 36(4):246–251.

54. Cutuli M, Cristiani S, Lipton JM, Catania A. Antimicrobial effects of alpha-MSH peptides. J Leukoc Biol 2000; 67(2):233–229.

55. Kew D, Kilpatrick DL. Widespread organ expression of the rat proenkephalin gene during early postnatal development. Mol Endocrinol 1990; 4(2):337–340.

56. Metz-Boutigue MH, Kieffer AE, Goumon Y, Aunis D. Innate immunity: involvement of new neuropeptides. Trends Microbiol 2003; 11(12):585–592.

57. Kapas S, Tenchini ML, Farthing PM. Regulation of adrenomedullin secretion in cultured human skin and oral keratinocytes. J Invest Dermatol 2001; 117(2):353–359.

58. Muller FB, Muller-Rover S, Korge BP, Kapas S, Hinson JP, Philpott MP. Adrenomedullin: expression and possible role in human skin and hair growth. Br J Dermatol 2003; 148(1):30–38.

59. Allaker RP, Zihni C, Kapas S. An investigation into the antimicrobial effects of adrenomedullin on members of the skin, oral, respiratory tract and gut microflora. FEMS Immunol Med Microbiol 1999; 23(4):289–293.

60. Thompson RC, Ohlsson K. Isolation, properties, and complete amino acid sequence of human secretory leukocyte protease inhibitor, a potent inhibitor of leukocyte elastase. Proc Natl Acad Sci U S A 1986; 83(18):6692–6696.

61. Fink E, Nettelbeck R, Fritz H. Inhibition of mast cell chymase by eglin c and antileukoprotease (HUSI-I). Indications for potential biological functions of these inhibitors. Biol Chem Hoppe Seyler 1986; 367(7):567–571.

62. Franzke CW, Baici A, Bartels J, Christophers E, Wiedow O. Antileukoprotease inhibits stratum corneum chymotryptic enzyme. Evidence for a regulative function in desquamation. J Biol Chem 1996; 271(36):21886–21890.
63. McNeely TB, Dealy M, Dripps DJ, Orenstein JM, Eisenberg SP, Wahl SM. Secretory leukocyte protease inhibitor: a human saliva protein exhibiting anti-human immunodeficiency virus 1 activity in vitro. J Clin Invest 1995; 96(1):456–464.
64. Hiemstra PS, Maassen RJ, Stolk J, Heinzel-Wieland R, Steffens GJ, Dijkman JH. Antibacterial activity of antileukoprotease. Infect Immun 1996; 64(11):4520–4524.
65. Darmstadt GL, Mentele L, Fleckman P, Rubens CE. Role of keratinocyte injury in adherence of Streptococcus pyogenes. Infect Immun 1999; 67(12):6707–6709.
66. Ruiz N, Wang B, Pentland A, Caparon M. Streptolysin O and adherence synergistically modulate proinflammatory responses of keratinocytes to group A streptococci. Mol Microbiol 1998; 27(2):337–346.
67. Freedberg IM, Tomic-Canic M, Komine M, Blumenberg M. Keratins and the keratinocyte activation cycle. J Invest Dermatol 2001; 116(5):633–640.
68. Murakami M, Lopez-Garcia B, Braff M, Dorschner RA, Gallo RL. Postsecretory processing generates multiple cathelicidins for enhanced topical antimicrobial defense. J Immunol 2004; 172(5):3070–3077.
69. Oppenheim JJ, Biragyn A, Kwak LW, Yang D. Roles of antimicrobial peptides such as defensins in innate and adaptive immunity. Ann Rheum Dis 2003; 62(Suppl 2):ii17–ii21.

23

The Epidermal Antioxidant Barrier

Jens J. Thiele
Department of Dermatology, Northwestern University, Chicago, Illinois, U.S.A.

INTRODUCTION

Located at the interface between the body and the environment, the stratum corneum (SC) is frequently and directly exposed to a pro-oxidative environment, including air-pollutants, ultraviolet solar radiation (UVR), chemical oxidants, and microorganisms (1–3). To counteract oxidative injury, the human skin is equipped with a network of enzymatic and non-enzymatic antioxidant systems (4). An imbalance between oxidative attack and antioxidant defense systems results in tissue-specific oxidative modifications of macromolecules and is referred to as "oxidative stress." The composition and structure of the SC lipid and protein play a key role in determining barrier integrity, which is essential for skin moisturization, normal desquamation, and healthy skin condition (5,6). As oxidative lipid and protein modifications commonly result in structural or functional loss, antioxidant barrier systems are believed to play an important role in maintaining barrier integrity. However, while many unique histological, biophysical, and biochemical features of the SC have been known for long, its redox properties have only recently become the subject of systematic basic research. Recent studies have revealed the existence of redox gradients in the human SC. The aim of this chapter is to provide a brief overview on the relevant data available on this emerging field of research.

GENERATION OF REACTIVE OXYGEN SPECIES AND OXIDATIVE STRESS

The formation of reactive oxygen species (ROS) during exposure to UVR represents the best characterized source of oxidative stress in skin. The cascade of ROS formation is initiated by UVR-absorption [predominantly ultraviolet A (UVA)] of endogenous or exogenous chromophores in the skin. Of the many skin constituents absorbing UVA, *trans*-urocanic acid, melanins, flavins, porphyrins, quinones, protein bound tryptophan, or advanced glycation end products are believed to be relevant photosensitizers initiating the ROS formation cascade. Following UVR absorption, the activated chromophore may react in two ways. In type I photoreactions, the excited chromophore directly reacts with a substrate molecule via electron or hydrogen atom transfer and gives rise to free radical formation. In the presence of molecular oxygen (minor type II reaction), this reaction may lead to the formation of the super-oxide anion radical ($^\bullet O_2^-$). Subsequently, $^\bullet O_2^-$ gives hydrogen peroxide (H_2O_2) by a dismutation reaction either spontaneously or catalyzed by cutaneous superoxide dismutase. Furthermore, in the presence of metal ions such as Fe(II) or Cu(II), H_2O_2 can be converted to the highly reactive hydroxyl radical ($^\bullet OH$). Otherwise (major type II reaction), electronically excited and reactive singlet oxygen ($^1O_2$) is formed by photo-energy transfer from UVR-excited chromophores in the presence of triplet oxygen $^3O_2$ (molecular oxygen in its ground state). Following their formation, ROS species including $^1O_2$, $^\bullet O_2^-$, $^\bullet OH$, and H_2O_2 react with an array of skin biomolecules including lipids, proteins, carbohydrates, and DNA. Unsaturated lipids react with ROS forming lipid peroxyl ($LOO^\bullet$) and alkoxyl radicals ($LO^\bullet$) which may initiate a chain-propagating autocatalytic reaction ("lipid peroxidation"). End products of lipid peroxidation, such as malondialdehyde (MDA) or 4-hydroxy-nonenal (4-HNE), induce a number of cellular stress responses and, at higher concentrations, are cytotoxic. Vitamin E is considered the "chain-breaking antioxidant" because it is able to terminate the chain-propagating lipid peroxidation reaction.

Oxidative Protein Modifications: General Mechanisms

A variety of proteins are important targets for oxidative modifications. Oxygen radicals and other activated oxygen species generated as by-products of cellular metabolism or from environmental sources cause modifications of the amino acids of proteins that generally result in functional changes in structural or enzymatic proteins. In addition to modification of amino acid side-chains, oxidation reactions can also mediate fragmentation of polypeptide chains and both intra- and inter-molecular crosslinking of peptides and proteins (7). Protein carbonyls may be formed either by oxidative cleavage of proteins or by direct oxidation of lysine, arginine, proline, and threonine residues. In addition, carbonyl groups may be intro-duced into proteins by reactions with aldehydes (4-hydroxy-2-nonenal, malondial-dehyde) produced during lipid peroxidation or with reactive carbonyl derivatives generated as a consequence of the reaction of reducing sugars or their oxidation pro-ducts with lysine residues of proteins (8). The presence of carbonyl groups in proteins has therefore been used as a marker of reactive oxygen mediated protein oxidation. As measured by the introduction of carbonyl groups, protein oxidation has been associated with aging, oxidative stress, and a number of diseases such as the prema-ture aging diseases, progeria, and Werner's syndrome (9). Importantly, ROS may cause specific "fingerprint" modifications of amino acids resulting in functional changes of structural or enzymic proteins. In particular, methionine residues in proteins are easily oxidized to methionine sulfoxide (MetO) and the repair of this damage appears to be essential for tissues to survive in the presence of ROS (10).

PHYSIOLOGICAL BARRIER ANTIOXIDANTS

Biosurfaces of plants and animals are directly exposed to an oxidative environment generating high levels of oxidative stress. Consequently, living organisms have devel-oped complex integrated extracellular and intracellular defense systems against stresses related to reactive oxygen and nitrogen species. Plant and animal epithelial surfaces and respiratory tract surfaces contain antioxidants that provide defense against environmental stress caused by ambient ROS, thus reducing their injurious effects on underlying cellular constituents (11). Upsetting the antioxidant systems at these biosurfaces may result in the formation of specific oxidation products, some of which have been identified as biomarkers of environmental oxidative stress. Moreover, secondary or tertiary reaction products may also induce injury to underlying cells or be involved in physiological tissue and site-specific responses, such as epidermal differentiation and desquamation.

Non-enzymic antioxidant concentrations as well as enzymic antioxidant activities are generally significantly higher in the epidermis than in the dermis of murine and human skin (12). This probably reflects the fact that the epidermis is more directly exposed to various exogenous sources of oxidative stress and thus requires a higher antioxidant defense capacity to maintain a physiological redox balance. On a molar basis, hydrophilic non-enzymic antioxidants including L-ascorbic acid, GSH, and uric acid appear to be the predominant antioxidants in human skin. Their overall dermal and epidermal concentrations are more than 10- to 100-fold greater than those found for vitamin E or ubiquinol. In contrast to uric acid, GSH, and ubiquinol, vitamins C and E cannot be synthesized by the human body and must be taken up by the diet. Consequently, the skin's antioxidant defense may be at least partially influenced by nutritive factors. However, to date little is known on the physiological regulation of antioxidant vitamins in human skin. While antioxidant concentration and activities of whole skin, dermis, and epidermis are reviewed in detail elsewhere (12), in this chapter information available on antioxidants investigated in the SC or skin surface lipids is summarized.

VITAMIN E

α-Tocopherol, the major biologically active vitamin E homologue, is generally regarded as the most important lipid-soluble antioxidant in human tissues (13). α-Tocopherol is known to efficiently scavenge lipid peroxyl and alkoxyl radicals by intercepting lipid chain propagation. The initial oxidation product of tocopherol is the meta-stable

Table 1 Physiological Levels of Ubiquinone/Ubiquinol ("Coenzyme Q10") in Skin

Skin layer	Species	Concentration	References
Total skin	Mouse	20 – 48 pmol ubiquinol-9/mg protein	77,78
		98 – 136 pmol ubiqinone-9/mg protein	
Epidermis	Mouse	1.9 ± 0.2 nmol ubiquinol-9/g tissue	33
		15.2 ± 1.1 nmol ubiuinone9/g tissue	
Dermis	Mouse	1.2 ± 0.2 nmol ubiquinol-9/g tissue	33
		10.0 ± 0.7 nmol ubiuinone9/g tissue	
Epidermis	Human	3.5 ± 0.8 nmol ubiqinol-10/g tissue	14
		4.1 ± 0.6 nmol ubiquinone-1/g tissue	
Dermis	Human	0.4 ± 0.1 nmol ubiqinol-10/g tissue	14
		2.9 ± 0.8 nmol ubiquinone-10/g tissue	
SC	Mouse	Ubiquinol-9 and ubiquinone-9: not detectable (<0.1 pmol/mg)	27
SC	Human	Ubiquinol-10 and ubiquinone-10: not detectable (<0.1 pmol/mg)	31

Abbreviation: SC, stratum corneum.

Table 2 Physiological Levels of α- and γ-Tocopherol in Cutaneous Tissues

Skin layer	Species	Concentration	References
Total skin	Mouse	200 pmol α-tocopherol/mg protein	77,78
Epidermis	Mouse	4.8 ± 0.5 nmol α-tocopherol/g tissue	33
Dermis	Mouse	3.3 ± 0.3 nmol α-tocopherol/g tissue	33
Epidermis	Human	31 ± 3.8 nmol α-tocopherol/g tissue; 3.3 ± 1 nmol γ-tocopherol/g tissue	14
Dermis	Human	16.2 ± 1.1 nmol α-tocopherol/g tissue; 1.8 ± 0.2 nmol γ-tocopherol/g tissue	14
SC	Mouse	8.4 ± 1.3 nmol α-tocopherol/g tissue; 2.9 ± 0.9 nmol γ-tocopherol/g tissue	27
SC	Human	33 ± 4 nmol α-tocopherol/g tissue; 4.8 ± 0.8 nmol γ-tocopherol/g tissue	31
Sebum	Human	76.5 ± 1.5 nmol α-tocopherol/g sebum; 8.7 ± 1.8 nmol γ-tocopherol/g sebum	49

Abbreviation: SC, stratum corneum.

tocopheroxyl radical, which can either react with another lipid radical leading to α-tocopherol consumption or abstract a hydrogen atom from polyunsaturated lipids to give α-tocopherol and lipid radical. In the second case, occurring preferentially at low lipid radical concentrations, the lipid radical may later react with oxygen to form a lipid peroxyl radical. As demonstrated in vitro in lipid and cellular systems, when ascorbic acid or ubiquinol ("Coenzyme Q10") is present, the tocopheroxyl radical is rapidly reduced and the active form of vitamin E, α-tocopherol, is regenerated (Table 1). Hence, the lack of such "co-antioxidants" from the antioxidant network may result in limited antioxidant protection of lipid bilayers or other lipophilic domains.

Remarkably, a vitamin E gradient is present in the SC of untreated, healthy human skin, with the lowest tocopherol concentrations at the surface and the highest in the deepest SC layers. In the human epidermis, the ratio of α- and γ-tocopherol was found to be about 10:1 (14). This is in accordance with the α- and γ-tocopherol ratio (Table 2) we have found in the deepest SC layer, with 10-fold higher α-tocopherol concentration compared with that of γ-tocopherol. The in vivo antioxidant activity of α-tocopherol is thought to be higher than that of γ-tocopherol.

Besides its protection against lipid peroxidation, vitamin E is suggested to stabilize lipid bilayers, which may also be of relevance for SC lipid bilayers, as the degree of disorder and the amount of lipids decrease over the outer cell layers of human SC (15). Thus, low levels of SC vitamin E correlate with a high degree of SC lipid disorder. However, a direct correlation between vitamin E levels and biophysical parameters of lipid bilayer arrangement in the human SC remains to be investigated.

VITAMIN C, GLUTATHIONE, AND URIC ACID

Baseline concentrations of hydrophilic SC antioxidants were investigated in healthy human upper arm skin (16). In analogy to the vitamin E gradients in the SC, the concentrations of ascorbate detected in human SC were the lowest in the outer SC and increasing to almost 10-fold in the lower SC. However, even lower SC ascorbate levels were between one and two orders of magnitude lower than epidermal ascorbate concentrations. Urate concentrations within human SC were distributed more

Table 3 Physiological Levels of Ascorbate in Cutaneous Tissues

Skin layer	Species	Concentration	References
Total skin	Rat	0.2 g/kg tissue	79
Total skin	Human	41 µg/g dry weight	80
Total skin	Mouse	6–7 nmol/mg protein	77,78
Epidermis	Mouse	1321 ± 77 nmol/g tissue	33
Dermis	Mouse	1064 ± 54 nmol/g tissue	33
Epidermis	Human	3798 ± 1016 nmol/g tissue	14
Dermis	Human	723 ± 320 nmol/g tissue	14
SC	Mouse	208 ± 82.5 pmol/10 tape strips	17
	Human	0.3 – 2.5 nmol/g tissue	16

Abbreviation: SC, stratum corneum.

evenly than those of ascorbate and tocopherols; urate concentration in the upper SC was more than 100-fold higher than that of ascorbate, and a small increase towards deeper layers was significant only when expressed per mg wet weight, not when expressed per extracted protein. Similar gradients with highest levels in basal SC layers were found for ascorbate, glutathione, and uric acid in the SC of the untreated hairless mouse (17) (Tables 3 and 4).

ENZYMATIC ANTIOXIDANTS IN THE STRATUM CORNEUM

Interceptive Antioxidant Enzymes

To date, the data available on the presence and activity of enzymatic antioxidants, such as catalase, superoxide dismutases (present in human skin as manganese and

Table 4 Physiological Levels of Glutathione in Cutaneous Tissues

Skin layer	Species	Concentration	References
Epidermis	Human	1.8 µmol/g tissue (GSH)	81
		0.09 µml/g tissue (GSSG)	
Total skin	Guinea pig	0.7–1.1 mol/g tissue (GSH)	82
		1.4–1.5 mol/g tissue (GSSG)	
Epidermis	Mouse	0.75 µmol/g tissue (GSH)	83
Dermis	Mouse	0.32 µmol/g tissue (GSH)	83
Epidermis	Human	1.2 µmol/g tissue (GSH)	84
Total skin	Mouse	3.9–6.3 µmol/g protein (GSH)	77,78
		1–1.5 µmol/g protein (GSSG)	
Epidermis	Mouse	1.16 µmol/g tissue (GSH)	33
		0.07 µmol/g tissue (GSSG)	
Dermis	Mouse	0.59 µmol/g tissue (GSH)	33
		0.16 µmol/g tissue (GSSG)	
Epidermis	Human	0.46 µmol/g tissue (GSH)	14
		0.02 µmol/g tissue (GSSG)	
Dermis	Human	0.08 µmol/g tissue (GSH)	14
		0.01 µmol/g tissue (GSSG)	
SC	Mouse	283.7 pmol/10 tape strips (GSH)	17

Abbreviation: SC, stratum corneum.

copper, zinc form), and glutathione peroxidases, in the SC is very few. Interestingly, recent publications point to a remarkable expression of catalase in human SC. Catalase is a tetrameric enzyme, which is expressed in all major body organs. Each of its four subunits contains a heme-group in its active site and one tightly bound molecule of NADPH. The highest catalase activity is found in the peroxisomes, where it constitutes about 50% of the peroxisomal protein. The major role of catalase as an antioxidant is to detoxify H_2O_2 by decomposing two H_2O_2 molecules to two molecules of water and one of oxygen. We have recently described remarkably high levels of catalase and, to some lesser extent, of superoxide dismutases in human SC (18). Remarkably, catalase levels were significantly decreased in acutely or chronically UV-exposed skin, as well as in intrinsically aged skin. These results were confirmed by Hellemans et al. on the activity level of the enzyme (19). The same authors also showed that SC catalase levels and activity are strongly affected by UVA, but remain unchanged upon ultraviolet B (UVB) exposure. Remarkably, lesional skin of patients with polymorphic light eruption displayed significantly decreased SC catalase levels (20). Today, UVA-induced photooxidation is considered to play an essential role in the pathogenesis of polymorphous light eruption (PLE), and topical pretreatment of skin with antioxidants was recently introduced as a new treatment approach for moderate-to-severe PLE (21).

Antioxidant Repair Enzymes

Besides "interceptive" antioxidant systems that intercept free radical accumulation and thus prevent oxidative damage, numerous human tissues are equipped with "repair enzymes" that are able to reverse and thus control protein oxidative damage. An antioxidant repair enzyme that has received considerable attention lately is the peptide methionine sulfoxide reductase (MSRA), which was initially identified in *Escherichia coli* and has meanwhile been identified in a number of different human tissues such as liver, cerebellum, and kidney (22). We have recently described the presence of MSRA in human skin, where it is most strongly expressed in basal and suprabasal epidermis (23). MSRA reverses the inactivation of many proteins due to oxidation of critical methionine (Met) residues by reducing methionine sulfoxide (MetO) to Met (Fig. 1). Unlike other antioxidant enzymes, its action is independent of metals or cofactors, but requires reducing equivalents from a thioredoxidin regenerating system. Such a system consists of thioredoxin and thioredoxin reductase and is present in the human epidermis (24). Our preliminary results point to a weak expression of MSRA in the human SC as well as in the dermis, which are the sites where the highest levels of protein oxidation are found in healthy as well as in UV-stressed skin (18).

IMPACT OF ENVIRONMENTAL FACTORS ON BARRIER ANTIOXIDANTS

Ozone

A series of studies investigating the effects of the air-pollutant ozone on antioxidants and lipids in skin have provoked an extensive interest in SC α-tocopherol and other SC antioxidants (1,17,25–27). These studies systematically led to the identification of the SC as the most susceptible skin layer to volatile environmental oxidants such as ozone. Ozone itself is too reactive to penetrate deeply into the skin and therefore reacts predominantly

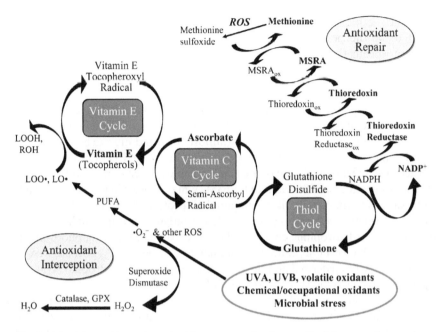

Figure 1 The epidermal antioxidant network: free radical interception and antioxidant repair. *Abbreviations*: ROS: reactive oxygen species; LOOH: lipid hydroperoxides; LOO•: lipid peroxyl radical; GPX: glutathione peroxidases; MSRA: methionine sulfoxide reductase.

with the skin barrier lipids and proteins in the outermost epidermis. However, while ozone might be of clinical relevance for the exacerbation of lung disorders, it does not appear to cause significant damage to murine or human skin, when used at relevant doses. The highly lipophilic SC barrier works as a very effective barrier to volatile oxidants, as opposed to the lung, which is covered by lining fluid that is able to dissolve ozone.

Comparison of transepidermal water loss levels detected in hairless mice after exposure with either solar simulated UVR (up to 3 MED) or high repetitive doses of ozone (5- to 10-fold the highest levels detected in photochemical smog) indicated that for skin, UVR represents a far more relevant source of barrier disturbance than ozone (28).

UVA and UVB

Photo-oxidative Stress in Skin

Exposure of mammalian skin to ultraviolet irradiation (UVIR) induces a spectrum of well-documented acute and chronic responses, including erythema, hyperproliferation, desquamation, and permeability barrier alterations. Diminished permeability barrier function has been demonstrated after single exposures to UVA and UVB (29). However, the underlying mechanisms of UVR-induced changes in SC barrier function remain unclear.

As it is well known that UVB and UVA irradiation induce the formation of reactive oxygen species in cutaneous tissues (30), numerous studies have focused on establishing baseline levels of antioxidants in the dermis and epidermis (14), the antioxidant response to UVB and UVA light in these, and the evaluation of photo-protective potential of topical antioxidant supplementation.

A prime mechanism of UVA- and UVB-induced damage to cutaneous tissues is thought to be the peroxidation of lipids. Vitamin E has been demonstrated to provide photo-protective effects in cell culture and in hairless mouse skin (12).

Effect on Vitamin E and Lipid Peroxidation

SC antioxidants are dramatically depleted by solar simulated UVR even at very low doses. A single suberythemogenic dose of solar simulated UV-light (SSUV; 0.75 MED) depleted human SC α-tocopherol by almost 50%, and murine SC α-tocopherol by 85% (31). In previous studies, SSUV doses equivalent to 3 MED or more were necessary to detect a significant depletion of α-tocopherol in whole epidermis and dermis (32–34). The high susceptibility of SC vitamin E to SSUV may, at least in part, be due to a lack of co-antioxidants in the SC. In vitro, ubiquinol-10 protects α-tocopherol from photo-oxidation by recycling mechanisms (35). In SSUV–irradiated murine skin homogenates, ascorbate, the major hydrophilic co-antioxidant, is capable of recycling photo-oxidized α-tocopherol (30). However, in murine and human SC, the levels of ascorbate were very low as compared with epidermal and dermal tissue. This lack of hydrophilic co-antioxidants is not surprising as the SC is a very hydrophobic environment. While α-tocopherol in murine SC is significantly depleted after suberythemogenic UVR, the lipid peroxidation parameter malondialdehyde (MDA) is increased only upon unphysiologically high doses. Similarly, in previous studies on the cutaneous effects of ozone we found that the dose necessary to detect increased MDA formation in the SC was five times higher than the one to deplete vitamin E (27). In theory, the observed SC tocopherol depletion could be caused either directly by absorption of short wave UVB and/or indirectly by excited-state singlet oxygen or reactive oxygen intermediates that are generated by photo-sensitizers upon UV absorption also in the UVA range. Our results indicate that both mechanisms may be relevant, as either UVB or UVA depleted murine SC α-tocopherol.

Photo-oxidation of Skin Surface Lipids

Of all the skin layers, the SC and skin surface lipids (SSL) are exposed to the highest intensities of solar UV radiation. It has been demonstrated by in vivo chemiluminescence that UVA exposure strongly increases the formation of reactive oxygen species in the skin's uppermost layers (36). Thus, SSL, which are covering the SC in sebaceous gland rich anatomical regions, such as the face, have to be considered as first-line-targets of solar UV exposure. SSL are derived from epidermal lipids as well as from sebaceous gland lipids (sebum). Squalene, an unsaturated lipid, which is generated in sebaceous glands, is one of the main components of human sebum (37).

Previously, in vitro studies suggested that both UVB and UVA radiation of squalene induce squalene hydroperoxides (38–41); however, in these studies unphysiologically high doses of UVB were applied. We have recently demonstrated that, under physiologically relevant conditions using suberythemogenic doses, UVA induces SqmOOH at rates at least one order of magnitude higher than UVB (37).

Accordingly, squalene levels in human sebum are depleted by suberythemogenic doses of UVA. Hence, it may be proposed that previously reported UVB-induced formation of squalene/SSL peroxidation products is due to "contaminating" UVA irradiation. In fact, nearly all "UVB lamps" used in photobiology will emit UVB and UVA (38). The inverse correlation between squalene depletion and SqmOOH formation further confirms that natural sebaceous gland squalene is the substrate for SqmOOH formation observed upon UVA exposure. As UVA-induced oxidative stress in skin is believed to be mediated via reactive oxygen species generated by photosensitizers, these data strongly point to an involvement of physiologic photo-sensitizers. Accordingly, exposure of purified squalene alone to suberythematogenic doses of UVB or UVA does not yield detectable levels of SqmOOH. In the presence of the photosensitizer rose Bengal or porphyrins, however, exposure to visible light yields high amounts of SqmOOH. As the latter finding points to photochemical reaction that involves singlet oxygen, it is likely that UVA-induced SqmOOH formation in vivo is also mediated via singlet oxygen. Intriguingly, in vitro data demonstrate that squalene itself is a good quencher of singlet oxygen (39). With respect to the pathophysiology of acne, bacterial porphyrins were proposed to mediate squalene oxidation in skin (40). Porphyrins are readily excited by light with a wavelength of about 400 nm (Soret band) and, in the presence of oxygen, will cause photodynamic effects mediated by singlet oxygen (41). The involvement of endogenous photosensitizers, such as porphyrins, and subsequent formation of singlet oxygen would explain the wavelength-dependent formation of SqmOOH with higher sensitivity in the UVA and rather a low sensitivity in the UVB range.

Notably, there is evidence that squalene oxidation products induce a number of harmful effects in skin cell cultures and in vivo. Low levels of UVB-peroxidated squalene increased the rates of DNA and protein synthesis in human keratinocytes, while high levels were cytotoxic (42). In the same study, similar histological changes were reported in guinea pig skin treated with UV-peroxidated squalene as with direct UV irradiation. Furthermore, similar to UV-induced immunosuppression, topically applied UV-peroxidated squalene was shown to inhibit the induction of contact hypersensitivity to dinitrofluorobenzene in mice. In the rabbit ear model, UVA-peroxidated squalene was highly comedogenic, while non-oxidized squalene was scarcely comedogenic (33).

Benzoyl Peroxide

Benzoyl peroxide (BPO) is widely used in the treatment of acne. As BPO is known to be a strong oxidant and to decompose within the SC, we investigated the impact of topical BPO application on the antioxidant defense capacity in the SC of human volunteers. A single 10% BPO treatment was found to strongly affect the antioxidant barrier, when compared with vehicle controls 24 hours after application. While the hydrophilic antioxidants, urate and ascorbate, showed differing susceptibility in upper and lower SC, α-tocopherol was most dramatically depleted by more than 90% throughout the entire SC thickness. We concluded that SC antioxidant depletion, particularly in the case of α-tocopherol, represents an early and very sensitive biomarker not only for ozone and UV-induced oxidation processes in the barrier, but also for cutaneous exposure to oxidizing chemicals. The BPO concentration used (10%) is available in many OTC products and the study design was vehicle controlled and performed in human volunteers. Therefore, it seems very likely that barrier α-tocopherol depletion occurs during BPO use in acne treatment. SC vitamin E depletion and/or oxidative stress may account, at least in part, for commonly observed BPO side effects such as dry and scaly skin

PHYSIOLOGICAL MECHANISMS OF BARRIER ANTIOXIDANT REPLETION

Human Sebum Contains High Amounts of Vitamin E

The first studies on sebum antioxidants were based on the rather unexpected observation that the upper SC layers of the environmentally exposed human facial skin contained several-fold higher levels of α-tocopherol than corresponding layers of the previously investigated, less exposed upper arm SC (44). It was suggested that this finding may be related to regional differences in the delivery pathway and/or regulation of vitamin E. In the environmentally highly exposed facial skin, the SC is covered by a film of SSL which consist of wax esters, triglycerides, and squalene, originating from sebum secretion by sebaceous glands. We hypothesized that sebaceous gland secretion is a physiological pathway of vitamin E delivery to the skin surface lipids and SC of facial skin. Using standardized techniques for SC tape stripping and sebum collection, followed by high performance liquid chromatography analysis of tocopherols and squalene, we found that (a) the ratio of facial versus upper arm α-tocopherol levels was 20:1 for the upper SC and decreased gradually with SC depth, (b) vitamin E (α- and γ-tocopherol forms) is a significant constituent of human sebum and is continuously secreted at cheek and forehead sites, and (c) vitamin E correlates very well with levels of co-secreted squalene ($r^2 = 0.86$, $p < 0.001$) (44).

Intriguingly, while a large body of evidence points to photo-protective effects of topically applied vitamin E against immunosuppression, DNA damage, and carcinogenesis, little is known about the role of physiological vitamin E regulation in cutaneous tissues. Remarkably, human sebum levels of α-tocopherol (moles/wet weight) are more than 3-fold higher than levels found in human blood plasma (45), human dermis, epidermis (14), and SC (31). Sebaceous α-tocopherol penetrates into subjacent SC layers, as was demonstrated for other sebum lipids (46). Thus, it accounts for the increased levels of α-tocopherol detected in the upper SC of the sebaceous gland regions of facial skin as compared to upper arm skin. These findings suggest that sebaceous gland secretion is a relevant physiological delivery pathway of α-tocopherol to sebaceous gland-rich skin regions, such as facial skin. Similarly, orally administered drugs have been reported to be transported to the skin surface and the SC by the sebaceous gland secretion route.

Dietary Supplementation of Vitamin E Increases Sebum Vitamin E Levels

While the effects of topical vitamin E have been studied extensively, little is known about the oral bioavailability of this important antioxidant in skin. The controversial results obtained from several studies on this issue are at least in part due to variations in the analysis of skin, in particular with respect to skin depth (whole epidermis, whole dermis, full skin with or without subcutaneous fat). Based on the high physiological concentrations of α-tocopherol in facial sebum and SSL, we hypothesized that the oral bioavailability of vitamin E in human skin is largely dependent on sebaceous gland secretion and thus should be site- and compartment-specific. To test this, 24 healthy volunteers (30 ± 9 years; means ± SD) were subjected to a randomized daily supplementation with either 400 mg RRR-α-tocopheryl acetate (RRR-α-toc) or 400 mg all-rac-α-tocopheryl acetate (all-rac-α-toc) for 14 days (47). Fasting blood samples, facial sebum samples, and SSL lipid extractions from a site with low density of sebaceous glands (lower arm) were taken at 0, 12 hours, 1, 2, 3, 7, 14, and 21 days after initiation of supplementation. Sebum and SSL samples were collected from the forehead of the volunteers using Sebutapes® (Cuderm, Dallas, Texas) and ethanol extraction, respectively. Serum, sebum, and SSL were analyzed by high performance liquid chromatography using electrochemical detection for α-tocopherol and UV-detection for squalene. Serum α-tocopherol levels were significantly increased as early as 12 hours after the first supplementation of RRR-α-toc or all-rac-α-toc and peaked on day 7 with an average increase of 76 and 79%, respectively. No significant changes were observed in lower arm SSL at any time point. Remarkably, while sebum levels remained unchanged during the first 14 days of supplementation, both the RRR-α-toc and the all-rac-α-toc group showed increased α-tocopherol levels in sebum of 87 and 92%, respectively. In conclusion, with respect to dietary supplementation of vitamin E and its bioavailability in human skin, these results suggest that (a) sebaceous gland secretion is a major mechanism leading to site-specific differences, (b) the bioavailability of RRR-α-toc and the all-rac-α-toc is comparable, and, (c) possible protective effects in the skin will not be achieved before a supplementation period of 2–3 weeks.

Other Mechanisms of Vitamin E Regulation

Other mechanisms of passive vitamin E regulation in skin may involve epidermal renewal and differentiation processes that lead to a gradual, passive transportation of epidermal membrane bound lipids including vitamin E. This movement alone would, however, not explain the vitamin E gradients found in facial skin with high amounts of vitamin E in the upper SC layers. Actively regulated pathways of epidermal vitamin E are currently not known. Recent experiments carried out by our own group point to the existence of an alpha;-tocopherol-transfer protein (TTP), which was demonstrated to regulate vitamin E plasma levels and so far only found in few body tissues, in particular liver tissue (13). Possibly, the expression of TTP in sebocytes may be involved in the high levels of alpha;-tocopherol found in sebum. However, the existence of TTP in cutaneous tissues needs further confirmation and should therefore not yet be considered a relevant regulation mechanism in skin.

CLINICAL IMPLICATIONS

Photo-Protection

The skin is equipped with at least two photo-protective barriers: a melanin barrier in the epidermis and a protein barrier in the SC. The SC is a major optically protective element of the epidermis, reflecting approximately 5% of the incident light and absorbing significant portions of UVB radiation (280–320 nm). With respect to erythema formation, the SC thickness was shown to be a main photo-protective factor, even more relevant than pigmentation and the thickness of viable epidermis (48). Only few studies on the mechanisms of action of the photo-protective properties of the SC are currently available. Recent studies on the redox properties of the SC point to the relevance of photo-oxidative changes in the barrier and the protective action of SC antioxidants. Topically applied antioxidants provide protection against UVB-induced oxidative damage in SC lipids (49). Even some systemically applied antioxidants accumulate in the SC and play an important role against UV-induced photodamage in skin. Studies on the photoprotective mechanisms of the antioxidant butylated hydroxytoluene (BHT) suggested that changes in the physico-chemical properties of SC keratins occurred, leading to increases in UV-absorption of underlying epidermal layers. These changes were proposed to be exerted via the anti-radical action of BHT that retards oxidation and prevents crosslinking of the keratin chains, resulting in a diminution of UVB radiation reaching potential epidermal target sites (50). Similar mechanisms of action are currently discussed for other lipophilic antioxidants like tocopherols and carotenoids (12). There is growing experimental evidence that cutaneous photoprotection should involve antioxidant strategies to prevent damage to SC lipids and proteins.

Vitamin E

Vitamin E esters, particularly vitamin E acetate, succinate, and linoleate, have been suggested as promising agents in reducing UVR-induced skin damage. However, their photo-protective effects appear to be less pronounced as compared with vitamin E; moreover, some studies failed to detect photo-protection provided by vitamin E esters. Vitamin E esters need to be hydrolyzed during skin absorption to show antioxidant activity, but it seems that the bioconversion of vitamin E acetate to its active antioxidative form, α-tocopherol, is slow and occurs only at rates of less than 1%. Some evidence exists that the epidermal bioconversion of vitamin E acetate into vitamin E may be enhanced by UV-exposure, possibly by an UVB-dependent increase in esterase activity in murine epidermis (51). Recent studies indicate that vitamin E acetate is not hydrolyzed in the SC and that the bioconversion into its active form only occurs as it penetrates beyond the SC into the nucleated epidermis (52). Thus, the controversial observations on photo-protective effects of topically applied vitamin E acetate may, consequently, be explained by the limited bioavailability of the active, ester-cleaved form during oxidative stress at the site of action.

Vitamin C

A limited number of studies on humans described photo-protective effects of vitamin C after topical application. Dreher et al. investigated 5% vitamin C incorporated into an alcoholic lotion and were unable to detect any photo-protective effects when applied at a dose of $2\,mg/cm^{-2}$, 30 min before UVR irradiation in humans (53). Unlike vitamin E, vitamin C does not absorb in the UV range and thus does not have sunscreen properties. On the other hand, using a porcine skin model, it was demonstrated that topically applied vitamin C is photo-protective when formulated at high concentrations in an appropriate vehicle (54). Vitamin C is preferentially absorbed into skin at low pH (55). The rather modest photo-protective effect of topically applied vitamin C in human skin may at least in part be explained by its instability and ease of oxidation in aqueous vehicles. Vitamin C can be protected from degradation by selecting appropriate vehicles such as emulsions (56). Furthermore, lipophilic and more stable vitamin C derivatives, such as its palmityl, succinyl, or phosphoryl esters, were reported to be promising compounds providing increased photoprotection as compared with vitamin C. As described for vitamin E esters, most of these compounds must be hydrolyzed to vitamin C to be effective as antioxidants, and thus are unlikely to be active in protecting the SC.

Protein Oxidation Gradients in the Skin Barrier and Possible Implications for Desquamation

In analogy to the high degree of saturation of fatty acids in the SC, the amount of disulfide crosslinks in human SC is known to be many-fold higher than in lower epidermal layers. Similarly, we found that keratins in human SC contain dramatically more carbonyl groups than the keratins present in keratinocytes, indicating that the baseline levels of keratin oxidation are considerably higher in the SC as compared with lower epidermal layers. By using sequential tape strippings, a steep gradient with lowest levels of carbonyl groups in keratins from lower layers and highest in the upper layers was found. Importantly, this protein oxidation gradient is inversely correlated with the gradients of the antioxidant vitamin E (31), and free thiols (57) in human SC. There is in vitro and in vivo evidence from other biological systems that protein oxidation can be counteracted by antioxidants such as vitamin E and thiols. The inverse correlation with SC antioxidant levels on the one hand and the positive correlation with the levels of oxygen and oxidizing xenobiotics within the SC on the other may account for the protein oxidation gradients in SC keratins.

We proposed that the protein oxidation gradient with increased levels towards outer SC layers may have implications for the regulation of desquamation (58). As proteins in corneodesmosomes play a crucial role in SC cell cohesion, and specific proteases have been identified in human SC, proteolysis is generally believed to be a key event in desquamation. However, as the SC consists of enucleated, "dead" cells, it is still unclear, how the onset of desquamation in the upper SC is regulated (59). Many common proteases degrade oxidized proteins more rapidly than non-oxidized forms (7). Thus, in addition to regulation by other factors, the higher levels of protein oxidation detected in the upper SC may account for an increased susceptibility of keratins and other macromolecules to be degraded by SC proteases, leading to desquamation in the superficial SC layers.

While protein oxidation increases proteolytic susceptibility up to a protein-specific degree, further damage actually causes a decrease in proteolytic susceptibility and leads to crosslinking and aggregation (60). Furthermore, protein-bound carbonyl groups are believed to be involved in intra- and intermolecular crosslinking. Although it is well accepted that crosslinking of SC keratins serves to improve the physical stability of the keratin network, very few biochemical details are known (61). The introduction of carbonyl groups into SC keratins is likely to have implications for keratin crosslinking, as protein crosslinking and aggregation is not limited to disulfide crosslinking, but extend to other forms of covalent crosslinks such as the formation of an intermolecular Schiff-base by reaction of a carbonyl group from one protein with an amino group from another. Possibly, transglutaminase, which catalyzes the formation of an amide bond between the γ-carbonyl group of glutamine and the ε-amino-group of lysine and plays an important role in the formation of the cornified envelope, is involved in this dimerization. Notably, eye lens proteins were shown to be far more susceptible to transglutaminase catalyzed reactions when preincubated with reactive oxygen species (62). The activity of cysteine proteases such as the SC thiol protease (SCTP), which was recently identified as cathepsin L2, is known to be regulated by the pH and the requirement for mild reducing conditions (63,64). In view of the complexity of the epidermal antioxidant network, it is therefore possible that other antioxidants than thiols contribute to the optimal reducing conditions in the SC in vivo.

Furthermore, as indicated above, specific protein oxidation repair enymes, such as MSRA, are expressed in the epidermis and may be involved in the redox regulation of particular proteins involved in epidermal differentiation and, possibly, desquamation.

Microbial Colonization and Infection

The healthy cutaneous barrier represents an effective defense mechanism against microbial infections. Predisposing factors such as mechanical injuries, abnormal humidity, immunodeficiency, or metabolic disorders can lead to severe microbial-associated skin disorders. The mechanisms of cellular damage caused by infectious and inflammatory processes in skin are complex. There is, however, a consensus that ROS generated by phagocytes migrating to injured tissues might be the main agents responsible for cellular damage in inflammatory processes (65). Intriguingly, phagocyte-generated ROS are necessary for an efficient clearance of pathogenic microor ganisms. Recent investigations have demonstrated that oxidative stress may be caused by the microbial flora of human skin. Common cutaneous pathogens, including dermatophytes and yeasts, or bacteria of the species *Streptococcus* or *Staphylococcus*, are aerobic organisms capable of generating remarkable amounts of reactive oxygen species (66). Furthermore, there is evidence that *Candida albicans*, the most important opportunistic fungal pathogen, releases hydrogen peroxide in a similar way as phago-cytes. Interestingly, the generation of ROS by *C. albicans* increases significantly during formation of hyphae, which occurs mostly during the pathophysiologically relevant penetration of the skin barrier into deeper skin layers (67). It seems likely that this mechanism involves oxidative stress in the skin barrier.

In conclusion, ROS play a crucial role in the pathophysiology of bacterial and fungal skin infections. However, while many basic research efforts have recently focused on antimicrobial factors and innate immunity, little is known on the redox control of cutaneous microorganisms by the epidermal antioxidant barrier.

Aging

It has been suggested that the aging process is dependent on the action of free radicals (7). Several key metabolic enzymes are oxidatively inactivated by a variety of mixed function oxidation systems. Many of the enzymes which are inactivated have been shown to accumulate as inactive or less active forms during cellular aging. Stadtman and co-workers have demonstrated that the levels of oxidatively modified proteins in cultured fibroblasts from normal donors increase only after the age of 60 (9). However, the levels of oxidatively modified proteins in fibroblasts from individuals with progeria or Werner's syndrome were significantly higher than age-matched controls. Moreover, treatment of glucose-6-phosphate dehydrogenase with a mixed function oxidation system was shown to lead to oxidative modification and increased heat lability of the enzyme. Taken together, these results suggest that loss of functional enzyme activity and increased heat lability of enzymes during aging may be due in part to oxi-dative modification by mixed function oxidation systems. Another recent study by Merker et al. demonstrated that old fibroblasts are much more vulnerable to the accu-mulation of oxidized proteins after oxidative stress and are not able to remove these oxidized proteins as efficiently as young fibroblasts (68).

There is the recent in vivo evidence that photoaging and solar elastosis corre-late well with different markers of oxidative stress including the accumulation of lipid peroxidation and glycation products (69,70), as well as protein oxidation (71). To investigate whether UV exposure is indeed capable of inducing protein oxidation in vivo, a human subject study mimicking extensive solar holiday exposure was performed (18). A significant increase of oxidatively modified proteins was observed within the papillary dermis as well as in the outermost layers of the SC, the latter confirming earlier reported findings obtained by the use of a different meth-odology (58). Nucleated epidermal layers were less affected by protein oxidation than dermal and SC layers, which is probably due to the far greater antioxidant capacity of the epidermis, including the expression of MSRA. In chronically UV-exposed human skin revealing typical features of photoaging, a significantly depleted expression of antioxidant enzymes (catalase, copper-zinc superoxide dismutase, and manganese superoxide dismutase) was found in SC, while dermal levels were not sig-nificantly reduced. These results indicate that oxidative stress is likely to be involved in the perturbation of the skin barrier following acute, and, possibly also, chronic UV exposures leading to photoaging.

Synopsis

Many clinical studies have reported beneficial effects obtained by the use of a variety of topical antioxidants. However, the underlying mechanisms are still not well described. To optimize the effects of *exogenously or systemically applied* antioxidants, it is important to better understand the *physiological* mechanisms that regulate the distribution and interplay of redox systems comprising the epidermal antioxidant barrier.

Our studies have demonstrated that α-tocopherol is, relative to the respective levels in the epidermis, the major antioxidant in the human SC, that α-tocopherol depletion is a very early and sensitive biomarker of environmentally induced oxidation, and that a physiologic mechanism exists to transport α-tocopherol to the skin surface via sebaceous gland secretion. With respect to interceptive antioxidant enzymes, catalase displays a remarkably high expression and activity in human SC. In contrast, the antioxidative repair enzyme MSRA is highly expressed in viable human epidermis, but not yet well investigated in human SC. While α-tocopherol depletion is a highly sensitive, but rather unspecific oxidative stress marker in the SC, the formation of the squalene oxidation product SqmOOH appears to be highly specific for photo-oxidative stress. In contrast, the introduction of carbonyl groups into human SC keratins is a less sensitive oxidative stress marker in the skin barrier, possibly because of the very high background levels predominantly found in the outer layers of human SC. Systematic analysis of antioxidants as well as of specific lipid- and protein-oxidation products in different layers of murine and human SC has led to the addition to the family gradients described in the skin barrier: the SC *redox gradient*. Specific redox gradients within the human SC may contribute to a better understanding of the complex biochemical processes of keratinization and desquamation. Taken together, the presented data suggest that, under conditions of environmentally challenged skin or during pro-oxidative dermatologic treatment, topical and/or systemical application of antioxidants could support physiologic mechanisms to maintain or restore a healthy skin barrier. Growing experimental evidence, rather than marketing-driven antioxidant strategies, may lead to the development of more powerful pharmaceutical and/or cosmetic formulations to protect cutaneous photodamage as well as to maintain or restore a healthy skin barrier function.

ACKNOWLEDGMENTS

This chapter is dedicated to my great scientific mentor, Lester Packer.

REFERENCES

1. Thiele JJ, Podda M, Packer L. Tropospheric ozone: an emerging environmental stress to skin. Biol Chem 1997; 378:1299–1305.
2. Cross CE, van der Vliet A, Louie S, et al. Oxidative stress and antioxidants at biosurfaces: plants, skin and respiratory tract surfaces. Environ Health Perspect 1998; 106: 1241–1251.
3. Thiele JJ. Oxidative targets in the stratum corneum: a new basis for antioxidative strategies. Skin Pharmacol Appl Skin Physiol 2001; 14(suppl 1):87–91.
4. Thiele JJ, Schroeter C, Hsieh SN, et al. The antioxidant network of the stratum corneum. Curr Probl Dermatol 2001; 29:26–42.
5. Rawlings AV, Scott IR, Harding CR, et al. Stratum corneum moisturization at the molecular level. J Invest Dermatol 1994; 103:731–740.

6. Elias PM. Epidermal lipids, barrier function, and desquamation. J Invest Dermatol 1983; 80:44–49.
7. Stadtman ER. Protein oxidation and aging. Science 1992; 257:1220–1224.
8. Berlett BS, Stadtman ER. Protein oxidation in aging, disease, and oxidative stress. J Biol Chem 1997; 272:20313–20316.
9. Oliver CN, Ahn B-W, Moerman EJ, et al. Age-related changes in oxidized proteins. J Biol Chem 1987; 262:5488.
10. Stadtman ER. Protein oxidation in aging and age-related diseases. Ann NY Acad Sci 2001; 928:22–38.
11. Cross CE, van der Vliet A, Louie S, et al. Oxidative stress and antioxidants at bio-surfaces: plants, skin, and respiratory tract surfaces. Environ Health Perspect 1998; 106(suppl 5):1241–1251.
12. Thiele JJ, Dreher F, Packer L. Antioxidant defense systems in skin. In: Elsner P, Maibach H, eds. Drugs vs Cosmetics: Cosmeceuticals? New York: Marcel Dekker, 2000:145–188.
13. Traber MG, Sies H. Vitamin E in humans—demand and delivery. Ann Rev Nutr 1996; 16:321–347.
14. Shindo Y, Witt E, Han D, et al. Enzymic and non-enzymic antioxidants in epidermis and dermis of human skin. J Invest Dermatol 1994; 102:122–124.
15. Bommannan D, Potts RO, Guy RH. Examination of stratum corneum barrier function in vivo by infrared spectroscopy. J Invest Dermatol 1990; 95:403–408.
16. Thiele JJ, Rallis M, Izquierdo-Pullido M, et al. Benzoyl peroxide depletes human stratum corneum antioxidants. J Invest Dermatol 1998; 110:675A.
17. Weber SU, Thiele JJ, Cross CE, et al. Vitamin C, uric acid and glutathione gradients in murine stratum corneum and their susceptibility to ozone exposure. J Invest Dermatol 1999; 113:1128–1132.
18. Sander CS, Chang H, Salzmann S, et al. Photoaging is associated with protein oxidation in human skin in vivo. J Invest Dermatol 2002; 118:618–625.
19. Hellemans L, Corstjens H, Neven A, et al. Antioxidant enzyme activity in human stratum corneum shows seasonal variation with an age-dependent recovery. J Invest Dermatol 2003; 120:434–439.
20. Guarrera M, Ferrari P, Rebora A. Catalase in the stratum corneum of patients with polymorphic light eruption. Acta Derm Venereol 1998; 78:335–336.
21. Fesq H, Ring J, Abeck D. Management of polymorphous light eruption: clinical course, pathogenesis, diagnosis and intervention. Am J Clin Dermatol 2003; 4:399–406.
22. Moskovitz J, Bar-Noy S, Williams WM, et al. Methionine sulfoxide reductase (MSRA) is a regulator of antioxidant defense and lifespan in mammals. Proc Natl Acad Sci USA 2001; 98:12920–12925.
23. Sander CS, Hansel A, Heinemann SH, et al. In vivo evidence for a link between photoaging and oxidative stress in human skin. J Invest Dermatol 2002; 119:331A.
24. Schallreuter KU, Wood JM. Thioredoxin reductase—its role in epidermal redox status. J Photochem Photobiol B 2001; 64:179–184.
25. Thiele JJ, Traber MG, Tsang KG, et al. In vivo exposure to ozone depletes vitamins C and E and induces lipid peroxidation in epidermal layers of murine skin. Free Radic Biol Med 1997; 23:385–391.
26. Thiele JJ, Traber MG, Podda M, et al. Ozone depletes tocopherols and tocotrienols topically applied to murine skin. FEBS Lett 1997; 401:167–170.
27. Thiele JJ, Traber MG, Polefka TG, et al. Ozone exposure depletes vitamin E and induces lipid peroxidation in murine stratum corneum. J Invest Dermatol 1997; 108:753–757.
28. Thiele JJ, Dreher F, Maibach HI, et al. Impact of ultraviolet radiation and ozone on the transepidermal water loss as a function of skin temperature in hairless mice. Skin Pharmacol Appl Skin Physiol 2003; 16:283–290.

29. Haratake A, Uchida Y, Mimura K, et al. Intrinsically aged epidermis displays diminished UVB-induced alterations in barrier function associated with decreased proliferation. J Invest Dermatol 1997; 108:319–323.
30. Kitazawa M, Podda M, Thiele JJ, et al. Interactions between vitamin E homologues and ascorbate free radicals in murine skin homogenates irradiated with ultraviolet light. Photochem Photobiol 1997; 355–365.
31. Thiele JJ, Traber MG, Packer L. Depletion of human stratum corneum vitamin E: an early and sensitive in vivo marker of UV-induced photooxidation. J Invest Dermatol 1998; 110:756–761.
32. Shindo Y, Witt E, Han D, et al. Dose-response effects of acute ultraviolet irradiation on antioxidants and molecular markers of oxidation in murine epidermis and dermis. J Invest Dermatol 1994; 102:470–475.
33. Shindo Y, Witt E, Packer L. Antioxidant defense mechanisms in murine epidermis and dermis and their responses to ultraviolet light. J Invest Dermatol 1993; 100:260–265.
34. Weber C, Podda M, Rallis M, et al. Efficacy of topically applied tocopherols and tocotrienols in protection of murine skin from oxidative damage induced by UV-irradiation. Free Radic Biol Med 1997; 22:761–769.
35. Stoyanovsky DA, Osipov AN, Quinn PJ, et al. Ubiquinone-dependent recycling of vitamin E radicals by superoxide. Arch Biochem Biophys 1995; 323:343–351.
36. Evelson P, Ordóñez CP, Llesuy S, et al. Oxidative stress and in vivo chemiluminescence in mouse skin exposed to UVA radiation. J Photochem Photobiol B Biol 1997; 38:215–219.
37. Wertz. 1991; 722.
38. Ohsawa. 1984; 2158.
39. Saint-Leger. 1986; 3939.
40. Dennis. 1989; 2862.
41. Kohno. 1995; 3397.
42. Ekanayake Mudiyanselage S, Hamburger M, Elsner P, et al. Ultraviolet a induces generation of squalene monohydroperoxide isomers in human sebum and skin surface lipids in vitro and in vivo. J Invest Dermatol 2003; 120:915–922.
43. Diffey B. Sources and measurement of ultraviolet radiation. Methods 2002; 28:4.
44. Kohno Y, Egawa Y, Itoh S, et al. Kinetic study of quenching reaction of singlet oxygen and scavenging reaction of free radical by squalene in n-butanol. Biochim Biophys Acta 1995; 1256:52–56.
45. Saint-Leger D, Bague A, Lefebvre E, et al. A possible role for squalene in the pathogenesis of acne. II. In vivo study of squalene oxides in skin surface and intra-comedonal lipids of acne patients. Br J Dermatol 1986; 114(5):543–552.
46. Spikes JD. Porphyrins and related compounds as photodynamic sensitizers. Ann NY Acad Sci 1975; 244:496–508.
47. Picardo M, Zompetta C, De Luca C, et al. Role of skin surface lipids in UV-induced epidermal cell changes. Arch Dermatol Res 1991; 283:191–197.
48. Chiba K, Yoshizawa K, Makino I, et al. Comedogenicity of squalene monohydroperoxide in the skin after topical application. J Toxicol Sci 2000; 25(2):77–83.
49. Thiele JJ, Weber SU, Packer L. Sebaceous gland secretion is a major physiological route of vitamin E delivery to skin. J Invest Dermatol 1999; 113:1006–1010.
50. Lang JK, Gohil K, Packer L. Simultaneous determination of tocopherols, ubiquinols, and ubiquinones in blood, plasma, tissue homogenates, and subcellular fractions. Anal Biochem 1986; 157:106–116.
51. Blanc D, Saint-Leger D, Brandt J. An original procedure for quantification of cutaneous resorption of sebum. Arch Dermatol Res 1989; 281:346–350.
52. Ekanayake Mudiyanselage S, Kraemer K, Thiele JJ. Dietary supplementation with 400 mg vitamin E: Delayed bioavailability in human skin and preferential accumulation of α-tocopherol in human sebum. In, Vol. Providence, RI: J Invest Dermatol, 2004. In press.

53. Gniadecka M, Wulf HC, Mortensen NN, et al. Photoprotection in vitiligo and normal skin. A quantititative assessment of the role of stratum corneum, viable epidermis and pigmentation. Acta Derm Venereol 1996; 76:429–432.

54. Pelle E, Muizzuddin N, Mammone T, et al. Protection against endogenous and UVB-induced oxidative damage in stratum corneum lipids by an antioxidant-containing cosmetic formulation. Photodermatol Photoimmunol Photomed 1999; 15:115–119.

55. Black HS, Mathews-Roth MM. Protective role of butylated hydroxytoluene and certain carotenoids in photocarcinogenesis. Photochem Photobiol 1991; 53:707–716.

56. Kramer-Stickland K, Liebler DC. Effect of UVB on hydrolysis of alpha-tocopherol acetate to alpha-tocopherol in mouse skin. J Invest Dermatol 1998; 111:302–307.

57. Baschong W, Artmann C, Hueglin D, et al. Direct evidence for bioconversion of vitamin E acetate into vitamin E: an ex vivo study in viable human skin. J Cosmet Sci 2001; 52:155–161.

58. Dreher F, Gabard B, Schwindt DA, et al. Topical melatonin in combination with vitamins E and C protects skin from ultraviolet-induced erythema: a human study in vivo. Br J Dermatol 1998; 139:332–339.

59. Darr D, Combs S, Dunston S, et al. Topical vitamin C protects porcine skin from ultraviolet radiation-induced damage. Br J Dermatol 1992; 127:247–253.

60. Pinnell SR, Yang H, Omar M, et al. Topical L-ascorbic acid: percutaneous absorption studies. Dermatol Surg 2001; 27:137–142.

61. Gallarate M, Carlotti ME, Trotta M, et al. On the stability of ascorbic acid in emulsified systems for topical and cosmetic use. Int J Pharm 1999; 188:233–241.

62. Broekaert D, Cooreman K, Coucke P, et al. A quantitative histochemical study of sulphydryl and disulphide content during normal epidermal keratinization. Histochem J 1982; 14:573–584.

63. Thiele JJ, Hsieh SN, Briviba K, et al. Protein oxidation in human stratum corneum: susceptibility of keratins to oxidation in vitro and presence of a keratin oxidation gradient in vivo. J Invest Dermatol 1999; 113:335–339.

64. Egelrud T, Lundstroem A, Sondell B. Stratum corneum cell cohesion and desquamation in maintenance of the skin barrier. In: Marzulli FN, Maibach HI, eds. Dermatotoxicology. Washington: Taylor & Francis, 1996:19–27.

65. Grune T, Reinheckel T, Davies KJ. Degradation of oxidized proteins in mammalian cells. FASEB J 1997; 11:526–534.

66. Pang Y-YS, Schermer A, Yu J, et al. Suprabasal change and subsequent formation of disulfide-stabilized homo- and heterodimers of keratins during esophageal epithelial differentiation. J Cell Sci 1993; 104:727–740.

67. Brossa O, Seccia M, Gravela E. Increased susceptibility to transglutaminase of eye lens proteins exposed to activated oxygen species produced in the glucose-glucose oxidase reaction. Free Radic Res Commun 1990; 11:223–229.

68. Watkinson A. Stratum corneum thiol protease (SCTP): a novel cysteine protease of late epidermal differentiation. Arch Dermatol Res 1999; 291:260–268.

69. Bernard D, Mehul B, Thomas-Collignon A, et al. Analysis of proteins with caseinolytic activity in a human stratum corneum extract revealed a yet unidentified cysteine protease and identified the so-called "stratum corneum thiol protease" as cathepsin l2. J Invest Dermatol 2003; 120:592–600.

70. Ginsburg I. Could synergistic interactions among reactive oxygen species, proteinases, membrane-perforating enzymes, hydrolases, microbial hemolysins and cytokines be the main cause of tissue damage in infectious and inflammatory conditions? Med Hypotheses 1998; 51:337–346.

71. Miller RA, Britigan BE. Role of oxidants in microbial pathophysiology. Clin Microbiol Rev 1997; 10:1–18.

72. Schroeter C, Hipler UC, Wilmer A, et al. Generation of reactive oxygen species by Candida albicans in relation to morphogenesis. Arch Dermatol Res 2000; 292:260–264.

73. Merker K, Sitte N, Grune T. Hydrogen peroxide-mediated protein oxidation in young and old human MRC-5 fibroblasts. Arch Biochem Biophys 2000; 375:50–54.

74. Jeanmaire C, Danoux L, Pauly G. Glycation during human dermal intrinsic and actinic ageing: an in vivo and in vitro model study. Br J Dermatol 2001; 145:10–18.
75. Tanaka N, Tajima S, Ishibashi A, et al. Immunohistochemical detection of lipid peroxidation products, protein-bound acrolein and 4-hydroxynonenal protein adducts, in actinic elastosis of photodamaged skin. Arch Dermatol Res 2001; 293:363–367.
76. Sander CS, Chang H, Salzmann S, et al. Photoaging is associated with protein oxidation in human skin in vivo. J Invest Dermatol 2002; 118:618–625.
77. Fuchs J, Huflejt ME, Rothfuss LM, et al. Impairment of enzymic and nonenzymic antioxidants in skin by UVB irradiation. J Invest Dermatol 1989; 93:769–773.
78. Fuchs J, Huflejt ME, Rothfuss LM, et al. Acute effects of near ultraviolet and visible light on the cutaneous antioxidant defense system. Photochem Photobiol 1989; 50: 739–744.
79. Salomon L, Stubbs DW. Some aspects of the metabolism of ascorbic acid in rats. Ann NY Acad Sci 1961; 92:128–140.
80. Stüttgen G, Schaefer E. Vitamine und Haut. In: Stüttgen G, Schaefer E, eds. Funktionelle Dermatologie. Berlin: Springer, 1974:78–79.
81. Halprin K, Ohkawara A. The measurement of glutathione in human epidermis using glutathione reductase. J Invest Dermatol 1967; 48:149–152.
82. Benedetto JP, Ortonne JP, Voulot C, et al. Role of thiol compounds in mammalian melanin pigmentation. J Invest Dermatol 1981; 77:402–405.
83. Wheeler LA, Aswad A, Connor MJ, et al. Depletion of cutaneous glutathione and the induction of inflammation by 8-methoxypsoralen plus UVA radiation. J Invest Dermatol 1986; 87:658–662.
84. Connor MJ, Wheeler LA. Depletion of cutaneous glutathione by ultraviolet radiation. Photochem Photobiol 1987; 47:239–245.

24

Sources and Role of Stratum Corneum Hydration

A. V. Rawlings
AVR Consulting Ltd, Northwich, Cheshire, U.K.

INTRODUCTION

Water is essential for life. All living cells require water to function but equally some "dead" cells also require water to be metabolically active. For humans to survive, the loss of water from the skin must be carefully regulated. This function of the epidermis is highly dependent on its sophisticated outer layer: the stratum corneum SC (1). However, this tissue must also retain sufficient water to allow it to function in arid and desiccating environments. Under normal circumstances this complex tissue must be as impermeable as possible except for a small amount of water loss to hydrate the outer layers of the stratum corneum to maintain its flexibility and to provide enough water to allow enzyme reactions that facilitate stratum corneum maturation events together with corneodesmolysis and ultimately desquamation (2–4). The water-retaining capacity of the stratum corneum is highly dependent upon the thickness of the SC, the precise phenotypes of the corneocytes and their organization, the precise composition and physical packing state of barrier lipids, and finally the presence of highly hygroscopic compounds largely found within the corneocytes (Fig. 1).

The primary function of the skin's barrier is to prevent water loss. However, hydration of the corneocytes is essential for SC function. Water acts as a plasticizer on corneocyte proteins giving elastic properties to the cells (1). If deprived of water dry skin is prone to crack open on mechanical stress. Since atmospheric conditions vary enormously, the corneocytes are hydrated from bodily water lost through the barrier. This imperfect barrier and inbuilt water loss is highly important for tissue functioning and flexibility, and certain metabolic processes.

Corneocytes have been described as very flat cells about 30 μm in diameter and 0.3 μm thick, filled with a fibrous keratin network located inside a protein envelope. Each corneocyte is derived from 1 of 20 basal keratinocytes. The keratin fibers span the interior of the corneocyte constituting an internal reinforced network ensuring that the cell in the plane of the skin remains virtually unchanged upon mechanical stress. In the vertical direction it is thought that there are less reinforcement fibrils and so the cells have a greater freedom to distend in this direction (5). As will be

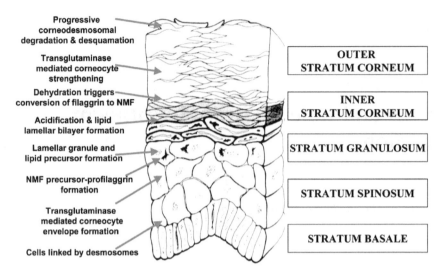

Progressive corneodesmosomal degradation & desquamation

Transglutaminase mediated corneocyte strengthening

Dehydration triggers conversion of filaggrin to NMF

Acidification & lipid lamellar bilayer formation

Lamellar granule and lipid precursor formation

NMF precursor-profilaggrin formation

Transglutaminase mediated corneocyte envelope formation

Cells linked by desmosomes

OUTER STRATUM CORNEUM

INNER STRATUM CORNEUM

STRATUM GRANULOSUM

STRATUM SPINOSUM

STRATUM BASALE

Figure 1 Typical structure of the epidermis and critical steps in formation of the stratum corneum. *Source*: Modified from Ref. 2.

discussed, however, the corneocyte swelling characteristics and the cellular reinforcement mechanisms are more complex than this.

The corneocytes contain a 15 μm thick layer of protein called the corneocyte envelope. This is highly insoluble due to extensive cross-linking of intermolecular disulphide bonds and gamma-glutamyl-lysine isopeptide bonds formed by the action of transglutaminases. Loricrin is the most abundant protein but involucrin is made hydrophobic by the transglutaminase-mediated esterification with ceramide and fatty acids. This forms a template to which the extracellular lipids, derived from precursor lipids secreted in the lamellar granules, form the primary barrier in the SC. Other proteins also exist and the small proline-rich proteins, in particular, influence the mechanical properties of the corneocyte envelope (6).

Corneocytes also contain hygroscopic compounds called natural moisturizing factors (NMFs). These are essential for maintaining tissue flexibility and, together with the extracellular lipids, tissue hydration (2).

Corneodesmosomes act as intercellular rivets effectively hindering the spatial movement of the corneocytes. In most circumstances these prevent shearing forces from disrupting the intercellular lipid matrix and thereby help to maintain SC barrier function and hydration (7).

Numerous techniques have been used to quantify the water content or hydration of the SC. However, as most of these methods are averaging techniques or also measure water found in the deeper layers of the skin, this review will be restricted to the more recent methods developed over the last decade to measure water gradients within the SC itself. In this respect new electron microscopic techniques have provided important ultrastructural information of the epidermis (8–11). However, these techniques have also shown that the SC is more homogeneous than originally thought. The whole of the SC appears to be compact and the intercellular spaces very narrow compared with the electron microscopic images of SC prepared by chemical fixation and dehydration. For instance the separation of the stratum compactum (the inner layers of the SC) and the stratum granulosum (the outer layers of the SC) appears to be artifactual and the stratum granulosum appears to contain fewer granules than originally perceived. Keratohyalin granules, the structures that contain the precursor protein to NMFs, are also not observed using these methods (10). Nevertheless, these methods have also been used to visualize corneocyte swelling and quantify SC water content ex vivo. New confocal methodologies have also been developed to quantify SC water gradients in vivo (12).

STRATUM CORNEUM HYDRATION AND WATER CONTENT

The importance of hydration for the SC and its functioning became apparent from studies in the 1950s. Gaul and Underwood (13) reported that skin chapping (flaking and irritation) occurred on days of low atmospheric dew points. As will be discussed later a factor that is equally important, however, is that each chapping event was initially preceded by high dew points and low barometric pressures, i.e., fluctuating atmospheric weather conditions were making the skin more susceptible to generating a dry and flaky phenotype.

At about the same time Blank (14) demonstrated that the lowered water content of the SC was probably the prime factor in causing the condition we commonly call "dry skin." In vitro, applications of oils did not influence SC softness and flexibility whereas water did. Although correct in principle, these early experiments were flawed as TEWL through the hydrated SC was not simulated where actually occlusive oils would have reduced TEWL and hydrated the SC by reducing water flux. Nevertheless, Blank was correct that water is the physiological plasticizer of the stratum corneum.

The state of SC hydration, however, depends on:

- the rate at which water reaches the SC from the tissue below,
- the rate at which water leaves the skin surface by evaporation,
- the ability of the SC to retain water.

Naturally, as water is being constantly lost from the skin surface, water gradients are established within the different layers of the SC. However, early experiments could only measure the mean averages of the different types of water found in the SC. From infrared spectroscopic measurements, three different classes of water were determined in the SC. At less than 10% w/w hydration, water is tightly bound to SC protein and was called primary bound water. At 10–40% w/w hydration, the additional water was less tightly bound, being bound probably to corneocyte osmolytes and the primary bound water. At 50% w/w hydration, the water found in the SC behaved like bulk liquid water (15). NMR studies (16) have also indicated that there is a single major pool of water which resides within a relatively homogeneous and large compartment of the SC, presumably within the corneocyte themselves. Based on NMR relaxation times it was also concluded that the water within the corneocyte interacts strongly with keratin.

Clearly, we need a greater understanding of the relative proportions of water within the SC to understand better its effect on SC functioning. Relative water gradients within the SC as a function of tape strip number were determined by Bommannan et al. (17) using FTIR. As expected, on removal of the SC, increased water levels were observed. However, this invasive method also increases TEWL as the different layers of the SC are removed. The increased TEWL can then also contribute to the apparent increased hydration as a new layer is exposed (Fig. 2).

It was not until the elegant work of Ronald Warner and his team at Procter & Gamble (8) that the first studies in truly measuring SC cellular water concentration

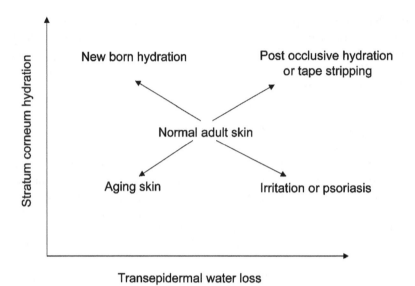

Figure 2 A simplified relationship between TEWL and skin hydration. *Source*: Modified from Loden M. The skin barrier and use of moisturizers in atopic dermatitis. Clin Dermatology 2003; 21:145–157.

gradients were conducted on human skin ex vivo using electron probe analysis. Even though the methodology could be criticized, as it still measures water content on ex vivo samples, it was pioneering at that time. A typical water concentration profile can be seen in Figure 3. The primary feature of the water gradient is the large discontinuity in the water content at the SC-granular interface. This gradient only starts after the last granular keratinocyte and this discontinuity accounts for approximately 50% of the water gradient across the skin. In these studies the shape of the concentration gradient within the SC appears to have a slight S-shape.

The variation in water content across the SC itself was found to be relatively small from 15% at the skin surface to 40% at the innermost layer compared with 80% within the granular layer, indicating that there is a significant barrier to water loss at the SC-granular interface. These data suggest that a barrier to water loss begins prior to the formation of the SC and is present within the granular layer. This may be a function of the tight junctions that have recently been demonstrated in the granular layer (18). Nevertheless, the SC takes up the role of reducing water flux from the skin as the granular cells are finally transformed into corneocytes.

In a further evolution of their method water content measurements were correlated with ultrastructural location and quantified using digitally acquired scanning transmission electron microscope images (STEM) (19). Figure 4 shows the STEM images of human skin with the pixels transformed into water content values; i.e., a quantitative water map. The discontinuity in cellular water content in the different regions of the SC is clearly visible.

The relative water binding capacities of individual corneocytes were also measured in porcine epidermis equilibrated at 97%RH (19). One can observe slightly thicker corneocytes in the suprabasal layers of the SC compared with the innermost corneocytes (Fig. 5). The suprabasal regions contain ~60% water compared with 53% for the remainder of the SC. The source of this cellular swelling

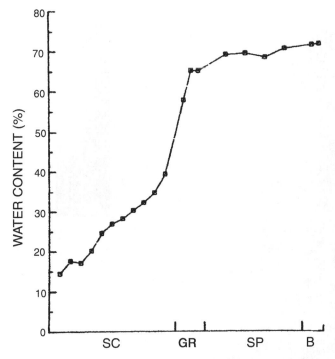

Figure 3 Water profile across human skin. The horizontal axis indicates the position within the tissue measured from the outer SC cell. *Abbreviations*: SC, stratum corneum; GR, stratum granulosum; SP, stratum spinosum; B, stratum basal. The widths of these morphological regions are not drawn to scale. *Source*: Modified from Ref. 8.

and increased water content must be related to a higher water binding capacity within these cells.

The water discontinuity within the different cellular compartments of human SC ex vivo was further elaborated using cryoelectron microscopy by Warner et al. (20) and also by Joke Bouwstra and her team of scientists from Leiden and Wageningen Universities, together with Johann Wiechers at Uniqema (9). This newer methodology has an advantage over the previous method in that water profiles can also be imaged in the intercellular spaces. Bouwstra et al. (9) demonstrated that at levels where only bound water is present (18–26% w/w) the corneocytes do not appear to swell but at 57–87% w/w the corneocytes were observed to be more swollen in the central portions of the SC compared with the superficial and deeper layers. When cell swelling was apparent, however, this was largely perpendicular to the skin surface (Fig. 6). Only at hydration levels of >300% w/w (9) or after occlusion (20) were extracellular pools of water observed. The minimal effect of hydration on the orthrorhombic-hexagonal lipid phase transitions indicate that under normal circumstances only a very small amount of water must be present in the intercellular lipid lamellae.

The results on the swelling characteristics of the SC concur with that of Norlen et al. (21) who used confocal laser scanning microscopy and observed a 26% increase in SC thickness upon tissue hydration. Richter et al. (22) also reported a 50% increase in the height and volume of isolated corneocytes with no such increases in the lateral dimensions and surface area. The unique arrangement of keratin fibers

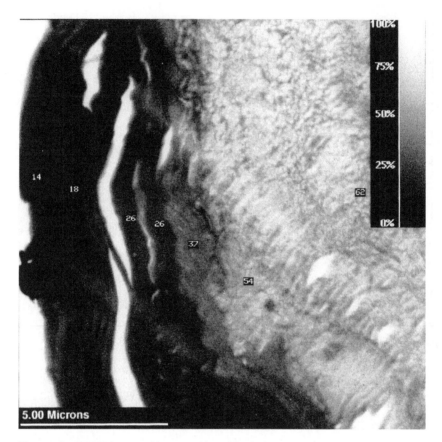

Figure 4 STEM image of human skin with pixels transformed to water content values. The grayscale, now in % water, is fixed and displayed in the upper right corner. Averaged values for water content from selected regions are superimposed on this image to provide a quantitative assessment of the water gradient across this tissue. *Source*: Modified from Ref. 19.

within the corneocytes oriented in the plane of the skin is believed to cause the reduced ability of the corneocytes for lateral expansion. Such reinforcing fibers are less in the vertical dimension and it has been argued that swelling in this direction might only be limited by the elasticity of the corneocyte envelope. However, as will be discussed later the biomechanics of the corneocytes are more heterogeneous than this simplistic view.

Recently, these ex vivo findings on SC water gradients have been proven non-invasively in vivo using the highly sophisticated but very elegant method of in vivo confocal Raman microspectroscopy. Caspers et al. (12) established that the natural hydration levels in the SC are between 15% and 45%. Typical in vivo water concentration profiles for non-palmoplantar and palmoplantar SC, respectively, can be seen in Figure 7. Currently, the spatial resolution (5 μm) is insufficient to measure individual corneocyte water contents but this method represents a tremendous advance for in vivo measurements.

Clearly, the SC has to retain a certain quantity of water in the tissue to function, and at the ultrastructural level different cellular compartments appear to bind differing quantities of water. So how do the individual cellular layers of the SC bind water differently?

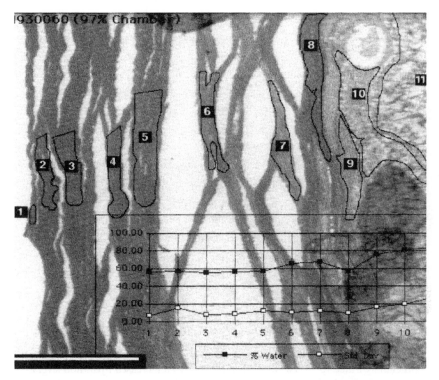

Figure 5 Image of water content from porcine epidermis equilibrated at 97% relative humidity. Water content was averaged within discrete regions identified by the drawn outlines across this image and the water values superimposed as a graph over the lower half of the image. *Source*: Modified from Ref. 19.

STRATUM CORNEUM WATER RETENTION CAPACITY

The capability of the SC to reduce bodily water loss and retain water within the corneocytes is due to its total composition and architecture. The precise phenotype of the corneocytes, their hydrophobicity, their volume, and their organization can influence water flux in the tissue. For example, for the same volume of SC, the diffusion path length of water diffusing through the SC lipids will be less if the corneocytes are smaller. However, within the deeper layers of the SC, corneodesmosomes tightly link together adjacent corneocytes all over the corneocyte surfaces, whereas in the higher levels of the tissue, corneodesmosomes only link corneocytes at the peripheral edges of the cells (23). This could be one of the reasons why corneocytes swell largely perpendicularly to the skin surface when the non-peripheral corneodesmosomes are degraded in the upper layers of the SC while the innermost corneocyte layer does not swell where the highest numbers of corneodesmosomes are found. Although the corneocytes may be more constrained in the lower layers of the SC, thereby potentially reducing any swelling behavior, this mechanism does not account for the lack of corneocyte swelling in the outermost SC layers.

Corneocytes also contain a covalently bound lipid layer which mixes with the extracellular lipid matrix between individual corneocytes and it is these lipid-enriched extracellular spaces of the stratum corneum that constitute the most important component of the barrier to water loss. The absolute concentration of the lipids,

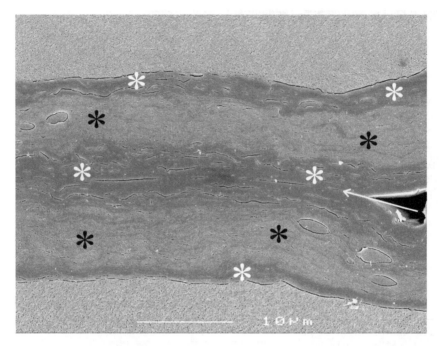

Figure 6 High magnification cryo-scanning electron microscopy images of two sheets of stratum corneum hydrated to 90% w/w. Both sheets show an increased hydration level in their central regions and a low hydration in the superficial and lowest part of the stratum corneum. *Source*: Modified from Ref. 9.

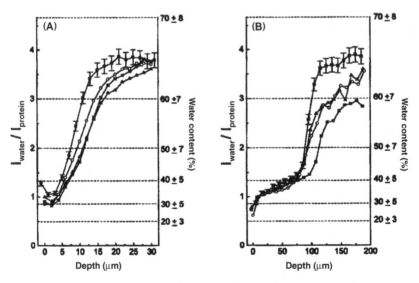

Figure 7 In vivo water concentration profiles of the SC. (A) Four water concentration profiles calculated from Raman measurements on the volar aspect of the forearm. (B) Four water concentration profiles based on Raman measurements on thenar. The left-hand coordinate is the ratio between the Raman signal intensities of water and protein. The right-hand ordinate represents the absolute water content. *Source*: Modified from Ref. 12.

the relative proportions of the different lipid species (ceramides, cholesterol, cholesterol sulfate, and fatty acids) and the physical organization of the lamellar lipid matrix is critical for the barrier function of the skin. The ceramides are a unique class of lipids and at least 10 different classes of ceramides have been described to date. The ceramides together with the other stratum corneum lipids form a solid, crystalline phase called an orthorhombic packing state which is the most tightly packed lipid state to provide optimal barrier function (23). However, just slowing down the rate of water lost through the tissue will not account for the apparent discontinuity in hydration between different corneocyte layers.

Selective retention of water in the different SC cellular layers is required to explain the apparent discontinuity in corneocyte swelling, which was highlighted by the works of Warner and Bouwstra and their respective teams (9,19,20). This function of the SC is believed to be largely dependent on the presence of SC osmolytes called the stratum corneum NMF.

Stratum corneum NMF is composed primarily of amino acids or their derivatives such as pyrrolidone carboxylic acid (PCA) and urocanic acid (UCA), together with lactic acid, urea, citrate, and sugars (24, Table 1). These compounds are present at high concentrations mostly within the corneocytes and may represent up to 20–30% of the dry weight of the SC (25). However, a fraction of the "NMF" is also probably extracellular to the corneocytes, e.g., the sugar fraction of NMF is probably derived from the processing of glucosylceramides whereas lactate and urea will be largely derived from sweat as described above. The intracellular and extracellular components of NMF may have different functions but the most advanced techniques available to date cannot image intercellular water pools in the SC except at very high hydration levels or after complete skin occlusion.

NMF is intensely hygroscopic and it is through this that corneocytes retain water intracellularly. Thus, corneocytes that retain more water and appear more swollen ultrastructurally also possess the highest concentration of these factors (9,19). Through cellular hygroscopicity, the outermost layers of the SC remain hydrated enough to function despite the desiccating action of the environment. However, NMF is much more important than this. By maintaining secondary bound water in the SC, the NMF also probably facilitates enzymic processing events. The coordinated activity of proteases, deglycosidases, and transglutaminases are essential for the maturation and optimum functioning of the SC (23). However

Table 1 The Chemical Composition of NMF

Free amino acids	40%
Pyrrolidone carboxylic acid	12%
Lactate	12%
Sugars	8.5%
Urea	7.0%
Chloride	6.0%
Sodium	5.0%
Potassium	4.0%
Ammonia, uric acid, glucosamine, and creatine	1.5%
Calcium	1.5%
Magnesium	1.5%
Phosphate	0.5%
Citrate, formate	0.5%

one of the most important events in SC maturation is the regulation of a number of proteases within the corneocytes which are responsible ultimately for the generation of the intracellular NMF itself.

The amino acids and their derivatives within the SC, which together represent over 50% of the NMF, are derived from a protein precursor system: the profilaggrin–filaggrin protein system (26–31, Fig. 8). Although the presence of keratohyalin granules in the stratum granulosum is now conjectural, following the study of the epidermis by using cryoelectron microscopy methods, profilaggrin is first expressed in the granular layer as a highly phosphorylated protein consisting of multiple filaggrin repeats joined by short hydrophobic linker peptides. As the corneocyte is formed from a granular cell, profilaggrin is rapidly dephosphorylated to form filaggrin which itself can be proteolyzed to NMF within the corneocytes themselves. The proteases involved are not completely known and the control mechanism for degrading filaggrin also is not completely understood. Nevertheless, the signal for proteolysis was found to be precise water activity within the SC itself (31). In normal adult skin filaggrin is only detected in the innermost layers of the SC whereas in newborn and fetal tissue there is no indication of any proteolytic breakdown of filaggrin even in the outer regions of the SC. However, within a few hours after birth, the breakdown of filaggrin is initiated in the outer regions of the tissue. This proteolysis of filaggrin could be prevented in a very humid environment, which indicated the possibility that the water activity of the SC was a critical factor in triggering these events. Subsequent studies on filaggrin breakdown in isolated SC revealed that hydrolysis occurred only if the SC was maintained within a certain RH range (80–95%) and total occlusion blocked proteolysis (31).

Thus, NMF is not produced in the lower layers of the SC and this together with the greater number of corneodesmosomes in this area of the tissue are probably the prime reasons for the lack of swelling of this cellular layer. When NMF is produced

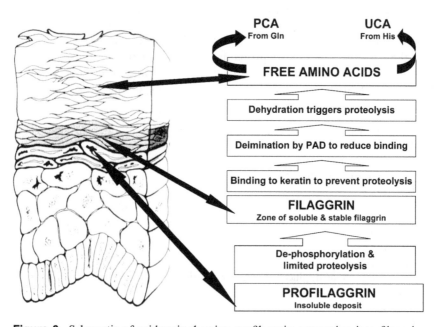

Figure 8 Schematic of epidermis showing profilaggrin conversion into filaggrin and PCA. *Source*: Modified from Ref. 2.

corneocyte swelling can occur perpendicularly to the skin surface as the corneodesmosomes no longer link adjacent corneocytes except at their peripheral edges. The unique arrangement of the keratin network explains the lack of lateral swelling of these corneocytes. However, these findings still do not explain the lack of swelling in the outermost cell layers of the SC. As will be described the reduced swelling of the outermost SC layer is probably due to a loss of NMF from the surface layers of the SC, together with a strengthening of the corneocyte envelope.

STRATUM CORNEUM LIPID AND NMF GRADIENTS

Like the gradation of water in the stratum corneum, there are also gradients in lipid composition, lipid ultrastructure, and NMF. The gradation of NMF within the SC, however, is more complicated than just through the biochemical synthesis routes outlined above and it is actually also related to bathing habits and to the changes in SC lipid composition and ultrastructure and ultimately barrier function.

Rawlings et al. (2) first reported the increasing NMF concentration profiles with increasing depth of stratum corneum obtained by sequential tape stripping of human skin. This diminution in NMF, or PCA in this example, toward the skin surface was considered to be due to NMF being leached out from the skin surface during bathing. More recently, Caspers et al. (12) measured the SC gradients of the other components of NMF in vivo using the confocal Raman microspectroscopy method. The typical in vivo profiles of the major NMF components can be seen in Figure 9. All of the NMF components generated from filaggrin decrease in concentration toward the surface of the SC. As expected, as lactate is derived from eccrine sweat, it shows a gradient different from the amino acid derived NMF components.

Depth profile changes in the levels of stratum corneum ceramides have also been observed with corresponding changes in lipid organization. Rawlings et al. (32) initially reported on the loss of ceramides and disruption of the lamellar ultrastructure in both normal and dry skin toward the surface layers of the SC (Fig. 10). Increasing levels of fatty acids were also observed at the skin surface. More recently, the lateral packing states of the SC lipids have also been shown to change toward the skin surface. In the upper layers of the SC a greater proportion of lipids in a hexagonal phase were observed, which is indicative of a weaker barrier. These changes in lipid organization can be complicated on skin sites where sebum is found in large quantities as can be seen in Figure 11 (33). These lipid gradients were confirmed in compositional studies by Bonte et al. (34). Greater quantities of fatty acids, particularly unsaturated fatty acids, were observed at the skin surface. Finally, cholesterol sulfate is hydrolyzed in the uppermost corneocyte cell layers which may contribute to these ultrastructural changes (35). These chemical and organizational changes will lead to a weaker barrier in the outer layers of the SC and it is, therefore, not too surprising that large quantities of NMF can be leached from the skin surface during cleansing. The weaker barrier in the superficial layers of the skin can lead to superficial dehydration at low absolute humidities which can then influence the differentiation of the underlying epidermis.

This loss of NMF from the superficial layers of the stratum corneum is probably the prime reason why corneocytes do not appear to swell in this area of the tissue. However, as will be discussed later, the corneocyte envelopes are further strengthened by protein cross-linking in the upper layers of the SC. The increased strength of these resilient corneocytes may also reduce their capability to swell.

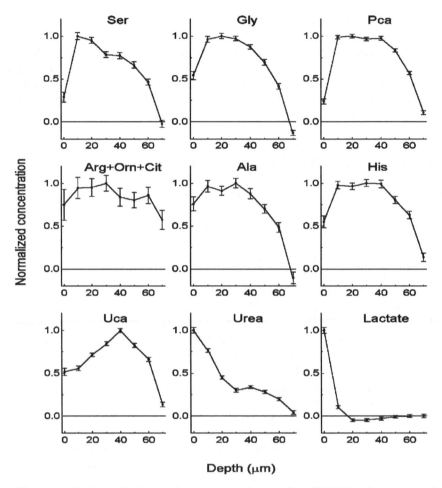

Figure 9 Semiquantitative in vivo concentration profiles of NMF and sweat constituents in the stratum corneum of the thenar as determined by Raman spectroscopy. *Source*: Modified from Ref. 12.

THE EFFECT OF THE SEASONS AND ATMOSPHERIC CONDITIONS ON THE STRATUM CORNEUM

Atmospheric conditions influence SC properties and, as initially reported by Gaul and Underwood (13), are the primary initiator of dry skin. More recently, changing humidity and temperature levels have also been reported to influence epidermal differentiation. Any disruption to the barrier of the skin of the stratum corneum elicits a homeostatic repair response in the epidermis that rapidly results in restoration of the natural moisture barrier. As will be discussed after conditioning to high humidity levels, the SC barrier is functionally weaker, there is less NMF present, and the SC water content is subsequently lower.

The effect of the weather on SC properties can be best exemplified by the changes in SC composition in different seasons. In studies conducted in summer and winter, Rogers et al. (36) demonstrated that there was a significant reduction in the levels of SC ceramides, fatty acids, together with linoleate-containing CER

Normal Skin   Grade 4 Dry Skin

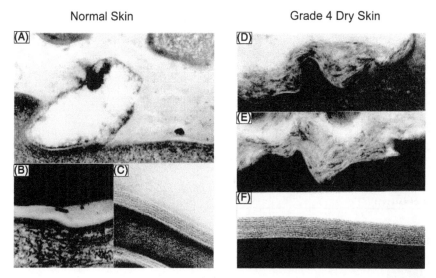

Figure 10 Organization of stratum corneum lipids and ultrastructural changes in lipid organization toward the surface of the stratum corneum, as seen in transmission electron micrographs of tape strippings from individuals with clinically normal skin (*left*) and severe xerosis (*right*). (A) First strip; absence of bilayers and presence of amorphous lipidic material. (B) Second strip; disruption of lipid lamellae. (C) Third strip; normal lipid lamellae (×200,000). (D) First strip; disorganized lipid lamellae. (E) Second strip; disorganized lipid lamellae. (F) Third strip; normal lipid lamellae (×200,000). *Source*: Modified from Ref. 32.

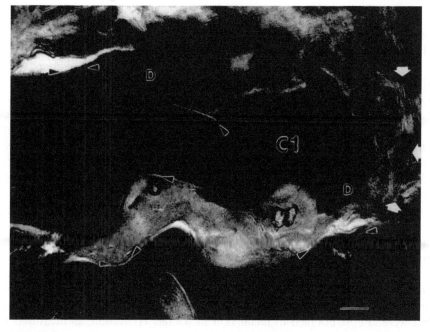

Figure 11 Amorphous sebum fills the intercellular spaces of the corneocytes. Lipid envelopes of corneocytes (*arrowheads*), deranged lipid lamellae (*white arrows*), corneodesmosome (D), and corneocyte (C1). *Source*: Modified from Ref. 33.

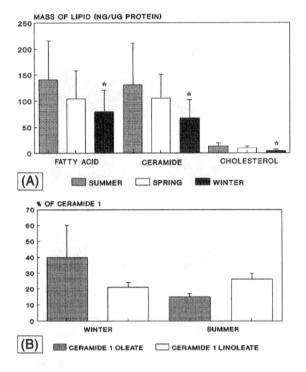

Figure 12 (A) Seasonal changes in the stratum corneum lipid levels of the face. (B) Seasonal changes in the levels of linoleate and oleate-containing CER EOS. *Source*: Modified from Ref. 36.

EOS in subjects living in a cold climates (Fig. 12). Similar differences in scalp lipid levels have been observed between the wet and dry seasons in Thailand (37). Black et al. (38) also reported reduced desquamatory potential in the winter. More recently, Declercq et al. (39) have reported an adaptive response in human barrier function. Subjects living in a dry climate like Arizona compared with a humid climate in New York had a much stronger barrier function due to increased ceramide levels. Their skin appeared less scaly probably also due to the increases in desquamatory enzyme levels. Although NMF was not measured in these experiments, SC hydration is clearly lower in winter compared with in summer even in normal skin (40). Corneocyte surface areas are usually larger in winter compared with in summer, indicating reduced epidermal proliferation (41). As TEWL levels are also normal, or sometimes increased in summer, reductions in NMF levels are the most likely explanation for the reduced SC hydration in winter.

The winter season has also been reported to more severely affect facial skin compared with forearm skin (41). Comparing SC turnover times the face shows a faster turnover compared with forearm skin. However, in winter, forearm skin showed a slower SC turnover compared with the exposed cheek where it was greater, resulting in even smaller corneocytes. TEWL levels were slightly elevated in forearm skin but were almost doubled in facial skin in winter. Hydration, as measured by conductance, was lower on forearm skin in winter suggesting a seasonal decline in NMF. However, this was not apparent on the face but this may be related to the barrier perturbation; i.e., higher TEWL leads to apparently higher hydration when measured by conductance. The skin surface temperature and skin redness were also higher on the cheek, indicating that inflammation was the cause of elevated TEWL levels and enhanced SC turnover. Increased inflammatory status can be measured by the increased SC interleukin-1 receptor antagonist protein/interleukin-1 ratio (IRAP/IL-1) (42). Reductions in the inflammatory status (SC IRAP/IL-1) have been demonstrated for creams that reduce TEWL (43).

Recently, the impact of changing experimental humidity conditions on skin barrier function was demonstrated by the elegant studies of Peter Elias and his collaborators (44,45,47). Over a two-week period, which is sufficient to allow full turnover of the stratum corneum, TEWL was reduced by approximately 30% in animals exposed to a dry (<10%RH) environment, due to increased lipid biosynthesis, increased lamellar body extrusion, and a slightly thicker SC layer. However, no significant differences in lipid composition were observed. At high humidity (80%RH) this induction of lipid biosynthesis was reduced (44). The barrier recovery following either acetone treatment or tape stripping treatments was accelerated in animals acclimated to the dry environment but delayed in those acclimated to the humid environment. Clearly, these findings support the findings in the human studies outlined above regarding the effect of season and geographical location.

Abrupt changes in environmental humidity can also influence stratum corneum moisturization. A humid exposure (80%RH) to dry (<10%RH) exposure transition induced a six-fold increase in TEWL. However, barrier function returned to normal within seven days due to the normal lipid repair processes. However, this did not occur in a normal-to-dry humidity transition (45). Similarly, abrupt changes in the environmental humidity affected the water holding capacity and free amino acid content of the stratum corneum. Katagiri et al. (46) at Shiseido demonstrated that exposing mice to a humid environment and transferring them to a dry one reduced skin conductance and amino acid levels even seven days after the transfer, whereas transferring them from a normal environment resulted in the amino acid levels recovering within three days. Filaggrin immunoreactivity also became faint in the mice that were transferred from a humid or normal to a dry environment. The finding of lower levels of filaggrin and NMF at higher humidity would be anticipated from the early results of Harding and Scott at Unilever (26–29,31).

Exposure to low humidity also increases epidermal DNA synthesis and amplifies the DNA synthetic response to barrier disruption. Mast cell hypertrophy, mast cell degranulation, and signs of inflammation also occur. These changes are attributable to changes in SC moisture content and provide evidence that changes in environmental humidities contribute to the seasonal exacerbation or amelioration of xerotic skin conditions which are characterized by a defective barrier, epidermal hyperplasia, and inflammation (47).

Interestingly, when the skin is fully occluded or when exposed to humid climates, stratum corneum skin surface pH rises (48). pH itself may have an effect on SC maturation processes and thereby SC water content. Indeed, by measuring barrier recovery it has been shown that barrier repair proceeds normally at an acidic skin pH whereas recovery is delayed at a neutral pH (49). However, this is not due to reduced lamellar body secretion; instead the post-secretory processing of newly secreted polar lipids (glucosylceramides) into mature lamellar bilayers (ceramides) is impeded at a neutral pH due to a reduction in the activity of beta-glucocerebrosidase in the lower stratum corneum. At these more alkaline pHs, increased proteolytic activities have been observed leading to increased corneodesmolysis and aberrations in corneocyte cohesion (50).

Ashida et al. at Shiseido have also demonstrated that exposure to a dry environment directly increased epidermal IL-1 levels and that the increased levels of this cytokine is greater on experimentally challenging the barrier (51). More recently, the same group also reported increased numbers of mast cells and increased dermal but not epidermal histamine levels (52). Others have reported increased SC nerve growth factor levels (53) and increased c-fibers in dry skin elicited by dry environments (54). These events would lead to increased itching in these conditions.

Clearly changes in SC lipid and NMF levels can occur under different atmospheric conditions. These changes explain the reduced SC hydration in winter compared with summer and it is not too surprising that xerotic skin conditions occur in the winter. Upon challenge to the skin using surfactants, the strength of the natural moisture barrier is further reduced. This will then further perturb the epidermal differentiation process and as such reduced SC NMF levels have been reported (55). However, as pointed out by Gaul and Underwood (13), atmospheric dew points and not relative humidity are important for inducing these changes. It is interesting, in these early studies, that a high dew point seemed to occur before a low dew point inducing skin chapping. From the work described above, at the high dew point filaggrin and glucosyl ceramide processing will be reduced making the SC more susceptible to challenge when the dew points subsequently decrease.

THE ROLE OF WATER IN THE STRATUM CORNEUM

From a mechanical viewpoint, the skin is a stratified composite material whose superficial layer, the SC, is the stiffest but yet it only represents approximately 1/100 of the total thickness of the skin. Clearly, hydration affects SC biomechanics. Blank estimated that 10 mgs of water per 100 mgs of dry SC was the critical moisture level for SC flexibility. This could be achieved at 60%RH (14). Singer and Vinson (56) demonstrated that the SC water content varied with RH with a logarithmic relationship (Fig. 13), which was also temperature related. The benefit of this

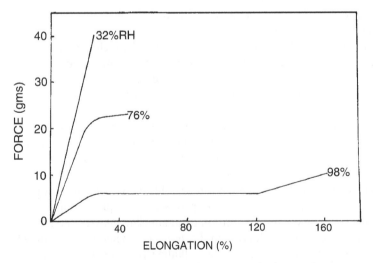

Figure 13 Plot of the logarithm of water uptake by newborn rat corneum versus relative humidity. *Source*: Modified from Ref. 56.

increased water content was initially quantified in vitro using SC extensibility measurements. The force required to elongate SC at various relative humidities in vitro is shown in Figure 15. As can be seen, hydration allows the SC to be extended more greatly. At reduced hydration the SC is less extendible and the forces required to stretch the skin are greater (57).

The structural features responsible for the mechanical characteristics of the SC during extension are obviously best observed during mechanical loading. Agache et al. (58) observed that the corneocytes of extended SC reduced in thickness and ruptured mainly at the corneocyte junctional edges namely at the corneodesmosomes. Leveque et al. (59) went on to further demonstrate that the elastic modulus of the corneocyte is greater than the corneocyte itself and suggested that SC extensibility occurs by plasticization of the intercellular medium and unfolding of the microrelief lines. Rawlings et al. (60) demonstrated that the intercellular lipids are indeed ruptured in vitro during mechanical extension of isolated SC; this was also associated with barrier disruption, which at the higher extensions was irreversible (Fig. 14).

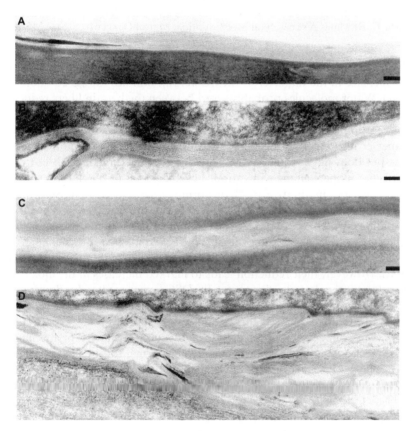

Figure 14 Electron microscopy of ruthenium tetroxide–fixed stratum corneum after (A) 0%, (B) 2%, (C) 5%, and (D) 8% extension of stratum corneum equilibrated to 97%RH. The intercellular lipid can be seen to be disrupted at 5 and 8% extensions (×200,000; bar 0.05 μm). Histogram of changes in stratum corneum water barrier function during in vitro extension. Note the large and irreversible increases in water vapor transport rate at 8% extension. *Source*: Modified from Ref. 60.

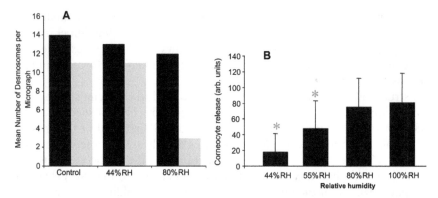

Figure 15 (A) Comparison of the number of corneodesmosomes in control SC incubated for 7 days at 44% and 80%RH. Note the decrease in intact corneodesmosomes in the 80%RH-treated samples. Total corneodesmosomes = gray box; intact corneodesmosomes = black box. (B) Relationship between corneocyte release and relative humidity ($^*P < 0.05$). Note the reduced corneocyte release at lower humidities. *Source*: Modified from Rawlings AV, Harding C, Watkinson A, Banks J, Ackerman C, Sabin R. The effect of glycerol and humidity on desmosome degradation in stratum corneum and Rawlings AV, Harding CR, Watkinson A, Chandar P, Scott IR. Humectants. In: Leyden JJ, Rawlings AV, eds. Skin Moisturization. Marcel Dekker Inc., 2002:245–266.

Clearly, hydration influences SC deformability. X-ray diffraction studies have shown a 10% increase in the diameter of the SC keratin bundles for SC equilibrated to 65%RH (61). Water molecules probably insert between the keratin fibers reducing the intermolecular keratin fiber forces making the SC more flexible. NMF in vivo is an important keratin plasticizer as on its extraction, the SC becomes less extendible.

Wildnauer et al. (57) reported that diethylether extraction of the SC, which extracts lipids but does not extract NMF, increased its breaking strength but only marginally affected its percentage elongation. Leveque et al. (62) demonstrated an increase in the elastic modulus for chloroform:methanol-extracted SC, which extracts both lipids and NMF, incubated at 56%RH but not at 73%RH. Therefore, at higher humidities, water can plasticize the SC, but in most circumstances, NMF plays an important role in plasticizing the SC. In fact, Imokawa in his chapter on "Ceramides as NMF" (63) has reported that SC amino acids do not function to hold water in the SC. However, their reduction leads to marked increases in the molecular interactions between the keratin filaments. In DSC experiments, Imokawa also demonstrated that extraction of NMF had no effect on the bound SC water. However, extraction of SC lipids reduced this bound water from 33% to 19.7% (64).

A variety of instruments have been used to study the effects on SC biomechanics in vivo but the most commonly used instrument is the dermal torque meter. A 1 mm guard ring is usually used to measure the SC/epidermal biomechanics. Using this type of instrument, a significant increase in skin flexibility (Ue) has been demonstrated following skin hydration. Moisturizers such as sodium lactate or sodium PCA and more recently glycerol have also been proven to increase stratum corneum flexibility. Using this method a decrease in stratum corneum elasticity is reported with aging, i.e., there is an increase in the modulus of elasticity and there is a notable decrease in the skin's ability to return to its original shape after being subjected to deformation. However, Batisse et al. (65) recently reported that the SC becomes less extendible with age (Ue decreased), but that it maintained its elasticity, i.e., Ur/Ue was the same in young and old subjects. This decrease in deformability is probably related to reduced

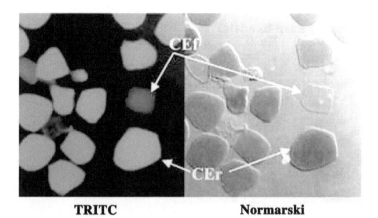

TRITC   **Normarski**

Figure 16 Cornified cell envelopes recovered from the surface layers of the volar forearm visualized by fluorescence of TRITC-stained envelopes and Normarski optics. The mature CEr shows increased fluorescence labeling compared to the immature CEf. *Source*: Modified from Ref. 71.

NMF levels and subsequently reduced SC water content. Like the age-related decline in SC ceramide levels (35,66), there is also an age-related diminution in the levels of NMF which probably reflects reduced epidermal synthesis of these ingredients (67,68).

Water, however, is also required for other stratum corneum properties. The exfoliation of corneocytes from the surface of the skin is facilitated by the action of specific hydrolases in the stratum corneum that degrade the glycoprotein complexes of corneodesmosomes and then allow cell loss from the surface of the skin (23). The effect of hydration on corneodesmolysis and desquamation can be seen in Figure 15. Glycosidases and proteases naturally require water for their activity and as a result the retention of water by barrier lipids and NMF is essential for their activity. Faulty desquamation occurs in dry flaky skin as a result of reduced corneodesmolysis due to reduced proteolytic enzyme activity, changes in ceramide biochemistry and structure, and reduced NMF levels. In these conditions the corneodesmosomes that occur on the non-peripheral edges of the corneocytes are not degraded effectively and corneocytes accumulate on the surface layers of the skin (23). These events initially occur in the superficial layers of the SC but this barrier perturbation leads to epidermal hyperproliferation and perturbed differentiation which produces an SC containing less NMF together with an imbalance in the types of SC ceramides. Decreased levels of SC phytosphingosine-containing ceramides and CER EOS have been observed (69,70).

Corneocytes also undergo further structural processing in the SC by the action of transglutaminases. The cornified cell envelope (CE) is formed by the transglutaminase-mediated gamma-glutamyl lysine crosslinking of corneocyte proteins but it is equally made hydrophobic by the esterification with ceramides and fatty acids by the same enzyme (71). This enzyme transforms soft or fragile corneocytes (CEf) into resilient corneocytes (CEr) (Fig. 16). Changes in the fragile corneocyte envelope (CEf) and rigid corneocyte envelope (CEr) levels also occur in dry skin, where CEf predominates in dry skin (Fig. 17). This appears to be related to the reduction in the level and activity of the enzyme, transglutaminase. This cellular strengthening mechanism could also contribute to the lack of cell swelling in the outer layers of the SC in normal skin observed by electron microscopy as well as due to a reduction in the total levels of NMF.

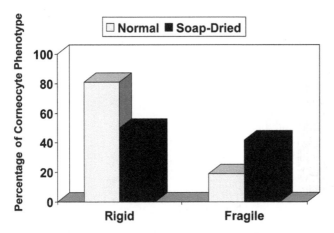

Figure 17 Percentage distribution of CEr and CEf in normal and soap dried dry skin. *Source*: Modified from Ref. 23.

The increased corneocyte strength in the outer layers of the SC has been further exemplified by the work of Kashibuchi et al. (72) at Pola. Using atomic force microscopy, volar forearm corneocytes were shown to exhibit a decrease in skin thickness, an increased surface area, and an increased flatness index toward the surface of the SC, i.e., the outermost corneocytes were less swollen than the inner corneocytes. These relative changes in corneocyte parameters were not apparent in facial skin corneocytes, which may be related to microinflammation, keratinocyte hyperproliferation, and heterogeneity of the corneocytes. Clearly, the individual corneocytes may possess differing water-holding or water-retaining capacities. Hirao et al. (73) at Shiseido used corneocyte hydrophobicity and involucrin immunoreactivity as markers of corneocyte maturation. In their studies immature corneocytes were found to be less hydrophobic as judged by Nile red staining and they are more easily bound by involucrin antibodies (Fig. 18). One would, therefore, expect the immature corneocytes to be leakier and to lose NMF more easily compared with the mature corneocytes due to reduced levels of covalently bound lipid. In this respect, aberrant

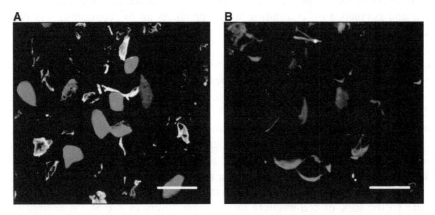

Figure 18 Double staining of CEs with Nile Red and anti-involucrin. (A) Face; (B) Upper arm. *Source*: Modified from Ref. 73.

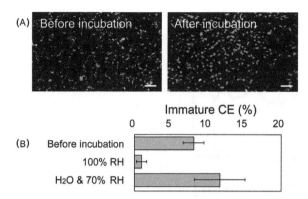

Figure 19 (A) Conversion of immature CEs in the SC of the face into mature CEs by ex vivo incubation at 100%RH and 37°C for four days. Scale bar = 100 μm. (B) Suppression of CE maturation ex vivo under low-humidity conditions and replenishment by hydration. **P < 0.01. *Source*: Modified from Ref. 75.

barrier function in scar tissue has been considered to be a function of the presence of immature corneocytes rather than lipid biochemical changes (74). The CE maturation is also suppressed in low humidity conditions, and, as can be seen from Figure 19, increased CE maturation can be induced by increasing SC hydration (75).

Thus, there is great heterogeneity in the proportions of these corneocyte envelope phenotypes and, therefore, probably great heterogeneity in the water content of these cells. These immature envelopes are present in greater numbers in xerotic skin (73) in a fashion similar to the increased presence of fragile envelopes reported by Harding et al. (71).

Facial skin appears to be the most heterogeneous with regard to barrier function, SC water content, and the type of corneocyte phenotype even on apparently healthy-looking skin. Increased levels of IRAP/IL-1 and other cytokines occur in facial SC, all of which are signs of sub-clinical inflammation. Variation in SC water content on different body sites needs careful consideration.

The biomechanics of the SC, the natural moisture barrier, the transglutaminase-mediated corneocyte strengthening, and corneodesmolysis are all reduced in dry skin. Low atmospheric dew points precipitate this condition. Temperature naturally has an impact on these processes but the wind and barometric pressure will also be important in determining the outcome of these processes. Rapidly changing atmospheric conditions influence epidermal differentiation, SC quality, and thereby SC water content. The barrier can be strengthened living in dry climates but presumably the dew point is large enough to prevent dry skin from occurring. In other geographical locations where a winter season occurs, the lower temperature and resulting lower dew points reduce the SC water content and lead to the production of a faulty SC. The need to humidify the air in winter was clearly exemplified by the studies of Gaul and Underwood (13). Also Hilliard and Dorogi (76) demonstrated that the impact of reduced temperature far outweighs the impact of just reduced humidity of SC properties (i.e., lower dew points). The reduced skin temperatures will also reduce TEWL and thus the SC is stressed even further as it loses water from the surface of the skin and now the water transport from the underlying tissue to the outer layers of the SC is further reduced. These changes can also lead to the formation of fine lines even before the generation of a flaky skin phenotype. Egawa et al. (77) demonstrated that a

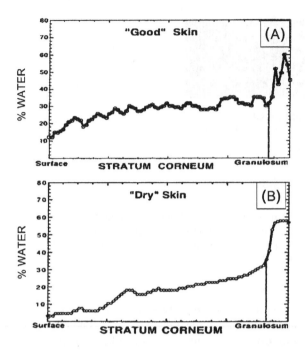

Figure 20 (A) Water profile averaged over a single rectangular region of a cryosection obtained from an individual with good skin, grade 0.5. The horizontal axis is the distance across the SC with the SC/granulosum junction indicated by a vertical line. (B) Water profile averaged over a single rectangular region of a cryosection obtained from an individual with dry skin, grade 4. *Source*: Modified from Ref. 19.

short exposure to a low humidity environment reduces SC hydration and changes the skin surface patterning leading to fine lines influenced by the dermal Langer's lines.

Nevertheless, so far the only study to quantitatively measure SC water profiles in relation to skin condition is that of Warner and Lilly (19). Figure 20 shows the average water profiles from a single cryosection from an individual with normal skin biopsied in summer. After the stratum granulosum, the SC water content drops to about 35% in the innermost corneocytes. This profile is largely maintained at over 25 to 35% water content except at the surface where it drops to 12%. In contrast, in a subject with dry skin biopsied in winter, the SC does not maintain the higher water content after the mid-layers of the SC and is finally less than 10% in the outermost layers. At this water content, according to the early studies of Blank (14), the SC will be dysfunctional and brittle. Although there are likely seasonal differences in the quality of the SC in these studies, it is clear that winter dry skin does not have the capacity to retain as much water as the normal-looking skin in summer. This is highly likely to be a result of the reduced barrier lipids, reduced NMF levels, and decreased corneocyte size induced by epidermopiosis in dry skin (78).

CONCLUSIONS

Ten years ago most of the research on SC water content was just related to SC biomechanics. Although vitally important for SC flexibility, it has become clearer over the last decade that water also has other roles in the SC. It is crucial in allowing lipid processing to form the barrier, corneodesmolysis to allow desquamation to proceed, corneocyte envelope strengthening, and in the generation of NMF itself. These structural and compositional changes in the SC influence water flux and water retention in the tissue. Ultimately, the SC controls the water gradient from the skin to the atmosphere.

Corneodesmosomes tightly bind adjacent corneocytes in the lower layers of the SC allowing the formation of an efficient barrier with corneocytes that appear not to swell. However, the non-peripheral corneodesmosomes are degraded in the upper layers of the SC, which allows corneocytes to swell at high water contents. At the same time NMF is formed from filaggrin, dictated by the SC water content itself. The additional water bound by this NMF allows corneodesmolysis to continue and transglutaminase activity to allow the formation of a fully mature corneocyte. Interestingly, the increased cellular hygroscopicity and increased swelling of the corneocytes occur in the central layers of the SC, but the outer and inner corneocytes do not swell as much. In the outer corneocytes this reduction in cellular swelling appears to be due to a combination of changes to the composition and ultrastructure of the barrier lipids, reduced NMF levels, and a strengthening of the corneocyte envelope, whereas in the lower layers of the SC it appears to be due to increased numbers of corneodesmosomes and a lack of filaggrin processing. If the barrier is not perturbed an optimally functioning SC is formed at the skin's surface. Soaps and surfactants can make the barrier weaker as they disrupt the lipid ultrastructure and leach ceramides from the skin surface. It is now possible to extract more NMF from the superficial layers of the SC and the initial visual signs of dry skin become apparent.

As the SC–epidermal–dermal interfaces are in physical contact, changes in SC water content can possibly lead to the secretion of different factors by the living cells. At high humidity somehow the epidermal biosynthetic machinery of lipids and NMF is switched off. When this skin is challenged, a dry skin state can be more easily induced. When the barrier becomes compromised, an ensuing series of events occur—a self perpetuating dry skin cycle.

Initially superficial dryness occurs in the SC and corneodesmolysis starts to be impaired—the first signs of dry skin. The reduction in NMF levels together with lipid compositional and organizational changes probably result in changes in the SC water gradients and barrier function, which leads to the local secretion of proinflammatory cytokines that can either directly or indirectly, by a double paracrine signaling with the dermis, lead to keratinocyte hyperproliferation and faulty desquamation further perturbing the barrier. At some point the skin is perceived to be tight and itchy, and subsequent scratching of the skin surface further compromises the barrier by mechanical disruption. In this state the epidermis is now also producing less filaggrin and thereby NMF together with reduced quantities of phytosphingosine-containing ceramides and acyl-ceramides. Thus, unless prevented, this dry skin cycle will continue to worsen the quality of the SC thereby further disrupting the natural moisture barrier of the skin. However, the most beneficial route to correcting this dysfunctional state is to repair the barrier itself which will break the dry skin cycle. Although outside the scope of this review, repair of the barrier by using a ceramide-dominant cream or by using agents to improve lipid biosynthesis, such as niacinamide, has been shown to be key in reducing the symptoms of a dry and flaky skin condition (79–81).

REFERENCES

1. Rawlings AV. Skin waxes: their composition, properties, structures and biological significance. In: Hamilton RJ, ed. Waxes: Chemistry, Molecular Biology & Functions. Chapter 6. Dundee, Scotland: The Oily Press, 1994:221–256.
2. Rawlings AV, Scott IR, Harding CR, Bowser PA. Stratum corneum moisturization at the molecular level. J Invest Dermatol 1994; 103:731–740.
3. Harding CR, Watkinson A, Rawlings AV. Dry skin, moisturization and corneodesmolysis. Int J Cosmet Sci 2000; 22:21–52.
4. Rawlings AV, Harding CR, Watkinson A, Scott IR. Dry & xerotic skin conditions. In: Leyden JJ, Rawlings AV, eds. Skin Moisturization. New York: 2002; 119–143.
5. Swanbeck G. On the keratin fibrils of the skin. An X-ray small angle scattering study of the horny layer. J Ultrastruct Res 1959; 3:51–57.
6. Downing DT, Lazo ND. Lipid & protein structures in the permeability barrier. In: Loden M, Maibach HI, eds. Dry Skin & Moisturizers Chemistry & Function. Florida: CRC Press LLC, 2000:39–44.
7. Lindberg M, Forslind B. The skin as a barrier. In: Loden M, Maibach HI, eds. Dry Skin & Moisturizers Chemistry & Function. Florida: CRC Press LLC, 2000:27–37.
8. Warner RR, Myers MC, Taylor DA. Electron probe analysis of human skin: determination of the water concentration profile. J Invest Dermatol 1988; 90:218–224.
9. Bouwstra JA, de Graaff A, Gooris GS, Nijsse J, Wiechers J, van Aelst AC. Water distribution and related morphology in human stratum corneum at different hydration levels. J Invest Dermatol 2003; 120:750–758.
10. Pfeiffer S, Vielhaber G, Vietzke JP, Wittern KP, Hintze U, Wepf R. High pressure freezing provides new information on human epidermis: simultaneous protein antigen & lamellar lipid structure preservation. Study on human epidermis by cryoimmobilization. J Invest Dermatol 2000; 114:1030–1038.
11. Norlen L. Skin barrier structure, function & formation-learning from cryo-electron microscopy of vitreous, fully hydrated native human epidermis. Int J Cosmet Sci 2003; 25:209–226.
12. Caspers PJ, Lucassen GW, Carter EA, Bruining HA, Puppels GJL. Semiquantitative in vivo concentration profiles of NMF and sweat constituents in the stratum corneum of the thenar as determined by Raman spectroscopy. J Invest Dermatol 2001; 116:434–442.
13. Gaul E, Underwood GB. Relation of dew point & barometric pressure to chapping of normal skin. J Invest Dermatol 1951; 19(1):9–19.
14. Blank IH. Factors which influence the water content of the stratum corneum. J Invest Dermatol 1952; 18:433–440.
15. Idson B. Water & the skin. J Soc Cosmet Chem 1973; 24:197–212.
16. Vavascour I, Kitson N, MacKay A. Whats water got to do with it? A nuclear magnetic resonance study of molecular motion in pig SC. J Invest Dermatol Symp Proc 1998; 3:101–104.
17. Bommannan D, Potts RO, Guy RH. Examination of stratum corneum barrier function in vivo by infrared spectroscopy. J Invest Dermatol 1990; 95:403–408.
18. Bazzoni G, Dejana E. Keratinocyte junctions & the epidermal barrier: how to make a skin tight dress. J Cell Biol 2002; 156:947–949.
19. Warner RR, Lilly NA. Correlation of water content with ultrastructure in the stratum corneum. In: Elsner P, Berardesca E, Maibach HI, eds. Bioengineering of the Skin: Water & the Stratum Corneum. Florida: CRC Press Inc., 1994:3–12.
20. Warner RR, Stone KJ, Biossy YL. Hydration disrupts human stratum corneum ultrastructure. J Invest Dermatol 2003; 120:275–284.
21. Norlen L, Emilson A, Forslind B. Stratum corneum swelling. Biophysical & computer assisted quantitative assessments. Arch Dermatol Res 1997; 289:506–513.
22. Richter T, Muller JH, Schwarz UD, Wepf R, Wiesendanger R. Investigation of the swelling of human skin cells in liquid media by tapping mode scanning forece microscopy. Appl Phys 2001; A72(Suppl):S125–S128.

23. Rawlings AV. Trends in stratum corneum research and the management of dry skin conditions. Int J Cosmet Sci 2003; 25:63–95.
24. Cler EJ, Fourtanier A. L'acide pyrrolidone carboxylique (PCA) et la peau. Int J Cosmet Sci 1981; 3:101.
25. Trianse SJ. The search for the ideal moisturizer. Cosmet Perfum 1974; 89:57.
26. Barratt JG, Scott IR. Pyrollidone carboxylic acid synthesis in guinea pig epidermis. J Invest Dermatol 1983; 81:122.
27. Scott IR, Harding CR. Studies on the synthesis and degradation of a histidine rich phosphoprotein from mammalian epidermis. Biochim Biophys Acta 1981; 669:65.
28. Scott IR, Harding CR, Barrett JG. Histidine rich proteins of the keratohyalin granule. Biochim Biophys Acta 1982; 719:110.
29. Harding CR, Scott IR. Histidine-rich proteins (filaggrins). Structural & functional heterogeneity during epidermal differentiation. J Mol Biol 1983; 170:651.
30. Angelin JH. Urocanic acid a natural sunscreen. Cosmet Toilet 1976; 91:47.
31. Scott IR, Harding CR. Filaggrin breakdown to water binding components during development of rat stratum corneum is controlled by the water activity of the environment. Dev Biol 1986; 115:84.
32. Rawlings AV, Watkinson A, Rogers J, Mayo AM, Hope J, Scott IR. Abnormalities in stratum corneum structure, lipid composition & desmosome degradation in sop-induced winter xerosis. J Soc Cosmet Chem 1994; 45:203–220.
33. Sheu H, Chao S, Wong T, Lee Y, Tsai J. Human skin surface lipid film: an ultrastructural study and interaction with corneocytes & intercellular lipid lamellae of the stratum corneum. Br J Dermatol 1999; 140:385–391.
34. Bonte F, Saunois A, Pinguet P, Meybeck A. Existence of a lipid gradient in the upper stratum corneum and its possible biological significance. Arch Dermatol Res 1995; 289:78–82.
35. Weerheim A, Ponec M. Determination of stratum corneum lipid profile by tape stripping in combination with high performance thin layer chromatrography. Arch Dermatol Res 2001; 293:191–199.
36. Rogers J, Harding CR, Mayo A, Banks J, Rawlings AV. Stratum corneums lipids: the effect of ageing & the seasons. Arch Dermatol Res 1996; 288:765–770.
37. Meldrum H, et al. The characteristic decrease in scalp stratum corneum lipids in dandruff is reversed by use of a ZnPTO containing shampoo. IFSCC Mag 2003; 6(1):3–6.
38. Black D, Pozo AD, Lagarde JM, Gall Y. Seasonal variability in the biophysical properties of stratum corneum from different anatomical sites. Skin Res Technol 2000; 6:70–76.
39. Declercq L, Muizzuddin N, Hellemans L, van Overloop L, Sparacio R, Marenus K, Maes D. Adaptation response in human skin barrier to a hot & dry environment. J Invest Dermatol 2002; 119:716.
40. Treffel P, Gabard B. Stratum corneum dynamic function measurements after moisturizer or irritant application. Arch Dermatol Res 1995; 287:474–479.
41. Kikuchi K, Kobayashi H, Le Fur I, Tschachler E, Tagami H. The winter season affects more severly the facial skin than the forearm skin: comparative biophysical studies conducted in the same Japanese females in later summer & winter. Exog Dermatol 2002; 1:32–38.
42. Hirao T, Aoki H, Yoshida T, Sato Y, Kamoda H. Elevation of interleukin 1 receptor antagonist in the stratum corneum of sun-exposed and UV-B irradiated human skin. J Invest Dermatol 1996; 106:1102–1107.
43. Kikutchi K, Kobayashi H, Hirao T, Ito A, Takahashi H, Tagami H. Improvement of mild inflammatory changes of the facial skin induced by winter environment with daily applications of a moisturizing cream. Dermatology 2003; 207:269–275.
44. Denda M, Sato J, Masuda Y, et al. Exposure to a dry environment enhances epidermal permeability barrier function. J Invest Dermatol 1998; 111:858–863.
45. Sato J, Denda M, Chang S, et al. Abrupt decreases in environmental humidity induce abnormalities in permeability barrier homeostasis. J Invest Dermatol 2002; 119:900–904.

46. Katagiri C, Sato J, Nomura J, et al. Changes in environmental humidity affect the water-holding capacity of the stratum corneum and its free amino acid content, and the expression of filaggrin in the epidermis of hairless mice. J Dermatol Sci 2003; 31:29–35.

47. Denda M, Sato J, Tsuchiya T, Elias PM, Feingold KR. Low humidity stimulates epidermal DNA synthesis & amplifies the hyperproliferative response to barrier disruption: implication for seasonal exacerbation of inflammatory dermatoses. J Invest Dermatol 1988; 111:873–878.

48. Fluhr JW, Elias PM. Stratum corneum pH: formation & function of the acid mantle. Exog Dermatol 2002; 1:163–175.

49. Mauro T, Grayson S, Gao WN, Man MQ, Kriehuber E, Behne M, Feingold KR, Elias PM. Barrier recovery is impeded at neutral pH, independent of ionic effects: implications for extracellular lipid processing. Arch Dermatol Res 1998; 290:215–222.

50. Fluhr JW, Kao J, Jain M, Sung K, Feingold KR, Elias PM. Generation of free fatty acids from phospholipids regulates stratum corneum acidification & integrity. J Invest Dermatol 2001; 117:44–51.

51. Ashida Y, Ogo M, Denda M. Epidermal interleukin-1 generation is amplified at low humidity: implications for the pathogenesis of inflammatory dermatoses. Br J Dermatol 2001; 144:238–243.

52. Ashida Y, Denda M. Dry environment increases mast cell number & histamine content in dermis in hairless mice. Br J Dermatol 2003; 149:240–247.

53. Yokota T, Matsumoto M, Sakamaki T, Hikima R, Hayashi S, Yanagisawa M, Kuwahara H, Yamazaki S, Ogawa T, Hayase M. Classification of sensitive skin & development of a treatment system appropriate for each group. Proceedings 22nd IFSCC Congress. Volume I: Podium 17 (2002).

54. Urashima R, Mihara M. Cutaneous nerves in atopic dermatitis. A histological, immuno-chemical & electron microscopic study. Virchows Arch 1998; 432:363–370.

55. Denda M, Hori J, Koyama J, et al. Stratum corneum sphingolipids & free amino acids in experimentally induced dry skin. Arch Dermatol Res 1992; 284:363.

56. Singer E, Vinson L. Water binding properties of skin. Proc Sci Sect Toilet Goods Assoc 1966; 46:29–36.

57. Wildnauer RH, Bothwell JW, Douglass AB. Stratum corneum biomechanical properties. I. Influence of relative humidity on normal & extracted human stratum corneum. J Invest Dermatol 1971; 56:72–78.

58. Agache P, Boyer JP, Laurent R. Biochemical properties & microscopic morphology of human stratum corneum incubated on a wet pad in vitro. Arch Derm Forsch 1973; 246:271–283.

59. Leveque JL, Poelman MC, de Rigal J, Kligman AM. Are corneocytes elastic? Dermatologica 1988; 176:65–69.

60. Rawlings AV, Watkinson A, Harding CR, Ackerman C, Banks J, Hope J, Scott IR. Changes in stratum corneum lipid & desmosome structure together with water barrier function during mechanical stress. J Soc Cosmet Chem 1995; 46:141–151.

61. Hey J, Taylor DJ, Derbishyre W. Water sorption by human callus. Biochem Biophys Acta 1978; 540:518–523.

62. Leveque JL, Escoubez M, Rasseneur L. Bioeng Skin 1987; 3:227–242.

63. Imokawa G. Ceramides as natural moisturizing factors & their efficacy in dry skin. In: Leyden JJ, Rawlings AV, eds. Skin Moisturization. New York: Marcel Dekker Inc., 2002:267–302.

64. Imokawa G, Kuno H, Kawai M. Stratum corneum lipids serve as a bound-water modulator. J Invest Dermatol 1991; 96:845–851.

65. Batisse D, Bazin R, Daldeweck T, Querleux B, Leveque JL. Influence of age on the wrinkling capacities of skin. Skin Res Technol 2002; 8:148–154.

66. Ghadially R, Brown BE, Sequeiramartin SM, et al. The aged epidermal permeability barrier-structural, functional and lipid biochemical abnormalities in humans and a senescent murine model. J Clin Invest 1995; 95:2281.

67. Hori I, Nakayama Y, Obata M, Tagami H. Stratum corneum hydration & amino acid content in xerotic skin. Br J Dermatol 1989; 121:587.
68. Tezuka T. Electron microscopal changes in xerotic senile epidermis. Dermatologica 1993; 166:57.
69. Chopart M, Castiel-Higounenc C, Arbey E, et al. Quantitative analysis of ceramides in stratum corneum of normal & dry skin. Poater at Stratum corneum III, Basel Switzerlans, 2001.
70. van Overloop L, Declercq L, Maes D. Visual scaling of human skin correlates to decreased ceramide levels and decreased stratum corneum protease activity. J Invest Dermatol 2001; 117:811.
71. Harding CR, Long S, Richardson J, Rogers J, Zhang Z, Bush A, Rawlings AV. The cornified cell envelope: an important marker of stratum corneum maturation in healthy and dry skin. Int J Cosmet Sci 2003; 25:1–11.
72. Kashibuchi N, Hirai Y, O'Goshi K, Tagami H. Three dimensional analyses of individual corneocytes with atomic force microscope: morphological changes related to age, location & to pathological skin conditions. Skin Res Technol 2002; 8:203–211.
73. Hirao T, Denda M, Takahashi M. Identification of immature cornified envelopes in barrier-impaired epidermis by characterization of their hydrophobicity and antigenicities of the components. Exp Dermatol 2001; 10:35–44.
74. Kunii T, Hirao T, Kikuchi K, Tagami H. Stratum corneum lipid profile & maturation pattern of corneocytes in the outermost layer of fresh scars: the presence of immature corneocytes plays a much more important role in barrier dysfunction than do changes in intercellular lipids. Br J Dermatol 2003; 149:749–756.
75. Hirao T. Involvement of transglutaminase in ex vivo maturation of cornified envelopes in the stratum corneum. Int J Cosmet Sci 2003; 25:245–257.
76. Hilliard PR, Dorogi PL. Investigation of temperature & water activity effects on pig skin in vitro. J Cosmet Chem 1989; 40:1–20.
77. Egawa M, Oguri M, Kuwahara T, Takahashi M. Effect of exposure of human skin to a dry environment. Skin Res Technol 2002; 8:212–218.
78. Leveque JL, Grove G, de Rigal J, Corcuff P, Kligman AM, Saint-Leger D. Biophysical characterization of dry facial skin. J Soc Cosmet Chem 1987; 82:171–177.
79. Chamlin SL, Kao J, Frieden IJ, Sheu MY, Fowler AJ, Fluhr JW, Williams ML, Elias PM. Ceramide-dominant barrier repair lipids alleviate childhood atopic dermatitis: changes in barrier function provide a sensitive indicator of disease activity. J Am Acad Dermatol 2002; 47:198–208.
80. Matts PJ, Oblong JE, Bissett DL. A review of the range of effects of niacinamide in human skin. IFSCC Mag 2002; 5:285–290.
81. Matts PJ, Gray J, Rawlings AV. The dray skin cycle – a new model of dry skin and mechanisms for intervention. International Congress & Symposum Series. The Royal Society of Medicine Press, Kent, UK 2005; 256:1–38.

25

Vitamin D and the Epidermis

Daniel D. Bikle

Professor of Medicine and Dermatology, Endocrine Research Unit, VA Medical Center, University of California, San Francisco, California, U.S.A.

INTRODUCTION

The epidermis is well known as the source of vitamin D_3 production in the body. Less well known is that epidermal cells (keratinocytes) also produce the active metabolite of vitamin D_3, 1,25 dihydroxyvitamin D_3 (1,25(OH)$_2$D$_3$) (1), contain 1,25(OH)$_2$D$_3$ receptors (VDR) (2–4), and respond to 1,25(OH)$_2$D$_3$ with changes in proliferation and differentiation (3,5,6). Calcium is an important modulator of these pathways. Calcium decreases 1,25(OH)$_2$D$_3$ production and regulates the effects of 1,25(OH)$_2$D$_3$ on proliferation and differentiation (7). Calcium is, by itself, an important regulator of keratinocyte proliferation and differentiation (8,9), the effects of which are, in turn, modulated by 1,25(OH)$_2$D$_3$. Although much of our information about the role of calcium and 1,25(OH)$_2$D$_3$ comes from in vitro studies, a calcium gradient exists in the epidermis that appears to be an important regulator of proliferation and differentiation in vivo. Animals lacking the ability to produce 1,25(OH)$_2$D$_3$ have difficulty restoring this gradient if disrupted, and such animals show abnormalities in terminal differentiation of the epidermis even when placed on a high-calcium diet. Similarly, animals lacking the vitamin D receptor (VDR) also have an abnormality in epidermal differentiation. Furthermore, these VDR-null animals have an abnormality in hair follicle cycling, not seen in vitamin D–deficient animals or in those lacking the capacity to produce 1,25(OH)$_2$D$_3$. Thus, the epidermis is not only an essential source of vitamin D, but is a source and target for its biologically active metabolite 1,25(OH)$_2$D$_3$, and can be uniquely regulated by the VDR in a ligand-independent manner.

VITAMIN D PRODUCTION AND METABOLISM IN THE EPIDERMIS

Vitamin D$_3$ Production

Vitamin D_3 is produced from 7-dehydrocholesterol (7-DHC) (Fig. 1). Although irradiation of 7-DHC was known to produce pre-D_3 (which subsequently undergoes a temperature rearrangement of the triene structure to form D_3), lumisterol, and tachysterol, the physiologic regulation of this pathway was not well understood until

Vitamin D Hydroxylations in keratinocytes

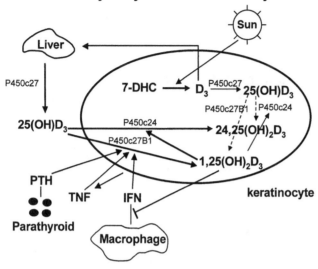

Figure 1 Vitamin D production and conversion to $1,25(OH)_2D_3$ in the keratinocyte. 7-dehydrocholesterol (7-DHC) is converted to vitamin D_3 by a photochemical reaction. The vitamin D_3 produced is either transported out of the keratinocyte to the liver, where it is converted to $25OHD_3$ or metabolized directly to $25OHD_3$ in the keratinocyte by the enzyme 25-hydroxylase (CYP27). $25OHD_3$ is metabolized either to $24,25(OH)_2D_3$ or to $1,25(OH)_2D_3$ by the enzymes 24-hydroxylase (CYP24) and 1α-hydroxylase (CYP27B1), respectively. Parathyroid hormone (PTH) secreted by the parathyroid gland (PTG) stimulates the production of $1,25(OH)_2D_3$, as does tumor necrosis factor-α (TNF) secreted by keratinocytes and interferon-γ (IFN) secreted by macrophages. $1,25(OH)_2D_3$ promotes its own catabolism by inducing the 24-hydroxylase [also responsible for $24,25(OH)_2D_3$ production], and decreasing IFN secretion by macrophages.

the studies of Holick et al. (10–12). They demonstrated that the formation of pre-D_3 under the influence of solar- or UVB irradiation (maximal effective wavelength between 290 and 310) is relatively rapid and reaches a maximum within hours. UV irradiation further converts pre-D_3 to lumisterol and tachysterol. Both the degree of epidermal pigmentation and the intensity of exposure correlate with the time required to achieve this maximal concentration of pre-D_3, but do not alter the maximal level achieved. Although pre-D_3 levels reach a maximum level, the biologically inactive lumisterol accumulates with continued UV exposure. Tachysterol is also formed, but like pre-D_3, does not accumulate with extended UV exposure. The formation of lumisterol is reversible and can be converted back to pre-D_3, as pre-D_3 levels fall. At 0°C, no D_3 is formed; however, at 37°C pre-D_3 is slowly converted to D_3. Thus, short exposure to sunlight would be expected to lead to a prolonged production of D_3 in the exposed skin because of the slow thermal conversion of pre-D_3 to D_3 and lumisterol to pre-D_3. Prolonged exposure to sunlight would not produce toxic amounts of D_3 because of the photoconversion of pre-D_3 to lumisterol and tachysterol, as well as the photoconversion of D_3 itself to suprasterols I and II and 5,6 transvitamin D_3 (13). Thus, stimulation of epidermal D_3 production is a safe way to provide D_3 to the body.

Melanin in the epidermis, by absorbing UV irradiation, can reduce the effectiveness of sunlight in producing D_3 in the skin. This may be one important reason for the lower 25OHD levels (a well-documented surrogate measure for vitamin D levels in the body) in Blacks and Hispanics living in temperate latitudes (14). Sunlight exposure increases melanin production, and so provides another mechanism by which excess D_3 production can be prevented. The intensity of UV irradiation is also important for effective D_3 production. The seasonal variation of 25OHD levels can be quite pronounced with higher levels during summer and with lower levels during winter. The extent of this seasonal variation depends on the latitude, and thus the intensity of the sunlight striking the exposed skin. In Edmonton, Canada (52°N) very little D_3 is produced in exposed skin from mid-October to mid-April; Boston (42°N) has a somewhat longer period for effective D_3 production, whereas in Los Angeles (34°N) and San Juan (18°N) the skin is able to produce D_3 all year long (15). Peak D_3 production occurs around noon, with D_3 being produced in the skin for a larger portion of the day during summer than other times of the year. Clothing (16) and sunscreens (17) effectively prevent D_3 production in the covered areas. This is one likely explanation for the observation that the Bedouins in the Middle East, who totally cover their bodies with clothing, are more prone to developing rickets and osteomalacia than the Israeli Jews with comparably more sunlight exposure.

Although in humans the D_3 produced in the epidermis is likely to enter the body primarily via the blood stream or lymphatics draining the skin, D_3 and its precursor 7-DHC may also be sloughed off onto the surface of the skin or fur. Here additional 7-DHC may be converted to D_3 under sunlight exposure and ingested by an animal grooming itself or others (18). Thus both the oral and parenteral routes may contribute to the bioavailability of D_3 produced in or on the epidermis.

Metabolism of D_3 to its Biologically Active Products

Keratinocytes are not only capable of producing D_3, but of metabolizing D_3, via the vitamin D-25 hydroxylase and the 25OHD-1α-hydroxylase steps, to its active metabolite $1,25(OH)_2D_3$ (1,19–21). Keratinocytes are the only cells in the body containing the entire pathway (Fig. 1). The vitamin D-25 hydroxylase in keratinocytes is the same mitochondrial enzyme (CYP27) that converts vitamin D_3 to $25OHD_3$ in the liver (22,23). Its expression is increased by vitamin D and UVB irradiation (22,23). Similarly the 25OHD-1α-hydroxylase in the epidermis, which is responsible for $1,25(OH)_2D_3$ production, is the same enzyme (CYP27B1) as that found in the kidney (24). Its expression and enzymatic activity are tightly regulated and coupled to the differentiation of these cells.

Most of the circulating $1,25(OH)_2D_3$ is produced by the kidneys. However, extrarenal production of $1,25(OH)_2D_3$ has been demonstrated in both anephric humans (25,26) and pigs (27). Although the tissue(s) responsible for the circulating levels of $1,25(OH)_2D_3$ in anephric animals has not been established, the epidermis is likely to contribute. Keratinocytes rapidly and extensively convert $25OHD_3$ to $1,25(OH)_2D_3$. In fact the expression of the 25OHD-1α-hydroxylase is higher in the keratinocyte than in any other cell including the cells of the proximal renal tubule. The apparent K_m for the enzyme (25OHD 1α-hydroxylase) metabolizing $25OHD_3$ to $1,25(OH)_2D_3$ is estimated to be 5×10^{-8} M, a value lower than that estimated for the kidney. The production of $1,25(OH)_2D_3$ by isolated keratinocytes in culture has been confirmed using intact pig skins perfused with $25OHD_3$ (28). However, when renal production of $1,25(OH)_2D_3$ is normal, the circulating levels of $1,25(OH)_2D_3$ are sufficient to limit the contribution from epidermal production. This is due to the induction of 25OHD-24 hydroxylase in the keratinocyte by

1,25(OH)$_2$D$_3$, the enzyme which catabolizes the endogenously produced 1,25(OH)$_2$D$_3$ before it leaves the cell in which it is produced (29).

Parathyroid hormone (PTH) exerts a modest stimulation of 1,25(OH)$_2$D production by keratinocytes. However, this involves a different mechanism from that resulting in stimulation of 1,25(OH)$_2$D$_3$ production by PTH in the kidney. The keratinocyte does not have a classic PTH receptor coupled to adenylate cyclase.

Furthermore, these effects of PTH are not reproduced by cAMP or its membrane-permeable derivatives, suggesting that the actions of PTH may be operating through a mechanism independent of cAMP (19). The effects of PTH are maximal after a four-hour incubation of cells with these agents before adding substrate (25OHD$_3$); that is, the effects are not immediate. In renal cells PTH exerts a more acute stimulation of 1,25(OH)$_2$D$_3$ production (30), and cAMP appears to play a second messenger role (31). The mechanism by which PTH stimulates 1,25(OH)$_2$D$_3$ production in the keratinocyte remains unclear.

1,25(OH)$_2$D$_3$ negatively regulates its own levels within the keratinocyte. This negative feedback loop is similar to that observed in the kidney, but it differs from that seen in the macrophage, in which 1,25(OH)$_2$D$_3$ fails to regulate 1,25(OH)$_2$D$_3$ production. In the keratinocyte, this feedback inhibition is not mediated by an effect on 1,25(OH)$_2$D$_3$ production, but is due solely to stimulation of 1,25(OH)$_2$D$_3$ catabolism. This is achieved by induction of the enzyme 25OHD-24-hydroxylase that converts 25OHD$_3$ and 1,25(OH)$_2$D$_3$ to 24,25(OH)$_2$D$_3$ and 1,24,25(OH)$_3$D$_3$, respectively (24). The exquisite responsiveness of the 25OHD-24-hydroxylase to 1,25(OH)$_2$D$_3$ in keratinocytes may explain why so little 1,25(OH)$_2$D$_3$ appear to enter the circulation from the skin when renal production of 1,25(OH)$_2$D$_3$ is intact.

The expression and activity of 25OHD-1α-hydroxylase change with differentiation (4). Enzymatic activity is greatest in the undifferentiated cells. Growing the cells in 0.1-mM calcium, which retards differentiation (32), permits them to maintain higher 1α-hydroxylase activity than growing in 1.2-mM calcium (7), although acute changes in calcium have little effect on 1,25(OH)$_2$D$_3$ production (19). These observations in vitro are consistent with the finding that 1α-hydroxylase expression is highest in the stratum basale of the epidermis in vivo (33).

Both tumor necrosis factor-α (TNFα) and interferon-γ (IFNγ) stimulate 1,25(OH)$_2$D$_3$ production by keratinocytes (7,34–36) (Fig. 1). These cells are exquisitely sensitive to IFNγ, with maximal stimulation of 1,25(OH)$_2$D$_3$ production at concentrations less than 10 pM. Higher concentrations are inhibitory, but such concentrations also profoundly inhibit the proliferation of these cells and limit their ability to differentiate. Although IFNγ is not made in keratinocytes, TNFα is produced by these cells, and its synthesis is stimulated by ultraviolet light (37) and barrier disruption (38). Thus, environmental perturbations could enhance 1,25(OH)$_2$D$_3$ production in the skin, and the increased levels of 1,25(OH)$_2$D$_3$ could play a role in the recovery from UV damage and/or barrier repair (39).

Keratinocytes from squamous cell carcinomas (SCC) do not differentiate normally in response to calcium (40) or 1,25(OH)$_2$D$_3$ (41) despite having genes for the differentiation markers that can be induced by serum (30). Nevertheless, these cells produce 1,25(OH)$_2$D$_3$ [and 24,25(OH)$_2$D$_3$], and in some cases the rates of production are comparable to those of normal keratinocytes (41). Furthermore, the SCC lines respond to exogenous 1,25(OH)$_2$D$_3$ with a reduction in 1,25(OH)$_2$D$_3$ production and an increase in 24,25(OH)$_2$D$_3$ production, although in some cases the sensitivity of the SCC line to 1,25(OH)$_2$D$_3$ is less than normal (41). The levels of the VDR mRNA and protein in SCC are comparable to those in normal keratinocytes (30), suggesting that the reason why $1,25(OH)_2D_3$ can regulate 25OHD metabolism but not differentiation in SCC lies in other transcription factors required for calcium and $1,25(OH)_2D_3$ regulation of the differentiation pathway. We (42) have recently demonstrated that the coactivator complex binding to the VDR in SCC and proliferating keratinocytes is the VDR interacting protein (DRIP) complex. As keratinocytes differentiate, components of the DRIP complex are no longer produced, whereas steroid receptor coactivator 3 (SRC3) increases in levels and binding from DRIP to SRC3 complex formation with VDR. This transition does not take place in SCC. The 24-hydroxylase gene appears to be activated by VDR bound to either DRIP or SRC3, whereas other vitamin D–regulated genes involved in differentiation (e.g., involucrin) prefer VDR bound to SRC3 (Oda and Bikle, unpublished).

ROLE OF VITAMIN D₃ IN EPIDERMAL DIFFERENTIATION

The Differentiation Process

The epidermis is composed of four layers of keratinocytes at different stages of differentiation. The basal layer (stratum basale) rests on the basal lamina separating the dermis and epidermis. These cells proliferate, providing the cells for the upper differentiating layers. They are large, columnar cells forming intercellular attachments with adjacent cells through desmosomes. An asymmetric distribution of integrins on their lateral and basal surfaces may also regulate their attachment to the basal lamina and adjacent cells (43–45). They contain an extensive keratin network comprising principally keratins K5 (58 kDa) and K14 (50 kDa) (46). By a process that we are only beginning to understand, cells migrate upward from this basal layer, acquiring the characteristics of a fully differentiated corneocyte, which is eventually sloughed off.

The layer above the basal cells is the spinous layer (stratum spinosum). These cells initiate the production of the keratins K1 and K10, which are characteristic of the more differentiated layers of the epidermis (47). Cornified envelope precursors, such as involucrin (48), also appear in the spinous layer as does the enzyme transglutaminase, responsible for the ε-(γ-glutamyl) lysine cross-linking of these substrates into the insoluble cornified envelope (49). The keratinocyte contains both the soluble (tissue, TG-C, or type II) and membrane-bound (particulate, TG-K, or type I) forms of transglutaminase. It is the membrane-bound form that correlates with differentiation and is thought to be responsible for the formation of the cornified envelope (49). The granular layer (stratum granulosum), lying above the spinous layer, is characterized by electron-dense keratohyalin granules. These are of two types (50). The larger of the two granules contains profilaggrin, the precursor of filaggrin, a protein thought to facilitate the aggregation of keratin filaments (51). The smaller granule contains loricrin, a major component of the cornified envelope (52). The granular layer also contains lamellar bodies, lipid-filled structures that fuse with the plasma membrane, divesting their contents into the extracellular space where the lipid contributes to the permeability barrier of skin (53). As the cells pass from the granular layer to the cornified layer (stratum corneum), they undergo destruction of their organelles with further maturation of the cornified envelope into an insoluble, highly resistant structure surrounding the keratin–filaggrin complex and linked to the extracellular lipid milieu (54). Calcium forms a steep gradient within the epidermis, with highest concentration in the stratum granulosum (55). Disruption of the permeability barrier by removing the stratum corneum or by extracting its lipids leads to a loss of this calcium gradient (56) resulting in increased lamellar body secretion, but reduced expression of the genes for loricrin, profilaggrin, and involucrin (57). Both calcium and 1,25(OH)$_2$D$_3$ play important and interacting roles in regulating this differentiation process.

Regulation of Differentiation by Calcium

Calcium is the best-studied pro-differentiating agent for keratinocytes (Fig. 2). In vivo, a calcium gradient exists in the epidermis such that in the basal and spinous layers calcium is primarily intracellular and in low amounts, but in the upper granular layers calcium accumulates in large amounts in the cell and the intercellular matrix (55). This gradient of calcium may provide the driving force for differentiation in intact epidermis (57). However, most of the information regarding calcium-induced differentiation comes from in vitro studies with cultured keratinocytes. In low calcium–containing medium, keratinocytes proliferate readily but differentiate slowly if at all, and remain as a monolayer in culture. On switching the cells to higher calcium concentrations (referred to as the calcium switch), keratinocytes undergo a coordinated set of responses at both the genomic and non-genomic levels that eventuates in a stratified culture in which the cells contain many of the features of the differentiated epidermis.

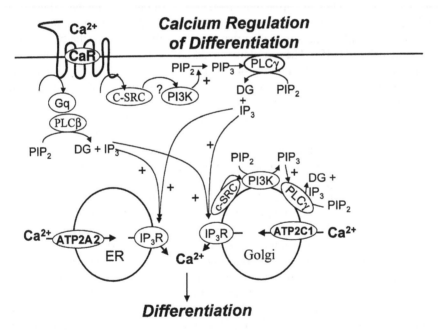

Figure 2 The calcium-sensing mechanism of the keratinocyte. The keratinocyte contains a calcium receptor that increases intracellular calcium by activating phospholipase C-β (PLC-β) via a G-protein–coupled process. Calcium also activates PLC-γ via a mechanism requiring src kinases and phosphatidyl inositol 3 kinase (PI3K). In addition to acutely activating these PLCs, calcium induces their synthesis. Both PLCs hydrolyze phosphatidylinositol bisphosphate (PIP$_2$) to inositol trisphosphate (IP$_3$) and diacylglycerol (DG). IP$_3$ releases calcium (Ca^{2+}) from intracellular stores such as the endoplasmic reticulum (ER) and Golgi apparatus by activating its receptor (IP$_3$R), which functions as a calcium channel in these organelles. Besides the IP$_3$R, the ER and Golgi apparatus each contain organelle-specific calcium pumps (CaATPases) that pump calcium into these organelles. The Golgi apparatus may be at least as critical for calcium signaling in the keratinocyte as the ER.

Response to the Calcium Switch

Within minutes to hours of the calcium switch, morphological changes are apparent, with rapid development of cell-to-cell contact (8), desmosome formation (58), and a realignment of actin and keratin bundles near the cell membrane at the point of intercellular contacts (59). Desmoplakin (a component of desmosomes), fodrin (an actin and calmodulin binding spectrin-like protein), and calmodulin are redistributed to the membrane shortly after the calcium switch by a mechanism that is blocked by cytochalasin, an agent that disrupts microfilament reorganization (59–61). These effects do not appear to be under genomic control, although this has not been tested rigorously. Within hours to days of the calcium switch, the cells begin to make involucrin (9,62,63), loricrin (64), transglutaminase (9,62,63), keratins K1 and K10 (65), and filaggrin (65), and they start to form cornified envelopes (9,65). The mRNA levels of these proteins increase following the calcium switch (62,64,65), indicating that these effects of calcium represent genomic actions, a conclusion confirmed by nuclear run on and promoter construct experiments for many of these genes. Calcium response regions have been identified in the involucrin (66) and K1 (67) genes. The redistribution of integrin isoforms within days following the calcium switch (43,45,68) contributes to the mechanism by which cells begin to stratify.

Regulation of Intracellular Calcium

The mechanisms by which calcium exerts its effects on keratinocyte differentiation are multiple. The intracellular free calcium ion concentration ($[Ca^{2+}]_i$) increases as keratinocytes differentiate, correlating closely with their ability to form cornified envelopes (6). Raising the extracellular calcium concentration ($[Ca^{2+}]_o$) increases $[Ca^{2+}]_i$ (6,61,62,65–67). This response is saturable (6). The response of $[Ca^{2+}]_i$ to $[Ca^{2+}]_o$ is multiphasic and changes with differentiation. In undifferentiated keratinocytes and in transformed keratinocytes that are unable to differentiate, the switch to higher $[Ca^{2+}]_o$ results in an initial spike of $[Ca^{2+}]_i$ that is followed by a plateau level that persists as long as the $[Ca^{2+}]_o$ remains elevated (69–71). As the cells differentiate, this acute response to $[Ca^{2+}]_o$ is lost (70,71). Lanthanum, which blocks calcium entry, blocks this response to $[Ca^{2+}]_o$, indicating that much of the rise in $[Ca^{2+}]_i$ following a change in $[Ca^{2+}]_o$ is dependent on calcium entry (71–74). L-type calcium channel blockers do not prevent the rise in calcium uptake (74). A number of other channels have been identified in the keratinocyte membrane that are candidates for mediating calcium-induced calcium influx (75–79) including trpc channels (Tu and Bikle, unpublished). The prolonged increase in $[Ca^{2+}]_i$ after elevation of $[Ca^{2+}]_o$ stands in contrast to the response of $[Ca^{2+}]_i$ to ATP (80–82). ATP increases $[Ca^{2+}]_i$ acutely and transiently from intracellular stores with less effect on calcium influx. As ATP inhibits rather than promotes keratinocyte differentiation (82), the sustained increase in $[Ca^{2+}]_i$ following the addition of calcium appears to be essential for the differentiation process. 1,25(OH)$_2$D$_3$ enhances the rise in $[Ca^{2+}]_i$ following the calcium switch (6) as will be discussed below.

The Role of the Calcium Receptor

The acute response of the keratinocyte to calcium resembles that of the parathyroid cell (83), which senses $[Ca^{2+}]_o$ via a seven-transmembrane domain, GTP binding protein-coupled calcium receptor (CaR) (84,85). This receptor was originally discovered in the parathyroid gland, but we have identified the same structure in the keratinocyte (71). We (86) also observed that the keratinocyte produces an alternatively spliced variant of the CaR (CaRalt) as it differentiates. CaRalt lacks exon 5 and so would be missing residues 461–537 in the extracellular domain. As mentioned above, keratinocytes lose their ability to sense calcium with differentiation. This change in calcium responsiveness is associated with the switch from the expression of the full-length calcium receptor (CaRfl) to the alternatively spliced form (CaRalt). The currently available mouse model in which CaRfl was knocked out by insertion of a neomycin cassette into exon 5 continues to produce CaRalt (87). The epidermis of this mouse is abnormal, contains markedly lower levels of the terminal differentiation markers loricrin and profilaggrin, and the keratinocytes from this mouse fail to respond to calcium with a substantial rise in Cai indicating that the full length CaR is required for normal epidermal differentiation and calcium signaling (87). These observations have been confirmed in human keratinocytes (88). Thus the switch from CaRfl to CaRalt may be a mechanism by which differentiation reduces the calcium responsiveness of the keratinocyte. $1,25(OH)_2D$ increases the CaR mRNA levels and prevents their decrease with time (89). Furthermore, $1,25(OH)_2D$ potentiates the ability of these cells to respond to $[Ca^{2+}]_o$ with a rise in $[Ca^{2+}]_i$ (6,89). Thus, the CaR appears to be important in mediating the acute response of undifferentiated keratinocytes to $[Ca^{2+}]_o$, one of the mechanisms by which $1,25(OH)_2D_3$ regulates calcium-induced epidermal differentiation.

The Role of Phospholipases

The calcium switch stimulates phospholipase C activity, which provides additional second messengers for mediating the effects of calcium on the keratinocyte (90–93). The main enzymes involved are phospholipase C (PLC)β and γ which hydrolyze phosphatidylinositol bisphosphate (PIP$_2$) to inositol trisphosphate (IP$_3$) and diacylglycerol (DAG). Both calcium and $1,25(OH)_2D$ induce these enzymes (94,95). In addition $1,25(OH)_2D_3$ induces phospholipase D1 (PLD), which hydrolyzes PIP$_2$ to DAG and phosphatidic acid (96). As for the response of $[Ca^{2+}]_i$ to $[Ca^{2+}]_o$, the rise in IP$_3$ and DAG is both immediate and prolonged following the calcium switch. Other agents such as ATP raise IP$_3$ levels at least as effectively as calcium and yet do not stimulate differentiation (82). Just as the rise in $[Ca^{2+}]_i$ after ATP is transient, so is the rise in IP$_3$. Conceivably, the prolonged rise in $[Ca^{2+}]_i$ and IP$_3$ after increases in $[Ca^{2+}]_o$, compared to the transient effects of ATP, contributes to the ability of $[Ca^{2+}]_o$ and not ATP to stimulate differentiation. This prolonged increase in IPs appears to be due to calcium activation of PLC-γ1 (97), although the initial increase in IP$_3$ and $[Ca^{2+}]_i$ after the calcium switch appears to be mediated by PLC-β. This extended activation of PLC-γ1 is mediated by a calcium-induced increase in src family tyrosine kinases (known activators of PLC-γ1) (98–100). The critical role for PLC-γ1 in mediating calcium-induced differentiation is demonstrated by the failure of calcium [or $1,25(OH)_2D_3$] to induce differentiation when PLC-γ1 production is inhibited (95,101). The induction of these phospholipases by $1,25(OH)_2D_3$ as well as by calcium provides another mechanism by which $1,25(OH)_2D_3$ regulates keratinocyte differentiation (94,102).

The Role of Protein Kinase C

The rise in DAG and $[Ca^{2+}]_i$ following the calcium switch results in protein kinase C (PKC) activation. PKC inhibitors block the ability of calcium to promote differentiation (103,104). However, the study of PKC in differentiation is complicated by the large number of isozymes of PKC in the epidermis, most of which are separate gene products and under different modes of regulation and distribution within the epidermis. Mouse and human keratinocytes contain PKC-α, -δ, -ε, -η, and -ζ (105–107). PKC-α is a classic PKC isozyme and is activated by calcium, phorbol esters, and DAG. PKC-δ, -ε, and -η are novel PKCs that are activated by phorbol esters and DAG like the classic PKCs, but are not activated by calcium. PKC-ζ is an atypical PKC that does not respond to calcium or phorbol esters. During the first 48 hours after the calcium switch in mouse keratinocytes, the translocation of PKC-α from the cytosol to the membrane parallels in time the induction of loricrin and profilaggrin (108,109). Blocking the expression of PKC-α with antisense oligonucleotides prevents calcium induction of a number of differentiation markers (108,109). Thus, PKC-α appears to be the major isozyme associated with calcium-induced differentiation, although PKC-δ has also been shown to have an important role (110), and other PKC isozymes have been implicated in the means by which other agents induce keratinocyte differentiation.

The actual mechanism by which PKC regulates differentiation is not clear (73,111–113), although a mechanism involving transcription factors in the fos and jun families acting on their AP-1 sites in the promoter regions of the genes involved with differentiation seems likely. PKC activation leads to a rapid increase in expression of c-fos and c-jun (81,82,114) and increased binding to AP-1 sites as assessed by gel-retardation studies (115). However, c-fos and c-jun are not the only transcription factors capable of binding to AP-1 sites. Other members of the fos and jun families (Fra-1, Fra-2, Jun B, Jun D) have been found in keratinocytes (116), and are differentially distributed throughout the epidermis. The distal AP-1 site in the promoter of the involucrin gene binds Fra-1, Jun B, and Jun D on gel-retardation analysis (117). A dominant negative mutant of c-jun (118), which blocks c-jun/fos-regulated transcriptional activity in AP-1–regulated genes such as prolactin, stimulates transcriptional activity of involucrin gene constructs (119) suggesting that some members of the fos and jun families are playing an inhibitory rather than a stimulatory role in involucrin gene transcription. As both keratin 1 and involucrin contain an AP-1 site within their calcium responsive regions, a role for members of the fos and jun families in calcium-induced differentiation appears likely. As will be discussed in the next section this AP-1 site also is close to the vitamin D response element in the involucrin gene, and when mutated blocks the ability of 1,25(OH)$_2$D$_3$ to induce this gene (120).

1,25(OH)$_2$D-Regulated Proliferation and Differentiation: Interactions with Calcium

The observation that 1,25(OH)$_2$D$_3$ induces keratinocyte differentiation was first made by Hosomi et al. (3), and provided a rationale for the previous and unexpected finding of 1,25(OH)$_2$D$_3$ receptors in the skin (2). As discussed earlier 1,25(OH)$_2$D$_3$ is likely to be an autocrine or a paracrine factor for epidermal differentiation since it is produced by the keratinocyte, but under normal circumstances keratinocyte production of 1,25(OH)$_2$D$_3$ does not appear to contribute to circulating levels (1,19). The receptors for and the production of 1,25(OH)$_2$D$_3$ vary with differentiation (4,121,122) in a manner that suggests feedback regulation; both are reduced in the later stages of differentiation. 1,25(OH)$_2$D$_3$ increases involucrin, transglutaminase activity, and cornified envelope formation at sub-nanomolar concentrations in preconfluent keratinocytes (3,5,6,41,123). At these concentrations, 1,25(OH)$_2$D$_3$

has been found to promote proliferation in some studies (124–126), although the antiproliferative actions are most frequently observed in vitro, especially when concentrations above 10^{-9} M are employed. However, when $1,25(OH)_2D_3$ is applied topically to normal mouse skin, a hyperproliferative response is readily observed (127,128). The mechanisms underlying the proliferative actions are not known. The antiproliferative effects are accompanied by a reduction in the mRNA levels for c-myc (129) and increases in the cell cycle inhibitors $p21^{cip}$ and $p27^{kip}$. Stimulation of differentiation is marked by the rise in mRNA and protein levels of the differentiation markers involucrin and transglutaminase (62).

The mechanisms by which $1,25(OH)_2D_3$ alters keratinocyte differentiation are multiple and overlap with the mechanisms by which calcium regulates differentiation (Fig. 3). The VDR is critical for the genomic actions of $1,25(OH)_2D_3$. An acute increase in $[Ca^{2+}]_i$ associated with an acute increase in phosphoinositide turnover (producing a rise in both IP_3 and DAG) following $1,25(OH)_2D_3$ administration has been observed in several studies (130–134). Not all investigators (including ourselves) have been able to reproduce these acute effects of $1,25(OH)_2D_3$ (71), although a gradual rise in $[Ca^{2+}]_i$ and cornified envelope formation is observed (6). The rise in $[Ca^{2+}]_i$, IP_3, and DAG is accompanied by translocation of PKC to the membrane

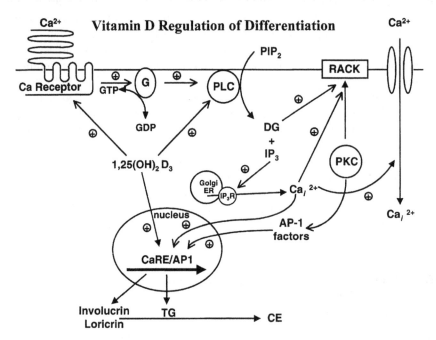

Figure 3 Regulation of keratinocyte differentiation by $1,25(OH)_2D_3$. The calcium receptor and the PLCs are induced by $1,25(OH)_2D_3$, which enhances the ability of calcium to raise intracellular calcium, IP_3, and diacylglycerol (DG) via the mechanisms described in Figure 2. The rise in these second messengers leads to protein kinase activation (PKC) in part by translocation of PKCs to their specific membrane receptors (RACK) and opening up of calcium channels in the plasma membrane. $1,25(OH)_2D_3$ in combination with the increase in intracellular calcium and the AP-1 transcription factors activated by PKC stimulates differentiation by inducing the substrates [e.g., involucrin (Inv) and loricrin] for cornified envelope (CE) formation as well as the enzyme transglutaminase (TG), which cross-links these substrates into the CE.

(132). Down-regulation of PKC and inhibition of its activity have been reported to block the ability of $1,25(OH)_2D_3$ to stimulate cornified envelope formation (132). However, the role of PKC in mediating or interacting with $1,25(OH)_2D_3$ in its effects on keratinocyte differentiation remains virtually unexplored.

Calcium and $1,25(OH)_2D_3$ interact in their ability to inhibit proliferation and stimulate involucrin and transglutaminase gene expression (62). The higher the $[Ca^{2+}]_o$, , the more sensitive is the keratinocyte to the antiproliferative effect of $1,25(OH)_2D_3$ (and vice versa) (123). The interaction on gene expression is more complex. Both calcium [in the absence of $1,25(OH)_2D_3$] and $1,25(OH)_2D_3$ (at $0.03\,\text{mM}$ Ca^{2+}) raise the mRNA levels for involucrin and transglutaminase in a dose-dependent fashion. The stimulation is synergistic at intermediate concentrations of calcium ($0.1\,\text{mM}$) and $1,25(OH)_2D_3$ ($10^{-10}\,\text{M}$), but inhibition is observed in combination at higher concentrations. The synergism is more apparent at earlier times after the calcium switch (four hours) than later (24–72 hours), when increased turnover of the mRNA by the higher combined concentrations of calcium and $1,25(OH)_2D_3$ becomes dominant. This provides a protective mechanism by which excess involucrin and transglutaminase production is prevented in the face of increased calcium and/or $1,25(OH)_2D_3$. At least one explanation for the synergism in the induction of involucrin is that the calcium response element (CaRE) and vitamin D response element (VDRE) in the involucrin promoter are quite close spatially (120). Mutations in the AP-1 site within the CaRE block both calcium and $1,25(OH)_2D_3$ induction of the involucrin gene, but mutations of the VDRE block only its response to $1,25(OH)_2D_3$. The molecular basis for the synergism with respect to transglutaminase induction has not been elucidated.

The recent availability of mice lacking either the VDR or the 25OHD-1α hydroxylase has expanded our understanding of the role of $1,25(OH)_2D_3$ in epidermal differentiation. Although the most striking feature of the VDR-null mouse is the development of alopecia (also found in many patients with mutations in the VDR), these mice also exhibit a defect in epidermal differentiation as shown by reduced levels of involucrin, profilaggrin, and loricrin and loss of keratohyalin granules (135). A different phenotype is observed in the 1α-hydroxylase–null mouse. These mice also show a reduction in levels of the epidermal differentiation markers, but 1α-hydroxylase–null animals do not have a defect in hair follicle cycling (39). Furthermore, the 1α-hydroxylase–null animals have a retarded recovery of barrier function when the barrier is disrupted, which on ultrastructural examination is found to be associated with an impaired re-establishment of the calcium gradient in the epidermis (39). This abnormality in barrier recovery or calcium-gradient formation has not been observed in VDR-null mice. The difference in phenotypes between these genotypes is surprising, and points to the possibility that the 1α-hydroxylase in the epidermis may be doing more than making $1,25(OH)_2D_3$, just as the phenotype in the VDR-null animal suggests that the VDR may have functions independent of $1,25(OH)_2D_3$.

REFERENCES

1. Bikle DD, Nemanic MK, Whitney JO, Elias PW. Neonatal human foreskin keratinocytes produce 1,25-dihydroxyvitamin D3. Biochemistry 1986; 25(7):1545–1548.
2. Stumpf WE, Sar M, Reid FA, Tanaka Y, DeLuca HF. Target cells for 1,25-dihydroxyvitamin D3 in intestinal tract, stomach, kidney, skin, pituitary, and parathyroid. Science 1979; 206(4423):1188–1190.

3. Hosomi J, Hosoi J, Abe E, Suda T, Kuroki T. Regulation of terminal differentiation of cultured mouse epidermal cells by 1 alpha,25-dihydroxyvitamin D3. Endocrinology 1983; 113(6):1950–1957.

4. Pillai S, Bikle DD, Elias PM. 1,25-Dihydroxyvitamin D production and receptor binding in human keratinocytes varies with differentiation. J Biol Chem 1988; 263(11): 5390–5395.

5. Smith EL, Walworth NC, Holick MF. Effect of 1 alpha,25-dihydroxyvitamin D3 on the morphologic and biochemical differentiation of cultured human epidermal keratinocytes grown in serum-free conditions. J Invest Dermatol 1986; 86(6):709–714.

6. Pillai S, Bikle DD. Role of intracellular-free calcium in the cornified envelope formation of keratinocytes: differences in the mode of action of extracellular calcium and 1,25 dihydroxyvitamin D3. J Cell Physiol 1991; 146(1):94–100.

7. Bikle DD, Pillai S, Gee E, Hincenbergs M. Regulation of 1,25-dihydroxyvitamin D production in human keratinocytes by interferon-gamma. Endocrinology 1989; 124(2):655–660.

8. Hennings H, Michael D, Cheng C, Steinert P, Holbrook K, Yuspa SH. Calcium regulation of growth and differentiation of mouse epidermal cells in culture. Cell 1980; 19(1): 245–254.

9. Pillai S, Bikle DD, Mancianti ML, Cline P, Hincenbergs M. Calcium regulation of growth and differentiation of normal human keratinocytes: modulation of differentiation competence by stages of growth and extracellular calcium. J Cell Physiol 1990; 143(2):294–302.

10. Holick MF, Richtand NM, McNeill SC, Holick SA, Henley JW, Potts JT. Isolation and identification of previtamin D3 from the skin of exposed to ultraviolet irradiation. Biochemistry 1979; 18:1003–1008.

11. Holick MF, McLaughlin JA, Clark MB, Holick SA, Potts JT, Anderson RR, Blank IH, Parrish JA, Elias P. Photosynthesis of previtamin D3 in human and the physiologic consequences. Science 1980; 210:203–205.

12. Holick MF, McLaughlin JA, Clark MB, Doppelt SH. Factors that influence the cutaneous photosynthesis of previtamin D3. Science 1981; 211:590–593.

13. Webb AR, DeCosta BR, Holick MF. Sunlight regulates the cutaneous production of vitamin D3 by causing its photodegradation. J Clin Endocrinol Metab 1989; 68(5): 882–887.

14. Bell NH, Greene A, Epstein S, Oexmann MJ, Shaw S, Shary J. Evidence for alteration of the vitamin D-endocrine system in blacks. J Clin Invest 1985; 76(2):470–473.

15. Webb AR, Kline L, Holick MF. Influence of season and latitude on the cutaneous synthesis of vitamin D3: exposure to winter sunlight in Boston and Edmonton will not promote vitamin D3 synthesis in human skin. J Clin Endocrinol Metab 1988; 67(2):373–378.

16. Matsuoka LY, Wortsman J, Dannenberg MJ, Hollis BW, Lu Z, Holick MF. Clothing prevents ultraviolet-B radiation-dependent photosynthesis of vitamin D3. J Clin Endocrinol Metab 1992; 75(4):1099–1103.

17. Matsuoka LY, Ide L, Wortsman J, MacLaughlin JA, Holick MF. Sunscreens suppress cutaneous vitamin D3 synthesis. J Clin Endocrinol Metab 1987; 64(6):1165–1168.

18. Silveira SR, Hadler WA. A histochemical study on the vitamin D synthesis into the epidermis. Acta Histochem 1985; 76(2):225–234.

19. Bikle DD, Nemanic MK, Gee E, Elias P. 1,25-Dihydroxyvitamin D3 production by human keratinocytes. Kinetics and regulation. J Clin Invest 1986; 78(2):557–566.

20. Matsumoto K, Azuma Y, Kiyoki M, Okumura H, Hashimoto K, Yoshikawa K. Involvement of endogenously produced 1,25-dihydroxyvitamin D-3 in the growth and differentiation of human keratinocytes. Biochim Biophys Acta 1991; 1092(3): 311–318.

21. Lehmann B, Genehr T, Knuschke P, Pietzsch J, Meurer M. UVB-induced conversion of 7-dehydrocholesterol to 1 alpha,25-dihydroxyvitamin D3 in an in vitro human skin equivalent model. J Invest Dermatol 2001; 117(5):1179–1185.

22. Lehmann B, Tiebel O, Meurer M. Expression of vitamin D3 25-hydroxylase (CYP27) mRNA after induction by vitamin D3 or UVB radiation in keratinocytes of human skin equivalents—a preliminary study. Arch Dermatol Res 1999; 291(9):507–510.

23. Masumoto O, Ohyama Y, Okuda K. Purification and characterization of vitamin D 25-hydroxylase from rat liver mitochondria. J Biol Chem 1988; 263(28):14256–14260.

24. Fu GK, Lin D, Zhang MY, Bikle DD, Shackleton CH, Miller WL, Portale AA. Cloning of human 25-hydroxyvitamin D-1 alpha-hydroxylase and mutations causing vitamin D-dependent rickets type 1. Mol Endocrinol 1997; 11(13):1961–1970.

25. Barbour GL, Coburn JW, Slatopolsky E, Norman AW, Horst RL. Hypercalcemia in an anephric patient with sarcoidosis: evidence for extrarenal generation of 1,25-dihydroxyvitamin D. N Engl J Med 1981; 305(8):440–443.

26. Lambert PW, Stern PH, Avioli RC, Brackett NC, Turner RT, Greene A, Fu IY, Bell NH. Evidence for extrarenal production of 1 alpha,25-dihydroxyvitamin D in man. J Clin Invest 1982; 69(3):722–725.

27. Littledike ET, Horst RL. Metabolism of vitamin D3 in nephrectomized pigs given pharmacological amounts of vitamin D3. Endocrinology 1982; 111(6):2008–2013.

28. Bikle DD, Halloran BP, Riviere JE. Production of 1,25 dihydroxyvitamin D3 by perfused pig skin. J Invest Dermatol 1994; 102(5):796–798.

29. Xie Z, Munson SJ, Huang N, Portale AA, Miller WL, Bikle DD. The mechanism of 1,25-dihydroxyvitamin D(3) autoregulation in keratinocytes. J Biol Chem 2002; 277(40): 36987–36990.

30. Rasmussen H, Wong M, Bikle D, Goodman DB. Hormonal control of the renal conversion of 25-hydroxycholecalciferol to 1,25-dihydroxycholecalciferol. J Clin Invest 1972; 51(9):2502–2504.

31. Rost CR, Bikle DD, Kaplan RA. In vitro stimulation of 25-hydroxycholecalciferol 1 alpha-hydroxylation by parathyroid hormone in chick kidney slices: evidence for a role for adenosine 3′,5′-monophosphate. Endocrinology 1981; 108(3):1002–1006.

32. Pillai S, Bikle DD, Hincenbergs M, Elias PM. Biochemical and morphological characterization of growth and differentiation of normal human neonatal keratinocytes in a serum-free medium. J Cell Physiol 1988; 134(2):229–237.

33. Zehnder D, Bland R, Williams MC, McNinch RW, Howie AJ, Stewart PM, Hewison M. Extrarenal expression of 25-hydroxyvitamin d(3)-1 alpha-hydroxylase. J Clin Endocrinol Metab 2001; 86(2):888–894.

34. Morhenn VB, Wood GS. Gamma interferon-induced expression of class II major histocompatibility complex antigens by human keratinocytes. Effects of conditions of culture. Ann NY Acad Sci 1988; 548:321–330.

35. Pillai S, Bikle DD, Eessalu TE, Aggarwal BB, Elias PM. Binding and biological effects of tumor necrosis factor alpha on cultured human neonatal foreskin keratinocytes. J Clin Invest 1989; 83(3):816–821.

36. Bikle DD, Pillai S, Gee E, Hincenbergs M. Tumor necrosis factor-alpha regulation of 1,25-dihydroxyvitamin D production by human keratinocytes. Endocrinology 1991; 129(1):33–38.

37. Trefzer U, Brockhaus M, Lotscher H, Parlow F, Budnik A, Grewe M, Christoph H, Kapp A, Schopf E, Luger TA, et al. The 55-kDa tumor necrosis factor receptor on human keratinocytes is regulated by tumor necrosis factor-alpha and by ultraviolet B radiation. J Clin Invest 1993; 92(1):462–470.

38. Wood LC, Elias PM, Sequeira-Martin SM, Grunfeld C, Feingold KR. Occlusion lowers cytokine mRNA levels in essential fatty acid-deficient and normal mouse epidermis, but not after acute barrier disruption. J Invest Dermatol 1994; 103(6):834–838.

39. Bikle DD, Chang S, Crumrine D, Elalieh H, Man MQ, Choi EH, Dardenne O, Xie Z, St-Arnaud R, Feingold K, Elias PM. 25 Hydroxyvitamin D 1 alpha-hydroxylase is required for optimal epidermal differentiation and permeability barrier homeostasis. J Invest Dermatol 2004; 122:984–992.

40. Rheinwald JG, Beckett MA. Defective terminal differentiation in culture as a consistent and selectable character of malignant human keratinocytes. Cell 1980; 22(2 Pt 2):629–632.

41. Bikle DD, Pillai S, Gee E. Squamous carcinoma cell lines produce 1,25 dihydroxy-vitamin D, but fail to respond to its prodifferentiating effect. J Invest Dermatol 1991; 97(3):435–441.

42. Oda Y, Sihlbom C, Huang L, Rachez C, Chang CP, Burlingame AL, Freedman LP, Bikle D. Sequential utilization of the VDR coactivators, DRIP/Mediator and SRC/p160, during keratinocyte differentiation. Mol Endocrinol 2003; 17:2329–2339.

43. Marchisio PC, Bondanza S, Cremona O, Cancedda R, De Luca M. Polarized expression of integrin receptors (alpha 6 beta 4, alpha 2 beta 1, alpha 3 beta 1, and alpha v beta 5) and their relationship with the cytoskeleton and basement membrane matrix in cultured human keratinocytes. J Cell Biol 1991; 112(4):761–773.

44. Peltonen J, Larjava H, Jaakkola S, Gralnick H, Akiyama SK, Yamada SS, Yamada KM, Uitto J. Localization of integrin receptors for fibronectin, collagen, and laminin in human skin. Variable expression in basal and squamous cell carcinomas. J Clin Invest 1989; 84(6):1916–1923.

45. Guo M, Kim LT, Akiyama SK, Gralnick HR, Yamada KM, Grinnell F. Altered processing of integrin receptors during keratinocyte activation. Exp Cell Res 1991; 195(2):315–322.

46. Moll R, Franke WW, Schiller DL, Geiger B, Krepler R. The catalog of human cyto-keratins: patterns of expression in normal epithelia, tumors and cultured cells. Cell 1982; 31(1):11–24.

47. Eichner R, Sun TT, Aebi U. The role of keratin subfamilies and keratin pairs in the formation of human epidermal intermediate filaments. J Cell Biol 1986; 102(5): 1767–1777.

48. Warhol MJ, Roth J, Lucocq JM, Pinkus GS, Rice RH. Immuno-ultrastructural locali-zation of involucrin in squamous epithelium and cultured keratinocytes. J Histochem Cytochem 1985; 33(2):141–149.

49. Thacher SM, Rice RH. Keratinocyte-specific transglutaminase of cultured human epidermal cells: relation to cross-linked envelope formation and terminal differentiation. Cell 1985; 40(3):685–695.

50. Steven AC, Bisher ME, Roop DR, Steinert PM. Biosynthetic pathways of filaggrin and loricrin—two major proteins expressed by terminally differentiated epidermal keratino-cytes. J Struct Biol 1990; 104(1–3):150–162.

51. Dale BA, Resing KA, Lonsdale-Eccles JD. Filaggrin: a keratin filament associated protein. Ann NY Acad Sci 1985; 455:330–342.

52. Mehrel T, Hohl D, Rothnagel JA, Longley MA, Bundman D, Cheng C, Lichti U, Bisher ME, Steven AC, Steinert PM, et al. Identification of a major keratinocyte cell envelope protein, loricrin. Cell 1990; 61(6):1103–1112.

53. Elias PM, Menon GK, Grayson S, Brown BE. Membrane structural alterations in murine stratum corneum: relationship to the localization of polar lipids and phospho-lipases. J Invest Dermatol 1988; 91(1):3–10.

54. Hohl D. Cornified cell envelope. Dermatologica 1990; 180(4):201–211.

55. Menon GK, Grayson S, Elias PM. Ionic calcium reservoirs in mammalian epidermis: ultrastructural localization by ion-capture cytochemistry. J Invest Dermatol 1985; 84(6): 508–512.

56. Mauro T, Bench G, Sidderas-Haddad E, Feingold K, Elias P, Cullander C. Acute barrier perturbation abolishes the Ca^{2+} and K^+ gradients in murine epidermis: quantitative measurement using PIXE. J Invest Dermatol 1998; 111(6):1198–1201.

57. Elias PM, Ahn SK, Denda M, Brown BE, Crumrine D, Kimutai LK, Komuves L, Lee SH, Feingold KR. Modulations in epidermal calcium regulate the expression of differentiation-specific markers. J Invest Dermatol 2002; 119(5):1128–1136.

58. Hennings H, Holbrook KA. Calcium regulation of cell–cell contact and differentiation of epidermal cells in culture. An ultrastructural study. Exp Cell Res 1983; 143(1):127–142.
59. Zamansky GB, Nguyen U, Chou IN. An immunofluorescence study of the calcium-induced coordinated reorganization of microfilaments, keratin intermediate filaments, and microtubules in cultured human epidermal keratinocytes. J Invest Dermatol 1991; 97(6):985–994.
60. Inohara S, Tatsumi Y, Cho H, Tanaka Y, Sagami S. Actin filament and desmosome formation in cultured human keratinocytes. Arch Dermatol Res 1990; 282(3):210–212.
61. Yoneda K, Fujimoto T, Imanura S, Ogawa K. Fodrin is localized in the cytoplasm of keratinocytes cultured in low calcium medium: immunoelectron microscopic study. Acta Histochem Cytochem 1990; 23:139–148.
62. Su MJ, Bikle DD, Mancianti ML, Pillai S. 1,25-Dihydroxyvitamin D3 potentiates the keratinocyte response to calcium. J Biol Chem 1994; 269(20):14723–14729.
63. Rubin AL, Parenteau NL, Rice RH. Coordination of keratinocyte programming in human SCC-13 squamous carcinoma and normal epidermal cells. J Cell Physiol 1989; 138(1):208–214.
64. Hohl D, Lichti U, Breitkreutz D, Steinert PM, Roop DR. Transcription of the human loricrin gene in vitro is induced by calcium and cell density and suppressed by retinoic acid. J Invest Dermatol 1991; 96(4):414–418.
65. Yuspa SH, Kilkenny AE, Steinert PM, Roop DR. Expression of murine epidermal differentiation markers is tightly regulated by restricted extracellular calcium concentrations in vitro. J Cell Biol 1989; 109(3):1207–1217.
66. Ng DC, Su MJ, Kim R, Bikle DD. Regulation of involucrin gene expression by calcium in normal human keratinocytes. Front Biosci 1996; 1:a16–a24.
67. Huff CA, Yuspa SH, Rosenthal D. Identification of control elements 3' to the human keratin 1 gene that regulate cell type and differentiation-specific expression. J Biol Chem 1993; 268(1):377–384.
68. Ryynanen J, Jaakkola S, Engvall E, Peltonen J, Uitto J. Expression of beta 4 integrins in human skin: comparison of epidermal distribution with beta 1-integrin epitopes, and modulation by calcium and vitamin D3 in cultured keratinocytes. J Invest Dermatol 1991; 97(3):562–567.
69. Hennings H, Kruszewski FH, Yuspa SH, Tucker RW. Intracellular calcium alterations in response to increased external calcium in normal and neoplastic keratinocytes. Carcinogenesis 1989; 10(4):777–780.
70. Kruszewski FH, Hennings H, Tucker RW, Yuspa SH. Differences in the regulation of intracellular calcium in normal and neoplastic keratinocytes are not caused by ras gene mutations. Cancer Res 1991; 51(16):4206–4212.
71. Bikle DD, Ratnam A, Mauro T, Harris J, Pillai S. Changes in calcium responsiveness and handling during keratinocyte differentiation. Potential role of the calcium receptor. J Clin Invest 1996; 97(4):1085–1093.
72. Pillai S, Bikle DD. Lanthanum influx into cultured human keratinocytes: effect on calcium flux and terminal differentiation. J Cell Physiol 1992; 151(3):623–629.
73. Schlessinger J. Allosteric regulation of the epidermal growth factor receptor kinase. J Cell Biol 1986; 103(6 Pt 1):2067–2072.
74. Reiss M, Lipsey LR, Zhou ZL. Extracellular calcium-dependent regulation of transmembrane calcium fluxes in murine keratinocytes. J Cell Physiol 1991; 147(2):281–291.
75. Galietta LJ, Barone V, De Luca M, Romeo G. Characterization of chloride and cation channels in cultured human keratinocytes. Pflugers Arch 1991; 418(1–2):18–25.
76. Mauro TM, Pappone PA, Isseroff RR. Extracellular calcium affects the membrane currents of cultured human keratinocytes. J Cell Physiol 1990; 143(1):13–20.
77. Mauro TM, Isseroff RR, Lasarow R, Pappone PA. Ion channels are linked to differentiation in keratinocytes. J Membr Biol 1993; 132(3):201–209.

78. Grando SA, Horton RM, Mauro TM, Kist DA, Lee TX, Dahl MV. Activation of keratinocyte nicotinic cholinergic receptors stimulates calcium influx and enhances cell differentiation. J Invest Dermatol 1996; 107(3):412–418.

79. Oda Y, Timpe LC, McKenzie RC, Sauder DN, Largman C, Mauro T. Alternatively spliced forms of the cGMP-gated channel in human keratinocytes. FEBS Lett 1997; 414(1):140–145.

80. Pillai S, Bikle DD, Mancianti ML, Hincenbergs M. Uncoupling of the calcium-sensing mechanism and differentiation in squamous carcinoma cell lines. Exp Cell Res 1991; 192(2):567–573.

81. Holladay K, Fujiki H, Bowden GT. Okadaic acid induces the expression of both early and secondary response genes in mouse keratinocytes. Mol Carcinog 1992; 5(1): 16–24.

82. Bollag WB, Xiong Y, Ducote J, Harmon CS. Regulation of fos-lacZ fusion gene expression in primary mouse epidermal keratinocytes isolated from transgenic mice. Biochem J 1994; 300(Pt 1):263–270.

83. Nemeth EF, Scarpa A. Rapid mobilization of cellular Ca^{2+} in bovine parathyroid cells evoked by extracellular divalent cations. Evidence for a cell surface calcium receptor. J Biol Chem 1987; 262(11):5188–5196.

84. Brown EM, Gamba G, Riccardi D, Lombardi M, Butters R, Kifor O, Sun A, Hediger MA, Lytton J, Hebert SC. Cloning and characterization of an extracellular Ca^{2+}-sensing receptor from bovine parathyroid. Nature 1993; 366(6455):575–580.

85. Garrett JE, Capuano IV, Hammerland LG, Hung BC, Brown EM, Hebert SC, Nemeth EF, Fuller F. Molecular cloning and functional expression of human parathyroid calcium receptor cDNAs. J Biol Chem 1995; 270(21):12919–12925.

86. Oda Y, Tu CL, Pillai S, Bikle DD. The calcium sensing receptor and its alternatively spliced form in keratinocyte differentiation. J Biol Chem 1998; 273(36): 23344–23352.

87. Oda Y, Tu CL, Chang W, Crumrine D, Kömüves L, Mauro T, Elias PM, Bikle DD. The calcium sensing receptor and its alternatively spliced form in murine epidermal differentiation. J Biol Chem 2000; 275(2):1183–1190.

88. Tu CL, Chang W, Bikle DD. The extracellular calcium-sensing receptor is required for calcium-induced differentiation in human keratinocytes. J Biol Chem 2001; 276(44): 41079–41085.

89. Ratnam AV, Cho JK, Bikle DD. 1,25-dihydroxyvitamin D3 enhances the calcium response of keratinocytes. J Invest Dermatol 1996; 106:910.

90. Jaken S, Yuspa SH. Early signals for keratinocyte differentiation: role of Ca^{2+}-mediated inositol lipid metabolism in normal and neoplastic epidermal cells. Carcinogenesis 1988; 9(6):1033–1038.

91. Tang W, Ziboh VA, Isseroff R, Martinez D. Turnover of inositol phospholipids in cultured murine keratinocytes: possible involvement of inositol triphosphate in cellular differentiation. J Invest Dermatol 1988; 90(1):37–43.

92. Moscat J, Fleming TP, Molloy CJ, Lopez-Barahona M, Aaronson SA. The calcium signal for Balb/MK keratinocyte terminal differentiation induces sustained alterations in phosphoinositide metabolism without detectable protein kinase C activation. J Biol Chem 1989; 264(19):11228–11235.

93. Lee E, Yuspa SH. Aluminum fluoride stimulates inositol phosphate metabolism and inhibits expression of differentiation markers in mouse keratinocytes. J Cell Physiol 1991; 148(1):106–115.

94. Pillai S, Bikle DD, Su MJ, Ratnam A, Abe J. 1,25-Dihydroxyvitamin D3 upregulates the phosphatidylinositol signaling pathway in human keratinocytes by increasing phospholipase C levels. J Clin Invest 1995; 96(1):602–609.

95. Xie Z, Bikle DD. Phospholipase C-gamma1 is required for calcium-induced keratinocyte differentiation. J Biol Chem 1999; 274(29):20421–20424.

96. Griner RD, Qin F, Jung E, Sue-Ling CK, Crawford KB, Mann-Blakeney R, Bollag RJ, Bollag WB. 1,25-dihydroxyvitamin D3 induces phospholipase D-1 expression in primary mouse epidermal keratinocytes. J Biol Chem 1999; 274(8):4663–4670.

97. Punnonen K, Denning M, Lee E, Li L, Rhee SG, Yuspa SH. Keratinocyte differentiation is associated with changes in the expression and regulation of phospholipase C isoenzymes. J Invest Dermatol 1993; 101(5):719–726.

98. Carpenter G, Ji Q. Phospholipase C-gamma as a signal-transducing element. Exp Cell Res 1999; 253(1):15–24.

99. Calautti E, Missero C, Stein PL, Ezzell RM, Dotto GP. Fyn tyrosine kinase is involved in keratinocyte differentiation control. Genes Dev 1995; 9(18):2279–2291.

100. Zhao Y, Sudol M, Hanafusa H, Krueger J. Increased tyrosine kinase activity of c-Src during calcium-induced keratinocyte differentiation. Proc Natl Acad Sci USA 1992; 89(17):8298–8302.

101. Xie Z, Bikle DD. Inhibition of 1,25-dihydroxyvitamin-D-induced keratinocyte differentiation by blocking the expression of phospholipase C-gamma1. J Invest Dermatol 2001; 117(5):1250–1254.

102. Xie Z, Bikle DD. Cloning of the human phospholipase C-gamma1 promoter and identification of a DR6-type vitamin D-responsive element. J Biol Chem 1997; 272(10): 6573–6577.

103. Dlugosz AA, Yuspa SH. Protein kinase C regulates keratinocyte transglutaminase (TG-K) gene expression in cultured primary mouse epidermal keratinocytes induced to terminally differentiate by calcium. J Invest Dermatol 1994; 102(4):409–414.

104. Matsui MS, Illarda I, Wang N, DeLeo VA. Protein kinase C agonist and antagonist effects in normal human epidermal keratinocytes. Exp Dermatol 1993; 2(6): 247–256.

105. Dlugosz AA, Mischak H, Mushinski JF, Yuspa SH. Transcripts encoding protein kinase C-alpha, -delta, -epsilon, -zeta, and -eta are expressed in basal and differentiating mouse keratinocytes in vitro and exhibit quantitative changes in neoplastic cells. Mol Carcinog 1992; 5(4):286–292.

106. Reynolds NJ, Baldassare JJ, Henderson PA, Shuler JL, Ballas LM, Burns DJ, Moomaw CR, Fisher GJ. Translocation and downregulation of protein kinase C isoenzymes-alpha and -epsilon by phorbol ester and bryostatin-1 in human keratinocytes and fibroblasts. J Invest Dermatol 1994; 103(3):364–369.

107. Fisher GJ, Tavakkol A, Leach K, Burns D, Basta P, Loomis C, Griffiths CE, Cooper KD, Reynolds NJ, Elder JT, et al. Differential expression of protein kinase C isoenzymes in normal and psoriatic adult human skin: reduced expression of protein kinase C-beta II in psoriasis. J Invest Dermatol 1993; 101(4):553–559.

108. Denning MF, Dlugosz AA, Williams EK, Szallasi Z, Blumberg PM, Yuspa SH. Specific protein kinase C isozymes mediate the induction of keratinocyte differentiation markers by calcium. Cell Growth Differ 1995; 6(2):149–157.

109. Yang LC, Ng DC, Bikle DD. Role of protein kinase C alpha in calcium induced keratinocyte differentiation: defective regulation in squamous cell carcinoma. J Cell Physiol 2003; 195(2):249–259.

110. Deucher A, Efimova T, Eckert RL. Calcium-dependent involucrin expression is inversely regulated by protein kinase C (PKC) alpha and PKC delta. J Biol Chem 2002; 277(19):17032–17040.

111. Downward J, Waterfield MD, Parker PJ. Autophosphorylation and protein kinase C phosphorylation of the epidermal growth factor receptor. Effect on tyrosine kinase activity and ligand binding affinity. J Biol Chem 1985; 260(27):14538–14546.

112. Kolch W, Heidecker G, Kochs G, Hummel R, Vahidi H, Mischak H, Finkenzeller G, Marme D, Rapp UR. Protein kinase C alpha activates RAF-1 by direct phosphorylation. Nature 1993; 364(6434):249–252.

113. Goode N, Hughes K, Woodgett JR, Parker PJ. Differential regulation of glycogen synthase kinase-3 beta by protein kinase C isotypes. J Biol Chem 1992; 267(24): 16878–16882.

114. Yaar M, Gilani A, DiBenedetto PJ, Harkness DD, Gilchrest BA. Gene modulation accompanying differentiation of normal versus malignant keratinocytes. Exp Cell Res 1993; 206(2):235–243.

115. Stanwell C, Denning MF, Rutberg SE, Cheng C, Yuspa SH, Dlugosz AA. Staurosporine induces a sequential program of mouse keratinocyte terminal differentiation through activation of PKC isozymes. J Invest Dermatol 1996; 106(3):482–489.

116. Welter JF, Eckert RL. Differential expression of the fos and jun family members c-fos, fosB, Fra-1, Fra-2, c-jun, junB and junD during human epidermal keratinocyte differentiation. Oncogene 1995; 11(12):2681–2687.

117. Welter JF, Crish JF, Agarwal C, Eckert RL. Fos-related antigen (Fra-1), junB, and junD activate human involucrin promoter transcription by binding to proximal and distal AP1 sites to mediate phorbol ester effects on promoter activity. J Biol Chem 1995; 270(21):12614–12622.

118. Forman BM, Casanova J, Raaka BM, Ghysdael J, Samuels HH. Half-site spacing and orientation determines whether thyroid hormone and retinoic acid receptors and related factors bind to DNA response elements as monomers, homodimers, or heterodimers. Mol Endocrinol 1992; 6(3):429–442.

119. Ng DC, Shafaee S, Lee D, Bikle DD. Requirement of an AP-1 site in the calcium response region of the involucrin promoter. J Biol Chem 2000; 275(31):24080–24088.

120. Bikle DD, Ng D, Oda Y, Hanley K, Feingold K, Xie Z. The vitamin D response element of the involucrin gene mediates its regulation by 1,25-dihydroxyvitamin D3. J Invest Dermatol 2002; 119(5):1109–1113.

121. Horiuchi N, Clemens TL, Schiller AL, Holick MF. Detection and developmental changes of the 1,25-(OH)2-D3 receptor concentration in mouse skin and intestine. J Invest Dermatol 1985; 84(6):461–464.

122. Merke J, Schwittay D, Furstenberger G, Gross M, Marks F, Ritz E. Demonstration and characterization of 1,25-dihydroxyvitamin D3 receptors in basal cells of epidermis of neonatal and adult mice. Calcif Tissue Int 1985; 37(3):257–267.

123. McLane JA, Katz M, Abdelkader N. Effect of 1,25-dihydroxyvitamin D3 on human keratinocytes grown under different culture conditions. In Vitro Cell Dev Biol 1990; 26(4):379–387.

124. Bollag WB, Ducote J, Harmon CS. Biphasic effect of 1,25-dihydroxyvitamin D3 on primary mouse epidermal keratinocyte proliferation. J Cell Physiol 1995; 163(2): 248–256.

125. Itin PH, Pittelkow MR, Kumar R. Effects of vitamin D metabolites on proliferation and differentiation of cultured human epidermal keratinocytes grown in serum-free or defined culture medium. Endocrinology 1994; 135(5):1793–1798.

126. Gniadecki R. Stimulation versus inhibition of keratinocyte growth by 1,25-Dihydroxyvitamin D3: dependence on cell culture conditions. J Invest Dermatol 1996; 106(3):510–516.

127. Gniadecki R, Gniadecka M, Serup J. The effects of KH 1060, a potent 20-epi analogue of the vitamin D3 hormone, on hairless mouse skin in vivo. Br J Dermatol 1995; 132(6):841–852.

128. Lutzow-Holm C, Heyden A, Huitfeldt HS, Brandtzaeg P, Clausen OP. Topical application of calcitriol alters expression of filaggrin but not keratin K1 in mouse epidermis. Arch Dermatol Res 1995; 287(5):480–487.

129. Matsumoto K, Hashimoto K, Nishida Y, Hashiro M, Yoshikawa K. Growth-inhibitory effects of 1,25-dihydroxyvitamin D3 on normal human keratinocytes cultured in serum-free medium. Biochem Biophys Res Commun 1990; 166(2):916–923.

130. Tang W, Ziboh VA, Isseroff RR, Martinez D. Novel regulatory actions of 1 alpha, 25-dihydroxyvitamin D3 on the metabolism of polyphosphoinositides in murine epidermal keratinocytes. J Cell Physiol 1987; 132(1):131–136.

131. McLaughlin JA, Cantley LC, Holick MF. 1,25(OH)2D3 increased calcium and phosphatidylinositol metabolism in differentiating cultured human keratinocytes. J Nutr Biochem 1990; 1:81–87.

132. Yada Y, Ozeki T, Meguro S, Mori S, Nozawa Y. Signal transduction in the onset of terminal keratinocyte differentiation induced by 1 alpha,25-dihydroxyvitamin D3: role of protein kinase C translocation. Biochem Biophys Res Commun 1989; 163(3): 1517–1522.

133. Tang W, Ziboh VA. Agonist/inositol trisphosphate-induced release of calcium from murine keratinocytes: a possible link with keratinocyte differentiation. J Invest Dermatol 1991; 96(1):134–138.

134. Bittiner B, Bleehen SS, MacNeil S. 1 alpha, 25(OH)2 vitamin D3 increases intracellular calcium in human keratinocytes. Br J Dermatol 1991; 124(3):230–235.

135. Xie Z, Komuves L, Yu QC, Elalieh H, Ng DC, Leary C, Chang S, Crumrine D, Yoshizawa T, Kato S, Bikle DD. Lack of the vitamin D receptor is associated with reduced epidermal differentiation and hair follicle growth. J Invest Dermatol 2002; 118(1):11–16.

26

Diseases That Affect Barrier Function

Hachiro Tagami and Katsuko Kikuchi
Department of Dermatology, Tohoku University School of Medicine, Sendai, Japan

INTRODUCTION

To sustain life, all of our body organs and tissues must be soaked in tissue fluid, and our body should be covered with a barrier that prevents water loss. The raison d'etre of the skin on our body surface is to produce the stratum corneum (SC) barrier that protects our body from desiccation (1). Just imagine clinical situations in which the skin surface is extensively lacking, such as pemphigus vulgaris, epidermolysis bullosa, toxic epidermal necrolysis, or burn. They all present a serious problem for survival.

In a similar fashion, our body is protected efficiently by this barrier from the invasion of various injurious agents such as pathogenic microorganisms, poisonous chemicals, air pollution, and even the ultraviolet (UV) rays of sunlight. Thus, the presence of SC is essential for our terrestrial life.

Despite its extremely thin structure with a thickness of less than $20\,\mu$, SC is such an efficient biological barrier that it allows even water passage only at a low level that is just slightly higher than that occurring through thin polyethylene film, which is used to protect fresh food from becoming dry in our daily life.

SC is comprised of a two-compartment system, i.e., corneocytes that are flattened dead cell bodies of keratinocytes covered by a tough, highly cross-linked protein, cornified envelope, and an extracellular matrix filled with lipid lamellae (2). The latter consists of roughly equimolar concentrations of ceramides, long-chain free fatty acids, and cholesterol released from lamellar bodies of the uppermost keratinocytes in the stratum granulosum. The ceramides are released as the precursors, glucocylceramides, from the lamellar bodies together with hydrolytic catabolic enzymes that are essential for subsequent establishment of structural and functional integrity of the SC.

Epidermosides are also released as precursors to ω-hydroxyceramides, the largest molecules among the ceramides that covalently bind to involucrin, composing the cornified envelopes of maturated corneocytes to form a hydrophobic cornified lipid envelope in the SC (3). The lipids bound to the cornified envelopes act as a template for lamellar lipid organization that endows the SC with an effective barrier function (4). For the production of a fully maturated cornified lipid envelope, quite a slow and steady differentiation process is required for the epidermis. However, in general, dermatoses are accompanied by enhanced proliferation of the epidermis, which accelerates its slow and steady keratinization process. Therefore, there develops an impairment in the SC barrier function in most skin diseases.

Because of the hydrophobic nature of the cornified lipid envelope which is highly impermeable to diffusing substances, a main penetration pathway of substances through the SC is located in the tortuous intercellular lipid matrix.

Most of the body regions are covered with SC composed of about 14 tightly stacked layers of corneocytes, except for certain locations such as the face and genitalia or the palms and soles; in the former the SC is extremely thin, less than 10 cell layers, and in the latter it is remarkably thick consisting of more than 50 cell layers (5). An effete fraction of the most superficial parts of the SC is shed daily at a rate that balances de novo production of functionally efficient corneocytes to keep the SC thickness fairly constant at a given body site. Because it takes about two weeks for the replacement of the whole SC layers in normal skin of the trunk and limbs (6), the desquamation proceeds there at a rate of more or less one cell layer per day. It occurs invisibly from a normal skin surface with shedding of individual cells, thus maintaining the smooth appearance of healthy skin. It is regulated by proteolytic enzyme degradation of corneodesmosomes that attach corneocytes to each other (7). If this desquamating process is affected in pathologic conditions, there develops a hyperkeratotic condition, which is observed in most skin diseases.

All the pathological events that are induced in the epidermis by skin diseases lead to an abnormal SC barrier function, which can now be evaluated easily in vivo by using biophysical measurements in a quantitative fashion.

IN VIVO FUNCTIONAL ASSESSMENT OF THE SC BARRIER

The SC of the trunk and limbs is such an efficient barrier that it hardly allows even the passage of small molecules like water. There is only 3 to $6 \, g/hour/m^2$ of transepidermal water loss (TEWL). In the skin lesions such as the completely tape-stripped skin surface that totally lack the SC, TEWL reaches a level of $70 \, g/hour/m^2$, which is comparable to the value recorded just above a water surface. Thus, TEWL measurement is a convenient way to evaluate the extent of SC barrier dysfunction.

TEWL can be measured with commercially available biophysical instruments that are equipped with an open chamber to estimate a water vapor pressure gradient present above the skin surface (8). The measurement should be conducted in a cool environment, of less than 22°C, to prevent sweating. When measured under such conditions, TEWL demonstrates a significant linear relationship with percutaneous absorption of various chemicals (9).

However, we should be careful of the data collection from areas such as the forehead, axilla, and palmo-plantar skin, because there may occur mental sweating even in a cool environment. In those who have localized hyperhidrosis in these areas, pretreatment with an antiperspirant, either topical or systemic, is required.

The SC barrier function is not uniform over the body, but there are great location-dependent differences. Among them, the face is unique, because it is covered with relatively thin SC (5). Its TEWL values range from 10 to $15 \, g/hour/m^2$ even in healthy individuals. These values are comparable to those recorded on moderately inflamed skin lesions of psoriasis or those of atopic dermatitis (AD) existing on the trunks and limbs. Thus, the facial skin easily develops visible or invisible contact dermatitis with various irritants or contact allergens from the environment. From the fact that the face is always exposed to a variety of environmental assaults such as the hot summer sunshine, cold and dry winter air, dust, and even cosmetics, the attenuation of the SC barrier function to this level does not seem to cause too much inconvenience in our daily life. It seems likely that this level of SC barrier function is sufficient for us to lead our terrestrial life.

It is also experimentally confirmed that whenever our SC sustains severe damage, the epidermis quickly restores its basal barrier function near to this level within four days (10).

However, when any potent topical agents are applied continuously on the skin equipped with such a level of barrier function, there is a possibility for the skin to develop a side effect. Hence, even in normal healthy individuals, the facial skin easily develops steroid rosacea or steroid acne after an inadvertently prolonged application of potent topical corticosteroids. Likewise, when patients' skin is diffusely covered with functionally deficient SC, serious systemic side effects may ensue after their extensive application. For example, adrenocortical suppression is observed in patients with erythroderma following prolonged application of potent topical steroids. Systemic intoxication of salicylate or lindane may occur after their diffuse application in neonates with lamellar ichthyosis.

A much poorer barrier function is observed at the sites where mucosal surfaces are directly exposed to the outside. For example, TEWL recorded on the vermilion border of the lip reaches a level almost three times higher than that of normal facial skin. It far exceeds those TEWL levels recorded on the lesional skin of acute and severe dermatitis (11). However, the area of the mucosal surfaces is too limited in our body surface to cause any serious problems in normal individuals.

Incidentally, the measurements of TEWL on the lips are only possible with the usage of an instrument that is equipped with a probe consisting of a closed chamber instead of the conventional open chamber, because the former is not influenced by the airflow caused by breathing. In general, TEWL values tend to decrease with age at any anatomic sites of the body. Such a tendency is much more prominent on the vermilion border of the lip (11).

MEASUREMENTS OF SKIN SURFACE HYDRATION STATE

The SC performs another important function on our skin surface. It keeps our skin smooth and flexible by holding water even in an extremely dry environment (12). This hydration also allows intracorneal enzymes to facilitate SC maturation and desquamation.

Poor water-holding capacity of pathologic SC easily allows the development of cracking or fissures in the dry and firm skin surface that permits permeation of even large proteinaceous molecules of aero-allergens or the invasion of microorganisms as noted in scratched skin.

There is a water gradient from the lowermost cell layer to the top one of the SC (13). The deepermost portion of the SC that faces the fully hydrated viable epidermal tissue is well hydrated, whereas the uppermost portion is much less hydrated because it is exposed to the dry atmosphere. We can instantly assess the skin surface hydration state in vivo by using a biophysical method that utilizes high frequency impedance measurements (13). High frequency conductometry is more suitable for measurements of a hydrated state of the skin such as that induced by the application of moisturizers. In contrast, capacitance measurements are more sensitive for dry skin conditions noted in various scaly dermatoses (14,15). Capacitance values recorded on the palms and soles or even on erosive lesions are remarkably low, despite the fact that their skin surface is well hydrated (13).

The components of the SC, especially highly hygroscopic glycerol derived from sebum, water-soluble amino acids (natural moisturizing factor) produced by enzymatic degradation of filaggrin, and keratin fibers, bind water, whereas the lamellar intercellular lipids prevent easy passage of water through the SC (12,16–18).

In general, inflammatory skin lesions involving the epidermis are covered with dry scales that show poor water-holding capacity in proportion to their severity (19). In such skin lesions, we can also detect an increase in TEWL depending on the severity of inflammation; there develops an inverse relationship between TEWL and high frequency impedance levels (10).

Nevertheless, these two functional properties of the SC, namely barrier function and water-holding capacity, are not always intercorrelated. One such example is found when the inflammatory changes affect only the dermal tissue as in fresh scars. In this case, there occurs an increase in both TEWL and skin surface hydration (20). Another example is observed when these measurements are performed on the palmo-plantar skin. These locations are distinct from other anatomic sites, because they are covered with remarkably thick but highly water-permeable SC as compared with that in other locations to prevent the skin surface from developing dry, hard, and friable changes which may easily produce deep painful fissures in dry ambient conditions. Therefore, the TEWL measured on the palm is much higher than that recorded on any other portions of the skin (21). It is certain that low lipid content noted in its SC is responsible for this high permeability (22). However, we cannot deny the possibility that its skin temperature as well as its highly functional sweat glands contribute to their high TEWL values.

Detergents are a well-known causative agent for irritant dermatitis. They induce damage to the proteinaceous components of the SC. Thus, skin irritation caused by sodium lauryl sulphate (SLS) induces an increase in TEWL on most bodily locations. In contrast, SLS produces a decrease in TEWL on the palmar skin (21). Such a phenomenon can only be explained by considering the functionally active sweat glands in the palmo-plantar skin. It is highly likely that normally patent intracorneal sweat ducts are occluded by SLS-induced structural changes in the remarkably thick palmar SC. Therefore, we cannot simply regard TEWL as a parameter for the skin barrier function as long as the palmo-plantar skin is concerned. To analyze the functional state of the SC in such skin areas, it is desirable to carry out simultaneous measurements of the SC hydration state.

ASSESSMENT OF SKIN BARRIER FUNCTION IN DERMATOSES

Any types of pathological conditions involving the epidermis may induce SC barrier disruption, which can be detected easily in vivo with biophysical instruments.

Inflammatory Dermatoses

Inflammatory skin diseases can be produced by either exogenous or endogenous causes. Stimuli inflicted on the skin from the environment leave damage not only in the SC but also in the underlying viable tissues. In contrast, endogenous proinflammatory stimuli that mostly result from the host immunological reactions against various agents, either external or internal, mainly produce damage on the viable skin tissues at first and secondarily induce acceleration of epidermal proliferation and differentiation which results in the production of functionally deficient SC. Most inflammatory skin lesions are covered with dry scales or scale-crusts due to the presence of SC with poor water-holding capacity. They also show an elevation in TEWL. Even in the absence of recognizable scaly changes, xerotic skin changes such as atopic xerosis, associated with clinically invisible inflammation, display mild impairment in SC barrier function that is only demonstrable with biophysical measurement (19).

Resistance of the SC to Drastic External Physical Insults

When the skin is exposed to various injurious agents from an environment that exceeds a certain threshold level, nobody can avoid the development of irritant dermatitis.

Harsh physical insults such as high-dose irradiation of UV light, ionic radiation, and heating or freezing always induce acute irritant dermatitis even with the formation of blisters covered with normally looking SC. These findings suggest that the SC is more resistant to the damaging effects of physical stimuli than the underlying viable epidermis. However, for ethical reasons, it is difficult to obtain direct evidence in vivo whether the SC actually retains its functional integrity even when drastic physical insults are inflicted on it.

To perform such an in vitro experiment, we can construct a simple simulation model of the in vivo SC (23). The model consists of a sheet of normal SC that tightly occludes the underlying water-saturated filter paper placed as in a diffusion chamber. In this model, it is possible to produce a concentration gradient of water between the surface and the lowermost portion of the SC as observed in vivo, in contrast to uniformly hydrated isolated SC samples. The upper surface of the SC in this model is exposed to the ambient atmosphere, whereas its lower surface faces water-saturated filter paper that is the water source for the overlying SC like the fluid-saturated skin tissues in vivo.

Using this model, we found that it is hard to produce any abnormality in the barrier function or in the water-holding capacity of the SC even after irradiation with high doses of UVB that can produce severe sunburn in normal human skin (24).

Because there occurs a significant decrease in the hydration levels of the skin surface or SC barrier disruption 24 hours after UVB irradiation in vivo (25,26), we can conclude that the functional disturbances of the SC observed in the UV-irradiated skin are not due to the direct effect of UV on the SC, but that they just reflect secondary changes in the SC produced by the UV-damaged epidermis. UVB induces a proliferative response in the epidermis and T lymphocyte–mediated events.

This is also the case with high-dose X-ray irradiation. Clinically, radiation therapy is conducted in a much milder pattern, where the SC functional damage evaluated with TEWL measurements occurs with a much more delayed pattern, starting after 10 days and reaching maximal values after 13 to 75 days (27). This SC barrier perturbation after irradiation also seems to reflect the delayed epidermal changes occurring in radiodermatitis.

The SC also retains its functional integrity after other drastic physical insults such as immersion in hot water, freezing with liquid nitrogen, or prolonged and repeated exposures to an excessively dry or humid environment, except for a transient and reversible change just after these assaults.

Because all of these environmental insults are well known to produce severe irritant dermatitis in vivo, eventual SC functional abnormalities observed after such physical insults seem to be a result of the damage produced in the underlying viable tissues rather than that of the SC damage. This functional derangement of the SC lasts until the homeostasis in the epidermis is restored.

In contrast to the rather innocuous effect of the physical stimuli on the SC, the effects of chemical substances, especially of organic solvents, are remarkable. It is because they can extract the intercellular lipids from the SC. Acetone/ether (1:1) application induces a moderate increase in TEWL as well as a decrease in high frequency conductance after two or four minutes. There occurs a much more prominent increase in TEWL together with a conspicuous decrease in high frequency conductance after the treatment with chloroform/methanol (1:1) mixture even for a few minutes. Among the studied lipid solvents, the effects of hexane on the SC seem to be the mildest. After treatment with hexane, there occurred only a minor decrease in high frequency conductance without any elevation in TEWL.

Application of the SC with detergents, e.g., 10% SLS aqueous solution for four minutes, induces an increase in TEWL afterward. However, in contrast to the organic solvents there occurs a moderate increase in high frequency conductance as reported before (28,29). Because SLS is an anionic surfactant, it is presumably due to the damage to the proteinaceous components such as keratin and matrix protein, which exposes new water-binding sites. Moreover, SLS is thought to increase the fluidity of the lipid lamellae of the SC, subsequently facilitating the desquamatory process.

All these findings in experiments conducted in vitro suggest that the SC is generally resistant to most of the physical insults from our environment, whereas it is vulnerable to some chemical insults that inflict damage to its structural components. Specifically, the irritant dermatitis caused by physical insults generally reflects the damage of the underlying viable tissues, whereas that induced by chemicals, especially by lipid solvents, may represent the results of complex damage not only to the viable tissues but also to the SC itself.

Influence of Traumatic Injuries on the Functions of the SC

Skin is always exposed to various mechanical traumas from the environment, which can easily damage the SC barrier function. Such mechanical insults include scratching that is unconsciously inflicted by ourselves. Even partial removal of the SC, produced by 10 times repeated tape-strippings that do not leave any skin changes afterward, allows easy demonstration of positive patch test reactions to large molecular allergens such as trichophytin released by dermatophytes, *Candida* antigens, or various aeroallergens in those who are sensitized to them (30). It is also the case with superficial scratching of the skin surface in a criss-cross pattern with a needle. These procedures are often utilized as pretreatment for skin testing in patients with AD (30–32).

When the viable epidermis is directly exposed to the air by totally removing the SC with tape-stripping, more than 80% of its impaired barrier function is quickly restored in the initial days as confirmed by TEWL measurements (20). There occurs a rapid increase in the synthesis and release of the intercellular lipids in the epidermis that is also exhibiting a profound increase in proliferation (33). The extent of the remaining elevation in TEWL attained after this initial rapid restoration phase is negligible as compared with the prominently high levels observed on the totally stripped skin. There are usually observed scaly skin changes, whose TEWL values are comparable to those recorded on the normal facial skin where no special complaint exists or to those obtained on the lesional skin of chronic dermatitis. As long as there remains a xerotic change, it is possible to demonstrate biochemically a reduction in the content of amino acids, which is a consistent feature in all the scaly skin lesions (34,35). In contrast, a decrease in the amount of intercellular ceramides is not observed any more after seven days (34). The eventual normalization of the SC barrier function with the normalization of the skin appearance takes place about two weeks later. Thus, the restoration of totally disrupted SC barrier takes place much slower in humans than in experimentally used mice.

The initial rapid restoration process of the SC barrier is delayed in the skin of the elderly (36). Their skin tends to be xerotic, developing pruritus more or less in dry winter on the lower half of the trunk and lower extremities where sebum excretion is much lower than that on the upper half of the body. Moreover, their epidermis is atrophic, being, however, accompanied by thicker SC than in young people. Their skin shows unimpaired water barrier function due to retention of corneocytes as a consequence of slower SC turnover time, unless there occurs secondarily a xerotic dermatitis or prominent cracking (37).

Patients with AD are also well known to suffer from pruritic dry skin, atopic xerosis, even on their uninvolved skin. Interestingly, the initial recovery process of the SC barrier function after tape-stripping of the SC is not delayed in atopic xerosis or is even faster than that noted in normal young individuals (38,39). This makes a sharp contrast to those findings observed in the aged skin (36). The epidermis is mildly acanthotic in atopic xerosis, which is accompanied by thicker SC that shows a higher turnover rate than that of normal individuals, in a fashion similar to that noted in lesional skin of dermatitis. In fact, histopathologically, we can find even the presence of mild inflammatory changes in the upper dermis (40). Therefore, their skin seems to be in a mildly activated state to facilitate the SC barrier recovery.

In contrast to the unaffected recovery process of the SC after mechanical disruption, the restoration of barrier function after a chemical injury such as that induced by the application of 1% SLS in petrolatum for 24 hours is much more prolonged and severe in the skin with atopic xerosis than in normal healthy skin (41). The damage is not confined to the SC and epidermis, but there are severe inflammatory changes in the dermis as well. Therefore, the persistence of the mild, clinically invisible inflammation in atopic xerosis seems to predispose to the development of a severe inflammatory response after chemical irritation.

Normal corneocytes retain a large amount of IL-1α that is constitutively produced by epidermal keratinocytes, which is released in response to all forms of acute barrier disruption, independent of new cytokine formation (42). In addition, there occurs a rapid increase in the mRNA levels and protein content of several downstream cytokines such as IL-1α, IL-1β, TNF-α, GM-CSF, and IL-6 in the epidermis that leads to further increases in inflammation and epidermal cell proliferation (43).

Under such an inflammatory process, there also occurs a control mechanism to regulate the proinflammatory activities of IL-1 in the epidermis by generating its inhibitor, IL-1 receptor antagonist (IL-1ra). IL-1ra functions as a specific and competitive inhibitor of IL-1, because it binds to the same receptors as IL-1α and β without eliciting any biological response. Thus, the balance between IL-1ra and IL-1 is important for maintaining homeostasis in the skin. An excess of 10 to 100 times more IL-1ra than IL-1 is required to abrogate the IL-1-induced biological response by 50%. The cutaneous response to acute or chronic barrier disruption includes mechanisms which increase IL-1 and IL-1ra mRNA levels in a coordinated manner. The net result provides a regulatory mechanism for controlling the biological effects of increased IL-1 production (44). Irradiation of the skin with UVB was also noted to result in striking elevation of IL-1ra in the desquamating scales (45). Furthermore, an increase in the ratio of IL-1ra to IL-1α was consistently observed in SC samples obtained from inflammatory dermatoses such as psoriasis and AD (46). Therefore, this increase in the ratio is a non-specific phenomenon that can occur in any kind of inflammatory skin diseases regardless of the characteristics of the inflammation.

We studied the influence of much more deep-reaching mechanical tissue damage on the restoration of SC barrier function (20). Because suction blisters are produced by separation at the lamina lucida of the basement membrane, we can produce erosive lesions lacking total epidermis by removing the top of suction blisters. In the erosive lesions, the restoration of the normal SC barrier function took three times longer (45 days) than that required for the normalization of the SC after total SC removal by tape-stripping (14 days). However, no scar formation occurs after the healing of the erosive lesions because there is little damage to the dermal fibrous tissues.

In contrast, injuries involving the dermal tissues always induce scar formation including hypertrophic scars or keloids depending on their depth and accompanying inflammation. To study the restoration of the SC function in mid-dermal wounds, we can use the donor sites for split-thickness skin grafts because a reproducible depth of the wound is attainable with a dermatome (20). Although re-epithelization of such wounds was completed within two weeks, abnormal SC functions expressed by elevated TEWL values persist beyond expectation. It ranged from about 150 to 500 days depending on the depth of the wound. There was a location-dependent difference. When the thigh and the lower abdominal were compared, the thigh skin appeared to take much longer to normalize.

Interestingly, the SC functional changes measured in hypertrophic skin and keloids were highly abnormal when compared with those of the split-thickness skin donor sites approximately 50 days after graft harvesting (20). Histologically, we can demonstrate a perivascular lymphoid infiltration in the dermis of such skin that is highly suggestive of persistence of inflammatory changes in addition to excessive formation of collagen fibers. Although the lipid content in the SC was not decreased, we found an increase in immature corneocytes in the SC that shows a higher turnover rate than that of normal skin, which may ensue insufficient formation of the lamellar lipid structure in the intercellular spaces (47).

Influences of Underlying Dermatitis on the SC Functions

All of the above-mentioned findings seem to indicate that the SC functions are greatly influenced by inflammation that secondarily occurs due to the damage produced in the living skin tissues as well as in the SC. Therefore, SC barrier dysfunction can be demonstrated sooner or later in the skin affected by any kind of dermatitis, including contact dermatitis, AD, various forms of eczematous dermatitis, superficial infections induced by various pathogens in a pattern reflecting the intensity of underlying inflammation, and body location. Facial lesions show much higher TEWL levels than those involving the lower legs even though the intensity of the inflammation looks similar objectively (48).

Enhanced epidermal proliferation and disorganized differentiation persist as long as there exists inflammation in the skin. They seem to remain much longer than skin redness, the clinically observable inflammatory sign. To confirm these clinical findings, we conducted analyses in two different types of experimentally induced dermatitis in guinea pigs that showed similar levels of erythematous changes. As a result, we found that the measurements of TEWL are a quite efficient method to evaluate the influence of inflammation on the epidermis as well as on the SC.

Analyses in an Experimentally Induced Model of Irritant Contact Dermatitis. By conducting various preliminary trials, we found that a diffusely bright erythematous reaction can be produced by the application of 10% SLS in petrolatum for 24 hours on the back skin of Hartley strain guinea pigs weighing 500 to 800 g after removing of their hair with an electric hair-clipper and electric shaver. We used these inflammatory lesions as a model to study the time course of different biophysical and biochemical parameters in irritant dermatitis. Biophysical measurements showed that the erythematous changes due to SLS irritation were highest at 24 hours and disappeared within five days. An analysis of the increase in epidermal proliferation in such skin by using FACS can revealed that the peak increase in DNA-synthesizing epidermal cells, which were in the S phase of the cell cycle, occurred on day 1, and then the level quickly returned to normal by day 4. In contrast, a maximal increase in TEWL occurred later than that of the erythematous change or that of the epidermal proliferation, being noted from day 3 to 5, followed by a gradual decrease that still showed a significant increase at least until day 9 with a return to normal levels after two weeks (24). Thus, the damage of the SC barrier function seemed to be restored much slower than the parameter of skin inflammation, redness, or that of epidermal proliferation. It lasts three to four times longer than redness or enhanced epidermal proliferation.

Analyses in an Experimentally Induced Model of Allergic Contact Dermatitis. To induce allergic contact dermatitis showing diffuse erythematous changes comparable to those found in the above-mentioned SLS dermatitis, we utilized positive patch test reactions noted in experimental candidiasis. In contrast to the dermatitis due to lipophilic compounds, water-soluble molecules from the environment such as those derived from various biological sources hardly permeate the SC. They penetrate through an alternative pathway of the SC, i.e., the openings of sweat glands and hair follicles where the SC barrier function is imperfect (49). However, the surface area of this alternative pathway amounts to only 0.1% of the total skin surface area. Nevertheless, in the case of contact allergens, even the penetration of a small amount can induce allergic contact dermatitis. Thus, *Candida albicans* allergen, which is not an irritant in non-immune guinea pigs, can induce diffuse erythematous inflammation on the skin of immune animals without any pretreatment of the SC such as scratching or stripping that compromises its barrier function performed on the skin of the volar forearm of humans (30–32). Similar phenomena are frequently observed in AD patients. The application of aeroallergens consisting of large proteinaceous molecules on non-lesional skin of the back can induce a positive patch test known as atopic patch test (50). The incidence of positive patch test is much lower on the mid–flexor forearm, where the presence of hair follicles is not prominent as compared with that of the seborrheic areas.

At first we experimentally produced allergic contact dermatitis with *C. albicans* antigen in five guinea pigs that had been made contact-sensitive to this antigen by the production of experimental cutaneous candidiasis one month before, as reported previously (31). Briefly, cutaneous candidiasis was induced by inoculation of 10^6 yeast cells of *C. albicans* to a 2 cm × 2 cm area under occlusion for 24 hours.

A 1:200 *Candida* antigen aqueous solution (Torii Pharmaceutical Co., Tokyo, Japan) was applied under occlusion for 24 hours on the back of the animals after removing their hair with an electric hair-clipper and electric shaver.

After two days, there was diffuse erythema with a redness slightly less than that induced by 10% SLS, which almost disappeared on day 4. We performed the analysis of epidermal proliferation in such skin by using FACScan. It revealed that the number of DNA-synthesizing epidermal cells remarkably increased from day 1, reaching a peak on day 2. Thereafter, it gradually decreased but tended to be higher than the control levels even on day 11, the last day of the examination (24).

Slightly behind the increased DNA synthesis in the epidermis, an increase in TEWL continuously occurred until day 4. Such a delayed increase in the barrier damage of the SC seemed to reflect the highly proliferative state of the epidermis, as observed in psoriasis, where it is difficult for keratinocytes to attain sufficient differentiation or maturation. Thereafter, the elevated TEWL values began to decrease but took more than two weeks for a significant increase to return to the control levels. Thus, the elevated TEWL reflects the prolonged course of the inflammation in allergic contact dermatitis that could not be detected by clinical observation of the skin inflammatory sign, redness. The total time course of TEWL abnormalities was much longer, at least by 1.5 times longer, than that in irritant contact dermatitis although the latter initially showed higher erythematous reactions.

These findings indicate that the barrier function of the SC is a quite sensitive indicator of the pathological changes taking place in the lesional skin of various types of dermatitis.

Immune-Mediated Inflammatory Dermatoses.   Skin functional changes in psoriasis and AD are the most documented and well studied among various dermatoses. In these diseases, the abnormalities in SC functions are suspected to trigger further exacerbation known as a Koebner phenomenon or to be responsible for sustaining their skin lesions.

Psoriasis.   Psoriasis is a chronic, generalized, and scaly erythematous dermatosis that is thought to occur due to a Th1 lymphocyte–mediated immune reaction against so far unidentified autoantigens in the skin tissue. Despite the presence of thick scales in lesional skin, its SC is well known to show impaired barrier function (51,52). The level of TEWL appears to be directly related to the clinical intensity of the lesion and closely reflects the disappearance of the lesions with effective treatment (52). Abnormalities in the SC intercellular lipids, especially a significant reduction in ceramide 1, are suggested to be responsible for the defect in skin barrier function (53,54). Electron microscopic studies disclosed severe structural alteration of the intercellular lipid lamellae (55).

There was also a significant negative correlation between TEWL and the size of coreocytes, a parameter for the proliferative activity of the underlying epidermis, which becomes smaller in the lesional skin with increased epidermal proliferation (56). Thus, in addition to the abnormal lipid component, an increase in the number of corneocytes with immature cornified envelope seems to be responsible for the incompetent SC function, because the latter cannot assist a sufficient assembly of intercellular lipids (57). Particularly, the extensive desquamation that is observed after acute generalized pustulation in pustular psoriasis seems to be due to the remarkably high epidermopoiesis caused by severe inflammation (58).

Atopic Dermatitis.   AD is a chronic systemic eczematous dermatitis based on Th1 and Th2 lymphocyte–mediated reactions against environmental proteinaceous allergens. It is well accepted that there exists a defect in skin permeability barrier function in AD (59). The extent of the barrier abnormality appears to correlate not only with the state of dermatitis but also with the affected anatomic sites (48,60). Therefore, TEWL levels recorded on lesional skin on the lower extremites are just comparable to those measured on the facial skin of normal individuals.

Many studies have indicated disrupted barrier function of the SC not only in their involved skin but also in their uninvolved dry skin (40,60–63). Thus, it is natural that attention has been focused on the intercellular lipids of the SC. It has been disclosed that there is a significant decrease in the ceramide fraction in AD patients (64). Di Nardo et al. (65) reported significantly lower levels of ceramides 1 and 3 in SC; the decrease in ceramide 3 was found to be correlated with the barrier impairment. Investigations on the lateral lipid packing in the intercellular matrix of SC in AD patients showed an increase in the hexagonal lattice (gel phase) with respect to the orthorhombic packing (crystalline phase), which is dependent on the presence of long-chain free fatty acids (66).

Murata et al. (67) reported an increased level of a novel enzyme, glycocylceramide/sphingomyelin deacylase, in the lesional and non-lesional skin of AD patients as a mechanism underlying the decreased ceramide content in the SC. In contrast, Ohnishi et al. (68) found that the skin of AD patients was colonized by ceramidase-secreting bacteria, which contributed to the ceramide deficiency in the SC. In addition to these enzymes degrading the ceramide precursors, Cui et al. (69) suggested that decreased levels of prosaposin, a large precursor protein that is proteolytically cleaved to form a family of sphingolipid activator proteins, might also be responsible for reduced enzyme activities for ceramide formation. Moreover, Fartasch and Diepgen (63) demonstrated a disturbance in the extrusion of lamellar bodies in the atopic dry skin.

The barrier function of the SC also depends on the presence of differentiated and mature corneocytes equipped with cornified envelope–associated proteins that can bind with ceramide-containing intercellular lipids. However, in contrast to lesional skin of AD, there is no prominent increase in the number of immature corneocytes with less hydrophobic CE in atopic xerosis (57). Similarly, Fartasch (55) found normal structural organization of the intercellular lipid lamellae in atopic xerosis.

The barrier function of the unaffected skin of AD seems to be restored eventually if there is no dermatitis for a long period of time. It seems to take at least a few years. For example, adult patients with hand eczema with a history of AD in childhood show normal TEWL levels on the non-involved volar forearm (70). Matsumoto et al. (71) found that, unlike atopic xerosis, the normal-appearing skin of their AD patients showed no decrease in their ceramide contents. Matsuda's group (72) demonstrated in their unique Nc/Nga mouse model that these animals never show any significant changes in skin surface hydration and TEWL or in the SC content of ceramides as long as they remain skin lesion–free in an air-regulated condition. In a conventional ventilation system, they develop severe dermatitis similar to human AD. They found that there occurred at first a decrease in high frequency conductance, due to decreased skin surface hydration, and later an increase in TEWL, due to barrier dysfunction together with a decrease in the lipid content including ceramides of the SC.

In a similar fashion, we followed human neonatal babies born from the mothers with atopic backgrounds (74). For the first two weeks, they showed neonatal xerosis that is associated with unimpaired SC barrier function as reported before (73). Those who developed AD around two to three months after the birth began to show increased TEWL at that time point. Therefore, during their neonatal period, their TEWL and skin surface hydration state were indistinguishable from those of the neonates whose skin remained lesion-free even in later life (74). These findings suggest that the barrier impairment found in AD is not inherent but represents a phenomenon secondary to dermatitic skin changes. In fact, there is no case of congenital AD.

Lichenoid Dermatoses.   Lichenoid tissue reactions are observed in lichen planus, lupus erythematosus (LE), and fixed drug eruption, in which, histopathologically, there is hydropic degeneration of the basal cell layer due to an immune-mediated cytotoxic attack. Because of this damage to the basal cell layer, there occurs a disorganization in epidermal proliferation and differentiation, which eventually leads to hyperkeratosis associated with hypergranulosis. In our preliminary studies conducted in the lesional skin present on the dorsa of the hands of two patients with discoid LE, we found a moderate increase in TEWL together with a moderately decreased hydration state of the skin surface. A facial lesion of a patient with systemic LE revealed only a slight increase in TEWL with no change in high frequency conductance. No biochemical analysis has been done on the SC of these dermatoses.

Bullous Dermatoses.   Bullous lesions or pustular lesions are observed in various dermatoses with different pathogenetic backgrounds, e.g., autoimmune bullous dermatoses such as pemphigus and bullous pemphigoid, epidermolysis bullosa, Stevens–Johnson syndrome, herpes virus infections, and irritant contact dermatitis including scalded skin. All of them do not show any special abnormalities in either SC barrier function or hydration state of the skin surface as long as they are covered with intact SC. Once it breaks to reveal an erosive skin surface, there results a total lack of skin barrier function. With the re-epithelization of the erosive wounds accompanied by the formation of crusts and scales, we can follow the restoration process with improvement in the barrier function in a fashion similar to that mentioned above.

Benign and Malignant Keratoses

Our unpublished data show that there are moderate abnormalities in their SC barrier function in both benign and malignant epidermal tumors. However, as compared with the inflammatory dermatoses, it is unlikely that any undesirable skin change is induced by the alteration in SC barrier function derived from the presence of skin tumors. Thus, so far no special studies have been conducted in them.

Hereditary Keratinization Disorders

Normal SC barrier function is produced only after the flawless formation of intact corneocytes and intercellular lipid domain. Therefore, any kinds of genetic defect in this process can result in the generation of pathologic SC that is associated with an abnormal barrier function as well as with an abnormal water-holding capacity of the SC (75). Most keratinization disorders are characterized by the presence of pathologic SC that clinically presents a dry scaly appearance. They have been recognized as a variety of ichthyosiform dermatoses. Recently, they also provide a nice model to analyze the production process of normal SC structure and function.

Autosomal Dominant Ichthyosis Vulgaris

Most cases of icthyosis vulgaris present a distinct ichthyosiform skin change mainly in dry and cold winter, because they have an autosomal dominant defect in the gene that encodes profilaggrin. The hydration state of the skin in ichthyosis vulgaris is much lower, together with a remarkably decreased content of water-soluble amino acids that is derived from filaggrin degradation rather than from senile xerosis, which also becomes evident in winter (16). The defective barrier function of the SC in it has been recognized for a long time (76). These patients show a mild but significant increase in TEWL on their volar forearm (77).

X-Linked Recessive Ichthyosis

Patients with this skin disorder also show a mild but significant increase in TEWL (77). They display not only an abnormal barrier but also a delay in barrier recovery after acute perturbation (78). However, no abnormal structural organization of the intercellular lipid lamellae has been found in their SC (55). There observed an accumulation of cholesterol sulfate and a deficiency of cholesterol in the SC due to a steroid sulfatase deficiency. Because experimentally applied cholesterol sulfate produces a barrier abnormality even in intact skin, its accumulation rather than the cholesterol deficiency is thought to be responsible for the barrier abnormality in this disorder.

Lamellar Ichthyosis and Non-Bullous Ichthyosisform Erythroderma

In contrast to ichthyosis vulgaris and X-linked ichthyosis, the group of autosomal congenital ichthyosis is characterized clinically by a severely ichthyotic appearance. Some of them may be associated with erythroderma (non-bullous ichthyosiform erythroderma). These patients exhibit markedly impaired skin barrier function, which is demonstrable by an elevation in TEWL by more than 2-fold when compared with normal individuals.

Lamellar ichthyosis is caused by mutations in the gene that encodes the enzyme transglutaminase, which is responsible for the assembly of the cornified envelope (79). Those mice lacking this gene show early neonatal death due to highly impaired barrier function (80). When the skin from these knockout mice is transplanted to normal mice, it develops severe ichthyosis with epidermal hyperplasia and marked hyperkeratosis. However, such a skin graft shows improvement of TEWL to control levels, suggesting that the ichthyosiform skin phenotype in transglutaminase 1 deficiency develops the massive hyperkeratosis as a physical compensation of the defective cutaneous permeability barrier required for survival in a terrestrial environment (81).

In addition to the defect in cornified envelope, prominent changes in SC lipid structure and composition have been observed in lamellar ichthyosis. There are significant differences in the relative amounts of ceramide fractions 2-3a-3b-4-5, free fatty acid/ceramide ratio, and free fatty acid/cholesterol ratio with smaller repeated distances of lipid bilayers in the SC (82). The SC of autosomal recessive lamellar ichthyosis is associated with remarkable alteration in the intercellular lipid lamellae. There are discontinuities of extracelluar membrane structures that account for the enhanced SC permeability (55,83). Lateral lipid packing of the SC lipids examined by using electron diffraction revealed that the hexagonal packing is predominantly present, whereas the orthorhombic packing is observed only occasionally, indicating a much more prominent abnormality than even that observed in the SC of AD (66). However, studies on permeability pathway of water-soluble tracer, colloidal lanthanum, across the SC clearly demonstrated the restriction of the tracer only to the SC interstices due to the presence of intact corneocyte–lipid envelope, despite the abnormalities in the cornified envelope (83).

Epidermolytic Hyperkeratosis

This dermatosis is a dominantly inherited ichthyosis, frequently associated with mutations in keratin 1 or 10 that result in disruption of the keratin filament ocytoskeleton leading to keratinocyte fragility. Despite the cell fragility, there is no evidence of defect in either the cornified envelope or the cornified-bound lipid envelope. However, its skin lesions show elevated baseline TEWL rates by 3-fold, because the intercellular domain shows decreased quantities and defective organization of extracellular lamellar bilayers due to incomplete lamellar body secretion (84). It is unique in that accelerated recovery is observed after barrier disruption in contrast to X-linked ichthyosis that shows delayed barrier recovery.

Type 2 Gaucher's Disease

A subset of type 2 Gaucher's disease patients who lack β-glucocerobrosidase activity exhibits ichthyosiform skin abnormalities. Because hydrolysis of glucosylceramide by β-glucocerobrosidase results in ceramide of the intercellular lamellae, the skin lacking the activities of this enzyme, such as that of infantile patients or that of transgenic Gaucher mice homozygous for a null allele, demonstrates incompletely processed, lamellar body–derived sheets throughout the SC interstices. They display severe barrier impairment. These findings clearly indicate the importance of this enzyme for the generation of functionally intact SC (85).

Netherton's Disease

Patients with Netherton's disease show generalized erythroderma indistinguishable from that of erythrodermic-psoriasis patients or that of lamellar-ichthyosis patients (86). In a similar pattern, they show the impairment of SC permeability barrier. However, in this disorder, premature lamellar body secretion and foci of electron-dense material are found in the intercellular spaces of SC. These morphological features constitute a unique diagnositic point to differentiate them from other clinically resembling ichthyosiform dermatoses in infantile cases before the appearance of characteristic hair shaft abnormality, trichorrhexis invaginata.

Other Keratinization Disorders

Patients with Darier's disease and those with erythrokeratoderma variablilis show a moderate but significant increase in TEWL only on their affected skin (77). No detailed studies have been performed on their SC morphology or functional properties. The fissured skin lesions observed in Darier's disease or in Hailey–Hailey disease totally lack the barrier function, allowing bacterial and viral invasion even to develop Kaposi's varicelliform eruption due to herpes simplex virus infection.

A patient with progressive symmetric erythrokeratoderma, who had heterozygous loricrin gene mutations with a mutant loricrin existing in the nuclei of differentiating keratinocyte (87), revealed impaired barrier function noted as an elevated TEWL (Ishida-Yamamoto A, personal communication).

SC CHANGES THAT OCCUR LATER IN LIFE IN THOSE WITH NORMAL HEALTHY SKIN

In general, systemic factors only minimally influence cutaneous lipid synthesis (88). Even thyroid, testosterone, and estrogen have little impact on cutaneous lipid synthesis or the resultant SC barrier function under day-to-day conditions. Only when potent topical corticosteroids are applied under occlusion, they induce local steroid atrophy together with mild barrier impairment (89).

There is no special barrier change in the SC of full-term newborn babies except for the presence of neonatal xerosis that lasts for two weeks after birth (73). However, when they begin to develop seborrheic dermatitis or AD, their SC demonstrates an increase in TEWL with a reduced hydration state of the skin surface on the lesional as well as on the non-lesional skin that shows a xerotic change (Kikuchi K and Tagami H, unpublished data). These functional abnormalities of their skin normalize eventually when the skin remains lesion-free for a long period of time after regression of the eczematous lesions (69). However, those individuals with a history of infantile AD may have a tendency to develop localized dermatitis such as lichen simplex chronicus on the neck or dry hand dermatitis even later in their life, whenever external physical or chemical insults are inflicted on such bodily sites. We can demonstrate abnormal SC functions in such lesions.

There is no difference in the SC barrier function between males and females. When moderate acne develops on the facial skin, there occurs a reduction in SC ceramide content together with SC barrier disruption in their affected skin (90). It seems to reflect mild dermatitis that accompanies the follicular inflammation.

We cannot reveal any impairment in barrier function in aged skin except for a reduction in SC water content. On the contrary, there is a tendency to show a slight decrease in TEWL with age, probably reflecting a mild increase in the number of cell layers in the SC with age (5). As mentioned above, such a tendency is most clearly observed on the vermilion border of the lip (11). With the biophysical measurements performed on the skin with senile xerosis, we can demonstrate a significant decrease in TEWL with an increase in the number of cell layers in the SC (37).

In contrast, photoaging of the skin does not exert any influence in the SC barrier function. We found no difference in TEWL between the exposed dorsal surface of the hands of long-time golf players and their contralateral, sun-protected side of the hand, although a significant decrease in hydration of the skin surface is found on their exposed skin (91).

TEWL demonstrates mild rhythms within a day even in the same individuals. Rhythms with periods of 8 and 12 hours were detected, possibly reflecting that of 8 hours for sebum excretion and that of 12 hours for skin temperature (92).

Much more prominent alterations are found when comparisons are made in the same individuals in the same environmental conditions of a climate-controlled chamber between summer and winter (93). TEWL and hydration state of the skin surface show a significant increase and decrease, respectively, in winter. Data from other biophysical measurements suggest that subclinical inflammation due to the exposure to the dry and cold environment of winter results in the enhanced turnover rate of the SC associated with elevated TEWL levels in winter. Such functional deteriorations taking place in the SC of normal individuals in winter can be restored at least to some extent by applying an effective moisturizer daily (94). In fact, higher irritability of the skin in winter is observed not only in the healthy subjects (95,96) but also in atopic subjects (97). It corresponds to the clinical observations indicating that skin disorders such as AD, psoriasis, and senile xerosis show a tendency to exacerbate in winter.

Experimentally induced severe diabetes mellitus in mice induces reduction in both the epidermal proliferation and SC water content (98) without any associated impairment in the SC barrier function, which is similar to that found in aged human skin. We can demonstrate a similar pattern of SC changes in those who have diabetes mellitus (99).

CONCLUDING REMARKS

The SC is such an efficient barrier that allows only 3 to 6 g/hour/m^2 of TEWL from normal skin of the trunk to protect our body from desiccation, enabling us to lead a terrestrial life. The efficiency of the SC as a skin barrier is totally dependent on the state of proliferation and differentiation of keratinocytes in the epidermis, because the SC is their final product. Thus, any kind of pathologic events that interferes with these processes eventually results in the production of abnormal SC, which can be functionally demonstrated with instrumental measurements. Experimentally it is demonstrable that TEWL is a far more sensitive parameter than the clinically observable skin changes.

All the dermatoses that affect the epidermis produce pathologic SC more or less associated with an abnormal barrier function. Its severe disruption, as noted in a baby with harlequin ichthyosis, a severe type of ichthyosiform erythroderma, or that with junctional epidermolysis bullosa, may even threaten survival. In a similar fashion, severe bullous dermatoses such as pemphigus vulgaris and toxic epidermal necrolysis can be fatal even in adult patients because they induce extensive loss of the skin barrier.

The abnormalities of the SC noted in hereditary keratinization disorders become an excellent model to analyze the normal SC function. It is of note that the continuously exposed facial skin exhibits moderately elevated TEWL values even

Table 1 Skin Conditions and Diseases that Affect Skin Barrier or Hydration State of the Skin Surface

(I) Those that show impairment in both barrier function and water-holding capacity of the SC
(A) Inflammation that affects the epidermis
Atopic dermatitis
Atopic xerosis
Psoriasis
Contact dermatitis
Eczema and prurigo
Dermatophytosis and other superficial microbial infections
Physical or chemical injuries
Autoimmune bullous dermatoses
Lichenoid dermatoses
Benign and malignant epidermal tumors
(B) Ichthyosiform dermatoses
Autosomal dominant ichthyosis vulgaris
X-linked ichthyosis
Lamellar ichthyosis
Epidermolytic hyperkeratosis
(II) Those that show impairment only in barrier function but rather exhibiting hydrated SC
(A) Keloid and fresh scars
(B) Retinoid-treated skin
(III) Those that show only decreased hydration state of the skin surface with normally retained barrier function
(A) Senile xerosis
(B) Photoaged skin
(C) Diabetes mellitus

in normal individuals, which are nearly twice as high as those of other body areas. Hence, the extent of barrier damage that is comparable to that of the facial skin does not cause so much inconvenience to the affected patients for leading a normal life. When the skin is totally removed of its SC by tape-strippings, it attains this level of barrier function in several days; thereafter a slow recovery process continues until the total resolution of the remaining inflammation. This initial recovery speed seems to be influenced by the underlying metabolic state of the epidermis. It is quicker in the skin of AD or in that of lamellar ichthyosis than in normal skin, whereas it is slower in elderly skin or in X-linked ichthyosis.

A moderately disrupted barrier function may present a threat to certain dermatoses such as AD, psoriasis, hypertrophic scars, and keloids that exacerbate easily by the stimulation from the environment (98). In such diseases, not only the treatment of the existing lesions but also pertinent and protective measures from the environment are urgently required to prevent further aggravation of the abnormal skin conditions (100,101). Even skin-care using an appropriate moisturizer is effective to restore a mildly disrupted barrier function such as noted on the facial skin of normal individuals in dry and cold winter.

Finally, we can loosely classify various dermatoses and skin conditions into three types based on the results of the above-mentioned biophysical measurements and their functional properties of the SC: (i) those associated with SC abnormalities both in barrier function and in water-holding capacity, (ii) those that show only impairment in barrier function but exhibit rather hydrated SC, and (iii) those that show only decreased hydration state of the skin surface with functionally retained barrier function (Table 1).

REFERENCES

1. Tagami H. What is the 'true' function of skin? Viewpoint 9. Exp Dermatol 2002; 11: 180–182.
2. Elias PM, Menon GK. Structural and lipid biochemical correlates of the epidermal permeability barrier. Ad Lipd Res 1991; 24:1–26.
3. Hamanaka S, Hara M, Nishio H, Otsuka F, Suzuki A, Uchida Y. Human epidermal glucocylceramides are major precursors of stratum corneum ceramides. J Invest Dermatol 2002; 119:416–423.
4. Downing DT, Stewart ME. Epidermal compsition. In Loden M, Maibach HI, eds. Dry Skin and Moisturizers. Chemistry and Function, CRC Press, Boca Raton, 2000:13–26.
5. Zhen Y-X, Suetake T, Tagami H. Number of cell layers of the stratum corneum in normal skin—relationship to the anatomical location on the body, age, sex and physical parameters. Arch Dermatol Res 1999; 291:555–559.
6 Baker H, Kligman AM. Technique for estimating turnover time of human stratum corneum. Arch Dermatol 1967; 195:408–411.
7. Egelrud T. Desquamation. In: Loden M, Maibach HI, eds. Dry Skin and Moisturizers. Chemistry and Function, CRC Press, Boca Raton, 2000:109–117.
8. Nilsson GE. Measurement of water exchange through skin. Med Biol Eng Comput 1997; 15:209–218.
9. Rougier A, Lotte C, Maibach HI. In vivo relationship between percutaneous absorption and transepidermal water loss. In: Bronaugh RL, Maibach HI, eds. Percutaneous Absorption: Drugs, Cosmetics, Mechanisms and Methodology. 3rd ed. New York: Marcel Dekker, 1999:117–132.

10. Tagami H, Yoshikuni K. Interrelationship between water-barrier and reservoir functions of pathologic stratum corneum. Arch Dermatol 1985; 121:642–645.
11. Kobayashi H, Tagami H. Unique functional properties of the vermilion zone of the lip. Br J Dermatol 2004; 150:563–567.
12. Rawlings AV, Scott IR, Harding CR, Bowser PA. Stratum corneum moisturization at molecular level. J Invest Dermatol 1994; 103:731–740.
13. Tagami H, Ohi M, Iwatsuki K, Kanamaru Y, Yamada M. Evaluation of the skin surface hydration in vivo by electrical measurement. J Invest Dermatol 1980; 75:500–507.
14. Hashimoto-Kumasaka K, Takahashi K, Tagami H. Electrical measurement of the water content of the stratum corneum in vivo and in vitro under various conditions. Comparison between skin surface Hygrometer and Corneometer in evaluation of the skin surface hydration state. Acta Derm Venereol (Stockh) 1993; 73:335–339.
15. Fluhr J, Gloor M, Lazzerini S, Kleesz P, Grieshaber R, Berardesca E. Comparative study of five instruments measuring stratum corneum hydration (Corneometer CM820 and CM 825, Skicon 200, Nova DPM 9003, DarmaLab). Part II. In vivo. Skin Res Technol 1999; 5:171–178.
16. Fluhr JW, Mao-Qiang M, Brown BE, Wertz PW, Crumrine D, Sundberg JP, Feingold KR, Elias PM. Glycerol regulates stratum corneum hydration in sebaceous gland deficient (asebia) mice. J Invest Dermatol 2003; 120:728–737.
17. Horii I, Nakayama Y, Obata M, Tagami H. Stratum corneum hydration and amino acid content in xerotic skin. Br J Dermatol 1989; 121:587–592.
18. Imokawa G, Kuno H, Kawai M. Stratum corneum lipids as a bound-water modulator. J Invest Dermatol 1991; 96:845–851.
19. Tagami H, Kanamaru Y, Inoue K, Suehisa S, Inoue F, Iwatsuki K, Yoshikuni K, Yamada M. Water sorption-desorption test of the skin in vivo for functional assessment of the stratum corneum. J Invest Dermatol 1982; 78:425–428.
20. Suetake T, Sasai S, Zhen Y-X, Ohi T, Tagami H. Functional analyses of the stratum corneum in scars. Sequential studies after injury and comparison among keloids, hypertrophic scars, and atrophic scars. Arch Dermatol 1996; 132:1453–1458.
21. Cua AB, Wilhelm KP, Maibach HI. Cutaneous sodium lauryl sulphate irritation potential: age and regional variability. Br J Dermatol 1990; 123:607–613.
22. Lampe MA, Burlingame AL, Whitney J, Williams ML, Brown BE, Roitman E, Elias PM. Human stratum corneum lipids: characterization and regional variations. J Lipid Res 1983; 24:120–130.
23. Obata M, Tagami H. Electrical determination of water content and concentration profile in a simulation model of in vivo stratum corneum. J Invest Dermatol 1989; 92:854–859.
24. Tagami H, Kobayashi H, Zhen X-Y, Kikuchi K. Environmental effects on the functions of the stratum corneum. J Invest Dermatol Symp Proc 2001; 6:87–94.
25. Miyauchi H, Horio T, Asada Y. The effect of ultraviolet radiation on the water-reservoir functions of the stratum corneum. Photodermatol Photoimmunol Photomed 1992–1993; 9:193–197.
26. Haratake A, Uchida Y, Schmuth M, Tanno O, Yasuda R, Epstein JH, Elias PM, Holleran WM. UVB-induced alterations in permeability barrier function; role for epidermal hyperproliferation and thymocyte-mediated response. J Invest Dermatol 1998; 108:769–775.
27. Schmuth M, Sztankay A, Weinlich G, Linder DM, Wimmer MA, Fritsch PO, Fritsch E. Permeability barrier function of skin exposed to ionizing radiation. Arch Dermatol 2001; 137:1019–1023.
28. Agner T, Serup J. Time course of occlusive effects on skin evaluated by measurement of transepidermal water loss (TEWL). Including patch test with sodium lauryl sulphate and water. Contact Dermatitis 1993; 28:6–9.
29. Leveque JL, de Rigal J, Saint-Leger D, Billy D. How does sodium lauryl sulfate alter the skin barrier function in man? A multiparametric approach. Skin Pharmacol 1993; 6:111–115.

30. Tagami H, Watanabe S, Ofuji S, Minami K. Trichophytin contact sensitivity in patients with dermatophytosis. Arch Dermatol 1977; 113:1409–1414.

31. Tagami H, Urano-Suehisa S, Hatchome N. Contact sensivity to *Candida albicans*— comparative studies in man and animals (guinea-pig). Br J Dermatol 1985; 113: 415–424.

32. Tanaka M, Aiba S, Matsumura N, Aoyama H, Tabata N, Sekita Y, Tagami H. IgE-mediated hypersensitivity and contact sensitivity to multiple environmental allergens in atopic dermatitis. Arch Dermatol 1994; 130:1393–1401.

33. Menon GK, Feingold KR, Elias PM. The lamellar secretory response to barrier disruption. J Invest Dermatol 1992; 98:279–289.

34. Denda M, Hori J, Koyama J, Yoshida S, Nanba R, Takahashi M, Horii I, Yamamoto A. Stratum corneum sphingolipids and free amino acids in experimentally-induced scaly skin. Arch Dermatol Res 1992; 284:363–367.

35. Takenouchi M, Suzuki H, Tagami H. Hydration characteristics of pathologic stratum corneum—evaluation of bound water. J Invest Dermatol 1986; 87:574–576.

36. Ghadially R, Brown BE, Hanley K, Reed JT, Feingold KR, Elias PM. Decreased epidermal lipid synthesis accounts for altered barrier function in aged mice. J Invest Dermatol 1996; 106:1064–1069.

37. Hara M, Kikuchi K, Watanabe M, Denda M, Koyama J, Nomura J, Horii I, Tagami H. Senile xerosis: functional, morphological, and biochemmical studies. J Geriatr Dermatol 1993; 1:111–120.

38. Tanaka M, Zhen YX, Tagami H. Normal recovery of the stratum corneum barrier function following damage induced by tape stripping in patients with atopic dermatitis. Br J Dermatol 1997; 136:966–967.

39. Gfesser M, Abeck D, Rugemer J, Schreiner V, Stab F, Disch R, Ring J. The early phase of epidermal barrier regeneration is faster in patients with atopic eczema. Dermatology 1997; 195:326–332.

40. Watanabe M, Tagami H, Horii I, Takahashi M, Kligman AM. Functional analyses of the superficial stratum corneum in atopic xerosis. Arch Dermatol 1991; 137:1689–1692.

41. Tabata N, Tagami H, Kligman AM. TI: a twenty-four-hour occlusive exposure to 1% sodium lauryl sulfate induces a unique histopathologic inflammatory response in the xerotic skin of atopic dermatitis patients. Acta Derm Venereol 1998; 78:244–247.

42. Wood LC, Elias PM, Calhoun C, Tsai JC, Grunfeld C, Feingold KR. Barrier disruption stimulates interleukin-1 alpha expression and release from a pre-formed pool in murine epidermis. J Invest Dermatol 1996; 106:397–403.

43. Menon GK, Price LF, Bommannan B, Elias PM, Feingold KR. Selective obliteration of the epidermal calcium gradient leads to enhanced lamellar body secretion. J Invest Dermatol 1994; 102:789–795.

44. Wood LC, Feingold KR, Seqeira-Martin SM, Elias PM, Grunfeld C. Barrier function coordinately regulates epidermal IL-1 and IL-1 receptor antagonist mRNA levels. Exp Dematol 1994; 3:56–60.

45. Hirao T, Aoki H, Yoshida T, Sato Y, Kamaoda H. Elevation of interleukin 1 receptor antagonist in the stratum corneum of sun-exposed and ultraviolet B-irradiated human skin. J Invest Dermatol 1996; 106:1102–1107.

46. Terui T, Hirao T, Sato Y, Uesugi T, Honda M, Iguchi M, Matsumura N, Kudoh K, Aiba S, Tagami H. An increased ratio of interleukin-1 receptor antagonist to interleukin-1 alpha in inflammatory skin diseases. Exp Dermatol 1998; 7:327–334.

47. Kunii T, Hirao T, Kikuchi K, Tagami H. Stratum corneum lipid profile and maturation pattern of corneocytes in the outermost layer of fresh scars: the presence of immature corneocytes plays a much more important role in the barrier dysfunction than do changes in intercellular lipids. Br J Dermatol 2003; 149:749–756.

48. O'goshi K, Okada M, Iguchi M, Tagami H. The predilection sites for chronic atopic dermatitis do not show any special functional uniqueness of the stratum corneum. Exog Dermatol 2002; 1:195–202.

49. Schaefer H, Redelmeier TE. Skin Barrier. Principles of Percutaneous Absorption. Karger, Basel, 1996.
50. Darsow U, Vieluf D, Ring J. Evaluating the relevance of aeroallergen sensitization in atopic eczema with the atopy patch test: a randomized, double-blind multicenter study. Atopy Patch Test Study Group. J Am Acad Dermatol 1999; 40:187–193.
51. Grice K, Satter H, Baker H. The cutaneous barrier to salts and water in psoriasis and in normal skin. Br J Dermatol 1973; 88:459–463.
52. Leveque JL. Mesurement of transepidermal water loss. In: Leveque JL, ed. Cutaneous Investigation in Health and Disease. Noninvasive Methods and Instrumentation. New York: Marcel Dekker, 1989:135–152.
53. Motta S, Monti M, Sesana S, Caputo R, Carelli S, Ghidoni R. Ceramide composition of the psoriatic scale. Biochim Biophys Acta 1993; 1182:147–151.
54. Motta S, Monti M, Sesana S, Mellesi L, Ghidoni R, Caputo R. Abnormality of water barrier function in psoriasis: role of ceramide fractions; Arch Dermatol 1994; 130: 452–456.
55. Fartasch M. Epidermal barrier in disorders of the skin. Microsc Res Tech 1997; 38: 361–372.
56. Kobayashi H, Tagami H. Functional analysis of the stratum corneum of patients with atopic dermatitis: comparison with psoriasis vulgaris. Exp Dermatol 2003; 2:33–40.
57. Hirao T, Terui T, Takeuchi I, Kobayashi H, Okada M, Takahashi M, Tagami H. The ratio of immature cornified envelopes does not correlate with parakeratosis in inflammatory skin disorders. Exp Dermatol 2003; 12:591–601.
58. De la Brassinne MF, Couteux-Dumont CM. Tritiated thymidine labelling of epidermis in pustular psoriasis. Arch Dermatol 1972; 106:768.
59. Proksch E, Elias PM. Epidermal barrier in atopic dermatitis. In: Bieber T, Leung DY, eds. Atopic Dermatitis. New York: Marcel Dekker 2002:123–143.
60. Seidenari S, Giusti G. Objective assessment of the skin of children affected by atopic dermatitis: a study of pH, capacitance and TEWL in eczematous and clinically uninvolved skin. Acta Derm Venereol 1995; 75:429–433.
61. Werner Y, Lindberg M. Transepidermal water loss in dry and clinically normal skin in patients with atopic dermatitis. Acta Derm Venereol (Stockh) 1985; 65:102–105.
62. Loden M, Olsson H, Axell T, Linde YW. Friction, capacitance and transepidermal water loss (TEWL) in dry atopic and normal skin. Br J Dermatol 1992; 126:137–141.
63. Fartasch M, Diepgen TL. The barrier function in atopic dry skin. Disturbance of membrane-coating granule exocytosis and formation of epidermal lipids? Acta Derm Venereol Suppl (Stockh) 1992; 176:26–31.
64. Melnik B, Hollmann J, Plewig G. Decreased stratum corneum ceramides in atopic individuals—a pathobiochemical factor in xerosis? Br J Dermatol 1988; 119:547–549.
65. Di Nardo A, Wertz P, Giannetti A, Seidenari S. Ceramide and cholesterol composition of the skin of patients with atopic dermatitis. Acta Derm Venereol 1998; 78:27–30.
66. Pilgram GS, Vissers DC, van der Meulen H, Pavel S, Lavrijsen SP, Bouwstra JA, Koerten HK. Aberrant lipid organization in stratum corneum of patients with atopic dermatitis and lamellar ichthyosis. J Invest Dermatol 2001; 117:710–717.
67. Murata Y, Ogata J, Higaki Y, Kawashima M, Yada Y, Higuchi K, Tsuchiya T, Kawainami S, Imokawa G. Abnormal expression of sphingomyelin acylase in atopic dermatitis: an etiologic factor for ceramide deficiency? J Invest Dermatol 1996; 106:1242–1249.
68. Ohnishi Y, Okino N, Ito M, Imayama S. Ceramidase activity in bacterial skin flora as a possible cause of ceramide deficiency in atopic dermatitis. Clin Diagn Lab Immunol 1999; 6:101–104.
69. Cui CY, Kusuda S, Seguchi T, Takahashi M, Aisu K, Tezuka T. Decreased level of prosaposin in atopic skin. J Invest Dermatol 1997; 109:319–323.
70. Agner T. Noninvasive measuring methods for the investigation of irritant patch test reactions. A study of patients with hand eczema, atopic dermatitis and controls. Acta Derm Venereol Suppl (Stockh) 1992; 173:1–26.

71. Matsumoto M, Sugiura H, Uehara M. Skin barrier function in patients with completely healed atopic dermatitis. J Dermatol Sci 2000; 23:178–182.

72. Aioi A, Tonogaito H, Suto H, Hamada K, Ra CR, Ogawa H, Maibach H, Matsuda H. Impairment of skin barrier function in NC/Nga Tnd mice as a possible model for atopic dermatitis. Br J Dermatol 2001; 144:12–18.

73. Saijo S, Tagami H. Dry skin of newborn infants: functional analysis of the stratum corneum. Pediatr Dermatol 1991; 8:155–159.

74. Kikuchi K, Kobayashi H, O'goshi K, Tagami H. The impairment of skin barrier function is not inherent in atopic dermatitis patients: A prospective study conducted in new borns. Pediatr Dermatol. In press.

75. Williams ML. Ichthyosis: mechanisms of disease. Pediatr Dermatol 1992; 9:365–368.

76. Frost P, Weinstein GD, Bothwell JW, Wildnauer R. Ichthyosiform dermatoses. III. Studies of transepidermal water loss. Arch Dermatol 1968; 98:230–233.

77. Lavrijsen AP, Oestmann E, Hermans J, Bodde HE, Vermeer BJ, Ponec M. Barrier function parameters in various keratinization disorders: transepidermal water loss and vascular response to hexyl nicotinate. Br J Dermatol 1993; 129:547–553.

78. Zettersten E, Man MQ, Sato J, Denda M, Farrell A, Ghadially R, Williams ML, Feingold KR, Elias PM. Recessive x-linked ichthyosis: role of cholesterol-sulfate accumulation in the barrier abnormality. J Invest Dermatol 1998; 111:784–789.

79. Huber M, Rettler I, Bernasconi K, Frenk E, Lavrijsen SP, Ponec M, Bon A, Lautenschlager S, Schorderet DF, Hohl D. Mutations of keratinocyte transglutaminase in lamellar ichthyosis. Science 1995; 267:525–528.

80. Matsuki M, Yamashita F, Ishida-Yamamoto A, Yamada K, Kinoshita C, Fushiki S, Ueda E, Morishima Y, Tabata K, Yasuno H, Hashida M, Iizuka H, Ikawa M, Okabe M, Kondoh G, Kinoshita T, Takeda J, Yamanishi K. Defective stratum corneum and early neonatal death in mice lacking the gene for transglutaminase 1 (keratinocyte transglutaminase). Proc Natl Acad Sci USA 1998; 95:1044–1049.

81. Kuramoto N, Takizawa T, Takizawa T, Matsuki M, Morioka H, Robinson JM, Yamanishi K. Development of ichthyosiform skin compensates for defective permeability barrier function in mice lacking transglutaminase 1. J Clin Invest 2002; 109: 243–250.

82. Lavrijsen AP, Bouwstra JA, Gooris GS, Weerheim A, Bodde HE, Ponec M. Reduced skin barrier function parallels abnormal stratum corneum lipid organization in patients with lamellar ichthyosis. J Invest Dermatol 1995; 105:619–624.

83. Elias PM, Schmuth M, Uchida Y, Rice RH, Behne M, Crumrine D, Feingold KR, Holleran WM, Pharm D. Basis for the permeability barrier abnormality in lamellar ichthyosis. Exp Dermatol 2002; 11:248–256.

84. Schmuth M, Yosipovitch G, Williams ML, Weber F, Hintner H, Ortiz-Urda S, Rappersberger K, Crumrine D, Feingold KR, Elias PM. Pathogenesis of the permeability barrier abnormality in epidermolytic hyperkeratosis. J Invest Dermatol 2001; 117:837–847.

85. Holleran WM, Ginns EI, Menon GK, Grundmann JU, Fartasch M, McKinney CE, Elias PM, Sidransky E. Consequences of beta-glucocerebrosidase deficiency in epidermis. Ultrastructure and permeability barrier alterations in Gaucher disease. J Clin Invest 1994; 93:1756–1764.

86. Fartasch M, Williams ML, Elias PM. Altered lamellar body secretion and stratum corneum membrane structure in Netherton syndrome: differentiation from other infantile erythrodermas and pathogenic implications. Arch Dermatol 1999; 135:823–832.

87. Ishida-Yamamoto A, Kato H, Kiyama H, Armstrong DK, Munro CS, Eady RA, Nakamura S, Kinouchi M, Takahashi H, Iizuka H. Mutant loricrin is not crosslinked into the cornified cell envelope but is translocated into the nucleus in loricrin keratoderma. J Invest Dermatol 2000; 115:1088–1094.

88. Feingold KR. The regulation and role of epidermal lipid synthesis. Adv Lipid Res 1991; 24:57–82.

89. Tagami H. Morphological and functional changes of the skin by topical corticosteroid application. Acta Dermatol (Kyoto) 1971; 66:1–2.
90. Yamamoto A, Takenouchi K, Ito M. Impaired water barrier function in acne vulgaris. Arch Dermatol Res 1995; 287:214–218.
91. Kikuchi-Numagami K, Suetake T, Yanai M, Tahahashi M, Tanaka M, Tagami H. Functional and morphological studies of photodamaged skin on the hands of middle-aged Japanese golfers. Eur J Dermatol 2000; 10:277–281.
92. Le Fur I, Reinberg A, Lopez S, Morizot F, Mechkouri M, Tschachler E. Analysis of circadian and ultradian rhythms of skin surface properties of face and forearm of healthy women. J Invest Dermatol 2001; 117:718–724.
93. Kikuchi K, Kobayashi K, le Fur I, Tschachler E, Tagami H. The winter season affects more severely the facial skin than the forearm skin: comparative biophysical studies conducted in the same Japanese females in later summer and winter Exog Dermatol 2002; 1:32–38.
94. Kikuchi K, Kobayashi H, Hirao T, Ito A, Takahashi H, Tagami H. Improvement of mild inflammatory changes of the facial skin induced by winter environment with daily applications of a moisturizing cream: a half-side test assessed by measurements of biophysical skin parameters, cytokine expression pattern and the formation of cornified envelope. Dermatology 2003; 207:269–275.
95. Agner T, Serup J. Seasonal variation in skin resistance to irritants. Br J Dermatol 1989; 121:323–328.
96. Frosch P, Duncan S, Kligman A. Cutaneous biometrics. I. The response of human skin to dimethyl sulphoxide. Br J Dermatol 1980; 102:263–274.
97. Tupker R, Coenraads P, Fidler V. Irritant susceptibility and weal and flare reactions to bioactive agents in atopic dermatitis. II. Influence of season. Br J Dermatol 1995; 133:365–370.
98. Sakai S, Endo Y, Ozawa N, Sugawara T, Kusaka A, Sayo T, Tagami H, Inoue S. Characteristics of the epidermis and stratum corneum of hairless mice with experimentally induced diabetes mellitus. J Invest Dermatol 2003; 120:79–85.
99. Sakai S, Kikuchi K, Satoh J, Tagami H, Inoue S. Functional Properties of the Stratum Corneum in Patients with Diabetes Mellitus: Similarities to Senile Xerosis. Br J Dermatol. In press.
100. Elias PM, Feingold KR, Fluhr JW. Skin as an organ of protection. In: Freedberg IM, Eisen AZ, Wolff K, Austen KF, Goldsmith LA, Katz SI, eds. Fitzpatrick's Dermatology in General Medicine. New York: McGraw Hill, 2003:107–118.
101. Suetake T, Sasai S, Zhaen YX, Tagami H. Effects of silicone gel sheet on the stratum corneum hydration. Br J Dermatol 2000; 53:503–507.

27

Pathogenesis of the Barrier Abnormalities in Disorders of Cornification

Matthias Schmuth
Department of Dermatology, Medical University Innsbruck, Innsbruck, Austria

Peter M. Elias
Dermatology Service, VA Medical Centre, and Department of Dermatology, University of California, San Francisco, California, U.S.A.

Mary L. Williams
Department of Paediatrics, VA Medical Centre, University of California, San Francisco, California, U.S.A.

INTRODUCTION

Normal Epidermal Differentiation and Cornification

The epidermis is a stratified epithelium. The bulk of epidermal cells consists of keratinocytes, which undergo a complex process of differentiation as they transit outwards from the basal, proliferative compartment. This sequence culminates in terminal cellular cornification and in the deposition of an extracellular lipid-enriched lamellar matrix to form the "two-compartment" stratum corneum (SC) (Fig. 1) (1–3). Terminal cornification involves: (i) extrusion of lamellar bodies (LBs) to deliver lipid precursors and their hydrolytic enzymes to the extracellular domain to form lamellar bilayers unit structures; (ii) dissolution of the nucleus and other organelles; (iii) hydrolysis of profilaggrin to filaggrin; (iv) aggregation of keratin filaments to form macrofibrils; (v) breakdown of filaggrin and other intracellular proteins to yield amino acids and other small molecules; and (vi) extensive cross-linking of loricrin, involucrin, and other structural proteins by transglutaminases to form the cornified envelope (CE), at the inner surface of the keratinocyte plasma membrane (4–10). As a result of these events (i) highly organized hydrophobic lamellar membranes in the extracellular domain form a barrier to the movement of water, electrolytes, and other molecules from the organism's interior to the skin surface and vice versa; (ii) intracellular keratin fibers and CEs, a rigid chemically resistant layer, provide a mechanical barrier to injury; and (iii) protcolysis of filaggrin generates a pool of osmotically active small molecules within the corneocyte to trap and hold water (corneocyte hydration) (11–16,19). Thus, the SC can be viewed as the end product of epidermal differentiation and as consisting of two interdependent compartments,

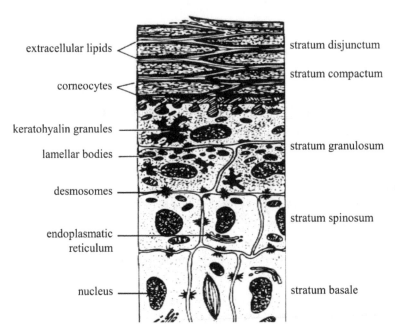

extracellular lipids — stratum disjunctum

corneocytes — stratum compactum

keratohyalin granules —

lamellar bodies — stratum granulosum

desmosomes —

endoplasmatic reticulum — stratum spinosum

nucleus — stratum basale

Figure 1 Structure of the epidermis.

the corneocytes (i.e., the "bricks") and the extracellular lipid membranes (i.e., the "mortar"). While the corneocytes are essential for the mechanical strength of the epidermis, the lipid-enriched matrix is primarily responsible for the permeability barrier to water and electrolyte transit (1).

Extracellular Compartment

   LBs. The lamellar membranes of the extracellular SC matrix, which subserves the barrier, derive from secretion of epidermal LBs, and these organelles in turn are generated by a highly active lipid-synthetic factory, operative in all of the nucleated cell layers of the epidermis. These secretory organelles are 0.3–0.4×0.25 μm structures that comprise about 10% of the cytosol of the stratum granulosum (SG) (17,18). Following secretion at the SG–SC interface, LB lipids are processed by co-secreted hydrolases from their polar lipid precursors into a more hydrophobic mixture of ceramides, free fatty acids (FFA), and cholesterol (in an ∼1:1:1 molar ratio), and organized into lamellar membrane unit structures. These lamellar membranes form the hydrophobic matrix in which corneocytes are embedded (19). If this system is experimentally disrupted, e.g., mechanically by tape stripping or chemically by solvent or detergent treatment, a homeostatic repair response ensues aimed at barrier recovery (20). The first step in the repair response following barrier disruption is rapid secretion (within minutes) of preformed LB contents from keratinocytes of the outer SG, leaving the cytosol of these cells largely depleted of LBs (12). Within hours, newly formed LBs appear in SG cells, and the quantities of secreted LB contents increase at the SG–SC interface, and new lamellar bilayers appear in the lower SC. The repair response continues with both accelerated formation and continued secretion of LB. The rapid LB formation by SG cells requires the availability of the major lipid components of LBs, namely cholesterol, glucosylceramides, and phospholipids. Permeability barrier disruption results in a rapid, marked increase in the synthesis of cholesterol, ceramides, and FFAs (a major component of both phospholipids and ceramides). The increase in cholesterol synthesis is associated with an increase in HMG CoA reductase activity, and other key enzymes in the cholesterol synthetic pathway, i.e., HMG CoA synthase, farnesyl diphosphate synthase, and squalene synthase. Whereas the increase in FA synthesis is due to an increased activity of both of the key enzymes of FA synthesis, acetyl CoA carboxylase and FA synthase, the increase in ceramide synthesis is due to an increased activity of serine palmitoyl transferase, the enzyme that catalyzes the initial and first committed step in ceramide synthesis. Since the activity of glucosylceramide synthase, the enzyme which synthesizes glucosylceramide, does not increase following barrier disruption, stimulation of glucosylceramide synthesis is dependent upon the availability of FAs for both sphingoid base formation and N-acylation. Thus, a specific, coordinate increase in the synthesis of the key lipid constituents of LBs provides the pool of lipids that is required for the formation of new LBs (21–25).

SC Lipids. The processing of secreted LB contents generates an approximately equimolar ratio of non-polar lipids. Lesser, but variable amounts of cholesterol esters, triglycerides, and diglycerides also persist, which may be, in part, of sebaceous gland origin (26–28). The FFA comprise a mixture of essential (EFA) and non-essential FFA (NEFA). NEFAs and EFAs are required separately as critical structural ingredients of the barrier (27). NEFAs derive largely, if not entirely, from the hydrolysis of phospholipids, which are co-secreted with their respective secretory phospholipases (sPLAs) at the SG–SC interface. These phospholipids-derived NEFAs are critical not only as structural ingredients for the barrier, but they also are key acidifiers of the SC interstices (28). The mortar lipids also contain abundant cholesterol, which is secreted unchanged from LBs. Lesser quantities of cholesterol for the barrier derive from the hydrolysis of cholesterol sulfate to cholesterol by the enzyme steroid sulfatase. The third key lipid constituent of the mortar is a family of seven ceramide species, which vary according to their (i) sphingosine versus phytosphingosine (extra-OH group) base; (ii) alpha- versus non-alpha-hydroxylated N-acyl FAs, which typically are ≥C30 in length; and (iii) the presence of an additional, omega-esterified linoleic acid residue. Ceramides 1 and 4 are the principal repositories for the EFAs, linoleic acid, a critical structural ingredient in the barrier. These epidermis-unique molecules appear to link adjacent bilayers through their highly elongated N-acyl chains. The esterified linoleate moiety is important for barrier function, because in EFA deficiency, the primary biochemical defect is a substitution of NEFA for linoleate, a biochemical alteration that results in a pronounced permeability barrier defect.

Corneocyte-Bound Lipid Envelope. A 10-nm, tightly apposed, electron-lucent plasma membrane–like structure represents the link between the extracellular lipids and the external aspect of the protein enriched mammalian corneocytes (14–16). The corneocyte-bound lipid envelope (CLE) comprises unique omega-hydroxyceramides with very long chain N-acyl FAs covalently bound to the CE. These omega-hydroxy FAs could either derive from the lipolytic hydrolysis of secreted acylceramides or from the insertion of the omega-glucosylhydroxyceramide-rich limiting membrane of the LB into the apical plasma membrane of the outer SG. The CLE appears to mediate several functions, including serving (i) as "molecular rivet" in SC cohesion and (ii) as a scaffold for extracellular lamellar membrane organization. Despite its extreme hydrophobicity, its ability to restrict water movement is unclear, since solvent extraction of SC leaves the CLE intact, but the SC is completely porous to transcutaneous water loss (29).

Corneodesmosomes. Cohesion between adjacent corneocytes is facilitated both by extracellular lipids, and by the "tongue-and-groove" arrangement of adjacent cells, by corneodesmosomes (CD) (= specialized desmosomes of the SC), which rivet together adjacent cells (30–33). Critical proteins mediating cell-to-cell adhesion in epithelia are the desmogleins and the desmocollins, desmosomal cadherins. Whereas desmosomes typically contain three isoforms of DSG and DSC, CD contain only the DSG1 and DSC1 isoforms (34), a modification that allows homophilic binding to their counterparts on adjacent corneocytes. A recently described 36- to 48-kDa differentiation product of the epidermis, corneodesmosin, is reportedly a secreted LB product, accounting for its localization to the extracellular surfaces of CD, where it appears to shield DSG1 and DSC1 from premature proteolysis. The cross-linking of additional CD constituents (e.g., envoplakin, periplakin) into the CE further stabilizes these structures.

The progressive changes that occur in CD and their constituent peptides point to a critical role for extracellular proteases in the orchestration of corneocyte shedding. Several types of serine, cysteine, and aspartate protease activities have been identified in SC, with the most convincing link to desquamation for two serine proteases, SC chymotryptic enzyme (SCCE) and SC tryptic enzyme (SCTE) (Table 1). Whereas SCCE is predominantly intercellular (34), SCTE occurs both in the SC interstices and the corneocyte cytosol (35). Based upon in vitro inhibitor studies, SCCE and SCTE appear to be the major regulators of desquamation. Endogenous serine and aspartate inhibitors are believed to critically balance this process. The serine protease inhibitors (SPI) present in the SC include secretory leukocyte protease inhibitor (SLPI), skin-derived antileukocyte proteinase (SKALP) or elafin, plasminogen activator inhibitor (PAI), and LEKTI (which is mutated in Netherton syndrome; see below). Cysteine protease inhibitors present in SC include cystatin-alpha and cystatin (M/E). Morphological evidence for loss of CD from the lower SC is paralleled by the progressive degradation of its constituent proteins, desmoglein 1 (DSG 1), and corneodesmosin (Table 1) (36).

Corneocyte Compartment

Whereas the importance of the extracellular lipid matrix for the permeability barrier is known, the role of the corneocyte in the permeability barrier is less clear. Its structural proteins have been studied intensively as markers of epidermal differentiation (7–10,37) and they are well known to perform other critical epidermal functions, i.e., mechanical resilience, UV filtration, and SC hydration. One of their contributions

Table 1 Protease and Anti-Protease Activity in SC

	Preferred substrate	Anti-proteases
Serine proteases		
SCTE	DSF1 pro-SCCE	LEKTI 1
SCCE	DSG1, DSC1, CDSN	SKALP, SLPI, LEKTI 1
Cysteine proteases		
SCCP	DSC1, CDSN	Cystatin M/E, Cystatin-α, SLPI
Aspartate proteases		
Cathepsin G	DSC1, CDSN	? SLPI

to the permeability barrier is to function as "spacers," i.e., they force water, microbes, and xenobiotics to transit via a tortuous extracellular pathway (38). Another important role relates to the CLE and the CE, which together comprise a critical scaffold for the deposition and organization of the extracellular lipid matrix (Fig. 2), as depicted above.

The CE. The CE is an insoluble proteinaceous layer, 10- to 15-nm thick, deposited subjacent to the plasma membrane, marking formation of the SC. The CE is composed of over 10 highly cross-linked cytosolic proteins, including involucrin, loricrin, elafin, desmoplakin, envoplakin, cytostatin-α, and pancornulins/cornifins [small proline-rich proteins (SPRRs)]. A distinctive feature of the CE is its stability to heat, reducing or chaotropic agents, and to mechanical trauma (39). Whereas involucrin predominates in the inner portion of the CE and accounts for 5% to 15% of the whole CE, loricrin accounts for up to 80% of CE protein mass, and is enriched in the outer portion of the CE (9,10,39).

Formation of the CE is catalyzed by the epidermal-specific, calcium-dependent enzyme, transglutaminase-1 (TG1), a 92-kDa protein, which catalyzes the formation of γ-glutamyl-ε-lysine isopeptide bonds between the precursor proteins of the CE. Although TG1 protein and mRNA are expressed in the cytosol of both the spinous and granular layers, enzymatic activity is expressed primarily in the outermost granular cell. At least two other TG isoforms, TG2 (82 kDa) and TG3 (77 kDa), are also present in the keratinocyte cytosol, and contribute variably to CE cross-linking. Biochemical studies on lamellar ichthyosis (LI) keratinocytes bearing mutations in TG1 have shown that virtually all cross-linked CEs are absent, suggesting that residual TG activities cannot compensate for TG1 deficiency. However, TG1 is not only the principal TG in the outer SG, but it is the only isoform that is anchored to the plasma membrane, hence other TGs' may be present in insufficient quantities and/or in the wrong locale to compensate for TG1 deficiency (39–41).

CE (Cornified Envelope)
Transglutaminase-1
Involucrin
Loricrin
Keratin
Profilaggrin/Filaggrin
Other Structural Proteins

CLE (Cornified Lipid Envelope)
Omega-Hydroxyceramides

ECM (Extracellular Matrix)
Lamellar Bilayers consisting of
    LB Lipids
(Serine/Cysteine/Aspartate-)
    Proteases
(Serine-) Protease Inhibitors
Other Enzymes

LB (Lamellar Body)
Cholesterol
Glycosylceramides
Sphingomyelin
Phospholipids
Hydrolases
Other Proteins

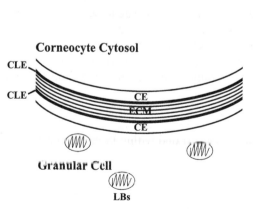

Corneocyte Cytosol
CLE
CLE
CE
ECM
CE
Granular Cell
LBs

Figure 2 Stratum granulosum (SG) — stratum corneum (SC) interface.

Involucrin is a 69-kDa rod-shaped molecule with a series of highly conserved 10 amino acid repeats containing three glutamine residues each as potential cross-linking sites. It is expressed in the upper spinous and SG layers, and appears to be the first envelope precursor that is cross-linked by TG1 in the outer SG. A defective scaffold presumably accounts for the minor barrier abnormality in involucrin knock-out mice that otherwise display a grossly normal phenotype (42).

Loricrin is a cysteine (7%)-, serine (22%)-, and glycine (55%)-enriched 38-kDa highly insoluble peptide, comprising one component of keratohyalin granules. Loricrin is expressed sequentially during differentiation after K1/10 and involucrin, just before profilaggrin, and is cross-linked to the CE immediately after LB secretion, coincident with cornification. Comprising up to 80% of CE proteins, loricrin accounts for much of its mechanical resistance (7,9,43,44). Yet, the CE not only protects against external injury, it also serves as a scaffold for the deposition of the extracellular lamellar bilayers. A mutation resulting in elongation of the C-terminal domain of one loricrin allele occurs in loricrin keratoderma. Patients with the loricrin defect display not only digital constrictions (pseudo-ainhum) and palmer keratoderma, but also a mild, generalized ichthyosis (Vohwinkel syndrome with ichthyosis) (45).

Keratins. Keratins (K) are the most abundant structural proteins of the epidermis and its appendages, maintaining the mechanical resilience of these epithelia, a role that is most vividly demonstrated in epidermis (46). Keratins are of two types, type I or acidic (K9–20) and type II or basic (K1–8), which are co-expressed in anti-parallel pairs under a variety of conditions. All keratins display a similar secondary structure, with a central rod domain comprising four α helices, and distinctive non-helical head and tail sequences. Whereas expression of keratins 5 and 14 is restricted to the basal cell compartment, keratins 1 and 10 are produced in all suprabasal nucleated cell layers, and keratin 2e is produced in the outermost nucleated layers (6,46).

Prior to cornification, these keratins are organized into filament bundles that loop between desmosomal plaques and the nuclear envelope providing a cytoskeleton that protects keratinocytes from mechanical injury (47). Deletions of as few as 10 amino acids from the rod domain of either pair result in keratin clumping, i.e., the defective allelic protein binds to its partner in a dominant-negative fashion, forming defective intermediate filaments, resulting in intracellular vacuolization and cellular fragility in the affected epidermal cell layers. For example, in epidermolysis bullosa simplex (EBS), caused by mutations in either K5 or K14, basal keratinocytes are less resilient to trauma, whereas in epidermolytic hyperkeratosis (EHK), due to mutations in either K1 or K10, both fragility of suprabasal keratinocytes and hyperkeratosis are evident (16,47,188,195).

Profilaggrin. Profilaggrin is a large, histidine-rich, highly cationic phospho-protein, consisting of filaggrin repeats, connected by peptide segments enriched in hydrophobic amino acids. Profilaggrin is concentrated within keratohyalin granules, where it may sequester loricrin, which also localizes to keratohyalin. During terminal differentiation, profilaggrin is both dephosphorylated and proteolytically processed by a Ca^{2+}-dependent protein convertase, furin, at the N-terminus to yield filaggrin, which ionically binds to K1/10, inducing collapse of associated intermediate filaments to form macrofibrils in the corneocyte cytosol. Filaggrin is attached to the inner surface of the CE in the lower SC, but it is proteolytically detached as corneocytes enter the stratum disjunctum (48,49). Thereafter, filaggrin undergoes proteolysis generating osmotically active small molecules that allow the corneocyte to attract water and maintain hydration; filaggrin hydrolysis is regulated by the relative humidity of the external environment (50).

Abnormal Cornification

When epidermal cornification proceeds incorrectly, the resulting skin phenotype frequently involves epidermal hyperplasia (acanthosis) and hyperkeratosis, with visible accumulation of squames (scales) on the skin's surface, and occasionally skin fragility or blistering.* The group of skin disorders with abnormalities in epidermal cornification resulting in excessive scaling has historically been termed ichthyosis (from Greek *ichthys* for fish). The ichthyoses comprise a large group of both hereditary and acquired disorders of cornification of diverse etiology (51–55). Mutations affecting a wide spectrum of epidermal structures and functions, including lipid metabolism enzymes, structural proteins, and cellular communication and signalling have been identified as causes of these disorders. Abnormalities in any of these factors seem to result in the rather stereotypic formation of excess SC with impaired functional properties; i.e., defects in a variety of critical SC components cause ichthyotic/hyperkeratotic skin phenotypes, indicating that excess SC formation, often accompanied by incomplete cornification, represents the inherent response of the epidermis to pleiotropic molecular insufficiencies. Pathological hyperkeratosis/ scaling of the skin can be due to increased keratinocyte proliferation, accelerated or abnormal differentiation, impaired or increased intercellular adhesion, defective composition, secretion or organization of the extracellular SC lipids, or the combination of one or more of these factors. In addition to the phenotypic characteristic of hyperkeratosis and scaling, most disorders of cornification also exhibit impaired permeability barrier function. As the SC serves as a biosensor, transmitting danger signals to the underlying nucleated, epidermal cell layers, any acute or sustained insult that results in barrier impairment stimulates a homeostatic repair response, including both increased synthesis and secretion of LB lipids and a mitogenic stimulus to the epidermis. Thus, the phenotype of hyperkeratosis and scaling might be the expression of this common response to a variety of pathophysiologic events. Other SC functions in addition to altered desquamation and an impaired barrier may be abnormal in these disorders. Increased susceptibility to cutaneous and systemic infections in several of these disorders suggests impairment of innate immune defense functions, but this has not been studied. Infants and children may have increased caloric requirements due to the energy losses that accompany excessive rates of transepidermal water loss (TEWL) (56,57). Some patients with more severe generalized ichthyoses [e.g., LI/congenital ichthyosiform erythroderma (CIE)] have decreased heat tolerance, attributed to obstruction of sweat ducts by the hyperkeratosis.

Pathogenesis—Permeability Barrier as End Product of Cornification

Traditionally the hereditary disorders of cornification have been classified according to inheritance pattern, clinical phenotype, and in a few instances, histopathological and biochemical criteria. With recent progress in the identification of the molecular basis of many ichthyoses, these classification schemes can now be put into new

---

* For example, epidermolytic hyperkeratosis.

perspectives (58). It is now possible to more precisely decipher the downstream con-sequences of defined alterations in the nucleic acid code for certain proteins based upon tissue morphology, biochemistry, and function (1,59–62). In some instances, the pathogenic sequence from gene defect to disease expression is quite straight-forward, while in others, a more complex sequence is operative. For example, in Gaucher's disease due to null mutations in the beta-glucocerebrosidase gene, inabil-ity to deglycosylate glucosylceramide to ceramide results in altered SC lamellar membrane structure and impaired barrier function (63). Yet in recessive X-linked ichthyosis, the pathway to altered SC function is considerably more complex than a mere effect of substitution of cholesterol sulfate for a portion of the bulk choles-terol in SC membranes (64). In addition to lipid metabolic defects that lead to altered lamellar membrane structure and function, abnormalities in the CE and even kera-tinocyte cytosol are accompanied by surprisingly severe barrier abnormalities. Yet these effects are mediated primarily by downstream effects on formation of the lamellar bilayer system, providing further support for the primacy of the extracellu-lar lipid bilayers in provision of the permeability barrier. For example, defects in the CE/CLE scaffold account for barrier abnormalities both in LI (61,65) and in loricrin keratoderma (45,62). Similarly, mutations in keratin 1 or 10 in EHK provoke a bar-rier abnormality by interfering with LB exocytosis (in this instance a cytoskeletal, rather than a scaffold abnormality) (60).

Complexity appears to be the unifying concept in the linkage between pheno-type and genotype in this family of disorders. Some disease phenotypes are geneti-cally heterogenous, e.g., LI/CIE, resulting from both lipid metabolic defects and CE abnormalities. And, despite the previous classification of the disorders of corni-fication into those with abnormalities in the "mortar" of the SC (i.e., barrier lipids and corneodesmosomes), and those with abnormalities in the "bricks" (i.e., CE pro-teins, keratins, filaggrin), recent studies have uncovered molecular defects in a num-ber of ichthyoses that do not fit either of these two categories. Indeed, the spectrum of defects that results in an ichthyotic phenotype has been astonishing, and includes gap junction proteins involved in intercellular communication [e.g., connexin muta-tions in Vohwinkel disease and erythrokeratodermia variabilis (EKV)], intracellular calcium transport involved in intracellular signaling (mutations in endoplasmic reti-culum), -Ca-ATPase in Darier's disease, and even enzymes of DNA excision repair (e.g., XPD, a $5'$ to $3'$ helicase that is a subunit of the transcription factor TFIIH) in Trichothiodystrophy (66,67). Moreover transgenic mouse models overexpressing growth factors [e.g., TGF-α (68)] similarly result in a hyperkeratotic, scaly pheno-type, suggesting that not only the components of the SC have all to be present, but that the coordination of the process is equally critical. The common denomina-tor of all these entities may be a general disturbance of epidermal differentiation, ultimately resulting in abnormalities in the two main components of the epidermal permeability barrier, the corneocytes and the extracellular lipid matrix. Thus, it appears, that disturbance in the formation and function of SC is the final common pathway of many mutations expressed in keratinocytes. Nevertheless, although this might be an oversimplification, for the purpose of this chapter we will group the disorders of cornification according to three categories: (i) abnormalities of extracel-lular lipid structures, (ii) abnormalities of corneocytes, and (iii) abnormalities in establishing/maintaining of the barrier. Elucidation of the pathogenic consequences of molecular defects leading to disorders of cornification will not only improve our understanding of ichthyoses, but also uncover processes required for normal skin function and elucidate the pathophysiology of other common cutaneous scaling disorders, including atopic dermatitis and psoriasis. Importantly, a better understanding of how the gene mutations/protein disruptions result in clinical disease will foster the development of rational therapeutic approaches (55,66,67).

ABNORMALITIES IN EXTRACELLULAR LIPID LAMELLAR STRUCTURES AND OTHER LIPID METABOLIC DEFECTS

Defects in extracellular lipid lamellar structures, LBs, or key enzymes of epidermal lipid synthesis can result in an ichthyotic skin phenotype and impaired epidermal permeability barrier function. For example, the barrier abnormalities in disorders, such as recessive X-linked ichthyosis (RXLI), essential fatty acid deficiency (EFAD), and neonatal Gaucher's disease result from changes in extracellular membrane architecture in SC due to abnormal membrane lipid composition as a result of discrete lipid biochemical defects (55,67,69–72). Because the permeability barrier to water and electrolyte movement resides in the extracellular, rather than in the corneocyte (brick), compartment of the SC, the impaired barrier function in these disorders can easily be explained. An expected consequence of impaired barrier function is epidermal hyperplasia (73,74), a common finding in the disorders of cornification.

Inherited Abnormalities of Lipid Metabolism

*Recessive X-Linked Ichthyosis (RXLI) (Steroid Sulfatase Deficiency, OMIM *308100)*

Clinical Characteristics. RXLI, due to its mode of inheritance, only affects males (approximately 1 in 2000–6000) (64,69,75,76). It is characterized by non-erythrodermic generalized scaling, which commonly is most prominent on the extensor surfaces of the extremities. One study reported involvement of the pre-auricular area in 93% of the affected individuals (77). There is typically no palmoplantar involvement. While asymptomatic corneal opacities represent common extracutaneous manifestations of RXLI, there have only been anecdotal reports about an increased incidence of cryptorchidism and undescended testes in young patients. The disorder usually manifests itself ~1 to 3 weeks of age with an exaggerated neonatal desquamation. By six months the mature phenotype is present and it tends not to remit with age. Mothers of infants with RXLI often display the placental sulfatase deficiency syndrome, which is characterized by an abnormal urinary sterol excretion pattern and has been associated with a failure of initiation and/or progression of labor. When an RXLI-like ichthyosis occurs in association with other abnormalities, e.g., developmental delay, Kallman's syndrome, short stature, chondrodysplasia punctata, albinism, etc., it is likely to be part of a contiguous gene syndrome called multiple sulfatase deficiency (OMIM #272200) This phenotype also includes features of metachromatic leukodystrophy and mucopolysaccharidosis.

Molecular Defect. RXLI is due to deletions/mutations in the steroid sulfatase (STS) gene, localized on the distal tip of the short arm of the X-chromosome (78–81). The majority (>90%) of RXLI cases are due to deletion of the STS gene, and the remainders are caused by point mutations within the gene. The diagnosis can be made by measurement of blood or scale cholesterol sulfate levels, serum lipid electrophoresis [increased mobility of beta-lipoproteins (LDL)], direct enzymatic assay, DNA sequencing, or fluorescence in situ hybridization (FISH) in cases due to gene deletion. The biochemical alterations associated with increased cholesterol sulfate contents in the SC are discussed in detail elsewhere in the book. Multiple sulfatase deficiency is an extremely rare autosomal recessive trait due to mutations in the formylglycine generating enzyme (FGE), encoded by the gene SUMF-1, which catalyzes the post-translational conversion of cysteine to Calpha-formylglycine in the catalytic site of sulfatases (82,83).

Morphological and Functional Consequences. Steroid sulfatase is secreted from LBs into the SC interstices, where it degrades cholesterol sulfate, generating cholesterol, one of three key lipid constituents of SC lamellar bilayers (64). Since cholesterol sulfate inhibits serine protease activity in keratinocytes (84), increased SC cholesterol sulfate levels in patients with RXLI result in CD retention, morphologically correlating with increased SC thickness, which has historically been termed retention hyperkeratosis. Functionally, increased SC thickness and generalized scaling in RXLI are accompanied by a moderate increase in basal TEWL (64,66,85–87). In line with these findings, topically applied cholesterol sulfate not only induces scaling (88,89), but also causes phase separation of SC lipids that form the extracellular lamellar bilayers, accounting for the barrier abnormality (64,87). Furthermore, in contrast to normal control skin, Ca^{2+} levels persist into the lower SC of RXLI epidermis, where they are restricted to the extracellular domains, preferentially localizing to CDs (64). Finally, cholesterol sulfate stimulates keratinocyte differentiation via AP-1–mediated induction of involucrin, which could also contribute to corneocyte retention in RXLI (90).

LI/CIE [Congenital Ichthyosiform Erythroderma, Lipoxygenase-3 (ALOXE3) Deficiency; 12R-Lipoxygenase (ALOX12B) Deficiency, ATP-Binding Cassette Transporter A12 Deficiency, OMIM #242100]

Clinical Characteristics. The terms LI/CIE denote a group of autosomal recessively inherited ichthyotic phenotypes with congenital onset as collodion babies, and generalized scaling of varying severity and variable degrees of erythroderma (estimated incidence 1 in 300,000–500,000). A spectrum of phenotypes is recognized, ranging from those with thick plate-like scales (LI phenotype) at one pole, to finer scaling, often with marked erythroderma (CIE) at the other, and with many intermediate phenotypes. Ectropion, eclabion, palmoplantar keratoderma, nail abnormalities, and scalp involvement are typically present. Recent discovery of several unrelated genetic defects in different kindreds exhibiting these phenotypic features confirm the long suspected heterogeneity of this group. A considerable degree of genetic overlap appears to exist among the phenotypes.

Molecular Defect. LI/CIE can result from both lipid abnormalities and CE abnormalities. Genetically, cases with this phenotype have been assigned to several different chromosomal susceptibility loci. At least one-third of LI cases is due to defective CE formation, caused by mutations in the cross-linking enzyme, TG-1 on chromosome 14 (40), and will be discussed further below with other CE abnormalities. Recent evidence indicates that another portion of LI cases is due to defects in lipid metabolism. Mutations in the 12R-lipoxygenase (ALOX12B) and lipoxygenase-3 (ALOXE3) on chromosome 17 have been reported in CIE (91–93). These lipoxygenases are sequential members of the same pathway. They catalyze the oxygenation of free and esterified polyunsaturated fatty acids to hydroxyperoxyderivates (HPETEs) or to epoxyalcohols, and are preferentially active in skin. Their endogenous substrates are unknown. Thus, the precise mechanism by which the deficiency in these lipoxygenases causes the phentoype is unclear. The clinical presentation in these cases seems to be similar to CIE in young patients and more like LI in adults. Another gene mutation recently described to cause LI/CIE affects another protein involved in cellular lipid metabolism. In an African family with the classical LI phenotype, mutations have been found in the ATP-binding cassette (ABC) transporter A12 on chromosome 2, belonging to a family of enzymes that are critical for the transmembrane transport of cellular lipids (91). Although the function of ABCA12 is unknown to date, in view of the abnormality of LB ultrastructure in CIE (see below), it is tempting to speculate that this protein may be required for importation of LB lipids. Interestingly, ABCA3 has been shown to be a membrane protein of the LBs of lung alveolar type II cells.[†] Moreover, mutations in yet another member, ABCA1, cause Tangier disease, characterized by cholesterol accumulation, decreased HDL, and atherosclerosis. Finally, within the known chromosomal susceptibility loci for LI/CIE several additional genes are likely candidates and can be expected to reveal further insights into disease pathogenesis.

Morphological and Functional Consequences. Prior to the delineation of the molecular defects underlying LI/CIE, ultrastructural findings described distinctive alterations in the SG and SC. Anton-Lamprecht (94) and Niemi (95–98) have described four subtypes based on ultrastructural findings. Type I is defined by intra-corneocyte droplets, type II by aggregates of "cholesterol clefts," type III by intra-corneocyte membranes, and type IV by lentiform areas filled with membrane inclusions. Types I and II appear to correlate with CIE and LI, respectively. However, the overall correlation with the clinical phenotypes remained obscure. Moreover, abnormalities in the LB and intercellular lamellar bilayer architecture were described among patients with LI versus CIE phenotypes (70,99–101). Nevertheless, in both phenotypic groups, desmosomes persist throughout the outer layers of the SC, indicative of impaired degradation.

Notably, in these studies, abnormal LBs were exclusively observed in CIE, antedating the recent discovery of defects in lipid metabolism in cases of CIE. Moreover, the CIE phenotype has been reported to display membranous inclusions with disorganization of lipid lamellae and lipid inclusions. In addition, a rise in ceramides and free sterols has been reported in some cases of LI/CIE (99). Increased basal TEWL has been reported in presumably heterogenous cohorts of patients before genotyping has become available (66,86).

*Sjögren–Larsson Syndrome (Fatty Aldehyde Dehydrogenase Deficiency, OMIM *270200)*

Clinical Characteristics. Sjögren-Larsson syndrome (SLS) is characterized by a "dandruff-like" hyperkeratosis with accentuation of flexural sites, the lower abdomen, and the sides and back of the neck, forming a ridged, hyperkeratotic pattern. It

[†] Lung LBs are distinct from epidermal LBs, differing by their larger size, fine structure, and different lipid, apoprotein, and hydrolytic enzymatic contents. However, they serve an analogous function, namely delivery of lipid to the extracellar compartment, and develop at the same time in utero. Some of the same regulatory signals accelerate (glucocorticoids, thyroid hormone, estrogens) and retard (androgens) their development, while other regulatory signals are tissue specific (e.g., EGF for lung but not skin; PPAR (α activators for skin but not lung).

is usually of moderate severity, and tends to spare the face, palms, soles, hair, and nails. Erythema can be minimal, but pruritus is usually striking. An exaggerated neonatal desquamation in the first days of life is typically the first sign of the disease. Extracutaneous manifestations include spastic diplegia or quadriplegia, mental retardation, and speech defects (53). Ocular abnormalities include corneal erosions or opacities, photophobia, juvenile macular dystrophy, and retinal "glistening white dots." The latter are pathognomonic, but may not develop until late childhood. There is a high prevalence of the disease in Sweden due to a founder effect in an inbred population, but cases have occurred worldwide.

Molecular Defect. SLS is an autosomal recessive trait due to the deficiency of fatty aldehyde dehydrogenase (FALDH) (102–104), encoded on the short arm of chromosome 17, a microsomal enzyme that catalyzes the oxidation of medium- and long-chain aliphatic aldehydes derived from metabolism of fatty alcohol, phytanic acid, ether, glycerolipids, and leukotriene B4.

More than 50 different mutations have been reported to date, the majority of them being unique to each family. Aside from mutational analysis, the diagnosis can be established by histochemical assay for epidermal alcohol dehydrogenase in skin biopsy specimens (104), or by an enzyme assay from fibroblasts, amniocytes, or peripheral blood leukocytes. Although the enzyme is active in the epidermis, the mechanism of disease may not involve a direct effect on the composition and structure of the SC extracellular lipid membranes. Fatty alcohols, substrates for the blocked enzymatic reaction, are constituents of certain lipids (e.g., plasmalogens and wax esters). Although cutaneous wax esters are synthesized predominantly by sebaceous glands, this site is unlikely to be the pathogenic locus for the disordered desquamation in SLS, because disease expression begins during infancy and continues during childhood, a time when sebaceous glands are normally quiescent. More recently, FALDH deficiency has been implicated in defective degradation of leukotriene B4 in SLS (105). This hypothesis is supported by evidence that administration of an inhibitor of LTB4 synthesis ameliorates the pruritus in SLS (106).

Morphological and Functional Consequences. The epidermis of SLS subjects is acanthotic with a prominent SG and an orthokeratosic SC. In the dermis, there usually is a moderate inflammatory infiltrate consisting of lymphocytes. Ultrastructurally, distinctive abnormalities in LBs have been described (107). Although they are normal in number, there is great variability in size and they contain abnormal internal structures. Yet, while the intercorneocyte spaces are abnormally wide, secretion appears to occur normally. In addition, abnormal configuration of the Golgi apparatus and increased numbers of mitochondria and keratin filaments have been described.

Refsum Disease (Syn. Heredopathia Atactica Polyneuritiformis, Phytanoyl-CoA Hydroxylase Deficiency, OMIM #266500); Rhizomelic Chondrodysplasia Punctata (OMIM #215100, 222765, 600121)

Clinical Characteristics. Refsum disease classically presents as a tetrad of retinitis pigmentosa, cerebellar ataxia, peripheral polyneuropathy, and elevated cerebrospinal fluid protein levels. Other frequently observed manifestations include anosmia, sensorineural deafness, skeletal abnormalities, renal dysfunction, and cardiomyopathy/cardiac arrhythmias. Ichthyotic skin changes are an infrequent and usually mild feature that typically develops after neurological symptoms, i.e., during late childhood or thereafter. The skin phenotype is characterized by generalized fine scaling resembling ichthyosis vulgaris and EFAD (see below) (108). Patients may display accentuated palmar creases and their melanocytic nevi have been described to exhibit a characteristic yellowish hue.

Rhizomelic chondrodysplasia punctata, a multisystem developmental disorder, in approximately one-third of the cases includes ichthyotic skin changes in addition to the characteristic stippled foci of calcification in hyaline cartilage, dwarfing, joint contractures, mental retardation, and cataracts.

Molecular Defect.   Refsum disease has an increased prevalence in Scandinavia. Adult or adolescent-onset Refsum disease is caused by an autosomal recessively inherited deficiency in phytanoyl-CoA hydroxylase, encoded by the PAHX gene on chromosome 10, a peroxisomal enzyme catalyzing the alpha-oxidation of phytanic acid (109). The deficiency results in the accumulation of phytanic acid (3,7,11,15-tetramethylhexadecanoic acid), a branched-chain fatty acid, which is present in many dietary vegetables (phytanic acid is tightly bound to chlorophyll, only released by ruminants) (110). Accordingly, in Refsum disease, in the phospholipid fraction of the epidermis, linoleic acid is largely replaced by phytanic acid (111). Other 3-alkyl-branched fatty acids also accumulate in patients with Refsum disease (112). Because Refsum disease results from the inability to brake down dietary phytanic acid, a diet poor in fish, beef, lamb, and dairy products is beneficial. Diagnosis can be made by detection of elevated levels of plasma phytanic acid or by measuring enzyme activity in cultured fibroblasts. Recent studies have demonstrated genetic heterogeneity in Refsum disease. Aside from PAHX/phytanoyl CoA hydroxylase, mutations affecting a protein, peroxin 7 receptor, required for the import of peroxisomal enzymes have been described (113). Mutations in this same gene also cause the more severe phenotype, rhizomelic chondrodysplasia punctata (RCDP). In addition to ichthyosis, the phenotype in RCDP has a congenital onset with limb reduction defects, cataracts, and profound developmental delay (114). However, these disorders should not be confused with Infantile Refsum disease, which is a genetically distinct disorder of more global peroxisome deficiency but without ichthyosis.

Morphological and Functional Consequences.   On histology, Refsum epidermis displays hyperkeratosis, acanthosis, and varying degrees of hyper- or hypogranulosis. Cytoplasmic lipid vacuoles have been described in the basal and suprabasal epidermal cells (115), and desmosomal structures abnormally persist into the outer SC. Special stains (Oil Red O) confirm the accumulation of lipids in the vacuoles. Thus, Refsum disease belongs to the few ichthyoses, in which light microscopy can aid the diagnosis (aside from EHK, Chanarin-Dorfman disease, and acquired ichthyosis of sarcoidosis). Phytanic acid accumulates in all acyl-lipid fractions of the epidermis in Refsum disease. Because it replaces linoleic acid in the phospholipid fraction, it is tempting to speculate that the epidermal phenotype is that of EFAD. However, it is also possible that substitution of phytanic acid for the other fatty acids in SC lipids may interfere with the formation and function of the SC intercellular lipid lamellae.

*X-Linked Dominant Ichthyosis: This category includes CHH (Conradi-Hünermann-Happle) syndrome (delta 8, delta 7, sterol isomerase imopamil-binding protein deficiency, EBP, OMIM #302960), and CHILD syndrome (syn. Congenital Hemidysplasia with Ichthyosiform Erythroderma and Limb Defects, NAD(P)H steroid dehydrogenase-like protein, NSDHL, OMIM *308050).*

Clinical Characteristics. CHILD and CHH syndromes are inherited as X-dominant, male-lethal traits. In both, radiographically stippled epiphyseal plates can be present during infancy. In CHH syndrome, skin lesions are distributed along the lines of Blaschko, reflecting morphogenic distribution of cells in which the X-chromosome bearing the CHH mutation is the active X. At birth, the affected skin exhibits an ichthyosiform erythroderma, which resolves during infancy leaving a distinctive form of scarring, follicular atrophoderma. Asymmetrical limb reduction defects, abnormal facies with frontal bossing and depressed nasal bridge, and focal cataracts are commonly present. In CHILD syndrome, the skin lesions typically involve one side of the body, sparing the face. It too is accompanied by ipsilateral limb reductions with chondrodysplasia, and often with ipsilateral hypoplasia of internal organs, including cardiac, renal, and CNS malformation. In both syndromes, alopecia and nail abnormalities are commonly seen. Usually, skin changes persist throughout life in CHILD syndrome, in contrast to the transient ichthyosiform erythroderma described in CHH syndrome. However, CHILD syndrome may also exhibit a tendency to resolve, at least partially (116).

Molecular Defect. CHH syndrome is attributed to mutations in delta 8, delta 7, sterol isomerase imopamil-binding protein (EBP) (117), resulting in increased levels of 8 dehydrocholesterol and 8(9)-cholestenol. In CHILD syndrome mutations have been found in the NSDHL gene encoding the proximal step in the biosynthetic pathway, 3-beta-hydroxysteroid dehydrogenase (118). Both enzymes are important for conversion of lanosterol to cholesterol.

Morphological and Functional Consequences. In CHH syndrome, there is acanthosis and hypogranulosis on histology. Calcifications can be visualized with special stains, particularly in the vicinity of hair follicle openings (119,120). Focal pigmentation of the basal layer and needle-like calcium inclusions in vacuoles may be seen ultrastructurally (121). In addition, follicular atrophoderma can be present, characterized by dilated ostia of pilosebaceous structures or atrophy of the hair follicles. Fibroblasts, cultured from patients with CHILD syndrome have been described to accumulate cytoplasmic lipids and exhibit fewer peroxisomes and decreased peroxisomal functions. This deficiency may be related to the role of peroxisomes in cholesterol biosynthesis. No ultrastructural or functional information related to the epidermal barrier is available. However, the SC membrane cholesterol derives largely if not entirely on de novo epidermal cholesterol synthesis, since only basal keratinocytes express LDL receptors, and thus spinous and granular layer keratinocytes that exhibit high rates of sterologenesis are not able to take up cholesterol from the circulation (122). Moreover, inhibitors of sterologenesis that similarly block the cholesterol biosynthetic pathway at distal points result in an ichthyotic phenotype, demonstrating that these sterols cannot substitute for cholesterol in the formation of SC membranes (123).

Harlequin Ichthyosis ATP-Binding Cassette Transporter A12 Deficiency (OMIM 242500)

Clinical Characteristics. Newborns with Harlequin ichthyosis display massive, restrictive plate-lake scaling, which can interfere with postnatal respiration and feeding, and result in perinatal death. Many are stillborn. In "survivors," the thick neonatal scales are replaced, shed, and the skin phenotype shifts to an intense, generalized exfoliative erythroderma, which is associated with ectropion. Longstanding disease commonly results in contractures, as a consequence of taut skin with restricted mobility. Underformed ears and loss of distal fingers and toes may be consequent to the severe intrauterine constrictions.

Molecular Defect. Mutations in ABCA12 on chromosome 2q3S have recently been described in Harlequin ichthyosis (124). Since mutations in the same gene have been implied in LI/CIE (c.f. page 478) this could either indicate that LI/CIE and Harlequin ichthyosis comprise a spectrum of the same pathogenetic process, or that there are discrepancies in the interpretatons of the phenotypes associated with this mutation.

Morphological and Functional Consequences. On histology, there is acanthosis and massive orthohyperkeratosis in neonates that is replaced by parakeratosis in "survivors." The ultrastructural hallmark of Harlequin ichthyosis is a paucity of LBs and their secreted contents. Rudimentary LB structures may be present within SG cells, but they do not display the characteristic membranes, and instead appear "empty." This results in the SC in a striking deficiency of lamellar membranes. The phenotypic shift to an ichthyosiform erythroderma in survivors of the neonatal period is postulated to be due to the shift from the aqueous intrauterine environment to the xeric atmosphere following birth, with a consequent requirement for a competent permeability barrier. Absence of lamellar membranes in the Harlequin ichthyosis neonate would result in a severely impaired permeability barrier with markedly increased rates of TEWL, that would in turn stimulate epidermal hyperproliferation. Dale et al. (125) have observed varying expression of the "hyperproliferative" keratins 6 and 16 and profilaggrin in Harlequin ichthyosis, and have proposed defining subgroups of HI based upon the expression of these epidermal differentiation markers. However, because keratins 6 and 16 are expressed in epidermis under conditions of hyperplasia, such as psoriasis or wound healing, these differences in keratin and profilaggrin expression may reflect the age of the patients at the time of study, rather than true disease subsets.

Gaucher's Disease (β-Glucocerebrosidase Deficiency, OMIM #231000, #230900, #230800)

Clinical Characteristics. Gaucher's disease is classified by its neurological symptoms: type I—the most common, mildest, and non-neuropathic form with adult onset; type II—a rapidly progressive, acute neuronopathic, infantile-onset form; and type III—a slowly progressive, neuronopathic, late childhood-onset form. Although most patients with Gaucher's disease do not have skin abnormalities, a subset of type II patients with severe neonatal onset of disease displays congenital ichthyosis, with a collodion baby or harlequin fetus phenotype. Extracutaneous manifestations are severe and include hepatosplenomegaly, hydrops fetalis, hypotonia, and apnea, with death in the perinatal period.

Molecular Defect. An autosomal recessive deficiency in β-glucocerebrosidase on chromosome 1q21 results in lysosomal accumulation of glucosylceramide. In the epidermis, β-glucocerebrosidase cleaves glucosylceramide to free ceramide, a step required for the final formation of the SC extracellular lamellar membrane structures. The three clinical subtypes arise from allelic mutations. Ichthyosis is only observed with homozygous null mutations, hence only in the lethal, neonatal onset group of type II disease. In other types, there is sufficient residual or compensatory enzymatic activity in SC to permit normal SC membrane function (63). Diagnosis is based on clinical symptoms, the presence of Gaucher cells containing large lysosomes on histology, enzyme assay and/or mutation analysis.

Morphological and Functional Consequences. In a Gaucher type II disease mouse model bearing homozygous null mutations of the β-glucocerebrosidase gene and with <1% of normal epidermal glucocerebrosidase activity, the lipid composition of SC membranes is altered, with elevated glucosylceramide and diminished ceramide content. This results in abnormal SC membrane ultrastructure with incompletely processed, LB-derived sheets throughout the SC interstices. The SC of a severely affected type II Gaucher's disease neonate with a collodion baby phenotype revealed a similarly abnormal SC membrane ultrastructure (63,72). Furthermore, the null-mutation Gaucher murine model demonstrates markedly elevated rates of TEWL (4.2 ± 0.6 Gaucher versus < 0.10 normal $g/m^2/hour$). Even in the complete absence of β-glucocerebrosidase activity, SC membranes still display at least 30% of normal ceramide levels (63,72). Hence, in Gaucher disease subtypes with residual enzyme activity, sufficient additional ceramide is generated to prevent development of a cutaneous phenotype.

Niemann Pick Disease (Sphingomyelinase Deficiency, OMIM #257200, #607616)

Clinical Characteristics. Traditionally, Niemann Pick disease types A (neurovisceral) and B (visceral) have been distinguished. More recently, types C–F have been described based upon variations in the clinical phenotype and the degree of the metabolic abnormality. The clinical findings in affected family members include short stature, hepatosplenomegaly, fine reticular infiltration of the lungs with recurrent respiratory infections, and neurologic deficits. Ocular changes include corneal and retinal opacifications, a macular cherry-red spot (type A) or a macular halo (type B). Niemann Pick patients commonly display a generalized, grayish-brown hyperpigmentation of the skin, but in most patients, ichthyosis is absent (126). Nevertheless, some (type B) Niemann Pick patients have been reported to display an ichthyosiform dermatosis, with a fine scale pattern (127).

Molecular Defect. Autosomal recessive mutations in the acid sphingomyelinase (aSM'ase) gene on chromosome 11p15 give rise to most types of Niemann Pick disease (except for types C and D), resulting in an accumulation of SM. In the epidermis, aSM'ase cleaves SM to free ceramide, a step that is required for the final formation of the SC extracellular lamellar membrane structures. Types C and D Niemann Pick disease are not due to sphingomyelinase deficiency, but rather to abnormalities in cholesterol metabolism.

Morphological and Functional Consequences. Although there is no abnormality of basal permeability barrier function in Niemann Pick subjects in non-scaly skin, the kinetics of barrier recovery after acute disruption (by tape stripping) are delayed. The absence of skin symptoms in most Niemann Pick patients could reflect either the presence of residual aSM'ase in the epidermis to suffice for basal conditions, and/or the compensatory generation of ceramide via the alternate glucosylceramide-to-ceramide pathway (63). Epidermal aSM'ase activity has been localized to both LBs and the SC interstices, using ultrastructural cytochemical and biochemical methods (128). Since epidermal LBs contain substantial SM (128,129), and since the plasma membrane disappears during terminal differentiation, both of these two sources of SM become available as potential pools for conversion of SM to Cer in the outer epidermis. To date, there is only indirect ultrastructural evidence about the consequences of aSM'ase deficiency in the epidermis. Mice, treated topically with an aSM'ase inhibitor, display elongated, incompletely processed SC lipid lamellae, which can be prevented by co-treatment with the inhibitor plus ceramide. Finally, application of inhibitors of both aSM'ase and the neutral pH-active isoform has impaired SC structure and function, demonstrating the importance of ceramide derived from SM for permeability barrier competence (127,130,131).

Chanarin Dorfman Disease (Syn. Neutral Lipid Storage Disease, Esterase–Thiolase–Lipase Deficiency, OMIM *604780)

Clinical Characteristics. Most cases of Chanarin Dorfman disease have been reported in Mediterranean countries. Individuals with Chanarin Dorfmann disease are born with erythroderma, associated with generalized, small, whitish scales. The postnatal phenotype most closely resembles CIE of mild to moderate severity. The face often has a taut appearance, and affected individuals may appear older than their actual age. All flexural surfaces are usually involved and prominent lichenification is frequently observed (71,132). The presence and severity of extracutaneous symptoms (myopathy, neurosensory deafness, cataracts, fatty liver, and in some cases developmental delay, growth retardation) are variable.

Molecular Defect. Chanarin Dorfman disease is an autosomal recessive trait due to mutations in CGI-58 on chromosome 3p21 (133), which codes for a protein that is homologous to several members of the esterase–thiolase–lipase subfamily, but differs in that its putative catalytic triad contains an asparagine in place of the usual serine residue. The precise function of CGI-58 is unknown. The stored lipid in Chanarin Dorfman disease is predominantly triacylglycerol (71,132,133). The defect is in intracellular TG metabolism; circulating lipoprotein-bound TG levels are normal. The disease does not appear to be secondary to a defect in uptake, transport, or beta oxidation of fatty acids (133–135), nor in a triacylglyceride lipase per se, but rather in the recycling of triglyceride-derived mono- or diacylglycerols to specific phospholipids, altering the synthetic and degradative rates of most cellular phospholipids (135,136). A diet poor in long chain fatty acids and enriched in medium chain fatty acids has been reported to improve skin changes (137,138).

Morphological and Functional Consequences. Besides mild acanthosis, Chanarin Dorfman epidermis displays cytoplasmic lipid droplets that are preferentially localized to the basal cell layer (special stains) and are also present in peripheral blood monocytes and leukocytes (Jordan's anomaly). In addition, the number of LBs appears to be increased in the SG, and their contents are distended by electron-lucent, non-lamellar material, which may represent accumulated triacylglycerol (71). After secretion into the intercellular spaces of the SC, these droplets coalesce, displacing the lamellar material. Vacuoles can also be within corneocytes (139).

Acquired Ichthyoses Due to Lipid Abnormalities

EFAD

Clinical Characteristics. Because humans and other mammals cannot insert a double bond in FA at the omega-6 position, these must be obtained from the diet and are termed "essential fatty acids." EFAD is rare in clinical practice, due, in part, to the extreme efficiency of uptake and utilization of linoleic acid (C16:2) by target tissues, including epidermis. A scaling skin phenotype is observed in both human EFAD (e.g., patients undergoing prolonged lipid-free parenteral nutrition, and infants with malnutrition), and animal models of EFAD. In rodents, the phenotype is an ichthyosiform erythroderma accompanied by poor growth.

Morphological and Functional Consequences. The scaling phenotype in EFAD is associated with increased basal TEWL and alopecia (140). It can be restored by topical linoleic acid and other di- and trienes (141). There is a distortion of LB architecture in EFAD mice, giving them an empty, "moth-eaten" appearance and absence/paucity of intercellular lipid lamellae (142). Other investigators did not observe similar changes in LB morphology and extracellular lipid lamellae. This may reflect a milder severity of the EFAD in their animals (143).

Hypocholesteronemic Drugs

Several drugs that lower serum cholesterol by inhibiting the distal steps in sterolo-genesis (e.g., nicotinic acid, 20,25 diazocholesterol, triparanol) can induce scaling skin or other cornifying disorders (144). The morphological alterations in an experimental mouse model given 20–25 diazocholesterol include increased SC thickness, fragmentations of intercellular lipid lamellae, and LBs that appear to be largely devoid of internal structures. Importantly, topical or systemic repletion with cholesterol can correct this scaling abnormality (145). The vulnerability of the epidermis to these agents derives from its requirement for cholesterol as a key lipid of the SC lamellar membranes (20), and from its dependency upon de novo sterologenesis to supply these needs, because suprabasal epidermis lacks LDL receptors for the uptake of circulating LDL-cholesterol (145–147).

ACQUIRED ICHTHYOSES DUE TO UNKNOWN MOLECULAR DEFECTS

There is a variety of acquired ichthyotic disorders, termed pseudo-ichthyoses, that present as a manifestation of systemic disease including HIV infection, cancer (e.g., Hodgkin disease), marasmus, endocrine and metabolic diseases, sarcoidosis, autoimmune disorders, graft versus host disease, drugs (other than lipid lowering drugs, e.g., tranquilizer, neuroleptics), or skin aging. The phenotype of acquired ichthyoses is usually mild, resembling ichthyosis vulgaris.

ABNORMALITIES OF CORNEOCYTES

Because the permeability barrier function of the epidermis resides in the extracellular lipid domains of the SC, it was anticipated that primary disorders of lipid metabolism that alter the extracellular (mortar) domains would inevitably be accompanied by permeability barrier abnormalities (147). Conversely, inherent attenuation of corneocytes in avian skin (148) or acquired CE attenuation in fetal rats after ligation of the uterine artery (149) does not result in gross barrier abnormalities. Hence, corneocyte structural proteins were expected to primarily provide mechanical resilience to the SC. Therefore it was somewhat surprising that several ichthyoses with structural protein abnormalities also displayed an abnormal barrier. Indeed, even in these disorders, due to primary corneocyte protein abnormalities, marked abnormalities in the quantities, morphology, and/or organization of extracellular lipid bilayer system are evident (60,62,150–153), demonstrating the dependency of the "mortar" on the integrity of the "bricks" for SC permeability barrier function.

Inherited Abnormalities of CE Proteins

Loricrin Keratoderma (Syn. Vohwinkel Syndrome with Ichthyosis, Camisa Variant of Vohwinkel Syndrome, Vohwinkel Disease Limited to the Skin, Loricrin Mutations, OMIM #604117)

Clinical Characteristics. Clinically, loricrin keratoderma exhibits a characteristic honeycomb-like palmoplantar keratoderma on the acral extremities including palms and soles, a generalized fine-scaling, hyperkeratotic knuckle pads on the dorsal surface of the fingers, and, often, constricting bands encircling the fingers and/or toes (pseudoainhum) (Fig. 3) (62,154–162). In the Camisa variant (loricrin keratoderma), a mild but generalized ichthyosis is present, while classic Vohwinkel syndrome as originally described in 1929 (161) is instead accompanied by neurosensory deafness and results from a distinct molecular defect (see below).

Molecular Defect. Loricrin keratoderma is caused by dominantly inherited mutations in the loricrin gene which is localized within the epidermal differentiation complex (EDC) encoded on chromosome 1q21, and that result in elongation of the C-terminal domain of the loricrin protein. Loricrin, along with profilaggrin, is the predominant constituent of keratohyalin granules. It is a glycine-serine-cysteine–rich protein, synthesized in the granular (SG) layer (45,162–164). In the outermost layer of the SG, loricrin migrates to the cell periphery, where it is deposited beneath the plasma membrane, and cross-linked to several other cytosolic proteins (e.g., involucrin, SPRRs, elafin, repetin, S100, and up to ≈20 other proteins) by TG1, forming the CE.

In loricrin keratoderma, the mutant loricrin is somehow translocated to the nuclei of the SG and SC layers, and fails to reach the CE (153). The relationship between the aberrant localization of the mutant loricrin and the phenotypic features of loricrin keratoderma remains unclear. While a dominant-negative interference of the mutant with the wild-type polypeptide has been proposed (45), alternatively, insufficient amounts of native protein (haploinsufficiency) may also account for the phenotype. Classical Vohwinkel disease (PPK with deafness) is caused by a mutation in gene encoding connexin 26 rather than by a loricrin defect (see below) (165).

Morphological and Functional Consequences. On histology, biopsies from loricrin keratoderma show epidermal hyperplasia, hypergranulosis, marked hyperkeratosis and parakeratosis with characteristic roundish rather than flattened nuclei in the lower SC (Fig. 3) (45,62). This hyper- and parakeratotic SC predisposes to cleavage of the SC from the outer granular layer, which can be induced by minimal trauma (Fig. 4). In concordance with these morphological findings, a high percentage of patients with loricrin keratoderma clinically display increased skin fragility to controlled friction (pseudo-Nikolskij sign). Moreover, impaired SC cohesion is also indicated by increased removal of SC proteins by tape stripping in loricrin keratoderma skin as compared to normal healthy skin. Functionally, there is a markedly reduced SC hydration in the hyperkeratotic/honeycomb-type skin sites, while the surface pH of the SC shows a trend towards being more acidic. Basal rates of TEWL are increased and lamellar bilayers are disorganized, but barrier repair kinetics are accelerated. Despite evidence of fragility, i.e., the increased susceptibility to mechanical (ultrasound) damage (153), and the penetration of small amounts of the water-soluble, electron-dense tracer, lanthanum, into the corneocyte cytosol (62), increased water loss occurs predominantly via extracellular domains, as demonstrated by the predominant pathway of lanthanum penetration

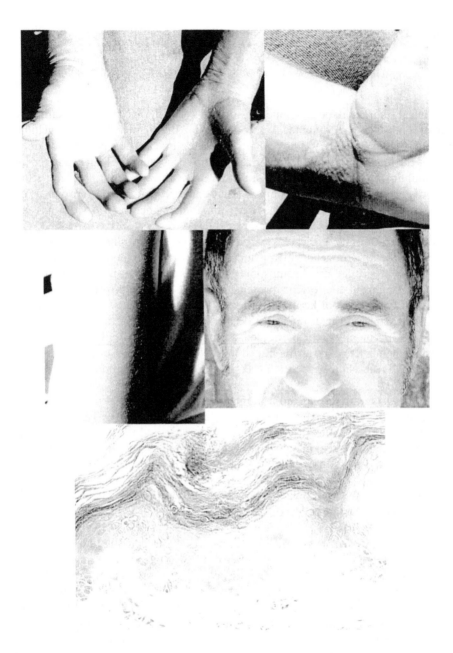

Figure 3 Clinical features of loricrin keratoderma (Vohwinkel syndrome with ichthyosis): Palmar keratoderma (*upper left panel*); honeycomb hyperkeratosis (*upper right*); fine scaling on limbs (*middle left*); erythema, fine scaling on face (*middle right*); hematoxylin & eosin section from skin biopsy showing hyperkeratosis with characteristic retained roundish retained nuclei in lower stratum corneum (SC), and acanthosis (*lower panel*). *Source*: Photos courtesy of Dr. Fluhn.

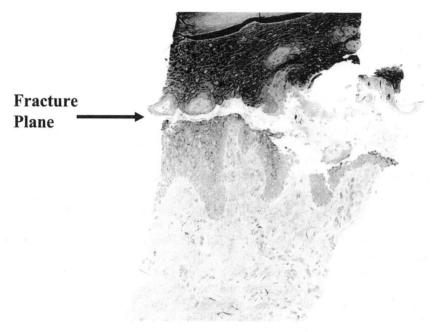

Fracture Plane

Figure 4 Fracture plane through SG — SC junction loricrin keratoderma (Vohwinkel syndrome with ichthyosis), semi-thin section, toluidine blue.

across the SC in loricrin keratoderma (62). Bilayer abnormalities are attributable to abnormal extracellular lipid processing, and occur adjacent to regions in the lower SC in which discontinuities and attenuation of the CE are present. However, CE dimensions partially normalize in the outer SC. This normalization correlates with persistence of abundant Ca^{++} in the extracellular spaces of the SC, where it would be in the correct location to activate TG1. The primary pathogenic role of the CE scaffold abnormality in loricrin keratoderma is underscored by the presence of a normal LB (LB) secretory system, with largely unimpeded secretion of LB contents and with a normal CLE and CLE-bound ceramides. The accelerated barrier recovery is explicable by amplified LB secretion. Thus, the permeability barrier abnormality in loricrin keratoderma is linked to a focally defective CE scaffold in the inner SC layers, resulting in increased extracellular permeability.

EHK (Mutations in Epidermal Keratins K1, K10, K2e, K9, , OMIM #113800, #146800, #144200, #193900)

Clinical Characteristic. A characteristic feature in many EHK patients is a phenotypic shift from predominant blistering in the newborn to prominent hyperkeratosis during later life. Due to the early blistering, EHK was previously termed bullous congental ichthyosiform erythroderma to distinguish it from the recessive, non-bullous CIE, which today is termed LI/CIE. Erythroderma is prominent in some patients, but absent in others. The hyperkeratoses in EHK often are generalized and may involve or spare the palms and soles. In the generalized variants, typically, involvement of flexural and extensor surfaces of large joints (elbows, knees) is accentuated, sometimes with massive hyperkeratosis, and typically giving a peculiar, ridged appearance (Fig. 5). Flexural scales often become secondarily colonized by bacteria, producing a foul odor. Variants with particularly widespread and thick porcupine-like (hystrix) hyperkeratosis (but lack of an early blistering phase) have been termed ichthyosis hystrix of Curth and Macklin. A milder variant of EHK, ichthyosis bullosa of Siemens (IBS), is characterized by blistering as well as annular, hyperkeratotic plaques preferentially over joints, shins, and the periumbilical region. There are also localized forms more limited to acral and flexural surfaces plus palms/soles or distributed in a linear pattern along the lines of Blaschko, with the clinical picture of an epidermal nevus. EHK strictly limited to palms and soles has been termed Vörner's PPK.

Molecular Defect. Mutations in keratin 1 (chromosome 12q13) and keratin 10 (chromosome 17q21-q22) have been identified as the cause of the classic generalized form of EHK and the forms presenting as epidermal nevi due to chromosomal mosaicism (166–188). The offspring of patients with mosaic or nevoid variants of EHK, due to K1 or K10 mutations, are at risk for generalized forms of the disease. There is a high frequency of spontaneous mutations. As many as one-half the cases have no family history, and there is a high degree of clinical variability, primarily between kindreds (185). In the milder variant of EHK, ichthyosis bullosa of Siemens (IBS), mutations in K2e have been identified. In families with the EHK limited to palms and soles (Vörner's PPK), mutations in keratin 9 have been identified (Table 2). Keratin mutations are inherited as autosomal dominant traits, and function in a dominant-negative manner to disrupt the keratin filament network within the keratinocyte cytosol. Filaments retract from their attachments to desmosomal plaques, and form clumps of perinuclear shells, disrupting the physiological intermediate filament scaffold that spans the cytosols of keratinocytes between desmosomal plaques and nucleus.

Keratins are the most abundant proteins produced during the vectorial process of epidermal differentiation. Prior to cornification, these keratins are organized into filament bundles that loop between desmosomal plaques and the nuclear envelope providing a cytoskeleton that protects keratinocytes from mechanical injury (189,190).

As the keratinocytes terminally differentiate, keratins aggregate in the presence of filaggrin to form a fibrous network that replaces the cytosol. Typically, one acidic (type I) keratin heterodimerizes with one basic (type II) keratin and two such dimers are arranged in an antiparallel and staggered configuration (protofilament) (191). In turn, two protofilaments comprise a protofibril, of which four assemble to form the 10-nm keratin intermediate filament. Within these filaments, the most abundant epidermal keratins, keratins 1 and 10, become linked to the CE (6,7,192,193). Skin fragility to mechanical trauma, which is most pronounced in the neonatal period, is an expected consequence of mutations in keratin 1 or 10, analogous to the fragile skin phenotype of epidermolysis bullosa, where mutations in K5 or 14 produce cytoskeletal defects in the epidermal basal layer (194–196) and result in a mechanobullous phenotype (Table 2).

Morphological and Functional Consequences. The histopathology of EHK is distinctive. Underlying a massive hyperkeratosis there is a characteristic vacuolar degeneration of the upper epidermal cell layers, which coined the term epidermolytic (Fig. 5). Large basophilic intracellular deposits are present in the upper epidermal layers that resemble enlarged keratohyalin granules, but which are instead composed of clumped keratin filaments. These changes are evident ultrastructurally in cases where the light microscopic features are mild and non-diagnostic.

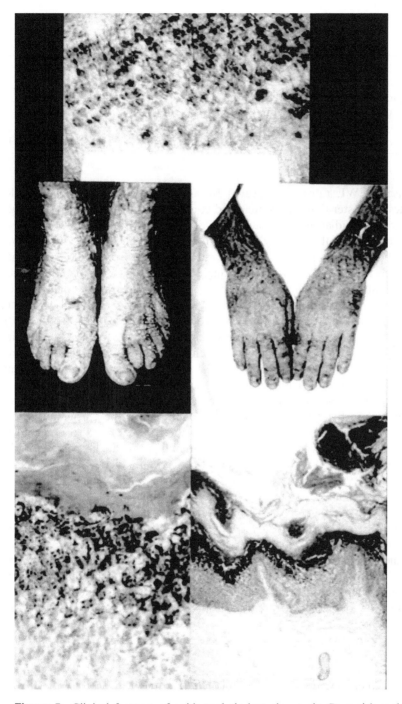

Figure 5 Clinical features of epidermolytic hyperkeratosis: Brownish scale (*upper panel*); hyperkeratotic and erosive changes on feet and hand (*middle panel*); hematoxylin & eosin section from skin biopsy showing prominent hyperkeratosis, vacuolization of the stratum granulosum (SG), and acanthosis.

Table 2 Keratin Mutations in Disorders of Cornification

Disease	Keratin
Epidermolytic hyperkeratosis (EHK)	K1, K10
Epidermolytic nevus	K1, K10
Ichthyosis bullosa (Siemens)	K2e
Epidermolytic palmoplantar keratoderma (Voerner)	K9
Non-epidermolytic palmoplantar keratoderma	K17
Pachyonychia congenita	K6, K16, K17

Whereas basal TEWL rates are elevated by approximately three-fold in EHK, recovery rates are faster than in age-matched control skin. There is no defect either in the CE, or in the adjacent CLE; hence, a corneocyte scaffold abnormality does not explain the barrier abnormality. Although the upper nucleated cell layers are unquestionably fragile in EHK, when the water-soluble tracer, colloidal lanthanum, is allowed to penetrate outwards through the epidermis, there is no evidence of tracer accumulation within corneocytes; i.e., despite the fragility of nucleated keratinocytes, the tracer does not move through an abnormal, intracellular route. Instead, as in normal SC, the tracer moves through the extracellular domains (60). Increased intercellular permeability in EHK correlates with decreased quantities and defective organization of extracellular lamellar bilayers, which in turn can be attributed to incompletely secreted LBs from SG cells, resulting in many "entombed" LB remnants in corneocytes. Yet, after acute barrier disruption, a rapid release of preformed LB contents is observed in conjunction with increased organelle contents in the extracellular spaces, accounting for the accelerated recovery kinetics in EHK. Loss of calcium from the outer SG cells is also observed in EHK following acute barrier disruption, which may provide the signal for the rapid exocytosis of LBs that results in accelerated repair kinetics (60). Thus, the baseline permeability barrier abnormality in EHK can be attributed to impaired LB secretion, rather than to corneocyte fragility or an abnormal CE/CLE scaffold, a defect that can be overcome in part by external applications of stimuli for barrier repair. The impaired LB secretion at baseline is likely to be caused by the disruption of the cytoskeletal framework (197), and suggests that a normal intermediate filament framework plays a role in LB secretion. As in Harlequin ichthyosis, there is a dramatic phenotypic shift in the neonatal period. In EHK the change is from a mechanobullous phenotype, where blistering from trauma predominates, to a hyperkeratotic phenotype. The resolution of mechanical blistering after the neonatal period may be due to stimulation of epidermal hyperplasia consequent to the barrier defect. Epidermal hyperplasia in turn would be accompanied by expression of the wound healing keratins, K6 and K16, as has previously been reported in the mouse model of EHK (198), which may ameliorate to some extent the disruption of the keratin filament system.

Ichthyosis Vulgaris (OMIM *146700)

Clinical Characteristics. Ichthyosis vulgaris represents the most common disorder of cornification. Its incidence has been estimated to comprise up to one in 250 in a British cohort of school children with dry skin (199). However, studies from adult cohorts (75,200) estimate lower incidences (i.e., $\leq$1:5300). Individuals with ichthyosis vulgaris commonly display rather mild generalized fine scaling with flexural sparing. The extensor surfaces of the extremities are usually most affected. Involvement of palms (scaling and palmar hyperlinearity) and soles is common and there is an association with keratosis pilaris and atopic dermatitis. It is difficult clinically to differentiate between individuals with mild ichthyosis vulgaris from the xerosis that accompanies atopic dermatitis. Thus, not only geographical variation, but also the clinical criteria for the diagnosis of ichthyosis vulgaris may account for the variations in incidence. The phenotype is rarely evident before three to six months after birth, but usually manifests during childhood and becomes severe with age.

Molecular Defect. A genetic mutation(s) underlying ichthyosis vulgaris has not been identified. Sybert et al. (201) demonstrated that profilaggrin and its proteolytic product, filaggrin, are reduced or absent in ichthyosis vulgaris, correlating with a paucity in keratohyalin within the SG. While linkage of the ichthyosis vulgaris phenotype to chromosome 1q, where the profilaggrin gene resides, has recently been reported (202,203), no mutation in the profilaggrin gene has been identified. Instability of the profilaggrin message underlies the reduced quantities of protein (204).

Keratohyalin granules in the outer nucleated layers of the epidermis, consisting primarily of phosphorylated profilaggrin, are responsible for the designation of this layer as the granular layer (SG) (49). Profilaggrin is a large histidine-rich, highly cationic phosphoprotein, consisting of filaggrin repeats, connected by peptide segments enriched in hydrophobic amino acids (163). Profilaggrin is concentrated within keratohyalin granules, where it may sequester newly synthesized loricrin, which then moves to the cell periphery. At the SG–SC interface, profilaggrin is both dephosphorylated and proteolytically processed by a Ca^{2+}-dependent protein convertase, furin, at the N-terminus to yield filaggrin, which ionically binds to keratin 1/10, inducing collapse of associated intermediate filaments into the macrofibrils of the corneocyte cytosol. Moreover, immunolocalization studies suggest that processed filaggrin peptides associate initially with the CE via their N-terminal domain in the lower SC. Above the stratum compactum, filaggrin is then released and proteolyzed further into its constituent amino acids. This step is thought to be catalyzed by an aspartate protease whose activity is up-regulated when relative humidity levels decline <80%, as occurs normally above the stratum compactum (48). Several of filaggrin's major amino acids are further de-aminated to acidic metabolites, which are thought to be major determinants of SC hydration (205).

Morphological and Functional Consequences. A histologic feature of ichthyosis vulgaris is a reduced or absent SG with a paucity of keratohyalin granules and reduced cellular profilaggrin content (206,207). Complete lack of a granular layer (SG) can be observed in approximately 50% of ichthyosis vulgaris patients, and using this criterion has been mapped to the epidermal differentiation complex on chromosome 1q (see above). Absence of the SG is independent of body site and season of the year, and it correlates with severity of the disease (207). Within kindreds both cases with reduced SG and keratohyalin granules, as well as cases with complete lack of SG have been observed. Ultrastructurally, keratohyalin granules, if present, have been described as poorly formed ("crumbly") (208) but these findings have recently been attributed to the use of osmic acid (rather than glutaraldehyde/paraformaldehyde) fixative. Moreover, somewhat surprisingly, corneocyte keratin macrofibers are normal ultrastructurally in ichthyosis vulgaris, suggesting that filaggrin is not required for their aggregation. The pathogenesis of the scaling abnormality in ichthyosis vulgaris has been attributed to deficiency of proteolytic products of filaggrin breakdown, which provide much of the osmotically active small molecules that regulate corneocyte hydration (205). Filaggrin hydrolysis has been shown to be regulated by environmental conditions with increased hydrolysis under conditions of xeric stress (50). In ichthyosis vulgaris, corneocytes would have reduced capacity to imbibe water when exposed to high humidity or during bathing. This would be anticipated to impair desquamation, since outer corneocytes would not "swell and slough" with the friction that accompanies bathing. We recently confirmed decreased corneocyte hydration in a cohort of ichthyosis vulgaris patients (M. Schmuth and P.M. Elias, unpublished observations). Moreover, although previously ichthyosis vulgaris has been reported to display normal rates of TEWL (66), we observed a delay in barrier recovery after acute disruption by tape stripping (M. Schmuth and P.M. Elias, unpublished observations). Preliminary ultrastructural findings suggest that LB contents in these patients are incompletely processed. It is possible that filaggrin participates in the linkage of keratins to the CE during cornification, and that impairment in this process improper conditions for lipid processing (M. Schmuth and P.M. Elias, unpublished observations).

Lamellar Ichthyosis (TG1 Deficiency, OMIM #242300)

Clinical Characteristics.   LI along with non-bullous CIE comprises a spectrum of phenotypes (see above). The classical LI phenotype with large, plate-like, pigmented scales without erythema appears to be primarily due to impaired CE crosslinking and is discussed here (Fig. 6). Other phenotypes from this spectrum are due to lipid abnormalities and are discussed above.

Molecular Defect.   At least one-third of LI cases appears to be due to defective CE formation, caused by mutations in the cross-linking enzyme, TG1, on chromosome 14 (40,41,209–211). To date, over 50 different mutations have been identified. As one possible mechanism, a destabilization of a hydrophobic pocket has been proposed, presumably distorting the active site of the enzyme, which results in loss of activity (210). As a consequence, the enzymatic cross-linking of CE proteins and of sphingolipids of the CLE to the CE is impaired (40,41). Ex vivo gene replacement of TG1, followed by transplantation to SCID mice, results in normalization of the classic LI phenotype (212).

Morphological and Functional Consequences.   We have recently studied a cohort of LI patients with defined deficiencies in TG1. In the SC of these patients, the CE is attenuated and the resilience of the CE to boiling in sodium dodecyl sulfate (SDS) and dithiothreitol (DTT) is diminished. Moreover, prominent abnormalities in extracellular lipid structures are evident ultrastructurally, showing truncation and fragmentation of extracellular lamellar membrane arrays (61). The resulting clefts in the SC interstices allow for increased movement of lanthanum tracer through the intercellular pathway, which functionally correlates to a moderately increased rate of TEWL under basal conditions. Abnormalities in lamellar spacing have been described by both electron microscopy (65) and x-ray diffraction (213), but these alone are not likely to account for the barrier abnormality. Although the lamellar membranes are abnormal in LI, CLE structure and bound omega-OH-ceramide content are unaffected (61). However, it is likely that despite a normal CLE, the extracellular lamellar membrane abnormalities are due to a lack of a proper CE scaffold.

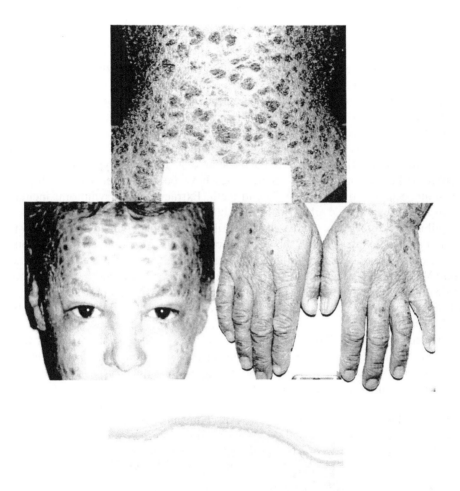

Figure 6 Clinical features of lamellar ichthyosis (transglutaminase-1 mutation): large, brownish scale on neck (*upper panel*), face (*middle left*), and hands (*middle right*); hematoxylin & eosin section from skin biopsy showing compact hyperkeratosis, and acanthosis.

ABNORMALITIES IN INTERCELLULAR COMMUNICATION (GAP JUNCTIONS)

As mentioned above, most disorders of cornification can be classified into abnormalities of the "mortar" lipids of the SC (i.e., barrier lipids), and abnormalities of the "bricks" (i.e., CE proteins, keratins, filaggrin). However, several disorders that show a scaly phenotype and abnormal barrier function do not fit the categorization into "mortar" or "brick" defects. Recent evidence points to a variety of pathomechanisms in these disorders including abnormal cell-to-cell communication, signaling, or proliferation.

KID Syndrome and (Classical) Vohwinkel Disease (PPK with Deafness,
Connexin 26 Mutations, OMIM #148210, #124500)

Clinical Characteristics. KID syndrome and (classical) Vohwinkel disease have been described in the literature as distinct entities. However, since the underlying molecular defects are alike, the cases described in the literature may represent the phenotypic spectrum of a single entity. The term KID syndrome has been coined to describe the triad of Keratitis (with corneal opacities), Ichthyosis, and Deafness. The ichthyotic skin lesions are described as erythematous plaques, preferentially on the face and the extremities, accompanied by a mild generalized hyperkeratosis and a pebbly or honey-combed PPK. Some cases have been reported to also display scaring alopecia and dystrophic nails and teeth. Extracutaneous symptoms include auditory, ophthalmologic abnormalities, abnormal dentition, and an increased susceptibility to infections. Increased susceptibility to mucocutaneous infections is common and sometimes fatal in the neonatal period. The development of squamous cell carcinomas has been reported in KID (including SCC occurring in trichilemmal cysts) (214,215). (Classical) Vohwinkel disease comprises honeycomb keratoderma and deafness. Aside from deafness, it differs from KID and loricrin keratoderma (Vohwinkel syndrome with ichthyosis, see above) by lack of the generalized fine-scaling (45,165).

Molecular Defect. Dominant mutations in the GJB2 gene, encoding for connexin 26 have been reported in KID syndrome. (Classical) Vohwinkel syndrome has been reported to be caused by mutations not only in the same gene on chromosome 13, but in the same first extracellular domain of the protein (165,216–218). Connexins are major proteins of gap junctions important in the process of intercellular communication. The phenotypic consequences of connexin mutations suggest a role in epidermal homeostasis. Decreased host defense and increased carcinogenic potential in KID illustrated that gap junction communication plays not only a crucial role in epithe lial homeostasis and differentiation but also in immune response and epidermal carcinogenesis.

Morphological and Functional Consequences. There is little published information on morphological characteristics of these disorders. Light microscopy shows acanthosis. On electron microscopy LBs appear normal. Dispersed keratohyaline granules have been described.

EKV (Connexin 31 Mutation, OMIM #133200)

Clinical Characteristics. Patients with EKV show patches of hyperkeratosis and erythema with a characteristic irregular outline and distribution (resembling the outline of a seacoast). The erythema can be migratory, varying in size from a few to many centimeters and can regress over minutes to hours. Skin lesions may be triggered by trauma or change in temperature. Lesions preferentially affect the face, buttocks, and extensor surfaces of the extremities. Palmoplantar keratoderma is present in about half of the cases. Hair, nails, and teeth are not affected. Several phenotypical variations have been clinically described. EKV Mendes de Costa is present at birth or during the first year of life and occurs in two distinct clinical presentations, a generalized brownish hyperkeratosis and a sharply demarcated, symmetrically distributed, localized type. Palmoplantar involvement has been described in this variant; hair, nails, and mucous membranes are unaffected. EKV associated with ataxia has been termed the Giroux-Barbeaux type. It presents during infancy. Lesions are typically accentuated over the extensor surface of the extremities. During adulthood the skin lesions typically diminish while a progressive spinocerebellar ataxia develops. Another symmetrical variant has been termed progressive symmetric erythrokeratoderma (Darier-Gottron disease).

Molecular Defect. EKV is due to autosomal dominant mutations in connexin 30.3 and connexin 31 on chromosome 1p34–35. These connexins, together with at least six other connexins, form gap junctions important for cell-to-cell communication.

Morphological and Functional Consequences. Light microscopy shows acanthosis and hyperkeratosis. The epidermis can acquire a marked papillomatosis with dilated capillaries and suprapapillary thinning, resulting in a "church spire" appearance. There are mild superficial perivascular lymphocytic infiltrates. Ultrastructurally, decreased numbers of LBs have been reported, but basal TEWL was normal (66,219).

ABNORMALITIES IN CORNEOCYTE COHESION DUE TO ABNORMAL PROTEOLYSIS OF DESMOSOMES

Netherton Syndrome (Syn. Ichthyosis Linearis Circumflexa or Comèl–Netherton Syndrome, LEKTI Deficiency, OMIM #256500)

Clinical Characteristics. Patients with Netherton syndrome display generalized scaling with inflammatory features, often with similarities to atopic dermatitis. At or shortly after birth, infants commonly present with generalized erythroderma. In older children and adults, a unique scaling pattern, termed ichthyosis linearis circumflexa, may develop in which migratory and surpiginous areas of double-edged scales are present. The skin abnormality is typically accompanied by pathognomonic hair shaft defects, called bamboo hair or trichorrhexis invaginata, in which the distal hair segment is telescoped into the proximal part. Only 20% to 50% of hair may be affected, and this feature may be absent in some patients. Atopy, with anaphylactic reactions to foods, is another feature of the disease triad.

Molecular Defect. NS is caused by autosomal recessive mutations in the SPINK5 gene, coding for the serine protease inhibitor LEKTI, and presumably resulting in unopposed serine protease activity. A large number of different mutations have been documented in the literature, many of them abolishing enzyme activity, a few mutations merely compromising enzyme function (220). LEKTI is expressed in skin, mucous membranes, tonsils, and thymus. It is cleaved into 15 active domains that suppress proteases like trypsin. However, the specific biological targets of LEKTI in human tissues are unknown. LEKTI may be important in the down-regulation of inflammatory processes, since the phenotypic finding of atopic manifestations in NS not seen in other congenital ichthyoses and polymorphisms in the SPINK5 gene (missense variants) has recently been associated with atopic disease (220–222). LEKTI may also play a role in terminal epidermal differentiation and/or corneocyte desquamation, as suggested by its restricted expression in the granular layer of the epidermis, and the severe cornification abnormality in NS. Among possible targets are the SC trypsin- and chymotrypsin-like enzymes (SCTE and SCCE, respectively), whose defective inhibition by LEKTI could result in both premature corneodesmosome degradation with premature desquamation as well as in the inactivation of other proteins, such as lipid hydrolases required for processing of LB lipids. Other putative targets are trypsin-like serine proteases, including the membrane-type serine protease 1 (MT-SP1), which could mediate inhibition of keratinocyte differentiation through activation of PAR-2 (protease-activated receptor-2) at the keratinocyte surface.

Morphological and Functional Consequences. Histological analysis shows acanthosis and a thin, variably parakeratotic SC in NS. Perivascular inflammation may be present, and neutrophils have also been described to invade the epidermis. The histological picture can be similar to psoriasis, particularly in infants. On EM, multilocular vesicles filled with an amorphous substance have been described at the level of the stratum spinosum (223), while premature secretion of LB contents is prominent at the SG–SC interface and LB-derived extracellular lamellae are disturbed and interspersed with foci of electron-dense material (224) in the SC.

Overall, SC thickness is reduced; hence in NS both the quantity and quality of SC membranes are abnormal. Moreover, a severe functional barrier defect is present in NS, as is predicted by these ultrastructural features (224). Growth failure can be very severe in infants with NS, who are also at risk for systemic infections, with consequent increased morbidity and mortality. The barrier defect, with loss of calories through heat of evaporation, appears to be the predominant cause of growth failure in NS (56,57). Patients with NS are also at risk for excessive systemic absorption of topical medications as a result of their severe barrier abnormality. An increased susceptibility to HPV infections, a presumed carcinogenic factor for the development of non-melanoma skin cancer, has also been reported (225), however, it seems unclear if this predisposition is related to the disease itself, to atopy, or to therapeutic exposure to UV-B irradiation.

REFERENCES

1. Elias PM, Kenneth R, Feingold, Joachim W, Fenhr. Skin as an organ of protection. In: Freedberg IM, Eisen AZ, Wolff K, Austen KF, Goldsmith LA, Katz SI, Fitzpatrick TB, eds. Dermatology in General Medicine. New York: Mc Graw-Hill, 2003:107–118.
2. Fuchs E. Epidermal differentiation: the bare essentials. J Cell Biol 1990; 111:2807–2814.
3. Eckert RL, Crish JF, Banks EB, Welter JF. The epidermis: genes on-genes off. J Invest Dermatol 1997; 109:501–509.
4. Downing DT. Lipid and protein structures in the permeability barrier of mammalian epidermis. J Lipid Res 1992; 33:301–313.
5. Elias PM. Epidermal lipids, membranes, and keratinization. Int J Dermatol 1981; 20:1–19.
6. Steinert PM, Marekov LN, Fraser RD, Parry DA. Keratin intermediate filament structure. Crosslinking studies yield quantitative information on molecular dimensions and mechanism of assembly. J Mol Biol 1993; 230:436–452.
7. Steinert PM, Marekov LN. The proteins elafin, filaggrin, keratin intermediate filaments, loricrin, and small proline-rich proteins 1 and 2 are isodipeptide cross-linked components of the human epidermal cornified cell envelope. J Biol Chem 1995; 270:17702–17711.
8. Steinert PM, Marekov LN. Direct evidence that involucrin is a major early isopeptide cross-linked component of the keratinocyte cornified envelope. J Biol Chem 1997; 17: 2021–2030.
9. Steinert PM, Marekov LN. Initiation of assembly of the cell envelope barrier structure of stratified squamous epithelia. Mol Biol Cell 1999; 10:4247–4261.
10. Steinert PM. The complexity and redundancy of epithelial barrier function. J Cell Biol 2000; 151:F5–F8.

11. Elias PM, Menon GK. Structural and lipid biochemical correlates of the epidermal permeability barrier. Adv Lipid Res 1991; 24:1–26.
12. Elias PM. Stratum corneum architecture, metabolic activity and interactivity with subjacent cell layers. Exp Dermatol 1996; 5:191–201.
13. Elias PM, Cullander C, Mauro T, Rassner U, Komuves L, Brown BE, Menon GK. The secretory granular cell: the outermost granular cell as a specialized secretory cell. J Investig Dermatol Symp Proc 1998; 3:87–100.
14. Swartzendruber DC, Wertz PW, Madison KC, Downing DT. Evidence that the corneocyte has a chemically bound lipid envelope. J Invest Dermatol 1987; 88:709–713.
15. Wertz PW, Swartzendruber DC, Kitko DJ, Madison KC, Downing DT. The role of the corneocyte lipid envelopes in cohesion of the stratum corneum. J Invest Dermatol 1989; 93:169–172.
16. Behne M, Uchida Y, Seki T, de Montellano PO, Elias PM, Holleran WM. Omega-hydroxyceramides are required for corneocyte lipid envelope (CLE) formation and normal epidermal permeability barrier function. J Invest Dermatol 2000; 114:185–192.
17. Odland GF, Holbrook K. The lamellar granules of epidermis. Curr Probl Dermatol 1981; 9:29–49.
18. Landmann L. The epidermal permeability barrier. Anat Embryol (Berl) 1988; 178:1–13.
19. Grubauer G, Elias PM, Feingold KR. Transepidermal water loss: the signal for recovery of barrier structure and function. J Lipid Res 1989; 30:323–333.
20. Grubauer G, Feingold KR, Elias PM. Relationship of epidermal lipogenesis to cutaneous barrier function. J of Lipid Research 1987; 28:746–752.
21. Proksch E, Elias PM, Feingold KR. Regulation of 3-hydroxy-3-methylglutaryl-coenzyme A reductase activity in murine epidermis. Modulation of enzyme content and activation state by barrier requirements. J Clin Invest 1990; 85:874–882.
22. Harris IR, Farrell AM, Grunfeld C, Holleran WM, Elias PM, Feingold KR. Permeability barrier disruption coordinately regulates mRNA levels for key enzymes of cholesterol, fatty acid, and ceramide synthesis in the epidermis. J Invest Dermatol 1997; 109:783–787.
23. Ottey KA, Wood LC, Grunfeld C, Elias PM, Feingold KR. Cutaneous permeability barrier disruption increases fatty acid synthetic enzyme activity in the epidermis of hairless mice. J Invest Dermatol 1995; 104:401–404.
24. Hanley K, Komuves LG, Ng DC, Schoonjans K, He SS, Lau P, Bikle DD, Williams ML, Elias PM, Auwerx J, Feingold KR. Farnesol stimulates differentiation in epidermal keratinocytes via PPARalpha. J Biol Chem 2000; 275:11484–11491.
25. Elias PM, Feingold KR. Lipids and the epidermal water barrier: metabolism, regulation, and pathophysiology. Semin Dermatol 1992; 11:176–182.
26. Schurer NY, Elias PM. The biochemistry and function of stratum corneum lipids. Adv Lipid Res 1991; 24:27–56.
27. Feingold KR. The regulation of epidermal lipid synthesis by permeability barrier requirements. Crit Rev Ther Drug Carrier Syst 1991; 8:193–210.
28. Fluhr JW, Kao J, Jain M, Ahn SK, Feingold KR, Elias PM. Generation of free fatty acids from phospholipids regulates stratum corneum acidification and integrity. J Invest Dermatol 2001; 117:44–51.
29. Elias PM, Fartasch M, Crumrine D, Behne M, Uchida Y, Holleran WM. Origin of the corneocyte lipid envelope (CLE): observations in harlequin ichthyosis and cultured human keratinocytes. J Invest Dermatol 2000; 115:765–769.
30. Chapman SJ, Walsh A, Jackson SM, Friedmann PS. Lipids, proteins and corneocyte adhesion. Arch Dermatol Res 1991; 283:167–173.
31. Serre G, Mils V, Haftek M, Vincent C, Croute F, Reano A, Ouhayoun JP, Bettinger S, Soleilhavoup JP. Identification of late differentiation antigens of human cornified epithelia, expressed in re-organized desmosomes and bound to cross-linked envelope. J Invest Dermatol 1991; 97:1061–1072.

32. Simon M, Montezin M, Guerrin M, Durieux JJ, Serre G. Characterization and purification of human corneodesmosin, an epidermal basic glycoprotein associated with corneocyte-specific modified desmosomes. J Biol Chem 1997; 272:31770–31776.

33. Elias PM, Matsuyoshi N, Wu H, Lin C, Wang ZH, Brown BE, Stanley JR. Desmoglein isoform distribution affects stratum corneum structure and function. J Cell Biol 2001; 153:243–249.

34. Sondell B, Thornell LE, Stigbrand T, Egelrud T. Immunolocalization of stratum corneum chymotryptic enzyme in human skin and oral epithelium with monoclonal antibodies: evidence of a proteinase specifically expressed in keratinizing squamous epithelia. J Histochem Cytochem 1994; 42:459–465.

35. Ekholm IE, Brattsand M, Egelrud T. Stratum corneum tryptic enzyme in normal epidermis: a missing link in the desquamation process? J Invest Dermatol 2000; 114:56–63.

36. Egelrud T. Desquamation in the stratum corneum. Acta Derm Venereol Suppl (Stockh) 2000; 208:44–45.

37. Hohl D. Cornified cell envelope. Dermatologica 1990; 180:201–211.

38. Potts RO, Mak VH, Guy RH, Francoeur ML. Strategies to enhance permeability via stratum corneum lipid pathways. Adv Lipid Res 1991; 24:173–210.

39. Candi E, Schmidt R, Melino G. The cornified envelope: a model of cell death in the skin. Nat Rev Mol Cell Biol 2005; 6:328–340.

40. Jeon S, Djian P, Green H. Inability of keratinocytes lacking their specific transglutaminase to form cross-linked envelopes: absence of envelopes as a simple diagnostic test for lamellar ichthyosis. Proc Natl Acad Sci USA 1998; 95:687–690.

41. Nemes Z, Marekov LN, Steinert PM. Involucrin cross-linking by transglutaminase 1. Binding to membranes directs residue specificity. J Biol Chem 1999; 274:11013–11021.

42. Djian P, Easley K, Green H. Targeted ablation of the murine involucrin gene. J Cell Biol 2000; 151:381–388.

43. DiSepio D, Bickenbach JR, Longley MA, Bundman DS, Rothnagel JA, Roop DR. Characterisation of loricrin regulation in vitro and in transgenic mice. Differentiation 1999; 64:225–235.

44. Bickenbach JR, Greer JM, Bundman DS, Rothnagel JA, Roop DR. Loricrin expression is coordinated with other epidermal proteins and the appearance of lipid lamellar granules in development. J Invest Dermatol 1995; 104:405–410.

45. Maestrini E, Monaco AP, McGrath JA, Ishida-Yamamoto A, Camisa C, Hovnanian A, Weeks DE, Lathrop M, Uitto J, Christiano AM. A molecular defect in loricrin, the major component of the cornified cell envelope, underlies Vohwinkel's syndrome. Nature Genetics 1996; 13:70–77.

46. Roop D. Defects in the barrier. Science 1995; 267:474–475.

47. Fuchs E, Cleveland DW. A structural scaffolding of intermediate filaments in health and disease. Science 1998; 279:514–519.

48. Rawlings AV, Scott IR, Harding CR, Bowser PA. Stratum corneum moisturization at the molecular level. J Invest Dermatol 1994; 103:731–741.

49. Kuechle MK, Thulin CD, Presland RB, Dale BA. Profilaggrin requires both linker and filaggrin peptide sequences to form granules: implications for profilaggrin processing in vivo. J Invest Dermatol 1999; 112:843–852.

50. Scott IR, Harding CR. Filaggrin breakdown to water binding compounds during development of the rat stratum corneum is controlled by the water activity of the environment. Dev Biol 1986; 115:84–92.

51. Traupe H. The ichthyoses: a guide to clinical diagnosis genetic counseling and therapy. Berlin: Springer, 1989.

52. Williams ML, Elias PM. From basket weave to barrier. Unifying concepts for the pathogenesis of the disorders of cornification. Arch Dermatol 1993; 129:626–629.

53. Williams M, LeBoit P. The ichthyoses: disorders of cornification. In: Arnd KK, LeBoit P, Robinson J, Wintroub B, eds. Cutaneous medicine and surgery: an integrated program in dermatology. Philadelphia: WB Saunders, 1996:1681–1711.

54. Vahlquist A, Ganemo A, Pigg M, Virtanen M, Westermark P. The clinical spectrum of congenital ichthyosis in Sweden: a review of 127 cases. Acta Derm Venereol Suppl (Stockh) 2003: 34–47.
55. Williams ML, Elias PM. Enlightened therapy of the disorders of cornification. Clin Dermatol 2003; 21:269–273.
56. Moskowitz DG, Fowler AJ, Heyman MB, Cohen SP, Crumrine D, Elias PM, Williams ML. Pathophysiologic basis for growth failure in children with ichthyosis: an evaluation of cutaneous ultrastructure, epidermal permeability barrier function, and energy expenditure. J Pediatr 2004; 145:82–92.
57. Fowler AJ, Moskowitz DG, Wong A, Cohen SP, Williams ML, Heyman MB. Nutritional status and gastrointestinal structure and function in children with ichthyosis and growth failure. J Pediatr Gastroenterol Nutr 2004; 38:164–169.
58. Bale SJ, Doyle SZ. The genetics of ichthyosis: a primer for epidemiologists. J Invest Dermatol 1994; 102:49S–50S.
59. Elias PM, McNutt NS, Friend DS. Membrane alterations during cornification of mammalian squamous epithelia: a freeze-fracture, tracer, and thin-section study. Anat Rec 1977; 189:577–594.
60. Schmuth M, Yosipovitch G, Williams ML, Weber F, Hintner H, Ortiz-Urda S, Rappersberger K, Crumrine D, Feingold KR, Elias PM. Pathogenesis of the permeability barrier abnormality in epidermolytic hyperkeratosis. J Invest Dermatol 2001; 117:837–847.
61. Elias PM, Schmuth M, Uchida Y, Rice RH, Behne M, Crumrine D, Feingold KR, Holleran WM. Basis for the permeability barrier abnormality in lamellar ichthyosis. Exp Dermatol 2002; 11(3):248–256.
62. Schmuth M, Fluhr JW, Crumrine DC, Uchida Y, Hachem JP, Behne M, Moskowitz DG, Christiano AM, Feingold KR, Elias PM. Structural and functional consequences of loricrin mutations in human loricrin keratoderma (Vohwinkel syndrome with ichthyosis). J Invest Dermatol 2004; 122:909–922.
63. Holleran WM, Ginns EI, Menon GK, Grundmann JU, Fartasch M, McKinney CE, Elias PM, Sidransky E. Consequences of beta-glucocerebrosidase deficiency in epidermis. Ultrastructure and permeability barrier alterations in Gaucher disease. J Clin Invest 1994; 93:1756–1764.
64. Elias PM, Crumrine D, Rassner U, Hachem JP, Menon GK, Man W, Choy MH, Leypoldt L, Feingold KR, Williams ML. Basis for abnormal desquamation and permeability barrier dysfunction in RXLI. J Invest Dermatol 2004; 122:314–319.
65. Ghadially R, Williams ML, Hou SY, Elias PM. Membrane structural abnormalities in the stratum corneum of the autosomal recessive ichthyoses. J Invest Dermatol 1992; 99:755–763.
66. Lavrijsen AP, Oestmann E, Hermans J, Boddé HE, Vermeer BJ, Ponec M. Barrier function parameters in various keratinization disorders: transepidermal water loss and vascular response to hexyl nicotinate. Br J Dermatol 1993; 129:547–553.
67. DiGiovanna JJ, Robinson-Bostom L. Ichthyosis: etiology, diagnosis, and management. Am J Clin Dermatol 2003; 4:81–95.
68. Dominey AM, Wang XJ, King LE, Jr., Nanney LB, Gagne TA, Sellheyer K, Bundman DS, Longley MA, Rothnagel JA, Greenhalgh DA, et al.: Targeted overexpression of transforming growth factor alpha in the epidermis of transgenic mice elicits hyperplasia, hyperkeratosis, and spontaneous, squamous papillomas. Cell Growth Differ 1993; 4:1071–1082.
69. Williams ML, Elias PM. Stratum corneum lipids in disorders of cornification: increased cholesterol sulfate content of stratum corneum in recessive x-linked ichthyosis. J Clin Invest 1981; 68:1404–1410.
70. Williams ML, Elias PM. Heterogeneity in autosomal recessive ichthyosis. Clinical and biochemical differentiation of lamellar ichthyosis and nonbullous congenital ichthyosiform erythroderma. Arch Dermatol 1985; 121:477–488.

71. Williams ML, Koch TK, O'Donnell JJ, Frost PH, Epstein LB, Grizzard WS, Epstein CJ. Ichthyosis and neutral lipid storage disease. Am J Med Genet 1985; 20:711–726.

72. Sidransky E, Fartasch M, Lee RE, Metlay LA, Abella S, Zimran A, Gao W, Elias PM, Ginns EI, Holleran WM. Epidermal abnormalities may distinguish type 2 from type 1 and type 3 of Gaucher disease. Pediatr Res 1996; 39:134–141.

73. Proksch E, Feingold KR, Man MQ, Elias PM. Barrier function regulates epidermal DNA synthesis. J Clin Invest 1991; 87:1668–1673.

74. Denda M, Wood LC, Emami S, Calhoun C, Brown BE, Elias PM, Feingold KR. The epidermal hyperplasia associated with repeated barrier disruption by acetone treatment or tape stripping cannot be attributed to increased water loss. Arch Dermatol Res 1996; 288:230–238.

75. Shwayder T, Ott F. All about ichthyosis. Pediatr Clin North Am 1991; 38:835–857.

76. Lykkesfeldt G, Nielsen MD, Lykkesfeldt AE. Placental steroid sulfatase deficiency: biochemical diagnosis and clinical review. Obstet Gynecol 1984; 64:49–54.

77. Okano M, Kitano Y, Yoshikawa K, Nakamura T, Matsuzawa Y, Yuasa T. X-linked ichthyosis and ichthyosis vulgaris: comparison of their clinical features based on biochemical analysis. Br J Dermatol 1988; 119:777–783.

78. Weiss MM. Wolff-Parkinson-White (Type B), Ebstein's anomaly, and congenital ichthyosis. Am Heart J 1978; 95:133.

79. Koppe G, Marinkovic-Ilsen A, Rijken Y, De Groot WP, Jobsis AC. X-linked icthyosis. A sulphatase deficiency. Arch Dis Child 1978; 53:803–806.

80. Marinkovic-Ilsen A, Koppe JG, Jobsis AC, de Groot WP. Enzymatic basis of typical X-linked ichthyosis. Lancet 1978; 2:1097.

81. Bonifas JM, Morley BJ, Oakey RE, Kan YW, Epstein EH, Jr. Cloning of a cDNA for steroid sulfatase: frequent occurrence of gene deletions in patients with recessive X chromosome-linked ichthyosis. Proc Natl Acad Sci USA 1987; 84:9248–9251.

82. Cosma MP, Pepe S, Annunziata I, Newbold RF, Grompe M, Parenti G, Ballabio A. The multiple sulfatase deficiency gene encodes an essential and limiting factor for the activity of sulfatases. Cell 2003; 113:445–456.

83. Dierks T, Schmidt B, Borissenko LV, Peng J, Preusser A, Mariappan M, von Figura K. Multiple sulfatase deficiency is caused by mutations in the gene encoding the human C(alpha)-formylglycine generating enzyme. Cell 2003; 113:435–444.

84. Sato J, Denda M, Nakanishi J, Nomura J, Koyama J. Cholesterol sulfate inhibits proteases that are involved in desquamation of stratum corneum. J Invest Dermatol 1998; 111:189–193.

85. Frost P, Weinstein GD, Van Scott EJ. The ichthyosiform dermatoses. II. Autoradiographic studies of epidermal proliferation. J Invest Dermatol 1966; 47:561–567.

86. Frost P, Weinstein GD, Bothwell JW, Wildnauer R. Ichthyosiform dermatoses. 3. Studies of transepidermal water loss. Arch Dermatol 1968; 98:230–233.

87. Elias PM, Williams ML, Maloney ME, Bonifas JA, Brown BE, Grayson S, Epstein EHJ. Stratum corneum lipids in disorders of cornification. Steroid sulfatase and cholesterol sulfate in normal desquamation and the pathogenesis of recessive X-linked ichthyosis. J Clin Invest 1984; 74:1414–1421.

88. Zettersten E, Man MQ, Sato J, Denda M, Farrell A, Ghadially R, Williams ML, Feingold KR, Elias PM. Recessive x-linked ichthyosis: role of cholesterol-sulfate accumulation in the barrier abnormality. J Invest Dermatol 1998; 111:784–790.

89. Maloney ME, Williams ML, Epstein EH, Jr., Law MY, Fritsch PO, Elias PM. Lipids in the pathogenesis of ichthyosis: topical cholesterol sulfate-induced scaling in hairless mice. J Invest Dermatol 1984; 83:252–256.

90. Hanley K, Wood L, Ng DC, He SS, Lau P, Moser A, Elias PM, Bikle DD, Williams ML, Feingold KR. Cholesterol sulfate stimulates involucrin transcription in keratinocytes by increasing Fra-1, Fra-2, and Jun D. J Lipid Res 2001; 42:390–398.

91. Lefevre C, Audebert S, Jobard F, Bouadjar B, Lakhdar H, Boughdene-Stambouli O, Blanchet-Bardon C, Heilig R, Foglio M, Weissenbach J, Lathrop M, Prud'homme

JF, Fischer J. Mutations in the transporter ABCA12 are associated with lamellar ichthyosis type 2. Hum Mol Genet 2003; 12:2369–2378.

92. Krebsova A, Kuster W, Lestringant GG, Schulze B, Hinz B, Frossard PM, Reis A, Hennies HC. Identification, by homozygosity mapping, of a novel locus for autosomal recessive congenital ichthyosis on chromosome 17p, and evidence for further genetic heterogeneity. Am J Hum Genet 2001; 69:216–222.

93. Jobard F, Lefevre C, Karaduman A, Blanchet-Bardon C, Emre S, Weissenbach J, Ozguc M, Lathrop M, Prud'homme JF, Fischer J. Lipoxygenase-3 (ALOXE3) and 12(R)-lipoxygenase (ALOX12B) are mutated in non-bullous congenital ichthyosiform erythroderma (NCIE) linked to chromosome 17p13.1. Hum Mol Genet 2002; 11:107–113.

94. Anton-Lamprecht I. Ultrastructural identification of basic abnormalities as clues to genetic disorders of the epidermis. J Invest Dermatol 1974; 103:6S–12S.

95. Niemi KM, Kanerva L, Wahlgren CF, Ignatius J. Clinical, light and electron microscopic features of recessive ichthyosis congenita type III. Arch Dermatol Res 1992; 284:259–265.

96. Niemi KM, Kanerva L, Kuokkanen K. Recessive ichthyosis congenita type II. Arch Dermatol Res 1991; 283:211–218.

97. Niemi KM, Kuokkanen K, Kanerva L, Ignatius J. Recessive ichthyosis congenita type IV. Am J Dermatopathol 1993; 15:224–228.

98. Niemi KM, Kanerva L, Kuokkanen K, Ignatius J. Clinical, light and electron microscopic features of recessive congenital ichthyosis type I. Br J Dermatol 1994; 130:626–633.

99. Williams ML, Elias PM. Elevated n-alkanes in congenital ichthyosiform erythroderma. Phenotypic differentiation of two types of autosomal recessive ichthyosis. J Clin Invest 1984; 74:296–300.

100. Holbrook KA, Dale BA, Williams ML, Perry TB, Hoff MS, Hamilton EF, Fisher C, Senikas V. The expression of congenital ichthyosiform erythroderma in second trimester fetuses of the same family: morphologic and biochemical studies. J Invest Dermatol 1988; 91:521–531.

101. Melnick B. Epidermal lipids and the biochemistry of keratinization. In: Traupe H, ed. The Ichtyoses a guide to clinical diagnosis, genetic counseling, and therapy. Heidelberg: Springer, 1989:14–42.

102. De Laurenzi V, Rogers GR, Hamrock DJ, Marekov LN, Steinert PM, Compton JG, Markova N, Rizzo WB. Sjogren-Larsson syndrome is caused by mutations in the fatty aldehyde dehydrogenase gene. Nat Genet 1996; 12:52–57.

103. Rizzo WB, Lin Z, Carney G. Fatty aldehyde dehydrogenase: genomic structure, expression and mutation analysis in Sjogren-Larsson syndrome. Chem Biol Interact 2001; 130–132:297–307.

104. Lake BD, Smith VV, Judge MR, Harper JI, Besley GT. Hexanol dehydrogenase activity shown by enzyme histochemistry on skin biopsies allows differentiation of Sjogren-Larsson syndrome from other ichthyoses. J Inherit Metab Dis 1991; 14:338–340.

105. Willemsen MA, de Jong JG, van Domburg PH, Rotteveel JJ, Wanders RJ, Mayatepek E. Defective inactivation of leukotriene B4 in patients with Sjogren-Larsson syndrome. J Pediatr 2000; 136:258–260.

106. Willemsen MA, Rotteveel JJ, Steijlen PM, Heerschap A, Mayatepek E. 5-Lipoxygenase inhibition: a new treatment strategy for Sjogren-Larsson syndrome. Neuropediatrics 2000; 31:1–3.

107. Koone MD, Rizzo WB, Elias PM, Williams ML, Lightner V, Pinnell SR. Ichthyosis, mental retardation, and asymptomatic spasticity. A new neurocutaneous syndrome with normal fatty alcohol:NAD+ oxidoreductase activity. Arch Dermatol 1990; 126:1485–1490.

108. Reynolds DJ, Marks R, Davies MG, Dykes PJ. The fatty acid composition of skin and plasma lipids in Refsum's disease. Clin Chim Acta 1978; 90:171–177.

109. Jansen GA, Ofman R, Ferdinandusse S, Ijlst L, Muijsers AO, Skjeldal OH, Stokke O, Jakobs C, Besley GT, Wraith JE, Wanders RJ. Refsum disease is caused by mutations in the phytanoyl-CoA hydroxylase gene. Nat Genet 1997; 17:190–193.

110. Klenk E, Kahike W. [on the Presence of 3,7,11,15-Tetramethylhexadecanoic Acid (Phytanic Acid) in the Cholesterol Esters and Other Lipoid Fractions of the Organs in a Case of a Disease of Unknown Origin (Possibly Heredopathia Atactica Polyneuritiformis, Refsum's Syndrome)]. Hoppe Seylers Z Physiol Chem 1963; 333:133–139.

111. Dykes PJ, Marks R, Davies MG, Reynolds DJ. Epidermal metabolism in heredopathia atactica polyneuritiformis (Refsum's disease). J Invest Dermatol 1978; 70:126–129.

112. Foulon V, Asselberghs S, Geens W, Mannaerts GP, Casteels M, Van Veldhoven PP. Further studies on the substrate spectrum of phytanoyl-CoA hydroxylase: implications for Refsum disease? J Lipid Res 2003; 44:2349–2355.

113. van den Brink DM, Brites P, Haasjes J, Wierzbicki AS, Mitchell J, Lambert-Hamill M, de Belleroche J, Jansen GA, Waterham HR, Wanders RJ. Identification of PEX7 as the second gene involved in Refsum disease. Am J Hum Genet 2003; 72:471–477.

114. Jansen GA, Mihalik SJ, Watkins PA, Moser HW, Jakobs C, Heijmans HS, Wanders RJ. Phytanoyl-CoA hydroxylase is not only deficient in classical Refsum disease but also in rhizomelic chondrodysplasia punctata. J Inherit Metab Dis 1997; 20:444–446.

115. Davies MG, Marks R, Dykes PJ, Reynolds D. Epidermal abnormalities in Refsum's disease. Br J Dermatol 1977; 97:401–406.

116. Happle R, Karlic D, Steijlen PM. [CHILD syndrome in a mother and daughter]. Hautarzt 1990; 41:105–108.

117. Becker K, Csikos M, Horvath A, Karpati S. Identification of a novel mutation in 3beta-hydroxysteroid-Delta8-Delta7-isomerase in a case of Conradi-Hunermann-Happle syndrome. Exp Dermatol 2001; 10:286–289.

118. Konig A, Happle R, Bornholdt D, Engel H, Grzeschik KH. Mutations in the *NSDHL* gene, encoding a 3beta-hydroxysteroid dehydrogenase, cause CHILD syndrome. Am J Med Genet 2000; 90:339–346.

119. Hamaguchi T, Bondar G, Siegfried E, Penneys NS. Cutaneous histopathology of Conradi-Hunermann syndrome. J Cutan Pathol 1995; 22:38–41.

120. Yanagihara M, Ueda K, Asano N, Ozawa T, Nakatani A, Hirose M. Usefulness of histopathologic examination of thick scales in the diagnosis of X-linked dominant chondrodysplasia punctata (Happle). Pediatric Derm 1996; 13:1–4.

121. Kolde G, Happle R. Histologic and ultrastructural features of the ichthyotic skin in X-linked dominant chondrodysplasia punctata. Acta Derm Venereol 1984; 64:389–394.

122. Mommaas M, Tada J, Ponec M. Distribution of low-density lipoprotein receptors and apolipoprotein B on normal and on reconstructed human epidermis. J Dermatol Sci 1991; 2:97–105.

123. Mao-Qiang M, Feingold KR, Elias PM. Inhibition of cholesterol sphingolipid synthesis causes paradoxical effects on permeability barrier homeostasis. J Invest Dermatol 1993; 101:185–190.

124. Kelsell DP, Norgett EE, Unsworth H, Teh MT, Cullup T, Mein CA, Dopping-Hepenstal PJ, Dale BA, Tadini G, Fleckman P, Stephens KG, Sybert VP, Mallory SB, North BV, Witt DR, Sprecher E, Taylor AE, Ilchyshyn A, Kennedy CT, Goodyear H, Moss C, Paige D, Harper JI, Young BD, Leigh IM, Eady RA, O'Toole EA. Mutations in ABCA12 underlie the severe congenital skin disease harlequin ichthyosis. Am J Hum Genet 2005; 76:794–803.

125. Dale BA, Holbrook KA, Fleckman P, Kimball JR, Brumbaugh S, Sybert VP. Heterogeneity in harlequin ichthyosis, an inborn error of epidermal keratinization: variable morphology and structural protein expression and a defect in lamellar granules. J Invest Dermatol 1990; 94:6–18.

126. Crocker AC, Farber S. Niemann-Pick disease: a review of eighteen patients. Medicine (Baltimore) 1958; 37:1–95.

127. Schmuth M, Man MQ, Weber F, Gao W, Feingold KR, Fritsch P, Elias PM, Holleran WM. Permeability barrier disorder in niemann-pick disease: sphingomyelin-ceramide processing required for normal barrier homeostasis. J Invest Dermatol 2000; 115:459–466.

128. Menon GK, Grayson S, Elias PM. Cytochemical and biochemical localization of lipase and sphingomyelinase activity in mammalian epidermis. J Invest Dermatol 1986; 86:591–597.

129. Grayson S, Johnson-Winegar AG, Wintroub BU, Isseroff RR, Epstein EH, Jr., Elias PM. Lamellar body-enriched fractions from neonatal mice: preparative techniques and partial characterization. J Invest Dermatol 1985; 85:289–294.

130. Jensen JM, Schutze S, Forl M, Kronke M, Proksch E. Roles for tumor necrosis factor receptor p55 and sphingomyelinase in repairing the cutaneous permeability barrier. J Clin Invest 1999; 104:1761–1770.

131. Kreder D, Krut O, Adam-Klages S, Wiegmann K, Scherer G, Plitz T, Jensen JM, Proksch E, Steinmann J, Pfeffer K, Kronke M. Impaired neutral sphingomyelinase activation and cutaneous barrier repair in FAN-deficient mice. Embo J 1999; 18:2472–2479.

132. Chanarin I, Patel A, Slavin G, Wills EJ, Andrews TM, Stewart G. Neutral-lipid storage disease: a new disorder of lipid metabolism. Br Med J 1975; 1:553–555.

133. Lefevre C, Jobard F, Caux F, Bouadjar B, Karaduman A, Heilig R, Lakhdar H, Wollenberg A, Verret JL, Weissenbach J, Ozguc M, Lathrop M, Prud'homme JF, Fischer J. Mutations in CGI-58, the gene encoding a new protein of the esterase/lipase/thioesterase subfamily, in Chanarin-Dorfman syndrome. Am J Hum Genet 2001; 69:1002–1012.

134. Williams ML, Monger DJ, Rutherford SL, Hincenbergs M, Rehfeld SJ, Grunfeld C. Neutral lipid storage disease with ichthyosis: lipid content and metabolism of fibroblasts. J Inherit Metab Dis 1988; 11:131–143.

135. Hilaire N, Salvayre R, Thiers JC, Bonnafe MJ, Negre-Salvayre A. The turnover of cytoplasmic triacylglycerols in human fibroblasts involves two separate acyl chain length-dependent degradation pathways. J Biol Chem 1995; 270:27027–27034.

136. Igal RA, Coleman RA. Acylglycerol recycling from triacylglycerol to phospholipid, not lipase activity, is defective in neutral lipid storage disease fibroblasts. J Biol Chem 1996; 271:16644–16651.

137. Igal RA, Coleman RA. Neutral lipid storage disease: a genetic disorder with abnormalities in the regulation of phospholipid metabolism. J Lipid Res 1998; 39:31–43.

138. Angelini C, Philippart M, Borrone C, Bresolin N, Cantini M, Lucke S. Multisystem triglyceride storage disorder with impaired long-chain fatty acid oxidation. Ann Neurol 1980; 7:5–10.

139. Akiyama M, Sawamura D, Nomura Y, Sugawara M, Shimizu H. Truncation of CGI-58 protein causes malformation of lamellar granules resulting in ichthyosis in Dorfman-Chanarin syndrome. J Invest Dermatol 2003; 121:1029–1034.

140. Yamanaka WK, Clemans GW, Hutchinson ML. Essential fatty acids deficiency in humans. Prog Lipid Res 1980; 19:187–215.

141. Hartop PJ, Prottey C. Changes in transepidermal water loss and the composition of epidermal lecithin after applications of pure fatty acid triglycerides to skin of essential fatty acid-deficient rats. Br J Dermatol 1976; 95:255–264.

142. Hou SY, Mitra AK, White SH, Menon GK, Ghadially R, Elias PM. Membrane structures in normal and essential fatty acid-deficient stratum corneum: characterization by ruthenium tetroxide staining and x-ray diffraction. J Invest Dermatol 1991; 96:215–223.

143. Melton JL, Wertz PW, Swartzendruber DC, Downing DT. Effects of essential fatty acid deficiency on epidermal O-acylsphingolipids and transepidermal water loss in young pigs. Biochim Biophys Acta 1987; 921:191–197.

144. Williams ML, Feingold KR, Grubauer G, Elias PM. Ichthyosis induced by cholesterol-lowering drugs. Implications for epidermal cholesterol homeostasis. Arch Dermatol 1987; 123:1535–1538.

145. Elias PM, Lampe MA, Chung JC, Williams ML. Diazacholesterol-induced ichthyosis in the hairless mouse. I. Morphologic, histochemical, and lipid biochemical characterization of a new animal model. Lab Invest 1983; 48:565–577.
146. Ponec M, Havekes L, Kempenaar J, Lavrijsen S, Wijsman M, Boonstra J, Vermeer BJ. Calcium-mediated regulation of the low density lipoprotein receptor and intracellular cholesterol synthesis in human epidermal keratinocytes. J Cell Physiol 1985; 125:98–106.
147. Williams ML. Lipids in normal and pathological desquamation. Adv In Lipid Res 1991; 24:211–262.
148. Menon GK, Brown BE, Elias PM. Avian epidermal differentiation: role of lipids in permeability barrier formation. Tissue Cell 1986; 18:71–82.
149. Williams ML, Aszterbaum M, Menon GK, Moser AH, Feingold KR, Hoath SB. Preservation of permeability barrier ontogenesis in the intrauterine growth-retarded fetal rat. Pediatr Res 1993; 33:418–424.
150. Elias P, Man MQ, Williams ML, Feingold KR, Magin T. Barrier function in K-10 heterozygote knockout mice. J Invest Dermatol 2000; 114:396–397.
151. Matsuki M, Yamashita F, Ishida-Yamamoto A, Yamada K, Kinoshita C, Fushiki S, Ueda E, Morishima Y, Tabata K, Yasuno H, Hashida M, Iizuka H, Ikawa M, Okabe M, Kondoh G, Kinoshita T, Takeda J, Yamanishi K. Defective stratum corneum and early neonatal death in mice lacking the gene for transglutaminase 1 (keratinocyte transglutaminase). Proc Natl Acad Sci USA 1998; 95:1044–1049.
152. Kuramoto N, Takizawa T, Matsuki M, Morioka H, Robinson JM, Yamanishi K. Development of ichthyosiform skin compensates for defective permeability barrier function in mice lacking transglutaminase 1. J Clin Invest 2002; 109:243–250.
153. Koch PJ, de Viragh PA, Scharer E, Bundman D, Longley MA, Bickenbach J, Kawachi Y, Suga Y, Zhou Z, Huber M, Hohl D, Kartasova T, Jarnik M, Steven AC, Roop DR. Lessons from loricrin-deficient mice. Compensatory mechanisms maintaining skin barrier function in the absence of a major cornified envelope protein. J Cell Biol 2000; 151:389–400.
154. Suga Y, Jarnik M, Attar PS, Longley MA, Bundman D, Steven AC, Koch PJ, Roop DR. Transgenic mice expressing a mutant form of loricrin reveal the molecular basis of the skin diseases, Vohwinkel syndrome and progressive symmetric erythrokeratoderma. J Cell Biol 2000; 151:401–412.
155. Camisa C, Rossana C. Variant of keratoderma hereditaria mutilans (Vohwinkel's syndrome). Treatment with orally administered isotretinoin. Arch Dermatol 1984; 120:1323–1328.
156. Camisa C, Hessel A, Rossana C, Parks A. Autosomal dominant keratoderma, ichthyosiform dermatosis and elevated serum beta-glucuronidase. Dermatologica 1988; 177:341–347.
157. Korge BP, Ishida-Yamamoto A, Punter C, Dopping-Hepenstal PJ, Iizuka H, Stephenson A, Eady RA, Munro CS. Loricrin mutation in Vohwinkel's keratoderma is unique to the variant with ichthyosis. J Invest Dermatol 1997; 109:604–610.
158. Armstrong DK, McKenna KE, Hughes AE. A novel insertional mutation in loricrin in Vohwinkel's Keratoderma. J Invest Dermatol 1998; 111:702–704.
159. Takahashi H, Ishida-Yamamoto A, Kishi A, Ohara K, Iizuka H. Loricrin gene mutation in a Japanese patient of Vohwinkel's syndrome. J Dermatol Sci 1999; 19:44–47.
160. O'Driscoll J, Muston GC, McGrath JA, Lam HM, Ashworth J, Christiano AM. A recurrent mutation in the loricrin gene underlies the ichthyotic variant of Vohwinkel syndrome. Clin Exp Dermatol 2002; 27:243–246.
161. Vohwinkel KH. Keratoderma hereditaria mutilans (Vohwinkel's syndrome). Arch Dermatol Syphil 1929; 158:354–364.
162. Mehrel T, Hohl D, Rothnagel JA, Longley MA, Bundman D, Cheng C, Lichti U, Bisher ME, Steven AC, Steinert PM, et al. Identification of a major keratinocyte cell envelope protein, loricrin. Cell 1990; 61:1103–1112.

163. Steven AC, Bisher ME, Roop DR, Steinert PM. Biosynthetic pathways of filaggrin and loricrin–two major proteins expressed by terminally differentiated epidermal keratinocytes. J Struct Biol 1990; 104:150–162.

164. Hohl D, Mehrel T, Lichti U, Turner ML, Roop DR, Steinert PM. Characterization of human loricrin. Structure and function of a new class of epidermal cell envelope proteins. J Biol Chem 1991; 266:6626–6636.

165. Maestrini E, Korge BP, Ocana-Sierra J, Calzolari E, Cambiaghi S, Scudder PM, Hovnanian A, Monaco AP, Munro CS. A missense mutation in connexin26, D66H, causes mutilating keratoderma with sensorineural deafness (Vohwinkel's syndrome) in three unrelated families. Hum Mol Genet 1999; 8:1237–1243.

166. Rothnagel JA, Dominey AM, Dempsey LD, Longley MA, Greenhalgh DA, Gagne TA, Huber M, Frenk E, Hohl D, Roop DR. Mutations in the rod domains of keratins 1 and 10 in epidermolytic hyperkeratosis. Science 1992; 257:1128–1130.

167. Cheng J, Syder AJ, Yu QC, Letai A, Paller AS, Fuchs E. The genetic basis of epidermolytic hyperkeratosis: a disorder of differentiation-specific epidermal keratin genes. Cell 1992; 70:811–819.

168. Chipev CC, Korge BP, Markova N, Bale SJ, DiGiovanna JJ, Compton JG, Steinert PM. A leucine–proline mutation in the H1 subdomain of keratin 1 causes epidermolytic hyperkeratosis. Cell 1992; 70:821–828.

169. Paller AS, Syder AJ, Chan YM, Yu QC, Hutton E, Tadini G, Fuchs E. Genetic and clinical mosaicism in a type of epidermal nevus. N Engl J Med 1994; 331:1408–1415.

170. Chipev CC, Yang JM, DiGiovanna JJ, Steinert PM, Marekov L, Compton JG, Bale SJ. Preferential sites in keratin 10 that are mutated in epidermolytic hyperkeratosis. American J Hum Gen 1994; 54:179–190.

171. Huber M, Scaletta C, Benathan M, Frenk E, Greenhalgh DA, Rothnagel JA, Roop DR, Hohl D. Abnormal keratin 1 and 10 cytoskeleton in cultured keratinocytes from epidermolytic hyperkeratosis caused by keratin 10 mutations. J Invest Dermatol 1994; 102:691–694.

172. Yang JM, Chipev CC, DiGiovanna JJ, Bale SJ, Marekov LN, Steinert PM, Compton JG. Mutations in the H1 and 1A domains in the keratin 1 gene in epidermolytic hyperkeratosis. J Invest Dermatol 1994; 102:17–23.

173. Syder AJ, Yu QC, Paller AS, Giudice G, Pearson R, Fuchs E. Genetic mutations in the K1 and K10 genes of patients with epidermolytic hyperkeratosis. Correlation between location and disease severity. J Clin Invest 1994; 93:1533–1542.

174. McLean WH, Eady RA, Dopping-Hepenstal PJ, McMillan JR, Leigh IM, Navsaria HA, Higgins C, Harper JI, Paige DG, Morley SM, al e Mutations in the rod 1A domain of keratins 1 and 10 in bullous congenital ichthyosiform erythroderma (BCIE). J Invest Dermatol 1994; 102:24–30.

175. Yang JM, Nam K, Park KB, Kim WS, Moon KC, Koh JK, Steinert PM, Lee ES. A novel H1 mutation in the keratin 1 chain in epidermolytic hyperkeratosis. J Invest Dermatol 1996; 107:439–441.

176. Yang JM, Yoneda K, Morita E, Imamura S, Nam K, Lee ES, Steinert PM. An alanine to proline mutation in the 1A rod domain of the keratin 10 chain in epidermolytic hyperkeratosis. J Invest Dermatol 1997; 109:692–694.

177. Joh GY, Traupe H, Metze D, Nashan D, Huber M, Hohl D, Longley MA, Rothnagel JA, Roop DR. A novel dinucleotide mutation in keratin 10 in the annular epidermolytic ichthyosis variant of bullous congenital ichthyosiform erythroderma. J Invest Dermatol 1997; 108:357–361.

178. Suga Y, Duncan KO, Heald PW, Roop DR. A novel helix termination mutation in keratin 10 in annular epidermolytic ichthyosis, a variant of bullous congenital ichthyosiform erythroderma. J Invest Dermatol 1998; 111:1220–1223.

179. Kremer H, Lavrijsen AP, McLean WH, Lane EB, Melchers D, Ruiter DJ, Mariman EC, Steijlen PM. An atypical form of bullous congenital ichthyosiform erythroderma

is caused by a mutation in the L12 linker region of keratin 1. J Invest Dermatol 1998; 111:1224–1226.

180. Michael EJ, Schneiderman P, Grossman ME, Christiano AM. Epidermolytic hyperkeratosis with polycyclic psoriasiform plaques resulting from a mutation in the keratin 1 gene. Exp Dermatol 1999; 8:501–503.

181. Arin MJ, Longley MA, Anton-Lamprecht I, Kurze G, Huber M, Hohl D, Rothnagel JA, Roop DR. A novel substition in keratin 10 in epidermolytic hyperkeratosis. J Invest Dermatol 1999; 112:506–508.

182. Arin MJ, Longley MA, Küster W, Huber M, Hohl D, Rothnagel JA, Roop DR. An asparagine to threonine substitution in the 1A domain of keratin 1: a novel mutation that causes epidermolytic hyperkeratosis. Exp Dermatol 1999; 8:124–127.

183. Yang JM, Nam K, Kim HC, Lee JH, Park JK, Wu K, Lee ES, Steinert PM. A novel glutamic acid to aspartic acid mutation near the end of the 2B rod domain in the keratin 1 chain in epidermolytic hyperkeratosis. J Invest Dermatol 1999; 112:376–379.

184. Sybert VP, Francis JS, Corden LD, Smith LT, Weaver M, Stephens K, McLean WH. Cyclic ichthyosis with epidermolytic hyperkeratosis: A phenotype conferred by mutations in the 2B domain of keratin K1. Am J Hum Genet 1999; 64:732–738.

185. McLean WH, Morley SM, Higgins C, Bowden PE, White M, Leigh IM, Lane EB. Novel and recurrent mutations in keratin 10 causing bullous congenital ichthyosiform erythroderma. Exp Dermatol 1999; 8:120–123.

186. Arin MJ, Longley MA, Epstein EH, Jr., Rothnagel JA, Roop DR. Identification of a novel mutation in keratin 1 in a family with epidermolytic hyperkeratosis. Exp Dermatol 2000; 9:16–19.

187. Cserhalmi-Friedman PB, Squeo R, Gordon D, Garzon M, Schneiderman P, Grossman ME, Christiano AM. Epidermolytic hyperkeratosis in a Hispanic family resulting from a mutation in the keratin 1 gene. Clin Exp Dermatol 2000; 25:241–243.

188. Irvine AD, McLean WH. Human keratin diseases: the increasing spectrum of disease and subtlety of the phenotype-genotype correlation. Br J Dermatol 1999; 140:815–828.

189. Ishida-Yamamoto A, Iizuka H, Manabe M, O'Guin WM, Hohl D, Kartasova T, Kuroki T, Roop DR, Eady RA. Altered distribution of keratinization markers in epidermolytic hyperkeratosis. Arch Dermatol Res 1995; 287:705–711.

190. Anton-Lamprecht I. Genetically induced abnormalities of epidermal differentiation and ultrastructure in ichthyoses and epidermolyses: pathogenesis, heterogeneity, fetal manifestation, and prenatal diagnosis. J Invest Dermatol 1983; 81:149s–156s.

191. Miller RK, Khuon S, Goldman RD. Dynamics of keratin assembly: exogenous type I keratin rapidly associates with type II keratin in vivo. J Cell Biol 1993; 122:123–135.

192. Ming ME, Daryanani HA, Roberts LP, Baden HP, Kvedar JC. Binding of keratin intermediate filaments (K10) to the cornified envelope in mouse epidermis: implications for barrier function. J Invest Dermatol 1994; 103:780–784.

193. Nemes Z, Steinert PM. Bricks and mortar of the epidermal barrier. Exp Mol Med 1999; 31:5–19.

194. Bonifas JM, Rothman AL, Epstein EH, Jr. Epidermolysis bullosa simplex: evidence in two families for keratin gene abnormalities. Science 1991; 254:1202–1205.

195. Coulombe PA, Hutton ME, Letai A, Hebert A, Paller AS, Fuchs E. Point mutations in human keratin 14 genes of epidermolysis bullosa simplex patients: genetic and functional analyses. Cell 1991; 66:1301–1311.

196. Lane EB, Rugg EL, Navsaria H, Leigh IM, Heagerty AH, Ishida-Yamamoto A, Eady RA. A mutation in the conserved helix termination peptide of keratin 5 in hereditary skin blistering. Nature 1992; 356:244–246.

197. Aunis D, Bader MF. The cytoskeleton as a barrier to exocytosis in secretory cells. J Exp Biol 1988; 139:253–266.

198. Porter RM, Reichelt J, Lunny DP, Magin TM, Lane EB. The relationship between hyperproliferation and epidermal thickening in a mouse model for BCIE. J Invest Dermatol 1998; 110:951–957.

199. Wells RS. Ichthyosis. Br Med J 1966; 2:1504–1506.
200. Cuevas-Covarrubias SA, Diaz-Zagoya JC, Rivera-Vega MR, Beirana A, Carrasco E, Orozco E, Kofman-Alfaro SH. Higher prevalence of X-linked ichthyosis versus ichthyosis vulgaris in Mexico. Int J Dermatol 1999; 38:555–556.
201. Sybert VP, Dale BA, Holbrook KA. Ichthyosis vulgaris: identification of a defect in synthesis of filaggrin correlated with an absence of keratohyaline granules. J Invest Dermatol 1985; 84:191–194.
202. Compton JG, DiGiovanna JJ, Johnston KA, Fleckman P, Bale S. Mapping of the associated phenotype of an absent granular layer in ichthyosis vulgaris to the epidermal differentiation complex on chromosome I. Exper Dermatol 2002:in press.
203. Zhong W, Cui B, Zhang Y, Jiang H, Wei S, Bu L, Zhao G, Hu L, Kong X. Linkage analysis suggests a locus of ichthyosis vulgaris on 1q22. J Hum Genet 2003; 48:390–392.
204. Nirunsuksiri W, Zhang SH, Fleckman P. Reduced stability and bi-allelic, coequal expression of profilaggrin mRNA in keratinocytes cultured from subjects with ichthyosis vulgaris. J Invest Dermatol 1998; 110:854–861.
205. Scott IR, Harding CR, Barrett JG. Histidine-rich protein of the keratohyalin granules. Source of the free amino acids, urocanic acid and pyrrolidone carboxylic acid in the stratum corneum. Biochim Biophys Acta 1982; 719:110–117.
206. Presland RB, Boggess D, Lewis SP, Hull C, Fleckman P, Sundberg JP. Loss of normal profilaggrin and filaggrin in flaky tail (ft/ft) mice: an animal model for the filaggrin-deficient skin disease ichthyosis vulgaris. J Invest Dermatol 2000; 115:1072–1081.
207. Fleckman P, Brumbaugh S. Absence of the granular layer and keratohyalin define a morphologically distinct subset of individuals with ichthyosis vulgaris. Exp Dermatol 2002; 11:327–336.
208. Anton-Lamprecht I, Hofbauer M. Ultrastructural distinction of autosomal dominant ichthyosis vulgaris and x-linked recessive ichthyosis. Humangenetik 1972; 15:261–264.
209. Russell LJ, DiGiovanna JJ, Rogers GR, Steinert PM, Hashem N, Compton JG, Bale SJ. Mutations in the gene for transglutaminase 1 in autosomal recessive lamellar ichthyosis. Nat Genet 1995; 9:279–283.
210. Kon A, Takeda H, Sasaki H, Yoneda K, Nomura K, Ahvazi B, Steinert PM, Hanada K, Hashimoto I. Novel transglutaminase 1 gene mutations (R348X/Y365D) in a Japanese family with lamellar ichthyosis. J Invest Dermatol 2003; 120:170–172.
211. Nemes Z, Marekov LN, Fesus L, Steinert PM. A novel function for transglutaminase 1: attachment of long-chain omega-hydroxyceramides to involucrin by ester bond formation. Proc Natl Acad Sci USA 1999; 96:8402–8407.
212. Choate KA, Kinsella TM, Williams ML, Nolan GP, Khavari PA. Transglutaminase 1 delivery to lamellar ichthyosis keratinocytes. Hum Gene Ther 1996; 7:2247–2253.
213. Lavrijsen AP, Bouwstra JA, Gooris GS, Weerheim A, Boddé HE, Ponec M. Reduced skin barrier function parallels abnormal stratum corneum lipid organization in patients with lamellar ichthyosis. J Invest Dermatol 1995; 105:619–624.
214. Grob JJ, Breton A, Bonafe JL, Sauvan-Ferdani M, Bonerandi JJ. Keratitis, ichthyosis, and deafness (KID) syndrome. Vertical transmission and death from multiple squamous cell carcinomas. Arch Dermatol 1987; 123:777–782.
215. Kim KH, Kim JS, Piao YJ, Kim YC, Shur KB, Lee JH, Park JK. Keratitis, ichthyosis and deafness syndrome with development of multiple hair follicle tumours. Br J Dermatol 2002; 147:139–143.
216. van Steensel MA, van Geel M, Nahuys M, Smitt JH, Steijlen PM. A novel connexin 26 mutation in a patient diagnosed with keratitis-ichthyosis-deafness syndrome. J Invest Dermatol 2002; 118:724–727.
217. Richard G, Rouan F, Willoughby CE, Brown N, Chung P, Ryynanen M, Jabs EW, Bale SJ, DiGiovanna JJ, Uitto J, Russell L. Missense mutations in GJB2 encoding connexin-26 cause the ectodermal dysplasia keratitis-ichthyosis-deafness syndrome. Am J Hum Genet 2002; 70:1341–1348.

218. Yotsumoto S, Hashiguchi T, Chen X, Ohtake N, Tomitaka A, Akamatsu H, Matsunaga K, Shiraishi S, Miura H, Adachi J, Kanzaki T. Novel mutations in GJB2 encoding connexin-26 in Japanese patients with keratitis-ichthyosis-deafness syndrome. Br J Dermatol 2003; 148:649–653.
219. McFadden N, Oppedal BR, Ree K, Brandtzaeg P. Erythrokeratodermia variabilis: immunohistochemical and ultrastructural studies of the epidermis. Acta Derm Venereol 1987; 67:284–288.
220. Walley AJ, Chavanas S, Moffatt MF, Esnouf RM, Ubhi B, Lawrence R, Wong K, Abecasis GR, Jones EY, Harper JI, Hovnanian A, Cookson WO. Gene polymorphism in Netherton and common atopic disease. Nat Genet 2001; 29:175–178.
221. Kato A, Fukai K, Oiso N, Hosomi N, Murakami T, Ishii M. Association of SPINK5 gene polymorphisms with atopic dermatitis in the Japanese population. Br J Dermatol 2003; 148:665–669.
222. Mevorah B, Frenk E, Brooke EM. Ichthyosis linearis circumflexa comel. A clinico-statistical approach to its relationship with Netherton's syndrome. Dermatologica 1974; 149:201–209.
223. Zina AM, Bundino S. Ichthyosis linearis circumflexa Comel.and Netherton's syndrome; an ultrastructural study. Dermatologica 1979; 158:404–412.
224. Fartasch M, Williams ML, Elias PM. Altered lamellar body secretion and stratum corneum membrane structure in Netherton syndrome: differentiation from other infantile erythrodermas and pathogenic implications. Archives Of Dermatol 1999; 135:823–832.
225. Weber F, Fuchs PG, Pfister HJ, Hintner H, Fritsch P, Hoepfl R. Human papillomavirus infection in Netherton's syndrome. Br J Dermatol 2001; 144:1044–1049.

28

Pathogenesis of Desquamation and Permeability Barrier Abnormalities in RXLI

Peter M. Elias, Debra Crumrine, Ulrich Rassner, Gopinathan K. Menon, and Kenneth R. Feingold

Department of Dermatology and Dermatology and Medical Service, University of California, San Francisco, and VAMC, San Francisco, California, U.S.A.

Mary L. Williams

Departments of Dermatology and Pediatrics, University of California, San Francisco, California, U.S.A.

THE MOLECULAR AND BIOCHEMICAL BASIS FOR RECESSIVE X-LINKED ICHTHYOSIS

In 1978, recessive X-linked ichthyosis (RXLI) was linked to deficiency of the microsomal enzyme, steroid sulfatase (SSase) (1,2). The SSase gene has been the subject of considerable research, because of its location on the distal tip of the short arm of the X chromosome (2–6). Patients with RXLI display gene mutations/deletions (7–11), resulting in ichthyosiform skin changes with occasional extracutaneous organ system involvement, due to contiguous gene syndromes (12,13).

SSase is a 62 kDa microsomal enzyme, responsible for hydrolyzing the 3β-sulfate esters from both cholesterol sulfate (CSO_4) and sulfated steroid hormones, generating their non-sulfated counterparts (14). As a result of the enzyme deficiency in RXLI, CSO_4 accumulates in skin, plasma, and red cell membranes [up to 10- to 20-fold increase (15,16)]. CSO_4 is carried in blood by the low-density (β-lipoprotein) fraction, producing diagnostic electrophoretic alterations (16,17). The fact that CSO_4 levels in skin are even higher than levels in blood presumably explains the prominence of skin involvement in RXLI (15,16,18).

To examine the regulation of epidermal CSO_4 content by SSase activity in relation to normal cohesion and desquamation, epidermal cell populations were prepared from normal and RXLI epidermis, and assayed for both SSase activity and CSO_4 content (19). Whereas SSase activity is low in the basal and spinous layers, its levels peak in the stratum granulosum (SG) (10–20 times higher), and persist at equally high levels in the stratum corneum (SC) (Fig. 1), where it is concentrated in membrane domains (19,20). In contrast, SSase activity is absent in both epidermal nucleated cell layers and the SC in RXLI (20,21). Normally, CSO_4 comprises about

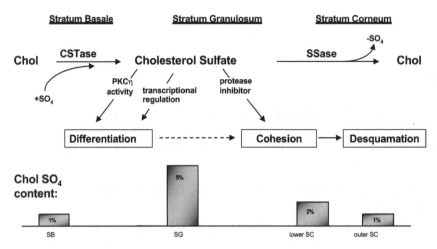

Figure 1 *Cholesterol sulfate cycle in normal epidermis.* Role of steroid sulfatase and cholesterol sulfate in normal epidermal physiology. *Abbreviations*: CSTase, cholesterol sulfotransferase; SSase, steroid sulfatase; Chol, cholesterol; PKC, protein kinase C; Chol SO_4, cholesterol
sulfate; SB, stratum basale; SG, stratum granulosum; SC, stratum corneum.

5% of the total lipid of human SG, declining to about 1% of lipid mass in the outer
SC through ongoing hydrolysis of CSO_4 during SC transit (Fig. 1). In RXLI, where
SSase activity is absent, the SC contains up to 12% CSO_4 by lipid weight ($\approx$1% of
total weight), a concentration that even exceeds that in hair, nail, and ungulate hoof,
where CSO_4 can account for 2–5% of total weight (18).

STEROID SULFATASE AND CHOLESTEROL SULFATE IN
NORMAL EPIDERMAL PHYSIOLOGY

Because cholesterol sulfotransferase activity predominates in lower nucleated cell
layers, while SSase peaks in the outer epidermis, Epstein et al. (22) proposed an
"epidermal cholesterol sulfate cycle," where cholesterol is first sulfurylated in the lower
epidermis, and then desulfated in outer epidermal layers, regenerating cholesterol
(Fig. 1). Moreover, CSO_4 levels are normally lower in the outer than in lower SC
(23,24), supporting the concept that ongoing hydrolysis of CSO_4 by SSase during
SC transit may be critical for normal desquamation (19,24). The "cholesterol sulfate
cycle," however, has a significance that extends well beyond desquamation (see below).
    Since SSase activity is reportedly not concentrated in lamellar body (LB)–
enriched fractions of whole SG (25), how the enzyme reaches membrane domains
has remained unresolved. Though it is a classic microsomal enzyme, ultrastructural
immunocytochemical studies have also localized the enzyme to the plasma membrane, where it localizes to coated pits (26,27). To address the question of SSase
delivery to SC, we developed a new cytochemical method, utilizing lead or barium
as the capture method, for the ultrastructural localization of SSase activity (20).
Using these techniques, we localized SSase not only to the cytosol (i.e., microsomes),
but also to LB contents (explaining the earlier presence of SSase in both LB and
homogenate functions). We further demonstrated the delivery of SSase to the SC
interstices following LB secretion, where its activity persists into the lower SC layers,
but disappears from the outer SC (20). Thus, like other lipid hydrolases that are

involved in the extracellular processing of secreted polar lipids (28), SSase utilizes the LB secretory system to reach sites where it participates in the regulation of barrier homeostasis and desquamation.

Like SSase, CSO_4 is concentrated in the SC interstices, but in contrast to other barrier lipid precursors, it is not concentrated in LB (25). Yet, its mode of delivery to the SC interstices can be explained readily by both its lipophilicity and its amphilicity. CSO_4, like many oxygenated sterols (but unlike cholesterol), readily diffuses across the keratinocyte plasma membrane (29). Therefore, in the absence of a lipid milieu within corneocytes, CSO_4 likely partitions preferentially to the highly hydrophobic, extracellular domains of the SC, based purely upon its solubility characteristics; i.e., it does not require delivery by a secretory organelle.

REGULATION OF DIFFERENTIATION BY CHOLESTEROL SULFATE

Sulfation of cholesterol by cholesterol sulfotransferase (SULT2B1b) is a step that is intimately linked to differentiation in keratinizing epithelia. For example, CSO_4 levels are several orders of magnitude higher in keratinizing than in mucosal epithelia, and induction of mucous metaplasia in keratinizing epithelia by application of exogenous retinoids induces a dramatic decline in CSO_4 levels. CSO_4 is known to stimulate epidermal differentiation by at least two related mechanisms (Fig. 2): (i) It activates the η isoform of protein kinase C (30), which in turn stimulates the phosphorylation of differentiation-linked proteins, assessed as increased cornified envelope (CE) formation (Fig. 2). (ii) CSO_4 is a transcriptional regulator of transglutaminase 1 (TG-1) and involucrin expression, operating through an AP-1 binding site in the promoter region (31,32). It is likely that these two mechanisms are linked as shown in Figure 2: PKC activation by CSO_4 could phosphorylate AP-1, leading to enhanced transcriptional regulation of TG-1 and involucrin. A key issue that remains unresolved, however, is whether the increased levels of

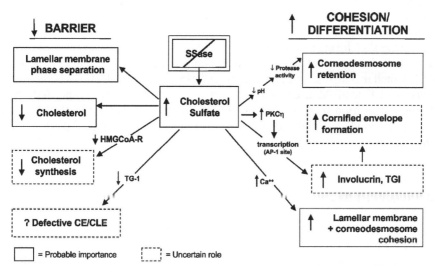

Figure 2 *Pathogenic mechanisms in RXLI. Abbreviations*: CE, cornified envelope; CLE, corneocyte-bound lipid envelope; TG-1, transglutaminase 1; HMGCoA-R, hydroxymethyl glutaryl Coenzyme A reductase (for others see legend to Fig. 1).

CSO_4 in RXLI not only cause increased corneocyte differentiation, but also whether such increased differentiation in turn provokes corneocyte retention. If operative, such a mechanism could explain the unique properties of hair, nail, and ungulate hooves, where CSO_4 levels are much higher than in normal SC ($\approx 5\%$).

MECHANISMS PROPOSED TO PERTURB PERMEABILITY BARRIER HOMEOSTASIS IN RXLI

Although patients with RXLI display only a minimal basal barrier abnormality (33), they demonstrate a pronounced delay in recovery kinetics following acute perturbations (34). Moreover, topically applied CSO_4 not only induces scaling, but also a barrier abnormality (35), lending further credence to the hypothesis that excess CSO_4 plays a destabilizing role in SC barrier function. Several mechanisms have been proposed to contribute to the barrier abnormality in RXLI (Fig. 2). First, CSO_4 fails to form eutectic mixtures with other SC lipids; hence, excess CSO_4 segregates into distinct non-lamellar domains in model lipid mixtures (=phase separation) (36). Indeed, ultrastructural images of SC in RXLI show extensive, but focal, non-lamellar domains, with disruption of the extracellular lamellae (34).

However, the barrier abnormality is probably less due to excess CSO_4 than to decreased cholesterol (the cholesterol content of the SC in RXLI is reduced by approximately 50%) (18); and decreased cholesterol alone can produce abnormal extracellular lamellar membranes (37). Two unrelated mechanisms have been invoked to explain the decrease in cholesterol in RXLI (Fig. 2): (i) Reduced generation of cholesterol from CSO_4 due to the enzyme deficiency, and (ii) CSO_4-mediated inhibition of hydroxymethyl glutaryl coenzyme A (HMGCoA) reductase, the rate-limiting enzyme of cholesterol synthesis (38). Thus, increased CSO_4 levels in RXLI could inhibit epidermal cholesterol synthesis, explaining the reduced levels of cholesterol in the SC of RXLI. Yet, topical cholesterol only partially improves clinical status and barrier function in RXLI, and it only partially reverses the barrier abnormality in CSO_4-treated mice (35), suggesting again that increased CSO_4 accounts in large part for the barrier abnormality in RXLI. Finally, CSO_4 inhibits transglutaminase 1 (TG-1)-mediated attachment of ω-hydroxyceramides to the CE in vitro, a step that forms the cornified-bound lipid envelope (CLE) (39). Together, the CE and CLE form a scaffold for the deposition and supramolecular organization of the SC lamellar bilayers, and in lamellar ichthyosis, decreased TG-1 activity leads to a defective CE scaffold, accounting in part for the barrier abnormality (40). Yet, despite the proposition that increased CSO_4 could alter the barrier in RXLI via an effect on TG-1-mediated scaffold function (39), no abnormalities of the CE/CLE scaffold have been found in RXLI.

MECHANISMS PROPOSED AS CAUSES OF ABNORMAL DESQUAMATION IN RXLI

The hyperkeratosis in RXLI is attributed to delayed desquamation rather than to excessive hyperproliferation (41). Both epidermal proliferation indices and transit times are normal, consistent with an absence of significant acanthosis in RXLI (42). Thus, RXLI is classified as a classic, retention-type ichthyosis, with delayed degradation of corneodesmosomes; i.e., these structures persist high into the SC (Fig. 2). Two key serine proteases, Kallikrein 7, the SC chymotryptic enzyme (SCCE) and Kallikrein 5, the SC tryptic enzyme (SCTE), are believed to mediate desquamation, because both can degrade corneodesmosomes in vitro (43). While the activity of these enzymes is restricted by the acidic pH of normal SC (SCCE and SCTE exhibit neutral pH optima), the pH of the SC in RXLI is lower than in normal SC (44). Hence, these serine proteases might be even less operative in RXLI than in normal SC. Although the basis for the decreased pH of SC in RXLI is not known, the negatively charged sulfate moiety could serve as a "sink" for protons generated by one or more endogenous acidifying mechanisms in SC (Fig. 2). Regardless of the mechanism, the reduced pH of SC alone could contribute to the abnormal cohesion in RXLI.

CSO_4 could also increase SC retention through its putative activity as a serine protease inhibitor (SPI). For example, CSO_4 inhibits sperm capacitation, a serine protease–catalyzed reaction [cited in Ref. 41], and it also inhibits serine protease activity in RXLI versus normal SC (20) and in vitro (45). However, the importance of CSO_4 in relation to other known SPI of the SC (e.g., elafin, secretory leukocyte protease inhibitor, or LEKTI 1) is not known.

A third, unrelated mechanism that could result in increased SC cohesion is that Ca^{++}, if present in sufficient quantities, could cross-link the highly anionic SO_4-group on adjacent lamellar bilayers (22). Indeed, CSO_4-containing liposomes aggregate avidly in the presence of calcium (46). Moreover, Ca^{++}, which is normally required for desmosome stabilization, could similarly stabilize attachments between opposing corneodesmosomes. To address this potential mechanism, we recently applied ion precipitation cytochemistry to localize Ca^{++} in RXLI versus normal SC. Whereas Ca^{++} is largely excluded from the intercellular spaces of normal SC, the lower SC in RXLI has abundant Ca^{++} in extracellular domains (20). Moreover, the Ca^{++} preferentially localizes along the external face of opposing corneodesmosomes, further suggesting a role for Ca^{++} in the increased cohesion in RXLI. Although Ca^{++} is largely excluded from normal SC, it presumably gains access to SC because of the barrier abnormality (34), i.e., barrier status regulates Ca^{++} levels in the outer epidermis (47). Thus, the delayed degradation of corneodesmosomes in RXLI correlates with increased Ca^{++} in the lower SC; and therefore, this mechanism, along with the Ca^{++} bridging of adjacent lamellar bilayers (22), could account for the increased corneocyte retention in RXLI.

In summary, RXLI is one of the best understood of all dermatological disease entities, extending from the gene to the SC intercellular spaces. Moreover, the elucidation of pathomechanisms in RXLI has led to new concepts about the normal regulation of epidermal differentiation, permeability barrier homeostasis, and cohesion/ desquamation.

REFERENCES

1. Koppe G, Marinkovic-Ilsen A, Rijken Y, De Groot WP, Jobsis AC. X-linked icthyosis A sulphatase deficiency. Arch Dis Child 1978; 53:803–806.
2. Webster D, France JT, Shapiro LJ, Weiss R. X-linked ichthyosis due to steroid-sulphatase deficiency. Lancet 1978; 1:70–72.
3. Tiepolo L, Zuffardi O, Rodewald A. Nullisomy for the distal portion of Xp in a male child with a X/Y translocation. Hum Genet 1977; 39:277–281.
4. Mohandas T, Shapiro LJ, Sparkes RS, Sparkes MC. Regional assignment of the steroid sulfatase-X-linked ichthyosis locus: implications for a noninactivated region on the short arm of human X chromosome. Proc Natl Acad Sci USA 1979; 76:5779–5783.

5. Li XM, Yen P, Mohandas T, Shapiro LJ. A long-range restriction map of the distal human X chromosome short arm around the steroid sulfatase locus. Nucleic Acids Res 1990; 18:2783–2788.

6. Shapiro LJ. Steroid sulfatase deficiency and the genetics of the short arm of the human X chromosome. Adv Hum Genet 1985; 14:331–388.

7. Ballabio A, Parenti G, Carrozzo R, Sebastio G, Andria G, Buckle V, Fraser N, Craig I, Rocchi M, Romeo G, Shapiro L. Isolation and characterization of a steroid sulfatase cDNA clone: genomic deletions in patients with X-chromosome-linked ichthyosis. Proc Natl Acad Sci USA 1987; 84:4519–4523.

8. Bonifas JM, Morley BJ, Oakey RE, Kan YW, Epstein EH Jr. Cloning of a cDNA for steroid sulfatase: frequent occurrence of gene deletions in patients with recessive X chromosome-linked ichthyosis. Proc Natl Acad Sci USA 1987; 84:9248–9251.

9. Conary JT, Lorkowski G, Schmidt B, Pohlmann R, Nagel G, Meyer HE, Krentler C, Cully J, Hasilik A, von Figura K. Genetic heterogeneity of steroid sulfatase deficiency revealed with cDNA for human steroid sulfatase. Biochem Biophys Res Commun 1987; 144:1010–1017.

10. Gillard EF, Affara NA, Yates JR, Goudie DR, Lambert J, Aitken DA, Ferguson-Smith MA. Deletion of a DNA sequence in eight of nine families with X-linked ichthyosis (steroid sulphatase deficiency). Nucleic Acids Res 1987; 15:3977–3985.

11. Shapiro LJ, Yen P, Pomerantz D, Martin E, Rolewic L, Mohandas T. Molecular studies of deletions at the human steroid sulfatase locus. Proc Natl Acad Sci USA 1989; 86:8477–8481.

12. Schmickel RD. Contiguous gene syndromes: a component of recognizable syndromes. J Pediatr 1986; 109:231–241.

13. Schnur RE, Trask BJ, van den Engh G, Punnett HH, Kistenmacher M, Tomeo MA, Naids RE, Nussbaum RL. An Xp22 microdeletion associated with ocular albinism and ichthyosis: approximation of breakpoints and estimation of deletion size by using cloned DNA probes and flow cytometry. Am J Hum Genet 1989; 45:706–720.

14. Roberts KD, Lieberman S. In: Chemical and Biological Aspects of Steroid Conjugation. New York: Springer-Verlag, 1970:219–290.

15. Bergner EA, Shapiro LJ. Metabolism of 3H-dehydroepiandrosterone sulphate by subjects with steroid sulphatase deficiency. J Inherit Metab Dis 1988; 11:403–415.

16. Epstein EH Jr, Krauss RM, Shackleton CH. X-linked ichthyosis: increased blood cholesterol sulfate and electrophoretic mobility of low-density lipoprotein. Science 1981; 214:659–660.

17. Ibsen HH, Brandrup F, Secher B. Topical cholesterol treatment of recessive X-linked ichthyosis. Lancet 1984; 2:645.

18. Williams ML, Elias PM. Stratum corneum lipids in disorders of cornification: increased cholesterol sulfate content of stratum corneum in recessive x-linked ichthyosis. J Clin Invest 1981; 68:1404–1410.

19. Elias PM, Williams ML, Maloney ME, Bonifas JA, Brown BE, Grayson S, Epstein EH Jr. Stratum corneum lipids in disorders of cornification. Steroid sulfatase and cholesterol sulfate in normal desquamation and the pathogenesis of recessive X-linked ichthyosis. J Clin Invest 1984; 74:1414–1421.

20. Elias P, Crumrine D, Rassner U, Menon GK, Mao-Qiang M, Leypoldt L, Williams ML. Basis for abnormal desquamation and barrier dysfunction in RXLI. J Invest Dermatol Sym Proc.

21. Kubilus J, Tarascio AJ, Baden HP. Steroid-sulfatase deficiency in sex-linked ichthyosis. Am J Hum Genet 1979; 31:50–53.

22. Epstein EH, Williams ML, Elias PM. The epidermal cholesterol sulfate cycle. J Am Acad Dermatol 1984; 10:866–868.

23. Long SA, Wertz PW, Strauss JS, Downing DT. Human stratum corneum polar lipids and desquamation. Arch Dermatol Res 1985; 277:284–287.

24. Ranasinghe AW, Wertz PW, Downing DT, Mackenzie IC. Lipid composition of cohesive and desquamated corneocytes from mouse ear skin. J Invest Dermatol 1986; 86:187–190.
25. Grayson S, Johnson-Winegar AG, Wintroub BU, Isseroff RR, Epstein EH Jr, Elias PM. Lamellar body-enriched fractions from neonatal mice: preparative techniques and partial characterization. J Invest Dermatol 1985; 85:289–294.
26. Willemsen R, Kroos M, Hoogeveen AT, van Dongen JM, Parenti G, van der Loos CM, Reuser AJ. Ultrastructural localization of steroid sulphatase in cultured human fibroblasts by immunocytochemistry: a comparative study with lysosomal enzymes and the mannose 6-phosphate receptor. Histochem J 1988; 20:41–51.
27. Dibbelt L, Herzog V, Kuss E. Human placental sterylsulfatase: immunocytochemical and biochemical localization. Biol Chem Hoppe Seyler 1989; 370:1093–1102.
28. Elias PM, Menon GK. Structural and lipid biochemical correlates of the epidermal permeability barrier. Adv Lipid Res 1991; 24:1–26.
29. Ponec M, Williams ML. Cholesterol sulfate uptake and outflux in cultured human keratinocytes. Arch Dermatol Res 1986; 279:32–36.
30. Denning MF, Dlugosz AA, Williams EK, Szallasi Z, Blumberg PM, Yuspa SH. Specific protein kinase C isozymes mediate the induction of keratinocyte differentiation markers by calcium. Cell Growth Differ 1995; 6:149–157.
31. Kawabe S, Ikuta T, Ohba M, Chida K, Ueda E, Yamanishi K, Kuroki T. Cholesterol sulfate activates transcription of transglutaminase 1 gene in normal human keratinocytes. J Invest Dermatol 1998; 111:1098–1102.
32. Hanley K, Wood L, Ng DC, He SS, Lau P, Moser A, Elias PM, Bikle DD, Williams ML, Feingold KR. Cholesterol sulfate stimulates involucrin transcription in keratinocytes by increasing Fra-1, Fra-2, and Jun D. J Lipid Res 2001; 42:390–398.
33. Lavrijsen AP, Oestmann E, Hermans J, Bodde HE, Vermeer BJ, Ponec M. Barrier function parameters in various keratinization disorders: transepidermal water loss and vascular response to hexyl nicotinate. Br J Dermatol 1993; 129:547–553.
34. Zettersten E, Man MQ, Sato J, Denda M, Farrell A, Ghadially R, Williams ML, Feingold KR, Elias PM. Recessive x-linked ichthyosis: role of cholesterol-sulfate accumulation in the barrier abnormality. J Invest Dermatol 1998; 111:784–790.
35. Maloney ME, Williams ML, Epstein EH Jr, Law MY, Fritsch PO, Elias PM. Lipids in the pathogenesis of ichthyosis: topical cholesterol sulfate-induced scaling in hairless mice. J Invest Dermatol 1984; 83:252–256.
36. Rehfeld SJ, Williams ML, Elias PM. Interactions of cholesterol and cholesterol sulfate with free fatty acids: possible relevance for the pathogenesis of recessive X-linked ichthyosis. Arch Dermatol Res 1986; 278:259–263.
37. Mao-Qiang M, Brown BE, Wu-Pong S, Feingold KR, Elias PM. Exogenous non-physiologic vs. physiologic lipids. Divergent mechanisms for correction of permeability barrier dysfunction. Arch Dermatol 1995; 131:809–816.
38. Williams ML, Rutherford SL, Feingold KR. Effects of cholesterol sulfate on lipid metabolism in cultured human keratinocytes and fibroblasts. J Lipid Res 1987; 28:955–967.
39. Nemes Z, Demeny M, Marekov LN, Fesus L, Steinert PM. Cholesterol 3-sulfate interferes with cornified envelope assembly by diverting transglutaminase 1 activity from the formation of cross-links and esters to the hydrolysis of glutamine. J Biol Chem 2000; 275: 2636–2646.
40. Elias PM, Schmuth M, Uchida Y, Rice RH, Behne M, Crumrine D, Feingold KR, Holleran WM, Pharm D. Basis for the permeability barrier abnormality in lamellar ichthyosis. Exp Dermatol 2002; 11:248–256.
41. Williams ML. Lipids in normal and pathological desquamation. Adv Lipid Res 1991; 24:211–262.
42. Frost P, Van Scott EJ. Ichthyosiform dermatoses. Classification based on anatomic and biometric observations. Arch Dermatol 1966; 94:113–126.

43. Ekholm IE, Brattsand M, Egelrud T. Stratum corneum tryptic enzyme in normal epidermis: a missing link in the desquamation process? J Invest Dermatol 2000; 114:56–63.

44. Ohman H, Vahlquist A. The pH gradient over the stratum corneum differs in X-linked recessive and autosomal dominant ichthyosis: a clue to the molecular origin of the "acid skin mantle?" J Invest Dermatol 1998; 111:674–677.

45. Sato J, Denda M, Nakanishi J, Nomura J, Koyama J. Cholesterol sulfate inhibits proteases that are involved in desquamation of stratum corneum. J Invest Dermatol 1998; 111:189–193.

46. Abraham W, Wertz PW, Landmann L, Downing DT. Stratum corneum lipid liposomes: calcium-induced transformation into lamellar sheets. J Invest Dermatol 1987; 88: 212–214.

47. Elias P, Ahn S, Brown B, Crumrine D, Feingold KR. Origin of the epidermal calcium gradient: regulation by barrier status and role of active vs. passive mechanisms. J Invest Dermatol 2002; 119:1269–1274.

29

Prevention and Repair of Barrier Disruption in Occupational Dermatology

Nanna Y. Schürer and Hans J. Schwanitz*
*Department of Dermatology, Environmental Medicine and Health Theory,
University of Osnabrück, Osnabrück, Germany*

INTRODUCTION

Hand dermatitis is recognized as one of the most common occupational diseases in the industrialized world (1). In occupational populations the one-year prevalence of hand dermatitis varies from 3% to 32% (2). Further epidemiological studies have identified wet-work professionals at high-risk of developing dermatitis of the hands (3). In these professions irritant contact dermatitis (ICD) results from frequent contact of the skin to irritants and humidity, and is more common than allergic contact dermatitis (ACD) (4).

Recent studies on occupational skin diseases (OSD) focus on (i) epidemiology (1,5,3), (ii) hazard identification (reviewed in Refs. 6 and 7), (iii) mechanisms of ICD (reviewed in Ref. 8), (iv) sensitization to work-related allergens (reviewed in Ref. 9), (v) mechanisms of ACD (reviewed in Ref. 10), and (vi) its prevention (reviewed in Ref. 11).

Despite the known fact that ICD of the human hand is more common than ACD and ICD follows barrier disruption (12,13), studies on the skin of the human hand, its specific anatomy, physiology, and epidermal barrier function are scarce. A recent study concentrates on the prevalence of hand dermatitis with respect to changes of exogenous work-related influences and genetic disposition (14). Trying to evaluate studies on the prevention of OSD with respect to epidermal barrier function, we must realize that

1. most biochemical studies on epidermal barrier function have been performed in murine and/or pig skin (15),
2. most studies on human skin physiology have been performed on the lower arm and not on the hand (see also Ref. 16),
3. barrier function differs between anatomical sites (17–19),
4. more than 90% of OSDs are hand dermatitis (3).

---

* Deceased.

Therefore, an evaluation of the present literature on epidermal barrier function with respect to OSD of the human hand remains hypothetical until studies address the above-mentioned needs.

Practical Aspects

So far at least in Germany, individuals suffering from hand dermatitis seek help at the dermatologist's office. If OSD is recognized, the dermatologist will inform the employers' liability insurance company in charge. In 2002 more than 18,000 initial reports of OSD were recorded [Hauptverband Berufsgenossenschaften (HVBG) "head of employers' liability insurance company," personal communication]. Over 90% of OSDs were indeed hand dermatitis (3). Treatments employing external corticosteroids are usually conducted in this outpatient setting. A study on 296 inpatients referred for tertiary prevention revealed that 40% used topical corticosteroids regularly for over one year prior to admission (Skudlik and Schwanitz, submitted 2004). This therapy may lead to an initial relief from symptoms; however, once the epidermal barrier is perturbed, modern work-leave does not allow sufficient time for corticosteroid-free barrier repair. Hence, inflammatory signs are only suppressed, and flare up reactions after steroid withdrawal required extensive measures of tertiary prevention in 30% of these 296 inpatients. However, if preventive measures are not employed, the consequence may be unemployment and early retirement. To counteract this unfortunate development, preventive measures in agreement with the WHO's definition of health promotion have been employed successfully (11).

Measurements of Prevention

While primary prevention is aimed at health maintenance, secondary prevention interferes with initial skin changes, with the intention to enable employees to remain employed, and tertiary prevention focuses on optimized rehabilitation of individuals suffering from long-term severe OSD. Studies on the prevention of OSD have been performed on an interdisciplinary and integrative level. These measures include:

1. correct diagnosis of the dermatological disorder,
2. early individualized preventive and therapeutic interventions,
3. altered individual behavior, i.e., increased self-determination and autonomy,
4. changes in work conditions,
5. social responsibilities of affected individuals.

Early individualized preventive and therapeutic interventions include:

1. elimination of irritants and/or allergens,
2. use of protective measures, i.e. gloves, barrier creams, skin care, and skin hardening,
3. therapy,
4. workers' education towards a health-conscious attitude (20).

These interventions led to a significant decrease in OSD among the hairdressers of Germany (11). Therefore, the German employers' liability insurance company for health and welfare (Berufsgenossenschaft für Gesundheitsdienst und Wohlfahrtspflege— BGW) has expressed increased interest in pursuing and supporting these strategies. Moreover, an interest in the integrity of the epidermal barrier has evolved in occupational dermatologists.

Table 1 Occurrence of OSD in Hairdressers' Trainees

Year	Number of trainees contacted	Response rate (*n*)	Response rate (%)	Manifestation of initial skin changes (%)	Seeking dermatological help (%)
1989	8256	4008	48.5	72	16
1994	4967	2505	50.8	58	48
1999	3741	2427	64.9	61	29

Initiation of the Program

The initial question in 1988 at the University of Osnabrück, Germany was: "How frequent is ICD in wet-work–related professions?" Questionnaires, addressing the incidence of OSDs in hairdresser trainees, were documented at five-year intervals in Lower Saxony, Germany (11). These questionnaires were sent out to hairdressers' training schools in 1989, 1994, and 1999 (Table 1).

In 1989 primary and secondary prevention of OSD was not established in the hairdressing profession. Seminars on skin care and protection were not conducted till then. Hairdressers had almost no knowledge of the skin's anatomy and, in particular, of the epidermal barrier function. Eighty percent of trainees used protective gloves only when hair colors were applied. Seventy percent of trainees noted changes of skin condition over their three-year training (Table 2), of which xerosis was the most frequent (21). Twenty percent of trainees were prepared to give up their training due to skin changes.

Five years of intervention and seminars on skin physiology, care, and protection revealed in 1994 a decrease in skin changes and an increase in seeking dermatological help (Table 1). This was achieved by the cooperation of hairdresser employers, BGW, training schools and the University of Osnabrück. Compared to 1994 fewer trainees consulted a dermatologist in 1999.

First we describe strategies of primary, secondary, and tertiary prevention with respect to the function and condition of the epidermal barrier, perturbation, and repair.

PRIMARY INDIVIDUAL PREVENTION

In 1992 (*n* = 2352) first year apprentices were examined by a dermatologist, involving 15 training schools in Northwest Germany (22). These trainees were interviewed

Table 2 Skin Changes of Hairdresser Trainees According to the 1989 Questionnaire in Lower Saxony, Germany

	Total *n* = 2813 (%)	Freshmen *n* = 1061 (%)	Junior *n* = 1028 (%)	Senior *n* = 724 (%)
Xerosis	85	86	91	75
Erythema	36	43	38	24
Scaling	17	22	16	12
Itch	43	50	41	37
Palmar hyperhidrosis	22	7	29	36

Table 3 Prospective Study of the Prevalence of Skin Changes and Hand Dermatitis in Hairdressers Trainees

Number of examination/year of training	Trainees examined (n)	Skin changes (%)	Hand dermatitis (%)
1	2352	36	13
2	1717	47	23
3	1134	55	24

about their history of atopy and intolerances as well as present forms of skin protection: Within the first six weeks of the training program 844 apprentices revealed skin changes of their hands (36%). Of these subjects, 679 suffered interdigital dermatitis (80% of 844). The prospective study continued. Prior to the second year a dermatologist examined 1717 of 2352 apprentices. After the third year of the training program 1134 apprentices could be retrieved and examined (Table 3).

Dermatological findings and standardized interviews revealed that the prevalence of OSD is influenced by

1. positive history of flexural eczema (OR 1.97),
2. optimized skin protection (OR 0.49).

Individuals with a history of atopic dermatitis appear to have an increased TEWL and enhanced sensitivity to irritants (23). However, one-fourth of atopic individuals do not experience problems even upon highly irritant exposures (24). The benefit of skin protection was comparable for non-atopics (48% without skin changes, OR 0.49) and atopics (38% without skin changes, OR 0.52). Therefore it was concluded that:

1. a positive history of flexural eczema is a risk factor for barrier perturbation and ICD,
2. unprotected wet work is a greater risk factor for barrier perturbation,
3. skin protection as a measure of primary individual prevention (PIP) is effective in both groups (5).

Skin Protection via Occlusion

In mice occlusive treatment of irritated skin results in a delay in barrier repair as reflected by TEWL-measurements (25). For wet-work professionals the use of protective and occlusive gloves is recommended. Clinical observations reflect the benefit of occlusive gloves as a measure of PIP. However, occlusion might interfere with barrier repair, if gloves are worn on irritated skin and potentially corticosteroid-treated skin. One controlled clinical study demonstrated the effect of occlusion on barrier repair of Sodium lauryl sulfate (SLS)-irritated or tape-stripped human skin on the lower arm (26). Experimental SLS irritation and tape stripping led to an increased TEWL, as a sign of barrier perturbation, followed by a TEWL decrease, as a sign of barrier repair, over the following days. Occlusion did not delay barrier repair of SLS-irritated skin, but it did delay recovery of tape-stripped skin. Further studies on the skin of the human hand are required to reveal whether occlusive membranes interfere with barrier repair in that area.

Skin Hardening

The hardening phenomenon has been ascribed to individuals subjected to repeated low-dose chemical (27) or physical irritation (28,29). While the stratum corneum thickness increases after repetitive UVB-irradiation (28), the mechanisms of chemical-induced hardening are speculative. Repeated SLS-irritations over a three-week irritation phase lead to an adaptation of irritation and initially increased TEWL (30). For this study SLS was chosen among other irritants because of its ability to penetrate and to impair the epidermal barrier. For quantification of SLS-induced barrier damage, TEWL measurements were found to be the most sensitive method. Furthermore, the SLS-induced hardening phenomenon was not restricted to the irritated area, but was measurable also on the contralateral site of irritation. The hardening phenomenon, which has been described as early as in 1967 (31), has been poorly studied with respect to OSDs so far (32). An increase of stratum corneum thickness, change of epidermal lipid content and composition, as well as "work-/irritant-specific" adaptation of barrier protection and repair mechanisms remain to be demonstrated for the human hand.

Hyper-Reactivity of the Skin

Atopic Disposition

Atopic disposition is a significant risk factor for developing skin changes in wet-work professions (14,33). In fact, 37% of OSD, within 24 occupational groups at high risk for developing OSD, present with an atopic skin diathesis (4). Further, TEWL values are increased at uninvolved sites in atopics, prone to develop skin changes (34). Therefore, PIP may require identification of atopic employees and/or optimized skin protection. A controlled prospective study of PIP in hairdresser trainees was performed at the University of Osnabrück, Germany (34). Seventy-three apprentices participated in a program of PIP (Tables 4 and 5) during their three-year apprenticeship, while 112 trainees remained untrained in this regard (control group, CG). To change an established behavior, consecutive interventions took place. At primary consultation, an intensive health pedagogic interview, as well as dermatological examination was conducted; theoretical and practical seminars concentrating on work-related disorders were also offered (Table 4). Participants gained practical experience about what they had theoretically learned.

At the beginning of their training the incidence and severity of skin changes were comparable in both groups. At the end of the three-year prospective study significant changes evolved: 80% of the trainees participating in PIP had no skin

Table 4 Program of PIP in Hairdressers' Trainees

Measures of primary prevention	Over a 3-year training period
Dermatologist examination	4 times
Seminars held by health educationalists (total of 15 hrs lesson on skin care management)	6 times
Supply of necessary skin care products	Continuous
Consultation concerning work environment	Upon demand
Knowledge of skin care management	6 times

Table 5 Controlled (CG) Prospective Study of PIP in Hairdressers'
Trainees Conducted between 1992 and 1996

	Intervention group (PIP) ($n=73$)	Control group (CG) ($n=112$)
Results in 1996	$n=41$	$n=56$
Skin change	7 (20%)	19 (35%)
Severity		
Mild	7 (20%)	11 (20%)
Moderate	0	7 (12%)
Severe	0	1 (2%)

changes, while 65% of CG were free of symptoms ($p < 0.05$). Of those affected,
20% of PIP and CG revealed mild hand dermatitis. However, moderate and severe
skin changes occurred only in the CG (12% and 2%) (Table 5). Ten percent of the
CG and none of the PIPs had to resign from work due to OSD.

This controlled study revealed that PIP of OSD is effective. Even though little
is yet known about the specificity of the epidermal barrier on the hand (see above),
this clinical study demonstrates that the resultant use of barrier creams and occlusive
gloves *prior* to occupation-related barrier disruption decreases the incidence of ICD
significantly.

Interdigital Contact Dermatitis

ICD occurred in 36% of 2352 examined hairdresser apprentices, and was initiated in
80% of cases in the interdigital space (IDS) (36). Interdigital contact dermatitis can
be regarded as a potential precursor of more severe hand dermatitis in hairdressers,
and probably ICD in wet-work occupations. For ethical reasons and practicability,
ΔTEWL measurements have not yet been performed on IDS, even though this would
seem to be a marker for barrier perturbation and ICD. However, on normal
volunteers baseline TEWL measurements of the IDS revealed 3-fold higher values
compared to data obtained from DAH (37). The high incidence of ICD within
the IDS led to skin physiological examinations with respect to the anatomy of the
epidermal barrier of the human hand.

Differential Irritation Test

According to most guidelines on non-invasive measurements of human skin
physiology, the TEWL is analyzed on the ventral aspect of the lower arm (VALA)
(Pinnagoda, 1990). However, with respect to OSD, data should be retrieved from
the hand, because the anatomy of the human hand differs significantly, revealing
(i) a thick SC, numerous sweat glands, and absence of sebaceous glands on the palmar surface (38,39), (ii) a thin SC and presence of both types of glands on the back of
the hand; and (iii) a newly recognized area of human skin physiology, i.e., the IDS.
These rough anatomical differences of skin surface lipids and barrier structure must
be respected when studying skin physiology of the human hand in the future.

So far, TEWL measurements were performed on the dorsal aspect of the hand
(DAH) and compared to data obtained from VALA. Two hundred thirty-seven individuals with a positive history of OSD participated in this study at the University of

Osnabrück (40). ΔTEWL measurements, employing irritation with 0.5 N NaOH for 2 × 10 minutes, distinguished atopics from non-atopics with a specificity and sensitivity of 75%. Clinical findings and increased ΔTEWL measurements after irritation on DAH reflects occupationally induced barrier perturbation, while on the VALA, a genetic-disposed irritability. Furthermore, this differential irritation test (DIT) was also employed on 237 wet-work professionals with cleared skin changes. Out of these workers, in 10% of cases ($n = 23$) a hyper-reactivity of the epidermal barrier of DAH was found, indicated by a high ΔTEWL and clinically obvious skin changes (erythema, vesicles, edema) after DIT. These as yet unpublished findings led to the conclusion that a small group of "hyper-reactors," i.e., patients with a positive history of an ex–barrier-damaging profession and consecutive unemployment and/or retirement, demonstrates long-term barrier hyper-reactivity on DAH, i.e., acquired hyper-irritability. These profound clinical differences must be addressed in future studies of the metabolic basis for epidermal barrier function on various aspects of the human hand.

Percutaneous Absorption

Understanding OSD and initial ICD, "percutaneous absorption" of a given irritant must also be taken into consideration (6). When a substance contacts the skin surface, the proportion penetrating into the viable epidermis will depend on:

1. the area of the skin contacted,
2. the duration and frequency of contact,
3. the chemical properties of the substance,
4. the vehicle,
5. the epidermal barrier function.

The barrier to penetration is located in the SC. Barrier disruption, as it occurs in OSD, increases the permeability of a given foreign substance. Absorption across the SC is believed to occur by passive diffusion. Hydration of the SC increases its permeability. The mechanism by which water elicits this change is not known, nor is the relationship between permeability and the extent of overhydration. After four hours of water exposure to VALA the SC expands up to three-fold (41). Further, intercellular water pools with disrupted lamellar delamination were detected (42). Corneosome degradation is known to be a function of the water content of the SC (42,43). Consequently, prolonged water contact, i.e., four hours (defined as 50% of one wet-work shift) facilitates the development of ICD (44). Moreover, these changes predominantly start in the IDS, where possible partial occlusion of the SC barrier differs from that of palms, DAH, and VALA. Once again the anatomical and physiological differences of the hand must be considered with respect to occupational-related percutaneous absorption.

Further, soaps and detergents facilitate penetration. Health care professionals repeatedly wash and disinfect their hands as required for hygienic reasons. Numerous studies have evaluated the effectiveness of different hand decontamination measures. However, the interaction between underlying skin condition and antimicrobial efficacy is rarely assessed. In practice, the issues of hygiene, disinfection, skin care, and protection are rarely studied at once. A clinical study on the skin tolerance of an alcohol-based disinfectant and a non-antiseptic soap for hand disinfection revealed better tolerability and effectiveness of the alcohol-based disinfectant (45). Further clinical and bioengineering studies are required to address this issue.

Palmar Hyperhidrosis

Epidemiologic studies revealed an increase of palmar hyperhidrosis in hairdresser trainees (21). Those who complained about an increased sweating of the palmar surface of the hand were 7% of freshmen, 29% of junior, and 36% of senior hairdresser trainees (Table 2). Further, dermatologic examination of 296 inpatients for tertiary prevention revealed palmar hyperhidrosis in 41% of cases (46). Moreover, of all hairdressers with severe OSD ($n = 58$), palmar hyperhidrosis was most frequent (62%). Hyperhidrosis seems to be a reaction of the numerous palmar eccrine sweat glands to exogenous repetitive chemical damages. This reaction seems to be enhanced when occlusive gloves are worn for several hours daily, followed possibly by barrier disturbances. Once palmar hyperhidrosis is induced, the long-term use of occlusive gloves for PIP might propagate the barrier perturbation—possibly due to hydration effects—and consequent ICD (see above), or even atopic palmar eczema (47). This interesting clinical observation requires further work-up, employing skin physiological and biochemical methods on the hand.

Relevance of an Acid Skin pH

A solution that increases the skin's pH not only results in ionization of a weak acid or base, which might penetrate more easily in its non-ionized form (6), but also perturbs epidermal barrier function (48). Recent achieved studies have demonstrated that a pH of 4.5–5.5 is required for optimal barrier function and restoration (49,50). However, these findings about epidermal physiology have not yet been included within strategies of PIP of OSD, or with respect to anatomical differences on the hand.

Epidermal Calcium Gradient

Murine and human studies have demonstrated the importance of the epidermal calcium gradient for proper barrier function (51). Disturbance of the calcium gradient leads to barrier perturbation (52). As damage accumulates, penetration of a given irritant can increase, and inflammation can develop (51,53). Although these important findings have not yet been extended to studies on the barrier function of the hand with respect to anatomical differences, i.e., DAH versus palmar surface versus IDS, especially for wet-work professionals an evaluation of the calcium gradient might be important, considering that the hand contacts numerous foreign substances with possible calcium-chelating properties.

Antioxidant

The skin of the dorsum of the hand (and the face) is directly exposed to a pro-oxidative environment. With respect to OSD, the hands also directly contact pro-oxidative substances, depending on the profession of the individual. The induction of oxidative damage by environmental stimuli, such as UV-light and ozone, was demonstrated to occur in lipids (54), proteins (55), and DNA (56) of mouse skin. To counteract these harmful effects, the skin is equipped with an antioxidant system that maintains an equilibrium between pro-oxidants and antioxidants (see Chapter 23). Vitamins E and C are such antioxidants, which must be supplied (systemically or topically), and are not synthesized by humans. Photoprotective effects of topically applied antioxidants have been demonstrated in mouse and human skin (57). Since skin damage of the hand is not solely dependent on photodamage, the protective effect of topical antioxidants against occupationally induced oxidative stress remains to be analyzed, once again with respect to the particular physiology of the epidermal barrier in that area.

Health Education

An understanding of epidermal function has already been successfully given to wet-work professionals, employing health educationalist skills (20). The education of employees towards a health-conscious attitude enables endangered individuals to continue to work with healthy hands in a hazardous occupational environment. It still remains to be determined whether protective, and therefore occlusive, gloves should be worn after (i) the skin contacts a given irritant, solvent, and/or detergent; (ii) perturbations of the epidermal calcium gradient, (iii) increased skin pH; and (iv) treatments with halogenated corticosteroids. Depending on the scientific data obtained, knowledge then needs to be transferred to the employee by health education.

In conclusion, the skin surface seems to be able to react to xenobiotics, irritants, and/or other exogenous substances in two main ways: (1) directly via barrier disruption, ICD and eventually barrier repair; and (2) indirectly, via an accommodation to long-term irritation, i.e., (i) an increased palmar hyperhidrosis, (ii) hypo-reactivity (hardening effect), or (iii) hyper-reactivity (acquired hyperirritability). In this context not only PIP, but also secondary prevention of ICD is required to prevent subsequent ACD.

SECONDARY INDIVIDUAL PREVENTION

The aim of secondary individual prevention (SIP) is to enable affected individuals to

1. remain employed,
2. reduce existing skin lesions, and eventually,
3. enable barrier repair.

A study on SIP of hand dermatitis in geriatric nurses (GNs) was conducted between 2000 and 2002. Inclusion criteria were employment and a positive history of OSD, reported by the dermatologist to the insurance company in charge. Two hundred and nine GNs with a history of hand dermatitis participated. Of these, 102 GNs volunteered for SIP and 107 participated in the control group (CG). For the CG participants there was no health educational intervention. Upon entry, 70% of the SIP and CG groups complained of hand dermatitis, and 90% of SIP hand dermatitis was diagnosed at the first dermatologist visit; yet after a training course of six months, including three more visits, hand dermatitis was diagnosed in only 40% of cases (Fig. 1).

Educative intervention, employing hands-on training in the correct use of appropriate protective gloves, barrier creams, and skin care was helpful in SIP. Altered barrier function affects the ability of an irritant to penetrate the SC, and produces deleterious effects on both SC and epidermis. Moreover, a damaged epidermis can be expected to produce a defective SC, thus resulting in a vicious cycle. High basal TEWL is not associated with skin symptoms and barrier impairment occurring during wet work, as evaluated in a follow-up study in baker and confectioner

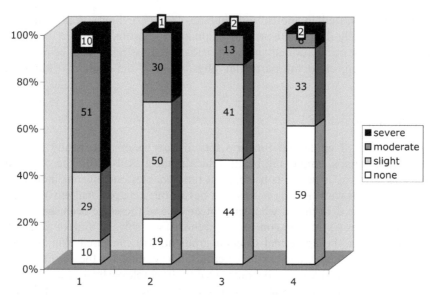

Figure 1   Severity of hand dermatitis upon clinical examination of SIP participants. The severity of hand dermatitis was documented at the start of a six-month intervention period (Column 1, $n = 102$), at the time of the first seminar, i.e., one month later (Column 2, $n = 94$), at the time of the voluntary consultation, i.e., three to four months later (Column 3, $n = 66$), and at the final visit, i.e., after six months (Column 4, $n = 102$).

apprentices (58). However, ΔTEWL values indicated the degree of irritability to the skin surface at a given point in time. Therefore, in this study TEWL measurements were taken before and after irritant challenge with 0.5 N NaOH on DAH upon each visit.

Studies on skin barrier function recovery in humans after mechanical irritation have found slow recovery rates (59,60). Here, repeated ΔTEWL measurements on DAH at more than monthly intervals seemed reasonable, considering the human skin's physiological epidermal turnover of about one month. SIP in GNs has a significant positive effect on sub-clinical skin changes assessed by ΔTEWL, these values being significantly higher initially than in subsequent visits (Fig. 2).

These findings are particularly important for those participants ($n = 10$) who entered the program without clinical skin manifestations due to prior long-term applications of halogenated corticosteroids. The lack of clinical manifestations may lead to the assumption that neither educational nor medical intervention is required. However, high ΔTEWL values will detect impaired barrier function in that group of long-term corticosteroid users, despite absence of skin changes (unpublished observations). Although the long-term use of corticosteroids may prevent inflammatory skin changes, barrier function is abnormal due to a depletion of intercellular lipid lamellae (61). Recently, the negative impact of short-term clobetasol treatment on epidermal barrier, including lipid-depletion, was shown in murine skin (62). For SIP in GNs, dermatological therapies have recommended against the long-term use of halogenated corticosteroids on the hands, whenever possible; and focused instead on the correct use of barrier creams and skin care ointments. Follow-up studies are planned to evaluate the employment rate in this professional subgroup.

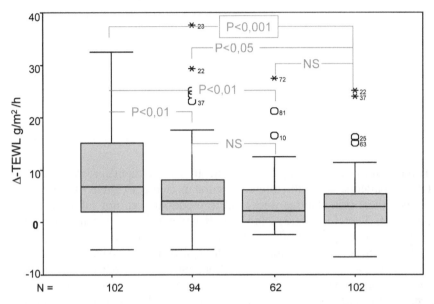

Figure 2 Boxplots represent the median of TEWL prior and subsequent to skin irritation with 0.5 N NaOH for 10 minutes on DAH of SIP participants [visit 1 (inclusion criteria) $n = 102$, visit 2 (first seminar) $n = 94$, visit 3 (optional visit) $n = 62$, and visit 4 (final seminar) $n = 102$ participants].

Another study addressed the question, of whether health education demonstrates a long-term benefit in SIP of ICD. A prospective controlled SIP study was performed with hairdresser trainees between 1994 and 1996. Five years later, i.e., in 2001, 172 of 215 contacted SIP and 55 of 85 contacted CG reported on their employment and skin condition. At that time 29% of the CG and 69% of SIP were still employed. Unemployment in the SIP group was in 30% of cases due to skin changes and that in the CG was in 41% of cases. From this long-term cohort study, we can infer that education provides long-term benefits for the proper care of the skin surface, and therefore of the epidermal barrier (63).

TERTIARY INDIVIDUAL PREVENTION

Tertiary individual prevention (TIP) focuses on the optimized rehabilitation and maintenance of the individual's employment. These individuals are treated for two to three weeks as inpatients, because outpatient treatments had been unsuccessful. At the University of Osnabrück the inpatient treatment course is usually followed by another three-week period of work leave and outpatient care. The total of a minimum six-week work leave is based on the finding that the perturbed barrier in humans requires a minimum of four weeks for restitution (64). During the inpatient period, primarily corticosteroid-free treatment, one-on-one consultations and seminars concentrate on skin protection, and work-relevant situations are targeted, i.e., handling of specific situations with preventive strategies. On an interdisciplinary level dermatologists, specialists for occupational medicine, ergotherapeutics, cosmeticians, health education, and psychologists are involved. The effects of such interventions are determined via interviewing the patient, the dermatologist in charge,

Table 6 Questionnaires One Year after an Inpatient Treatment Course at the University of Osnabrück

Number of questionnaires (n)	Response rate (n)	Remain employed (%)	Job change due to OSD (%)	Job change due to other circumstances (%)
490	352	66	23	11

and the relevant insurance company one year after the patient's hospital admission (65). Of 352 patients, 232 still suffered from skin changes (Table 6). However, in 72% of cases these skin changes were mild to moderate, i.e., not sufficient to cause unemployment. Therefore, of 352 individuals endangered to become unemployed due to OSD, tertiary prevention was effective in two-thirds of cases.

These findings reflect the ability of the epidermis to repair itself, even after long-term irritation and barrier perturbation, and it also reflects the ability to continue to work in a hazardous occupational environment, if one employs skin protective measures, despite ongoing minor to moderate skin changes, and therefore, most likely an unresolved barrier perturbation.

As a consequence of these studies in Osnabrück, clinical and epidemiologic studies reveal the success of PIP, SIP, and TIP interventions in professionals working in a hazardous environment. With respect to the prevention of OSD, as well as barrier perturbation and repair, TIP and SIP are more challenging than PIP.

1. Prior to SIP- and TIP-measures, skin changes are present, primarily on the hand, preferably in the IDS.
2. Before SIP- and TIP-measures are employed, perturbation of the epidermal barrier has already occurred.
3. For SIP and TIP skin protection—and barrier occlusion—is initiated after barrier perturbation.
4. SIP- and TIP-measures balance between employment, usually in a barrier hazardous environment, and barrier perturbation and repair.

Focusing on the prevention of OSD with respect to epidermal barrier function of the hand, we realize that health education has shown important clinical benefits within the last 15 years. However, to understand, and therefore to further improve measures of prevention of OSD, bioengineering and biochemical studies on epidermal barrier function of the hand are urgently required.

REFERENCES

1. Diepgen TL, Coenraads PJ. The epidemiology of occupational contact dermatitis. In: Kanerva L, Elsner P, Wahlberg JE, Maibach HI, eds. Handbook of Occupational Dermatology. 1st ed. Berlin, Heidelberg, New York: Springer-Verlag, 2000:3–16.
2. Sustitaival P, Flyholm MA, Meding B, Kanerva L, Lindberg M, Svensson A, Ólafs JH. Nordic occupational skin questionnaire (NOSQ-2002): a new tool for surveying occupational skin disease and exposure, 2003.
3. Dickel H, Kuss O, Blesius CR, Schmidt A, Diepgen TL. Occupational skin diseases in northern Bavaria between 1990 and 1999: a population-based study. Br J Dermatol 2001; 145:453–462.

4. Dickel H, Bruckner TM, Schmidt A, Diepgen TL. Impact of atopic skin disease on occupational skin diseases: incidence in a working population. J Invest Dermatol 2003; 121:37–40.

5. Uter W, Pfahlberg A, Gefeller O, Schwanitz HJ. Hand dermatitis in a prospectively-followed cohort of hairdressing apprentices: final results of the POSH study. Prevention of occupational skin disease in hairdressers. Contact Dermat 1999:280–286.

6. Emmett EA. Occupational contact dermatitis II: risk assessment and prognosis. Am J Contact Dermat 2003; 14:21–30.

7. Drexler H. Skin protection and percutaneous absorption of chemical hazards. Int Arch Occup Environ Health 2003; 76:359–361.

8. Chew AL, Maibach HI. Occupational issues of irritant contact dermatitis. Int Arch Occup Environ Health 2003; 76:339–346.

9. Andersen KE. Occupational issues of allergic contact dermatitis. Int Arch Occup Environ Health 2003; 76:347–351.

10. Enk AH, Knop J. T cell receptor mimic peptides and their potential application in T-cell-mediated disease. Int Arch Allergy Immunol 2000; 123:275–281.

11. Schwanitz HJ, Riehl U, Schlesinger T, Bock M, Skudlik C, Wulfhorst B. Skin care management: educational aspects. Int Arch Occup Environ Health 2003; 76:374–381.

12. Nickoloff BJ, Naidu Y. Pertubation of epidermal barrier function correlates with irritation of cytokine cascade in human skin. J Am Acad Dermatol 1994; 30:535–546.

13. Tur E, Eshkol Z, Breener S, Maibach HI. Cumulative effect of subthreshold concentrations of irritants in humans. Am J Contact Dermat 1995; 6:216–220.

14. Meding B, Järvholm. Hand eczema in Swedish adults—changes in prevalence between 1983 and 1996. J Invest Dermatol 2002; 118:719–723.

15. Elias PM, Feingold KR. Coordinate regulation of epidermal differentiation and barrier homeostasis. Skin Pharmacol Appl Skin Physiol 2001; 14:28–34.

16. Coenraads PJ, Diepgen TL. Problems with trials and intervention studies on barrier creams and emollients at the workplace. Int Arch Occup Environ Health 2003; 76:362–366.

17. Lampe MA, Burlingame AL, Whitney J, Williams ML, Brown BE, Roitman E, Elias PM. Human stratum corneum lipids: characterization and regional variations. J Lipid Res 1983; 24:120–130.

18. Greene RS, Downing DT, Pochi PE, Strauss JS. Anatomical variation in the amount and composition of human skin surface. J Invest Dermatol 1970; 54:240–247.

19. Schwindt DA, Wilhelm KP, Maibach HI. Water diffusion characteristics of human stratum corneum at different anatomical sites in vivo. J Invest Dermatol 1998; 111:385–389.

20. Schwanitz HJ, Wulfhorst B. Workers' education. In: Kanerva L, Elsner P, Wahlberg JE, Maibach HI, eds. Handbook of Occupational Dermatology. 1st ed. Berlin, Heidelberg. New York: Springer-Verlag, 2000:441–443.

21. Budde U, Schwanitz HJ. Kontaktdermatitiden bei auszubildenden des friseurhandwerks in niedersachsen. Dermatosen 1991; 39:41–48.

22. Uter W, Gefeller O, Schwanitz HJ. Occupational dermatitis in hairdressing apprentices: early onset irritant skin damage. In: Elsner P, Maibach HI, eds. Irritant Dermatitis, New Clinical and Experimental Aspects. Basel, Switzerland: Karger, 1995:49–55.

23. Agner T, Serup J. Sodium lauryl sulfate for irritant patch testing: a dose response study using bioengineering methods for determining skin irritation. J Invest Dermatol 1995; 95:543–547.

24. Rystedt I. Hand eczema and long.term prognosis in atopic dermatitis. Acta Derm Venereol Suppl 1985; 117:1–59.

25. Grubauer G, Elias PM, Feingold KR. Transepidermal water loss: the signal for recovery of barrier structure and function. J Lipid Res 1989; 30:323–333.

26. Welzel J, Wilhelm KP, Wolff HH. Skin permeability barrier and occlusion: no delay of repair in irritated human skin. Contact Dermat 1996; 35:163–168.

27. Widmer J, Elsner P, Burg G. Skin irritant reactivity following experimental cumulative irritant contact dermatitis. Contact Dermat 1994; 30:35–39.

28. Lehmann P, Hölzle E, Plewig G. Effects of ultraviolet A and B on the skin barrier: a functional, electron microscopic and lipid biochemical study. Photodermatol Photoimmunol Photomed 1991; 8:129–134.
29. Pearse AD, Gaskell SA, Marks R. Epidermal changes in human skin following irradiation with either UVB or UVB. J Invest Dermatol 1987; 88:83–87.
30. Wulfhorst B. Skin hardening in occupational dermatology. In: Kanerva L, Elsner P, Wahlberg JE, Maibach HI, eds. Handbook of Occupational Dermatology. 1st ed. Berlin, Heidelberg, New York: Springer-Verlag, 2000:115–121.
31. McOsker DE, Beck LW. Characteristics of accommodated (hardened) skin. J Invest Dermatol 1967; 48(4):372–383.
32. Seidenari S. Evaluation of barrier function and skin reactivity of occupational dermatoses. In: Kanerva L, Elsner P, Wahlberg JE, Maibach HI, eds. Handbook of Occupational Dermatology. 1st ed. Berlin, Heidelberg, New York: Springer-Verlag, 2000:64–75.
33. Tacke J, Schmidt A, Fartasch M, Diepgen TL. Occupational contact dermatitis in bakers, confectioners and cooks. A population-based study. Contact Dermat 1995; 33:112–117.
34. Seidenari S, Giusti G. Objective assessment of the skin of children affected by atopic dermatitis: a study of pH, capacitance and TEWL in eczematous and clinically uninvolved skin. Acta Derm Venereol 1995; 75:429–433.
35. Rhiel U. Interventionsstudie zur Prävention von Hauterkrankungen bei Auszubildenden des Friseurhandwerks. Universitätsverlag Rasch Osnabrück, 2001.
36. Schwanitz JH, Uter W. Interdigital dermatitis: sentinel skin changes in hairdressers. Br J Dermatol 2000; 142:1011–1012.
37. Bock M. Topographische unterschiede hauphysiologischer parameter an den Händen (Abstr.) Allergologic 1997; 20:427
38. Benfenati A, Brillanti F. Sulla distribuzione delle ghiandole sebacee nelle cute del corpo umano. Arch Ital Dermatol 1939; 15:33.
39. Sato K, Dobson RL. Regional and individual variations in the function of the human eccrine sweat gland. J Invest Dermatol 1970; 54:443.
40. John SM, Schwanitz HJ. Evidence for the phenomenon of aquired cutaneous hyperirritability after previous eczema. Skin Res Technol 2003; 9:179.
41. Warner RR, Boissy YL, Lilly NA, Spears MJ, McKillop K, Marshall JL, Stone KJ. Water disrupts stratum corneum lipid lamellae: damage is similar to surfactants. J Invest Dermatol 1999; 113:960–966.
42. Warner RR, Stone KJ, Boissy YL. Hydration disrupts human stratum corneum ultrastructure. J Invest Dermatol 2003; 120:275–284.
43. Rawlings AV, Scott IR, Harding CG, Bowser PA. Stratum corneum moisturizing at the molecular level. J Invest Dermatol 1994:731–740.
44. Meding B. Differences between the sexes with regard to work-related skin disease. Contact Dermat 2000; 43:65–71.
45. Winnefled D, Richard MA, Drancourt M, Grob JJ. Skin tolerance and effectiveness of two hand decontamination procedures in everyday hospital use. Br J Dermatol 2000; 143:546–550.
46. Skudlik C, Schwanitz HJ. Tertiary prevention of occupational dermatoses. JDDG (submitted), 2003.
47. Schwanitz HJ. The Atopic Palmoplantar Eczema. Heidelberg, Berlin, Tokio, New York: Springer, 1988.
48. Mauro T, Grayson S, Gao WN, Mao-Qiang M, Kriehuber E, Behne M, Feingold KR, Elias PM. Barrier recovery is impeded at neutral pH, independent of ionic effects: implications for extracellular lipid processing. Arch Dermatol Res 1998; 290:215–222.
49. Fluhr JW. Impact of anatomical location on barrier recovery, surface pH and stratum corneum hydration after acute barrier disruption. Br J Dermatol 2002; 146:770–776.

50. Hachem JP, Crumrine D, Fluhr J, Brown BE, Feingold KR, Elias PM. pH directly regulates epidermal permeability barrier homeostasis, and stratum corneum integrity/cohesion. J Invest Dermatol 2003; 121:345–353.

51. Elias PM, et al. Modulations in epidermal calcium regulate the expression of differentiation-specific markers. J Invest Dermatol 2002; 119:1128–1136.

52. Menon GK, Elias PM, Feingold KR. Integrity of the permeablity barrier is crucial for maintenance of the epidermal calcium gradient. Br J Dermatol 1994; 130:139–147.

53. Elias PM, Ahn S, Brown B, Crumrine D, Feingold KR. Origin of the epidermal calcium gradient: regulation by barrier status and role of active vs passive mechanisms. J Invest Dermatol 2002; 119:1269–1274.

54. Thiele JJ, Traber MG, Polefka TG, Cross CE, Packer LP. Ozone exposure depletes vitamin E and induces lipid peroxidation in murine stratum corneum. J Invest Dermatol 1997; 108:753–757.

55. Thiele JJ, Hsieh SN, Briviba K, Sies H. Protein oxidation in human stratum corneum, susceptibility of keratins to oxidation in vitro and presence of a keratin oxidation gradient in vivo. J Invest Dermatol 1999; 113:335–339.

56. McVean M, Liebler DC. Inhibition of UVB induced DNA photodamage in mouse epidermis by topically applied alpha-tocopherol. Carcinogenesis 1997; 18:1617–1622.

57. Thiele JJ, Dreher F, Elsner P. Antioxidant defense systems in skin. In: Elsner P, Maibach HI, eds. Cosmeceuticals. 2001:145–188.

58. Bauer A, Bartsch R, Stadler M, Schneider W, Grieshaber R, Wollina U, Gebhardt M. Development of occupational skin diseases during vocational training in baker and confectioner apprentices: a follow up study. Contact Dermat 1998; 39:307–311.

59. Fluhr JW, Gloor M, Lehmann L, Lazzerini S, Distante F, Beradesca E. Glycerol accelerates recovery of barrier function in vivo. Acta Derm Venereol 1999; 79:418–419.

60. Ghadially R, Brown BE, Sequeria-Martin SM, Feingold KR, Elias PM. The aged epidermal permeability barrier. J Clin Invest 1995; 95:2281–2290.

61. Sheu HM, Lee JYY, Chai CY, Kuo DW. Depletion of stratum corneum intercellular lipid lamellae and barrier function abnormalities after long-term topical corticosteroids. Br J Dermatol 1997; 136:884–890.

62. Kao JS, Fluhr JW, Man MQ, Fowler AJ, Hachem J-P, Crumrine D, Ahn SK, Brown BE, Elias PM, Feingold KR. Short-term glucocorticoid treatment compromises both permeability barrier homeostasis and stratum corneum integrity: inhibition of epidermal lipid synthesis accounts for functional abnormalities. J Invest Dermatol 2003; 120:456–464.

63. Wulfhorst B. Langzeiteffektivität von Schulungsprogrammen für Patienten mit berufsbedingten Hauterkrankungen. JDDG 2003; 1:S154.

64. Fartasch M, Hüner A, Tepe A, Funke U, Diepgen TL. Hautphysiologische untersuchungsmethoden in der berufsdermatologie. Allergologie 1993; 1:25–34.

65. Schwanitz HJ. Tertiäre Prävention von Berufsdermatosen. Occup Environ Dermatol 2002; 50:212–217.

66. Chacko LW, Vaidya MC. The dermal papillae and ridge patterns in human volar skin. Acta Anat 1968; 70:99–108.

67. Smit HA, Burdorf A, Coenraads PJ. The prevalence of hand dermatitis in different occupations. Int J Epidemiol 1993; 22:288–293.

68. Smith HR, Basketter DA, McFadden JP. Irritant dermatitis, irritancy and its role in allergic contact dermatitis. Clin Exp Dermatol 2002; 27:138–146.

69. Stingeni L, Lapomarda V, Lisi P. Occupational hand dermatitis in hospital environments. Contact Dermat 1995; 33:172–176.

70. Wahlberg JE. Prevention and rehabilitation. In: Kanerva L, Elsner P, Wahlberg JE, Maibach HI, eds. Handbook of Occupational Dermatology. 1st ed. Berlin, Heidelberg, New York: Springer-Verlag, 2000:412–416.

71. Van der Walle HB, Brunsveld VM. Dermatitis in hairdressers (I). The experience of the past 4 years. Contact Dermat 1994; 30:217–221.

30

The Aged Epidermal Permeability Barrier: Basis for Functional Abnormalities

Chantal O. Barland, Peter M. Elias, and Ruby Ghadially
Department of Dermatology, and Dermatology Service, VA Medical Center, University of California, San Francisco, California, U.S.A.

STRUCTURE, FUNCTION, LIPID COMPOSITION, AND METABOLISM OF THE BARRIER

The cutaneous permeability barrier, which allows life in a terrestrial environment, resides in the outer layer of the epidermis, the stratum corneum (SC). The lipid-depleted cells (corneocytes) of the SC are embedded in a continuous, lipid-enriched, extracellular matrix organized into characteristic lamellar membrane unit structures. This lipid-enriched matrix mediates permeability barrier function by a variety of mechanisms (Table 1). SC lipids consist predominantly of ceramides (Cer) (approximately 50% by weight) with lesser amounts of cholesterol (Chol) and free fatty acids (FA) (108). Importantly, these three species comprise about 10% of the dry weight of the SC, and they are present in about a 1:1:1 molar ratio. Although the SC traditionally is viewed as inert, recent studies have shown that it is both *metabolically active*, and *interactive* with the underlying nucleated cell layers of the epidermis (23).

Chol and FA Syntheses

The epidermal lipid synthetic apparatus is highly active and relatively autonomous from circulating influences (41,84,120). Yet, epidermal lipid synthesis can be regulated by changes in barrier function; barrier perturbations result in increased synthesis of all three key lipids (22,26,54,74,82), which fuel the formation and accelerated secretion of new lamellar bodies (LBs) with rapid replenishment of lipid in the SC interstices and barrier restoration (LB formation and lipid replenishment are blocked by occlusion).

Acute barrier disruption coordinately increases the mRNA levels of several enzymes required for Chol [HMG-CoA reductase, HMG-CoA synthase, farnesol pyrophosphase synthase (FPPS), and squalene synthase], FA (ACC and FAs), and Cer [serine palmitoyl transferase (SPT)] syntheses (49,50). As discussed in Chapters 5 and 17, the coordinate increase in the mRNA levels of the enzymes for Chol and FA syntheses is due to regulation of these genes by sterol regulatory element binding

Table 1 How Lipids Mediate Barrier Function

1. Extracellular localization (only intercellular lipids play role)
2. Amount of lipid (lipid wt %)
3. Elongated, tortuous pathway (increases diffusion length)
4. Organization into lamellar membrane structures
5. Hydrophobic composition (absence of polar lipids and presence of very long chain, saturated fatty acids)
6. Correct molar ratio (approximately 1:1:1 of three key lipids: ceramides, cholesterol, and free fatty acids)
7. Unique molecular structures (e.g., acylceramides)

protein-2 (SREBP-2) (50). In contrast, although SPT, the rate-limiting enzyme for Cer synthesis, is not regulated by SREBP (50), Cer levels could be regulated indirectly through SREBPs by the availability of bulk FAs for formation of either the sphingoid base and/or N-acyl FA moieties of Cer.

Regulation of Sphingolipid Metabolism

SPT, a 56- to 60-kDa protein, which has been sequenced recently (85), is a functional heterodimer in which the SPT1 and SPT2 subunits combine (4,43) and catalyze the initial rate-limiting step in the synthesis of Cer, i.e., condensation of L-serine and palmitoyl CoA. The mRNA levels of SPT are regulated by barrier requirements, independent of SREBPs (50). In addition, SPT mRNA protein expression (25) and activity (53) increase in response to inflammatory stimuli, such as UV light, endotoxin, and cytokines (TNF and IL-1) (25). Increased SPT activity in response to these mediators of inflammation reflects the role of Cer in regulating cell functions other than barrier homeostasis, including induction of apoptosis and programmed cell death (reviewed in Ref. 83). Pertinent to the discussion of epidermal aging, excess

Table 2 Potential Signaling Molecules in Relation to Barrier Repair

	Changes with acute barrier disruption	Change inhibited by occlusion
Cytokines		
IL-1α	Increases	No
IL-1β	Increases	No
IL-1ra	Increases	No
TNFα	Increases	No
GM-CSF	Increases	ND
IL6	No change	ND
IFNγ	No change	ND
Growth factors		
TGFα	No change	ND
AR	Increases	Yes
NGF	Increases	Yes
TGFβ1	Decreases (tape-stripping)	ND

Abbreviation: ND, not determined.

Cer-mediated apoptosis of keratinocytes, through up-regulation of SPT activity, can negatively impact barrier homeostasis and interfere with normal barrier function.

Regulation of Epidermal DNA and Protein Syntheses

Barrier requirements also regulate epidermal DNA synthesis. Barrier perturbations stimulate DNA synthesis in a manner that is partially ($\approx 70\%$) blocked by occlusion (94). Pertinent to this proposal, both IL-1α and amphiregulin (AR) stimulate proliferation in cultured human keratinocytes (14,44,58,92,100,104). Thus, an age-related diminution in either or both of these factors could alter the number of cells available to synthesize barrier lipids. In contrast, epidermal bulk protein synthesis is not up-regulated, nor does inhibition of protein synthesis interfere with the dynamics of barrier recovery (10).

REGULATION OF THE NORMAL EPIDERMAL BARRIER

Earlier in the book, the role of cell-signaling pathways, including the IL-1 and EGF families, in maintaining the proper function of the epidermal permeability barrier is described. Important to this discussion are the changes in these signaling molecules that occur with aging, and their resultant effects on the cutaneous permeability barrier.

Interleukin-1 Family

Aged epidermis is characterized by both decreased proliferation and decreased lipid synthesis. Since IL-1α induces a wide variety of keratinocyte responses, it has been our hypothesis that abnormal cytokine signaling in general, and IL-1, in particular, could contribute to the barrier abnormality in aged epidermis (123). IL-1α stimulates keratinocyte proliferation (44,50,100,104). Finally, IL-1α can initiate a cytokine cascade whose net biological outcomes may be mediated by cytokines that are expressed distal to IL-1α itself, and IL-1α stimulates epidermal lipid synthesis in cultured human keratinocytes (5).

The effects of IL-1α are initiated by its binding to the type 1 IL-1 receptor (IL-1RT1), whose levels are very low in keratinocytes. In contrast, a second IL-1 receptor, IL-1RT2, predominates in keratinocytes, where it is thought to mitigate IL-1 signaling by serving as a "decoy receptor." IL-1ra, a protein that displays 19% homology with IL-1α, binds to the IL-1RT1 with approximately the same affinity as IL-1α; however, it lacks a signal peptide, and thereby acts to inhibit IL-1α activity, as well. Thus, net responses to IL-1α in skin and other tissues are mediated by the net balance of agonists (IL-1α, IL-1RT1) and antagonists (IL-1ra, IL-1RT2) (64).

Growth Factors

Keratinocytes synthesize diverse growth factors, including several members of the EGF family, platelet-derived growth factor, NGF, and VEGF which function as autocrine regulators of growth and differentiation (60,69). The downstream effects of EGF, TGFα, and AR include stimulation of DNA synthesis and the phosphorylation of several cytoplasmic proteins, including the ribosomal protein, S6 (115). The receptor's tyrosine kinase activity has been shown to be essential for such cellular responses as enhanced expression of c-fos and c-myc, morphological changes, and increased DNA synthesis (91). Although the EGFR is restricted to the basal layer and eccrine sweat ducts in normal epidermis (76,86), its levels increase suprabasally in hyperplastic epidermis and following mild epidermal trauma, including tape-stripping (87), which disrupts the barrier, while inducing epidermal hyperplasia.

AR is a potent autocrine stimulator of keratinocyte proliferation, a process that is regulated by cell surface glycosaminoglycans, i.e., heparin inhibits the mitogenic response of cultured cells to exogenous AR (14,92). Since the EGF-related proteins share certain biological activities, e.g., stimulation of cell growth, great redundancy probably exists. Extensive overlapping regulation of protein/gene expression has been reported via transcriptional and posttranscriptional mechanisms (13,14). Yet, AR could be unique among the EGF family for its apparent link to barrier homeostasis, i.e., it is the only member of the EGF family that is down-regulated by occlusion (67), and pertinently, AR expression appears to be abnormal (reduced) in aged epidermis (123).

THE AGED EPIDERMAL BARRIER

Functional Changes in Chronologic and Photoaged Skin

As in other organs, the functional status of the skin is best assessed under dynamic, rather than static conditions. Cutaneous barrier function, as assessed by TEWL rates and xenobiote penetration rates, is normal or even supernormal under basal conditions in aged skin. In contrast, the functional pathology of the epidermis is revealed only after an active insult. For example, after acute barrier disruption with either acetone or cellophane tape strippings, recovery rates are slower in aged mice (>18 months) and in aged humans (>75 years) than in normals (36). Whereas these alterations are detectable in chronologically aged skin, they are further aggravated (by about 20%) in human skin sites with superimposed photoaging (96) (Fig. 1). In addition, tape-stripping studies reveal that aged epidermis is less cohesive, i.e., disrupted with fewer strippings, than is younger skin (36,96). Paradoxically, the epidermal response to acute UV-B challenge is less robust in aging skin (47). Hence, the

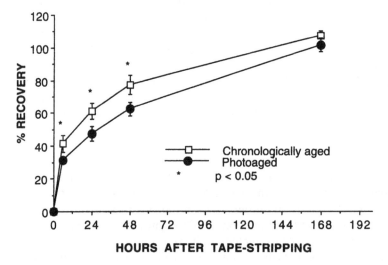

Figure 1 Barrier recovery in chronological vs. photoaged slain.

transient barrier abnormality that occurs two to three days after UV-B exposure is attenuated in aged versus young skin, presumably as a result of a decreased mitotic response (56). Whether these changes in function occur suddenly, or incrementally above a certain threshold age, is not known.

Finally, a number of other factors also are known to impact barrier homeostasis negatively in young skin, including psychological stress, high ambient humidity, and androgen excess (Table 3). Whether these factors, when present, impose an extra burden on the aged barrier is not known. However, similar assessments of environmental and hormonal factors on aged skin have been performed. A dry environment has been shown to induce epidermal proliferation and scaling in both young and old murine skin, but it does not affect barrier recovery in aged skin (11). Conversely, the age-associated decrease in female hormone levels may affect barrier function in elderly women, as estrogens have been reported to significantly influence SC sphingolipid composition (17).

In addition to its role in barrier homeostasis, the lipid-enriched matrix of the SC mediates several other defensive functions of the skin. As outlined throughout this text, key factors important to barrier maintenance and function include hydration, pH, integrity/cohesion (= "desquamation"), antioxidant defense, and antimicrobial properties. All of these are compromised to some degree in aging, in part as a result of the faulty lipid synthetic pathway (Fig. 2).

Maintenance of an optimal level of hydration is an important function of the epidermis and is dependent on several factors. These include (i) the lamellar bilayer structure of intercellular lipids which aids in water trapping within the corneocyte; (ii) the amount of Natural Moisturizing Factor (NMF), a complex mixture of low molecular weight downstream products from filaggrin degradation, produced within corneocytes and (iii) SC glycerol content (30). In aged epidermis, all three of these factors are compromised.

The hydration level of the aged epidermis is influenced by characteristic SC structural abnormalities. The decreased lipid content in aged SC coupled with the disorganized lamellar network and enlarged corneocytes, impair SC water retention. As well, NMF is decreased in aged SC, likely as a result of reduced synthesis of profilaggrin (96). Finally, aged SC exhibits a decreased glycerol content. Although the mechanism underlying the low glycerol level in aged SC is still under investigation, at least two possible explanations exist. First, the known decrease in sebaceous lipid production and turnover in aged skin could result in decreased glycerol generation from triglycerides. A recent study assessing the role of glycerol in SC hydration supports this theory, as sebaceous gland–derived glycerol was shown to be a major contributor to SC hydration in a murine model, lacking sebaceous glands (30).

Table 3 Effects of Physiologic Lipid Mixtures on Barrier Recovery in Young vs. Aged Skin

Physiologic lipids[a]	Young	Aged
Single lipid	Delay	Accelerates (cholesterol only)
Triple lipids		
Equimolar	No change	Accelerates
Fatty acid-dominant	Accelerates	Delays
Ceramide-dominant	Accelerates	Not studied
Cholesterol-dominant	Accelerates	Accelerates

[a]Physiologic lipids: free fatty acids, cholesterol, and ceramides.

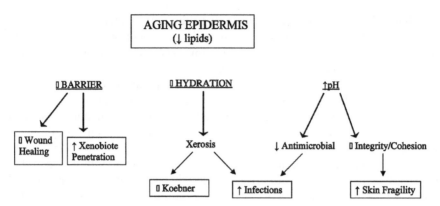

Figure 2 Effects of decreased lipids on aged epidermal function.

A second possibility is that aged skin may exhibit decreased levels of the epidermal water/glycerol transporter, aquaporin-3 (AQP3). Basal keratinocytes express AQP3 that delivers both water and glycerol to the epidermis and SC (45). AQP3-deficient mice display defective skin hydration, elasticity, and barrier function (69,45), which is corrected by glycerol replacement, suggesting that diminished glycerol transport to the SC generates the observed functional defects of the skin (46). In summary, decreased hydration of aged epidermis and SC is largely influenced by functional abnormalities, including decreased levels of endogenous humectants, NMF, and glycerol, and by structural anomalies resulting from faulty lipid processing.

Dysfunctional lipid processing also results from the elevated pH level in aged skin. An acidic pH is essential for permeability barrier homeostasis, SC integrity/cohesion, and for certain antimicrobial properties of the epidermis. In aged skin, pH levels increase. While the specific underlying defect causing this increase is still under investigation, the deleterious effects on the epidermis of a more neutral pH are well characterized. Beta-glucocerebrosidase and acidic sphingomyelinase, two key enzymes which generate the formation of Cer from glucosylceramide and sphingomyelin precursors, respectively, exhibit low pH optima (55,59,107). When pH is increased, as in aged skin, the enzymes do not function properly, resulting in defective Cer synthesis, which further compromises barrier function.

Conversely, SC chymotryptic enzyme (SCCE) and SC tryptic enzyme (SCTE), two serine proteases that regulate desquamation, should be activated at the increased pH of aged skin (112,57,18,21). As a result, elevations of extracellular pH could impact SC integrity/cohesion through acceleration of serine protease–mediated degradation of corneodesmosomes (= desquamation) (29). Activation of SCCE and SCTE is tightly controlled under basal conditions and influenced by a number of factors, including hydration, pH[6], and the co-localization of certain SC lipids (111), all of which are abnormal in aged SC. For example, SCCE activity is inhibited by micromolar concentrations of cholesterol sulfate and FFA. Furthermore, it was recently demonstrated that the rate of desquamation can be increased by mevalonic acid–induced alteration of the cholesterol sulfate:cholesterol ratio, as mevalonic acid is a known inducer of cholesterologenesis (see below) (47). In summary, alterations in any of the control mechanisms, such as increased pH or a change in the cholesterol sulfate:cholesterol ratio—both features of aged skin—alter the integrity/cohesion of aged epidermis.

Finally, the acidic milieu of the SC aids in its antimicrobial function (2,95). Nonetheless, the antimicrobial function of the SC does not rely solely on the maintenance of an acidic pH. Antimicrobial peptides have been demonstrated in the intercellular compartment of the permeability barrier (33,90). Human ß-defensin 2 (HBD-2) is stored in the LBs of stimulated keratinocytes in the spinous layer of the epidermis as well as in the intercellular spaces, suggesting that HBD-2 is released along with the contents of LB to provide an antibiotic shield for the epidermis (90). Alterations in HBD-2 and other antimicrobial peptides with aging have not been studied; however, as HBD-2 is under transcriptional control of IL-1α and IL-1β (68), alterations in IL-1α signaling with aging could decrease the efficacy of peptide up-regulation. Moreover, the decreased IL-1 signaling in aged epidermis reduces the inflammatory response exhibited by aged skin. Therefore, the defective IL-1α signaling in aged epidermis could increase the risk of infections by altering not only the antimicrobial properties of the barrier, but also by diminishing the inflammatory response to pathogens.

In summary, aging imposes structural and functional changes on the epidermis, which, in turn, influence the integrity of the permeability barrier. These functional changes are closely related to lipid processing abnormalities in aged skin and, thus, become more pronounced when the skin is challenged than under basal conditions.

Structural Basis for the Aged Permeability Barrier

The phenotypic appearance of aged skin results from a combination of functional alterations associated with intrinsic (chronologic) aging and the morphologic and physiologic changes that occur as a result of chronic sun damage (photoaging) (121,28) (Fig. 3). These processes are cumulative and affect the constituents of the skin on a cellular level (28). A histopathologic analysis of sun-protected skin and sun-exposed sites designed to separate the effects of intrinsic aging from those of photoaging found that while epidermal thickness was constant in different decades in both sun-exposed and -protected skin, it was significantly greater in sun-exposed skin (19). Light microscopy further reveals a wide range of additional alterations in aged epidermis, including a decreased number of nucleated cell layers, flattening of the rete ridges, and variable orthohyperkeratosis (see elsewhere in this volume). In addition, on the cellular level, the epidermis of sun-exposed skin displays

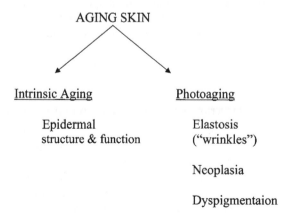

Figure 3 Age-related changes in the epidermis.

disorganized cellular maturation with some cytologic atypia, a significant decrease in the number of Langerhans cells, and an uneven distribution of melanocytes in the basal layer (121). Functionally, the latter two changes explain the decreased cutaneous immune responsiveness associated with aging and reduced protection to UV irradiation (121), respectively, which become more evident when the skin is stressed.

None of these features, however, explains the permeability barrier abnormality, which instead, can be attributed to the reduced delivery of secreted lipids to the SC (28). The decrement in secretion, in turn, results in a reduction in the number of extracellular lamellar bilayers in the SC, as visualized by electron microscopy, utilizing ruthenium tetroxide post-fixation (28). As a result, the extracellular matrix of SC may be more porous in aged than in young epidermis, although direct evidence for an intercellular defect, in the form of tracer-perfusion studies with aging, is still lacking.

While the mechanism responsible for this decreased LB secretion is not known, it has been postulated that loss of the epidermal calcium gradient may be at the root of this deficiency (16). This gradient serves many functions in the epidermis, which include the induction of terminal differentiation (117), formation of the cornified envelope (88), epidermal lipid synthesis (116), exocytosis of LBs (82), and regulation of the late events of terminal differentiation that together form the barrier (20). The calcium gradient in normal, young skin is characterized by low levels of calcium in both the basal and spinous layers, with an increase in extracellular and intracellular calcium that peaks in the outer stratum granulosum (16). In aged epidermis, the normal calcium distribution is lost, becoming abnormally broad, with calcium distributed more evenly throughout the epidermis (80,31). Loss of the calcium gradient may be due to a decreased number of ion pumps, ion channels, or ionotropic receptors in aged skin (16). The calcium abnormality, then, negatively influences the aged permeability barrier by impeding the delivery of LBs to the SC, which results in a decrease in extracellular lipid bilayers.

Metabolic and Regulatory Basis for the Aged Barrier Abnormality

Several laboratories have described lipid biochemical abnormalities in aged epidermis, most commonly a reduction in the Cer content of the SC. The reduced Cer content has, in turn, been linked to increased activity of ceramidase and/or reduced generation of Cer from sphingomyelin due to reduced acid sphingomyelinase activity. Whereas our laboratory also showed that the Cer content of aged murine SC is reduced, we found that the content of the two other major lipid species, free sterols and free FAs, were reduced at least comparably (36). The membrane structural abnormality, then, is best explained by a global reduction in aged SC lipids (about 1/3 less lipid weight % than in young SC).

We then pursued the metabolic basis for the barrier abnormality, and found a decline in Cer, Chol, and FA syntheses, attributable in turn, to reduced activity of the key (rate limiting) enzymes for each of these lipids [SPT, HMGCoA reductase, and acetyl CoA carboxylase (ACC)] (35). Moreover, the most profound synthetic abnormality was in Chol rather than in Cer or FA synthesis. Finally, lipid synthesis and enzyme activities not only were reduced under basal conditions, but they also failed to upregulate sufficiently after acute barrier disruption (35). Thus, epidermal lipid synthesis does not "catch-up" to young epidermis after comparable insults.

Recent studies have demonstrated a role for topical mevalonic acid in acute barrier repair in aged, but not young, epidermis. Mevalonic acid is an intermediate substrate generated early in Chol biosynthesis. Similar to Chol, application of mevalonic acid to aged murine epidermis enhances the rate of barrier repair after acute disruption.

Moreover, the amount of mevalonate required to achieve this effect is much less than that of Chol. These effects on cholesterologenesis are mediated through acceleration of Chol synthesis from mevalonic acid, stimulation of de novo Chol biosynthesis (47), and perhaps other effects of mevalonate (e.g., acidification).

While the molecular basis for the lipid synthetic abnormality is partially understood, the complete picture is still under investigation. One mechanism under exploration is that the content or activation of the SREBPs, which transcriptionally regulate several key enzymes of Chol and FA syntheses (see above), may be abnormal. Recent studies have revealed that abnormal autocrine/paracrine signaling is, at least in part, responsible for the faulty lipid metabolic pathway (Fig. 4). Cytokines alter lipid metabolism in liver and other tissues. For example, systemic administration of TNFα, IL-1α, IL-6, and IFNα increases de novo FA and Chol syntheses in liver (42). Moreover, TNFα, IL-1, and IL-6 acutely stimulate hepatic FA synthesis by increasing hepatic levels of citrate, an allosteric activator of ACC, a key enzyme in FA synthesis (27,42). TNFα also increases the quantity of ACC and fatty acid synthetase (FAS) in the liver (42). The TNFα-mediated increase in Chol synthesis is due to an increase in the activity of HMG CoA reductase (42). In addition, systemic administration of NGF increases serum triglyceride and free FA levels in rats (89). Moreover, it was shown that TNFα and IL-1α stimulate Cer synthesis, and SPT-, mRNA-, and enzyme levels in liver and isolated hepatocytes (81). Recently, we have demonstrated that addition of IL-1α to cultured human keratinocytes stimulates epidermal lipid synthesis (3). These studies highlight the importance of certain cytokines/growth factors in the regulation of lipid synthesis in various

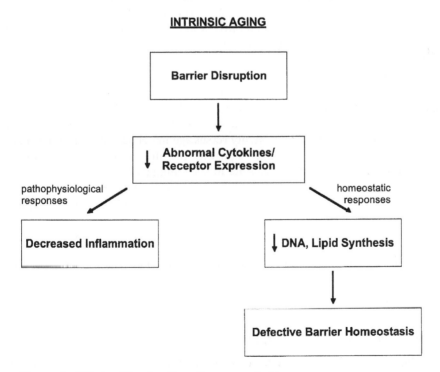

Figure 4 Effects of barrier disruption on aged skin.

organ systems, support their fundamental role in epidermal lipid synthesis, and provide further evidence for the role of reduced IL-1α signaling in the decline of permeability function in aged skin.

Aging is paralleled by a decline in immune competence, manifest by increased susceptibility to certain infections, autoimmune and immune complex–mediated diseases, and cancer (114). Studies have shown abnormalities in cytokine production with aging. However, aged tissues maintain the capacity to produce cytokines in response to stimuli, and some cytokines either do not change or even increase with aging (24,40,53,61,99,101,118). There are few studies on local cytokine levels in the skin during aging. In multiple studies IL-1α has been shown to decrease in various tissues of the aged, including a decrease in cytokine protein in aged humans' keratinocytes in culture (105) and lower mRNA levels in aged mice (106) and humans (38). Moreover, one study demonstrated increased expression of IL-1ra in aging human keratinocytes in culture, but a decrease in photoaging (33). Furthermore, in a study by Piepkorn et al. (93) a decrease in AR was evident in the epidermis of single sample of middle-aged versus newborn skin. Finally, there are not only age-dependent changes in cytokine expression, but also a decreased response to cytokines with aging (8,39,79,101). These results suggest that dysregulation of cytokine production and/or downstream biological reactivity are a general feature of aging tissues that could impact on the functional abnormalities in aging skin (Fig. 4).

Finally, studies of growth factors in the skin suggest similar dysregulation. Human diploid fibroblasts elaborate decreased active TGF-β1 during replicative senescence (125), whereas TGFα gene expression in cultured human keratinocytes is unaffected by donor age (13). With increasing donor age, cultured human fibroblasts also expressed fewer EGFR (98). Induction of keratinocyte growth factor mRNA by various cytokines was unchanged with age (112), and the mitogenic response to cytokine stimulation and protein synthesis following TGFβ stimulation was preserved with aging (31). However, a diminished proliferative response of advanced passage human diploid fibroblasts to TNF, IL-1, and fibroblast growth factor (1), as well as decreased mitogenic responsiveness to epidermal growth factor was also observed. Several cytokines and growth factors, produced by keratinocytes, are known mitogens for keratinocytes, and they are known to stimulate lipid synthesis in extracutaneous tissues. We have shown that expression of two of these factors, IL-1α and AR, is reduced in aged epidermis (120). Moreover, aged transgenic mice with a knockout of the functional IL-1α receptor display a barrier abnormality versus age-matched, wild-type littermates (123). Finally, topical treatment of aged skin with the immomodulator, imiquimod, enhances (normalizes) barrier recovery rates in aged animals (3).

A third regulatory mechanism, namely glucosylceramide (GlcCer) signaling, could account, in part, for the lipid synthetic abnormality. GlcCer, whether applied exogenously or enhanced by inhibition of β-glucocerebrosidase, is mitogenic for young and aged epidermis (76,78). However, comparable levels of GlcCer fail to induce an equivalent mitotic response in aged epidermis (76). Hence, defective GlcCer signaling could decrease the pool of keratinocytes available for lipid synthesis in aged epidermis. Further studies will be needed to distinguish the relative role and importance of these potential signaling mechanisms in the aged barrier.

Molecular Mechanisms Mediating Epidermal Aging

On the cellular level, apoptosis and decreased proliferative capacity, two key features of the aging process, also impact the epidermis and epidermal permeability barrier.

While the specific mechanisms that may induce changes in the permeability barrier have not been elucidated, the molecular mechanisms responsible for the characteristic structural and functional changes of chronologic and photoaging in the skin, are beginning to be elucidated. Reactive oxygen species (ROS) are the primary mediators of UV damage, while telomere shortening characterizes the process of intrinsic chronologic aging (121,28). The emerging information reveals that these processes share fundamental molecular pathways, some of which are initiated in the epidermis (28).

UV irradiation damages the epidermis through the generation of ROS including the superoxide anion, peroxide, and singlet oxygen. Ultraviolet-induced ROS cause deleterious modifications through chemical oxidation of cellular components, including DNA, proteins, and lipids (28). Interestingly, excess ROS from mitochondrial oxidative metabolism mediate some of the same effects seen in chronologic aging, although ROS-mediated injury is not the primary mediator of cellular damage intrinsic to this process. In both chronologic and photoaging, oxidation of DNA leads to mutations, while oxidation of proteins leads to reduced function (28). More pertinent to the alterations of the aged epidermal permeability barrier, lipid oxidation results in reduced transport efficiency (28), and may be yet another key factor in the altered transmembrane signaling that impacts permeability barrier function.

Although ROS play a role in photoaging, telomere shortening appears to be the primary mediator of intrinsic aging. Telomeres are repetitive DNA sequences that cap the ends of chromosomes. The terminal base pairs of these sequences are lost with each round of mitosis, resulting in progressive chromosome shortening with each somatic cell division, which is, therefore, more pronounced in aged cells (121). Importantly, there is a molecular connection between UV-induced DNA damage from photoaging and replication-induced telomere shortening from chronologic aging (121,122). Both pathways lead to telomere destabilization and exposure of a 3′ overhang of telomeric DNA, which is normally sequestered in a loop structure and stabilized by a binding factor.

Destabilization of the loop structure by DNA damage due to UV irradiation or gradual erosion during aging exposes this single-stranded 3′ overhang of the telomeric repeat sequence. An as yet unidentified sensing mechanism interacts with the overhang to initiate a cascade of events that can lead to cell cycle arrest, senescence, apoptosis, or differentiation (reviewed in Ref. 122). Thus, the internal and external insults causing DNA damage can ultimately lead to cellular senescence and apoptosis (both fundamental to the aging process) through a common pathway (121).

In summary, all of the mechanisms outlined in this section, from altered cytokine profiles and the dysfunctional calcium gradient to loss of cells and loss of proliferative capacity, influence cellular responsiveness and mediate the structural, functional, and metabolic deficiencies which characterize aged epidermis.

BARRIER REPAIR STRATEGIES FOR AGED EPIDERMIS

Based upon the lipid biochemical abnormality in aged epidermis, we assessed whether one or more SC lipids could correct the functional abnormality. In young murine or human skin, any incomplete mixture of one or two of the three major lipid species (Chol, Cer, and free FAs) worsens barrier function (Table 3) (75). In contrast, equimolar mixtures of the three key lipids allow normal rates of barrier recovery in young skin (Table 3) (75). Further adjustment of the three-component mixtures to 3:1:1 molar ratios actually accelerates barrier recovery significantly (72,73), and in young skin, any of the three key species can predominate (Table 3) (72). In contrast, in aged epidermis, with its global decline in lipid synthesis and profound abnormality in Chol synthesis, the requirements for barrier repair are quite different. Topical Chol alone, which delays barrier recovery in young skin, accelerates barrier recovery in aged murine and human skin (Table 3) (36). Moreover, equimolar mixtures of the three key lipids also accelerate barrier recovery, and optimized ratios only accelerate recovery if Chol is the predominant lipid (Fig. 5) (126). Finally, the Chol-dominant mixture shown to repair the barrier of aged human skin (126) is available commercially (Crème de l'Extrème, Osmotics). These results underscore the selective (profound) abnormality in Chol synthesis that characterizes the aged epidermal permeability barrier.

CLINICAL IMPLICATIONS

Aged patients suffer from a variety of cutaneous problems due to alterations in barrier function, including dryness, pruritus, scaling, and abnormal transdermal drug delivery. Furthermore, the consequences of epidermal aging are also important in terms of altered responses to inflammatory/infectious insults (Fig. 3). Whereas most research on skin aging has focused on the effects of photoaging on the dermis (66), epidermis also undergoes several important functional alterations that could be linked to a defective barrier, including (i) altered drug permeability (51,102), (ii) decreased susceptibility to irritant contact dermatitis (62,110), (iii) severe xerosis (7,62), (iv) an altered threshold to pro-inflammatory and immunogenic stimuli (37,114), (v) decreased cell renewal rates, (vi) decreased SC water content, (vii) decreased vitamin D generation (71), and (viii) abnormal desquamation. However, there are more serious consequences of epidermal aging, including altered transdermal absorption and abnormal susceptibility to exogenous pro-inflammatory and infectious agents. We have examined aged epidermis in humans and in a murine model of senescence. Profound abnormalities in barrier function occurred not under

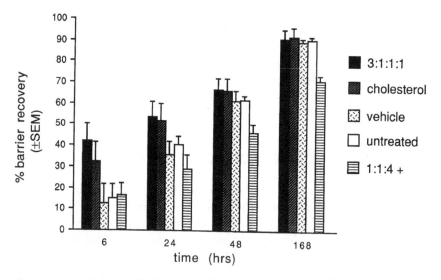

Figure 5 Physiological lipids improve barrier recovery in aged humans.

basal conditions, but only when the skin was stressed. The structural and lipid biochemical basis for the functional abnormalities is now known, and faulty IL-1α signaling is, at least partly, responsible for the defective epidermal permeability barrier in aged skin. Whether other faulty mechanisms of lipid synthesis or transport exist in the aged epidermis and add to the functional abnormality is still under investigation.

REFERENCES

1. Schurer NY, Elias PM. The biochemistry and function of stratum corneum lipids. Adv Lipid Res 1991; 24:27–56.
2. Elias PM, Wood LC, Feingold KR. Epidermal pathogenesis of inflammatory dermatoses. Am J Contact Dermat 1999; 10:119–126.
3. Grubauer G, Feingold KR, Elias PM. The relationship of epidermal lipogenesis to cutaneous barrier function. J Lipid Res 1987; 28:746–752.
4. Mommaas-Kienhuis AM, Grayson S, Wijsman MC, et al. Low density lipoprotein receptor expression on keratinocytes in normal and psoriatic epidermis. J Invest Dermatol 1987; 89:513–517.
5. Williams ML, Mommaas-Kienhuis AM, Rutherford SL, et al. Free sterol metabolism and low density lipoprotein receptor expression as differentiation markers in cultured human keratinocytes. J Cell Physiol 1987; 132:428–440.
6. Elias PM, Menon GK. Structural and lipid biochemical correlates of the epidermal permeability barrier. Adv Lipid Res 1991; 24:1–23.
7. Feingold KR, Brown BE, Lear SR, et al. The effect of essential fatty acid deficiency on cutaneous sterol synthesis. J Invest Dermatol 1986; 87:588–591.
8. Holleran WM, Feingold KR, Mao-Qiang M, et al. Regulation of epidermal sphingolipid synthesis by permeability barrier function. J Lipid Res 1991a; 32:1151–1158.
9. Mao-Qiang M, Elias PM, Feingold KR. Fatty acids are required for epidermal permeability barrier function. J Clin Invest 1993a; 92:791–798.
10. Menon GK, Feingold KR, Moser AH, et al. De novo sterologenesis in the skin. II. Regulation by cutaneous barrier requirements. J Lipid Res 1985; 26:418–427.
11. Harris IR, Farrell AM, Grunfeld C, et al. Permeability barrier disruption coordinately regulates mRNA levels for key enzymes of cholesterol, fatty acid, and ceramide synthesis in the epidermis. J Invest Dermatol 1997; 109:783–787.
12. Harris IR, Farrell AM, Holleran WM, et al. Parallel regulation of sterol regulatory element binding protein-2 and the enzymes of cholesterol and fatty acid synthesis but not ceramide synthesis in cultured human keratinocytes and murine epidermis. J Lipid Res 1998; 39:412–422.
13. Nagiec MM, Baltisberger JA, Wells GB, et al. The LCB2 gene of Saccharomyces and the related LCB1 gene encode subunits of serine palmitoyltransferase, the initial enzyme in sphingolipid synthesis. Proc Natl Acad Sci USA 1994; 91:7899–7902.
14. Bejaoui K, Uchida Y, Yasuda S, et al. Hereditary sensory neuropathy type 1 mutations confer dominant negative effects on serine palmitoyltransferase, critical for sphingolipid synthesis. J Clin Invest 2002; 110:1301–1308.
15. Hanada K, Hara T, Nishijima M. Purification of the serine palmitoyltransferase complex responsible for sphingoid base synthesis by using affinity peptide chromatography techniques. J Biol Chem 2000; 275:8409–8415.
16. Farrell AM, Uchida Y, Nagiec MM, et al. UVB irradiation up-regulates serine palmitoyltransferase in cultured human keratinocytes. J Lipid Res 1998; 39:2031–2038.
17. Hobbs M, Weigle WO, Noonan DJ, et al. Patterns of cytokine gene expression b CD4+ T cells from young and old mice. J Immunol 1993; 150:3602–3614.
18. Mimeault M. New advances on structural and biological functions of ceramide in apoptotic/necrotic cell death and cancer. FEBS Lett 2002; 530:9–16.

19. Proksch E, Feingold KR, Man MQ, et al. Barrier function regulates epidermal DNA synthesis. J Clin Invest 1991; 87:1668–1673.
20. Cook PW, Mattox PA, Keeble WW, et al. Inhibition of autonomous human keratinocyte proliferation and amphiregulin mitogenic activity by sulfated polysaccharides. In Vitro Cell Dev Biol 1992b; 28A:218–222.
21. Hancock GE, Kaplan G, Cohn Z. Keratinocyte growth regulation by the products of immune cells. J Exp Med 1988; 168:1395–1402.
22. Hua X, Yokoyama C, Wu J, et al. SREBP-2, a second basic-helix-loop-helix-leucine zipper protein that stimulates transcription by binding to a sterol regulatory element. Proc Natl Acad Sci USA 1993; 90:11603–11607.
23. Piepkorn M, Lo C, Plowman G. Amphiregulin-dependent proliferation of cultured human keratinocytes: autocrine growth, the effects of exogenous recombinant cytokine and apparent requirement for heparin-like glycosaminoglycans. J Cell Physiol 1994; 159:114–120.
24. Ristow HJ. A major factor contributing to epidermal proliferation in inflammatory skin diseases appears to be interleukin-1 or a related protein. Proc Natl Acad Sci USA 1987; 84:1940–1944.
25. Sauder DN. Biological properties of epidermal thymocyte activity factor (ETAF). J Invest Dermatol 1985; 85:176S–182S.
26. Choi S-J, Jackson SM, Elias PM, et al. The role of protein synthesis in permeability barrier homeostasis. In: Ohkawara A, McGuire JS, and Kobayashi H, eds. The Biology of the Epidermis: Molecular and Functional Aspects. Amsterdam, Elsevier, 1992: 11–19.
27. Ye J, Calhoun CF, Feingold K, et al. Age-related changes in the IL-1 gene family and their receptors before and after barrier abrogation. J Invest Dermatol 1999; 112:543.
28. Bell T, Harley C, Stetsko D, et al. Expression of mRNA homologous to interleukin-1 in human epidermal cells. J Invest Dermatol 1987; 92:809–816.
29. Kupper TS, Groves RW. The interleukin-1 axis and cutaneous inflammation. J Invest Dermatol 1995; 105:62S–66S.
30. Karvinen S, Pasonen-Seppanen S, Hyttinen JM, et al. Keratinocyte growth factor stimulates migration and hyaluronan synthesis in the epidermis by activation of keratinocyte hyaluronan synthases 2 and 3. J Biol Chem 2003; 278:49495–49504.
31. Ma T, Hara M, Sougrat R, et al. Impaired stratum corneum hydration in mice lacking epidermal water channel aquaporin-3. J Biol Chem 2002; 277:17147–17153.
32. Ullrich A, Schlessinger J. Signal transduction by receptors with tyrosine kinase activity. Cell 1990; 61:203–222.
33. Pawson T, Schlessinger J. SH2 and SH3 domains. Curr Biol 1993; 3:434–442.
34. Marchell NL, Uchida Y, Brown BE, et al. Glucosylceramides stimulate mitogenesis in aged murine epidermis. J Invest Dermatol 1998; 110:383–387.
35. Nanney LB, McKanna JA, Stoscheck CM, et al. Visualization of epidermal growth factor receptors in human epidermis. J Invest Dermatol 1984; 82:165–170.
36. Nanney LB, Sundberg JP, King LE. Increased epidermal growth factor receptor in fsn/fsn mice. J Invest Dermatol 1996; 106:1169–1174.
37. Compton CC, Tong Y, Rookman N, et al. Transforming growth factor alpha gene expression in cultured human keratinocytes is unaffected by cellular aging. Arch Dermatol 1995; 131:683–690.
38. Liou A, Elias PM, Grunfeld C, et al. Amphiregulin and nerve growth factor expression are regulated by barrier status in murine epidermis. J Invest Dermatol 1997; 108: 73–77.
39. Ghadially R, Brown BE, Sequeira-Martin SM, et al. The aged epidermal permeability barrier. Structural, functional, and lipid biochemical abnormalities in humans and a senescent murine model. J Clin Invest 1995; 95:2281–2290.
40. Rawlings AV, Harding CR. Moisturization and skin barrier function. Dermatol Ther 2004; 17(suppl 1):43–48.

41. Haratake A, Komiya A, Horikoshi T, et al. Acceleration of de novo cholesterol synthesis in epidermis influences desqumation of stratum corneum in aged mice. J Invest Dermatol. In press.

42. Holleran WM, Uchida Y, Halkier-Sorensen L, et al. Structural and biochemical basis for the UVB-induced alterations in epidermal barrier function. Photodermatol Photoimmunol Photomed 13:117–128.

43. Coffey RJ, Derynck R, Wilcox JN, et al. Production and auto-induction of transforming growth factor alpha in human keratinocytes. Nature 1987; 238:817–820.

44. Didierjean L, Salomon D, Mérot Y, et al. Localization and characterization of the interleukin-1 immunoreactive pool (IL-1 alpha and beta forms) in normal human epidermis. J Invest Dermatol 1989; 92:809–816.

45. Fluhr JW, Mao-Qiang M, Brown BE, et al. Glycerol regulates stratum corneum hydration in sebaceous gland deficient (asebia) mice. J Invest Dermatol 2003; 120(5):728–737.

46. Hara M, Ma T, Verkman AS. Selectively reduced glycerol in skin of aquaporin-3-deficient mice may account for impaired skin hydration, elasticity, and barrier recovery. J Biol Chem 2002; 277:46616–46621.

47. Hara M, Verkman AS. Glycerol replacement corrects defective skin hydration, elasticity, and barrier function in aquaporin-3-deficient mice. Proc Natl Acad Sci USA 2003; 100:7360–7365.

48. Holleran WM, Takagi Y, Menon GK, et al. Processing of epidermal glucosylceramides is required for optimal mammalian cutaneous permeability barrier function. J Clin Invest 1993; 91:1656–1664.

49. Jensen JM, Schutze S, Forl M, et al. Roles for tumor necrosis factor receptor p55 and sphingomyelinase in repairing the cutaneous permeability barrier. J Clin Invest 1999; 104:1761–1770.

50. Schmuth M, Man MQ, Weber F, et al. Permeability barrier disorder in Niemann-Pick disease: sphingomyelin-ceramide processing required for normal barrier homeostasis. J Invest Dermatol 2000; 115:459–466.

51. Suzuki Y, Nomura J, Hori J, et al. Detection and characterization of endogenous protease associated with desquamation of stratum corneum. Arch Dermatol Res 1993; 285:372–377.

52. Horikoshi T, Igarashi S, Uchiwa H, et al. Role of endogenous cathepsin D-like and chymotrypsin-like proteolysis in human epidermal desquamation. Br J Dermatol 1999; 141:453–459.

53. Ekholm IE, Brattsand M, Egelrud T. Stratum corneum tryptic enzyme in normal epidermis: a missing link in the desquamation process? J Invest Dermatol 2000; 114:56–63.

54. Elias PM, Matsuyoshi N, Wu H, Lin C, Wang ZH, Brown BE, Stanley JR. Desmoglein isoform distribution affects stratum corneum structure and function. J Cell Biol 2001; 153:243–249.

55. Fluhr JW, Kao J, Jain M, et al. Generation of free fatty acids from phospholipids regulates stratum corneum acidification and integrity. J Invest Dermatol 2001; 117:44–51.

56. Bouwstra JA, de Graaff A, Gooris GS, et al. Water distribution and related morphology in human stratum corneum at different hydration levels. J Invest Dermatol 2003; 120:750–758.

57. Suzuki Y, Koyama J, Moro O, et al. The role of two endogenous proteases of the stratum corneum in degradation of desmoglein-1 and their reduced activity in the skin of ichthyotic patients. Br J Dermatol 1996; 134:460–464.

58. Aly R, Maibach HI, Rahman R, et al. Correlation of human in vivo and in vitro cutaneous antimicrobial factors. J Infect Dis 1975; 13:579–583.

59. Puhvel SM, Reisner RM, Sakamoto M. Analysis of lipid composition of isolated human sebaceous gland homogenates after incubation with coetaneous bacteria. Thin-layer chromatography. J Invest Dermatol 1975; 64:406–411.

60. Ganz T, Liu L, Valore EV, et al. Defensins; microbicidal and cytotoxic peptides of mammalian host defense cells. Med Microbiol Immunol Berl 1992; 18:275–281.

61. Oren A, Ganz T, Liu L, Meerloo T. In human epidermis, beta-defensin 2 is packaged in lamellar bodies. Exp Mol Pathol 2003; 74:180–182.

62. Liu AY, Destoumieux D, Wong AV, et al. Human beta-defensin-2 production in keratinocytes is regulated by interleukin-1, bacteria, and the state of differentiation. J Invest Dermatol 2002; 118:275–281.

63. Yaar M, Eller MS. Mechanisms of aging. Arch Dermatol 2002; 138:1429–1430.

64. Fisher G, Kang S, Varani J, et al. Mechanisms of photoaging and chronological skin aging. Arch Dermatol 2002; 138:1462–1470.

65. El-Domyati M, Attia S, Saleh S, et al. Intrinsic aging vs. photoaging: a comparative histopathological, immunohistochemical, and ultrastructural study of skin. Exp Dermatol 2002; 11:398–405.

66. Denda M, Tomitaka A, Akamatsu H, et al. Altered distribution of calcium in facial epidermis of aged adults. J Invest Dermatol 2003; 121:1557–1558.

67. Watt FM. Terminal differentiation of epidermal keratinocytes. Curr Opin Cell Biol 1989; 1:1107–1115.

68. Nemes Z, Steinert PM. Bricks and mortar of the epidermal barrier. Exp Mol Med 1999; 31:5–19.

69. Watanabe R, Wu K, Paul P, et al. Up-regulation of glucosylceramide synthase expression and activity during human keratinocyte differentiation. J Biol Chem 1998; 273:9651–9655.

70. Elias PM, Ahn SK, Denda M, et al. Modulations in epidermal calcium concentration regulate the expression of differentiation-specific markers. 2002; 119:1128–1136.

71. Mauro T, Bench G, Sidderas-Haddad E, et al. Acute barrier perturbation abolishes the $Ca+2$ and $K+$ gradients in murine epidermis: quantitative measurement using PIXE. J Invest Dermatol 1998; 111:1198–1201.

72. Forslind B, Werner-Linde Y, Lindber M, et al. Elemental analysis mirrors epidermal differentiation. Acta Derm Venereol (Stockh) 1999; 79:12–17.

73. Ghadially R, Brown BE, Hanley K, et al. Decreased epidermal lipid synthesis accounts for altered barrier function in chronologically aged murine epidermis. J Invest Dermatol 1996a; 106:1064–1069.

74. Grunfeld C, Soued M, Adi S, et al. Evidence for two cleasses of cytokines that stimulate heptic lipogenesis: relationships among tumor necrosis factor, interleukin-1 and interferon-alpha. Endocrinology 1990; 127:46–54.

75. Feingold KR, Soued M, Serio MK, et al. Multiple cytokines stimulate hepatic lipid synthesis in vivo. Endocrinology 1989; 125:267–274.

76. Nonogaki K, Moser AH, Shigenaga J, et al. b-nerve growth factor as a mediator of the acute phase response in vivo. Biochem Biophys Res Commun 1996; 219:956–961.

77. Memon RA, Holleran WM, Moser AH, et al. Endotoxin and cytokines increase hepatic sphingolipid biosynthesis and produce lipoproteins enriched in ceramides and sphingomyelin. Arterioscler Thromb Vasc Biol 1998; 18:1257–1265.

78. Barland CO, Zettersten E, Brown BS, et al. Imiquimod-induced interleukin-1 alpha stimulation improves barrier homeostasis in aged murine epidermis. J Invest Dermatol 2004; 122:330–336.

79. Thivolet J, Nicolas JF. Skin aging and immune competence. Br J Dermatol 1990; 122:77–81.

80. Fagiolo U, Cossarizza A, Scala E, et al. Increased cytokine production in mononuclear cells of healthy elderly people. Eur J Immunol 1993; 23:2375–2378.

81. Goonewardene IM, Murasko DM. Age associated changes in mitogen induced proliferation and cytokine production by lymphocytes of the long-lived Brown Norway rat. Mech Age Dev 1993; 71:199–212.

82. Khansari DN, Gustad T. Effects of long-term, low-dose growth hormone therapy on immune function and life expectancy of mice. Mech Age Dev 1991; 57:87–100.

83. Riancho JA, Zarrabeitia MT, Amado JA, et al. Age-related differences in cytokine secretion. Gerontology 1994; 40:8–12.

84. Rosenberg JS, Gilman SC, Feldman JD. Effects of aging on cell cooperation and lymphocyte responsiveness to cytokines. J Immunol 1983; 130:1754–1758.

85. Weksler ME. Immune senescence and adrenal steroids: immune dysregulation and the action of dehydroepiandrosterone (DHEA) in old animals. Eur J Clin Pharm 1993; 45(suppl 1):S21–S23.

86. Sauder DN, Ponnappan U, Cinader B. Effect of age on cutaneous interleukin 1 expression. Immunol Lett 1989; 20:111–114.

87. Sauder DN, Stanulis-Praeger BM, Gilchrest BA. Autocrine growth stimulation of human keratinocytes by epidermal cell-derived thymocyte-activating factor: implications for skin aging. Arch Dermatol Res 1988b; 280:71–76.

88. Gilchrest BA, Garmyn M, Yaar M. Aging and photoaging affect gene expression in cultured human keratinocytes. Arch Dermatol 1994; 130:82–86.

89. Piepkorn M, Underwood RA, Henneman C, et al. Expression of amphiregulin is regulated in cultured human keratinocytes and in developing fetal skin. J Invest Dermatol 1995; 105:802–809.

90. Chen YQ, Mauviel A, Ryynanen J, et al. Type VII collagen gene expression by human skin fibroblasts and keratinocytes in culture: influence of donor age and cytokine responses. J Invest Dermatol 1994; 102:205–209.

91. Gilhar A, Aizen E, Pillar T, et al. Response of aged versus young skin to intradermal administration of interferon gamma. J Am Acad Dermatol 1992; 27:710–716.

92. Martin LW, Deeter LB, Lipton JM. Acute-phase response to endogenous pyrogen in rabbit: effects of age and route of adminstration. Am J Physiol 1989; 257:R189–R193.

93. Zeng G, McCue HM, Mastrangelo L, et al. Endogenous TGF-beta activity is modified during cellular aging: effects on metalloproteinase and TIMP-1 expression. Exp Cell Res 1996; 228:271–276.

94. Reenstra WR, Yaar M, Gilchrest BA. Aging affects epidermal growth factor receptor phosphorylation and traffic kinetics. Exp Cell Res 1996; 227:252–255.

95. Aggarwal BB, Totpal K, LaPushin R, et al. Diminished responsiveness of senescent normal human fibroblasts to TNF-dependent proliferation and interleukin production is not due to its effect on the receptors or on the activation of a nuclear factor NF-kappa B. Exp Cell Res 1995; 218:381–388.

96. Marsh NL, Elias PM, Holleran WM. Glucosylceramides stimulate mitogenesis in murine epidermis. J Clin Invest 1995; 95:2903–2909.

97. Yaar M, Eller MS, Gilchrest B. Fifty years of skin aging. J Invest Dermatol 2002; 7:51–58.

98. Mao-Qiang M, Feingold KR, Elias PM. Exogenous lipids influence permeability barrier recovery in acetone-treated murine skin. Arch Dermatol 1993b; 129:728–738.

99. Man MM, Feingold KR, Thornfeldt CR, et al. Optimization of physiological lipid mixtures for barrier repair. J Invest Dermatol 1996; 106:1096–1101.

100. Mao-Qiang M, Brown BE, Wu-Pong S, et al. Exogenous nonphysiologic vs physiologic lipids. Divergent mechanisms for correction of permeability barrier dysfunction. Arch Dermatol 1995; 131:809–816.

101. Zettersten EM, Ghadially R, Feingold KR, et al. Optimal ratios of topical stratum corneum lipids improve barrier recovery in chronologically aged skin. J Am Acad Dermatol 1997; 37:403–408.

102. Lavker RM. Structural alterations in exposed and unexposed aged skin. J Invest Dermatol 1979; 73:59 66.

103. Harvell JD, Maibach HI. Percutaneous absorption and inflammation in aged skin: a review. J Am Acad Dermatol 1994; 31:1015–1021.

104. Roskos KV, Guy RH, Maibach HI. Percutaneous absorption in the aged. Dermatol Clin 1986; 4:455–465.

105. Kleinsmith DM, Perricone NV. Common skin problems in the elderly. Dermatol Clin 1986; 4:485–499.

106. Suter-Widmer J, Elsner P. Age and irritation. In: van der Valk PGM, Maibach HI, eds. The Irritant Contact Dermatitis Syndrome. Boca Raton: CRC Press, 1996:257–261.

107. Carter DM, Balin AK. Dermatological aspects of aging. Med Clin N Am 1983; 67: 531–543.
108. Gilchrest B, Stoff J, Soter N. Chronologic aging alters the response to ultraviolet-induced inflammation in human skin. J Invest Dermatol 1982; 79:47–53.
109. MacLaughlin JA, Holick MF. Aging decreases the capacity of human skin to produce vitamin D3. J Clin Invest 1985; 76:1536–1538.
110. Chen EH, Kim MJ, Ahn SK, et al. The skin barrier state of aged hairless mice in a dry environment. Br J Dermatol 2002; 147:244–249.
111. Coffey RJ, Graves-Deal R, Dempsey PJ, et al. Differential regulation of transforming factor alpha autoinduction in a nontransformed and transformed epithelial cell. Cell Growth-Differ 1992; 3:347–354.
112. Denda M, Koyama J, Hori J, et al. Age- and sex-dependent changes in stratum corneum sphingolipids. Arch Dermatol Res 1993; 285:415–417.
113. Freedland M, Karmiol S, Rodriguez J, et al. Fibroblast responses to cytokines are maintained during aging. Ann Plast Surg 1995; 35:290–296.
114. Garmyn M, Yaar M, Boileau N, et al. Effect of aging and habitual sun exposure on the genetic response of cultured human keratinocytes to solar-simulated irradiation. J Invest Dermatol 1992; 99:743–748.
115. Haratake A, Uchida Y, Schmuth M. UVB-induced alterations in permeability barrier function: roles for epidermal hyperproliferation and thymocyte-mediated response. J Invest Dermatol 1997; 108:769–775.
116. Hauser C, Saurat JH, Schmitt A, et al. Interleukin-1 is present in normal human epidermis. J Immunol 1986; 16:3317–3323.
117. Kubilus J, Tarascio AJ, Baden HP. Steroid-sulfatase deficiency in sex-linked ichthyosis. Am J Hum Genet 1979; 3:50–53.
118. Larson CJ, Oppenheim JJ, Matsushima K. IL-1 or TNF alpha stimulate the production of MAP/IL-8 by normal fibroblasts and keratinocytes. J Invest Dermatol 1989; 92: 467–471.
119. Maas-Szabowski N, Starker A, Fusenig NE. Epidermal tissue regeneration and stromal interaction in HaCaT cells is initiated by TGF-alpha. J Cell Sci 2003 15; 116(Pt 14): 2937—2948.
120. Marinus FW, Ponec M. Differentiation of keratinocytes and the expression of receptors for epidermal growth factor and low density lipoproteins. J Invest Dermatol 1988; 89:342–346.
121. Reed JT, Elias PM, Ghadially R. Integrity and permeability barrier function of photo-aged human epidermis [letter]. Arch Dermatol 1997; 133:395–396.
122. Sato J, Denda M, Nakanishi J, et al. Cholesterol sulfate inhibits proteases that are involved in desquamation of stratum corneum. J Invest Dermatol 1998; 111:189–193.
123. Shapiro LJ, Weiss R, Buxman MM, et al. Enzymatic basis of typical X-linked icthyosis. Lancet 1978; 2:756–757.
124. Tang A, Gilchrest BA. Regulation of keratinocyte growth factor gene expression in human skin fibroblasts. J Dermatol Sci 1996; 11:41–50.
125. Williams ML, Elias PM. Stratum corneum lipids in disorders of cornification: increased cholesterol sulfate content of stratum corneum in recessive x-linked ichthyosis. J Clin Invest 1978; 68:1404–1410.
126. Ye J, Garg A, Calhoun C, et al. Alterations in cytokine regulation in aged epidermis: implications for permeability barrier homeostasis and inflammation. Exp Dermatol 2002; 11:209–216.

31

Psychological Stress and the Barrier: The Psychosensory Interface

Mitsuhiro Denda
Shiseido Life Science Research Center, Yokohama, Japan

INTRODUCTION

Skin permeability barrier function is a self-regulatory system. When the barrier is damaged, normal function is rapidly restored. On the other hand, abnormalities in skin barrier function are present in many inflammatory and non-inflammatory skin conditions, such as psoriasis and atopic dermatitis (1); i.e., normal function is never restored. Previous reports suggest that even a single barrier insult can induce cytokine activation secretion (2), and or increased epidermal DNA synthesis (3). Moreover, even though barrier function is normally restored quickly, when the damage is repeated or when it occurs under low environmental humidity, epidermal hyperplasia or inflammation can result (4,5). Thus, the skin barrier recovery response is clinically important for disease pathogenesis.

In modern society, various factors can cause excessive psychological stress that can affect human health. For example, sustained psychological stress is associated with alterations in both humoral and cellular immune responses (6–13). Moreover, psychological stresses influence the progress and survival of patients with cancer (9,14–17).

Many reports have suggested that psychological stress also causes the onset or exacerbation of both psoriasis and adult atopic dermatitis (18–21). Al'abadie et al. (22) reported that psoriasis patients were more likely to have experienced stress immediately before disease onset or exacerbations of their condition than patients with other skin diseases. For psoriatic patients, the most common stressful factors in daily life were new family problems and recent work or school demands, but chronic stress was also commonly essential for diseases flares to occur.

Kodama et al. (23) demonstrated the effect of stress on atopic dermatitis after the Great Hanshin earthquake.

They analyzed 457 patients with atopic dermatitis, immediately after the patients experienced the earthquake. They divided them into three groups according to the severity of damage: severe damage to buildings and houses (area A), mild damage (area B), and no damage (control area). Exacerbation of skin symptoms occurred in 38% and 34% of patients in areas A and B, while similar symptoms were found in only 7% of the control group.

These epidemiological reports suggest that increased stress induced by drastic alterations of living condition is significantly correlated with the skin pathology. However, scientific and experimental research on the relationship between skin homeostasis and psychological factors is limited. Recently, several trials have evaluated the effects of psychological stress on skin barrier homeostasis. In the next section, we will describe those trials that demonstrated the relationship between psychological stress and barrier function in experimental models. Moreover, confirmatory human experiments are also described and discussed.

ANIMAL MODEL

Experiments using humans are difficult to control, and it is also hard to obtain endocrinological information. Moreover, one should carry out experiments using human subjects under similar physiological conditions, but each human experiences different levels of stress to standard stressors. Here, several different experimental models of stress in animals have been developed. In these studies, endocrinological factors under different types of stress have also been evaluated. Thus, to obtain an initial outline of the relationship between psychological, endocrinological, and dermatological factors, an animal model would be useful.

Immobilization-Induced Stress (24)

Immobilization-induced stress is a technique extensively used in the field of neurophysiology, neuropathology, and neuropharmacology (25). In Syrian hamsters, immobilization stress simultaneously decreased plasma testosterone levels, lipogenesis in sebaceous glands, and epidermal DNA synthesis simultaneously (26,27). Thus, one could expect an influence of psychological factors on skin metabolism and function.

To examine the effects of the stress in this model, we evaluated the skin barrier recovery rates in male rats. For transepidermal water loss (TEWL) measurements in this study, we utilized the ears of the rats. Seventeen hours after immobilization stress, the basal TEWL and skin surface temperatures did not change in the stressed rats even after they received three consecutive days of immobilization stress in comparison with non-stressed controls. On the other hand, three hours after tape stripping, the percentage of barrier recovery was significantly lower in stressed animals than in the controls (Fig. 1). The effects of three days of stress were similar in female animals; i.e., barrier homeostasis gradually deteriorated over the following days. Both diazepam and chlorpromazine suppressed the electron cephalogram changes induced by immobilization stress in the rat (28) and chlorpromazine markedly inhibited the development of stress ulcer in pylorus-ligated rats (29). Application of the tranquilizers, chlorpromazine and diazepam, reverted the delay in barrier recovery in the immobilized animals. In contrast, the tranquilizers had no observable effect in control animals; i.e., basal TEWL levels in the tranquilized animals were the same as in untreated controls. These results suggest that emotional factors relate directly or indirectly to cutaneous barrier homeostasis.

The influence of immobilization stress on barrier recovery became more obvious with longer stress exposures (6 hrs/day for 3 days) than a short exposure

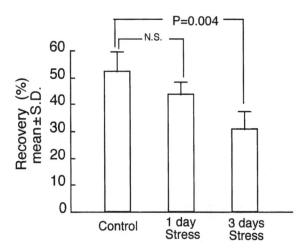

Figure 1   Three days of immobilization stress delayed barrier recovery in male rat ear skin 3 hrs after barrier disruption. On animals stressed for 1 day, the mean percentage barrier recovery was lower than in controls; however, no significant difference was observed. The ear skin was treated with tape stripping until transepidermal water loss reached $8.5 \pm 1.5\,\text{mg/cm}^2/\text{h}$. Values are mean $\pm$ SD. n $= 4$.

(6 hrs for 1 day, Fig. 1). These results suggest that the degree of stress produces a quantitative dose–response effect in barrier function.

Crowded Environment-Induced Stress

The crowded condition (i.e., high population density) has also been used as a psychological stress model. Lin et al. (30). demonstrated that it affected mouse plasma lipids and the development of very low-density lipoprotein (VLDL) + low-density (LDL) cholesterol levels by increasing the VLDL + LDL/high-density lipoprotein ratio and lesion severity. Their findings suggest that housing density can affect peripheral pathology.

Experiments were performed on the ears of the mice, assigned to three groups. One, five, or 10 mice were housed per cage ($22.5 \times 33.8\,\text{cm}$) for two weeks.

Whereas basal TEWL levels remained the same in each group, barrier recovery rates were significantly lower in the group in which 10 animals were kept together in the same cage for two weeks, than in animals kept under less-crowded conditions. In contrast, no significant difference was observed between group 1 (one animal per cage) and group 5 (five animals per cage) (Fig. 2). In hairless mice, housed five to a cage for 10 days, barrier recovery at three hours was very similar to animals housed one per cage for 10 days. In contrast, mice kept 10 to a cage for 10 days had a delay in barrier recovery. These results demonstrate that a prolonged crowded condition can alter permeability barrier homeostasis, as described above.

These results suggest that crowded living or working conditions can be psychologically stressful and can affect skin pathophysiology.

New Environment-Induced Stress (31)

As described above, both immobilization stress and crowded-environment stress affect skin barrier homeostasis. Here we describe another stress model, i.e., transfer

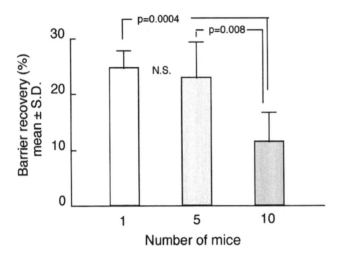

Figure 2 Population density affected barrier homeostasis in male mouse ear skin 3 hrs after tape stripping. The barrier recovery percentage in group 3 (10 animals per cage) was lower than that in group 2 (five animals per cage) and group 1 (one animal per cage). No significant difference was observed between groups 1 and 2. The ear skin was treated with tape stripping until transepidermal water loss reached $8.5 \pm 1.5 \, \mathrm{mg/cm^2/h}$. Values are mean $\pm$ SD. $n = 4$.

of mice to a new cage environment. Because this method is more convenient than the previous two methods described above, more in-depth investigations are possible into the responsible pathophysiology and mechanisms.

Five hairless mice were kept in the same cage ($22.5 \times 33.8 \, \mathrm{cm}$) together for 10–14 days under the same conditions. The animals were then moved to a different cage of the same size, material, and structure in the same room. Mice in the control group were handled in the same way and then returned to the same cage in which they had been kept initially.

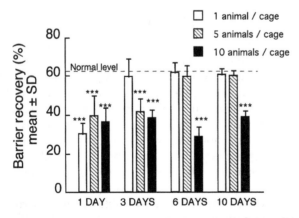

Figure 3 Delay of skin barrier recovery after tape stripping was induced by transferring hairless mice to a new cage. Hairless mice were kept five animals per cage for 10 days. Then one (open bars), five (hatched bars), or 10 (solid bars) mice were housed in an identical new cage for 1, 3, 6, or 10 days. Barrier disruption was achieved by tape stripping, and percent barrier recovery was measured at 3 hrs. Results are mean $\pm$SD. Dotted line indicates barrier recovery in mice kept five per cage for 11 days (normal recovery). $n = 5$–10, ***$P < 0.001$.

Basal TEWL did not change in any of the groups during the experimental period. In contrast, barrier recovery was delayed one day after transfer to a new cage, independent of the number of animals (Fig. 3). Yet the rate of normalization of barrier recovery after introduction to a new environment was influenced by the number of animals per cage. Whereas animals housed one per cage displayed normal barrier recovery by three days, animals housed five per cage required six days, and animals housed ten per cage did not display normal barrier recovery even after 10 days. After that, the delay in barrier recovery was dependent on purely the population density in the cage (Fig. 3).

Pre-treatment with chlorpromazine reversed the delay in barrier recovery induced by transferring animals to a new cage (Fig. 4). Hairless mice kept five animals per cage for 10 days were transferred to individual cages for one day. Thirty or forty minutes before changing cages, either chlorpromazine or saline (control) was injected intraperitoneally. Twenty-four hours after changing cages, barrier recovery rates were compared. Together these results suggest that even a change of environment can be sufficiently stressful to affect skin barrier homeostasis.

Metabolic Bases for the Barrier Abnormality

Psychological stress is well recognized to increase the plasma glucocorticoid levels in rodents. Here, we next evaluated plasma corticosterone levels of the mice in the experiments described in the section on new environment-induced stress. One day after transfer of animals to a new cage environment, plasma corticosterone levels were increased, and in animals maintained under crowded conditions, this increase persisted at least for six days (Fig. 5). Not only the stress-induced delay of barrier repair, but also the increase in plasma corticosterone could be blocked by pre-treatment with chlorpromazine, a tranquilizer (Fig. 6). Systemic administration of

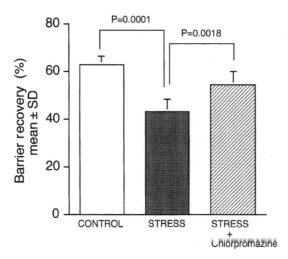

Figure 4 Pre-treatment with chlorpromazine reduced delay of barrier recovery induced by transferring animals to a new cage. Hairless mice were kept five animals per cage for 10 days and then transferred to individual cages for one day. Control animals were kept five animals per cage throughout the experiment. Thirty to forty minutes before changing animals to another cage, animals were injected intraperitoneally with either 8 mg/kg chlorpromazine or saline. Twenty-four hours after changing animals to a new cage, barrier was disrupted by tape stripping and percent barrier recovery was measured at 3 hrs. Results are mean ± SD. n = 5.

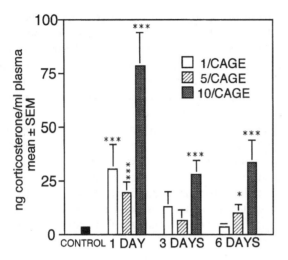

Figure 5 Plasma corticosterone levels in hairless mice increased one day after a change in environment. Hairless mice were kept five animals per cage for 10 days. Then one (open bars), five (hatched bars), or 10 (solid bars) mice were housed in an identical new cage for 1, 3, 6, or 10 days. Control animals were kept five animals per cage throughout the experiment. Data are presented as mean ± SE. n = 9–23, *P < 0.05, ***P < 0.001.

glucocorticoids also delay the barrier recovery. These results suggest that the stress-induced increase in corticosterone could be the metabolic basis for the alterations in barrier homeostasis.

To determine whether increased corticosterone production accounts for altered barrier homeostasis, we next treated animals with the glucocorticoid receptor

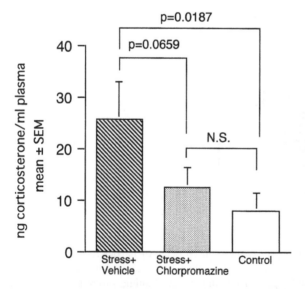

Figure 6 Chlorpromazine reduced the increase of plasma corticosterone levels in hairless mice after a change in environment. Control animals were kept five animals to a cage throughout the experiment. Plasma was obtained for corticosterone measurements 24 hrs after changing to a new cage. Data are presented as mean ± SE. n = 10.

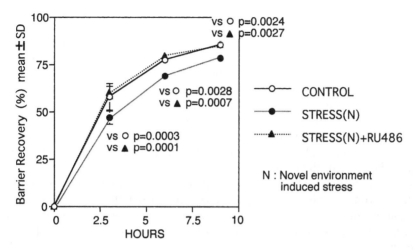

Figure 7 Glucocorticoid receptor antagonist, RU-486, blocked the delay of barrier recovery by novel environmental induced stress. Control animals were kept five animals per cage throughout the experiment. Barrier was disrupted by tape stripping. Results are mean ± SD. n = 5.

antagonist, RU-486. Systemic RU-486 administration did not alter either baseline TEWL or barrier recovery rate. However, RU-486 treatment blocked the delay of the barrier repair induced both by systemic corticosterone administration and by psychological stress induced by the change to a new cage (31) (Fig. 7). These results further suggest that glucocorticoids are an important mediator of the alterations in barrier homeostasis due to environment-induced psychological stress.

Recently, Kao et al. (32) demonstrated that short-term administration of either systemic or topical glucocorticoids to mice induced not only a delay in barrier recovery, but also abnormal stratum corneum intensity and cohesion. In steroid-treated mouse skin, decreased extracellular lamellar bilayers, corneodesmosome density, and lipid synthesis were observed. Topical co-applications of an equimolar mixture of ceramide, cholesterol, and free fatty acids, however, corrected the abnormality in barrier homeostasis, and to a large extent, the abnormality in stratum corneum intensity as well (32). These results suggest that even short-term exposure to a potent glucocorticoid detrimentally affects both barrier homeostasis and integrity of the stratum corneum, and that the metabolism basis is a decrease in epidermal lipid synthesis. Since increased endogenous glucocorticoid production is induced by a variety of different stressors, including trauma, surgery, infection, and inflammation, it is likely that barrier homeostasis, and its clinical corollaries such as wound healing, will be compromised in a wide variety of situations.

HUMAN EXPERIMENTS (33)

The animal models described above demonstrate the outline of the relationship between psychological stress and skin barrier homeostasis. However, to investigate the effects of prolonged psychological stress in humans, one should carry out analogous experiments with appropriate forms of stress. In the following two sections, two different types of human experiments are introduced.

Short Period of Stress

As a short period of mental stress for humans, the Stroop color–word conflict test was selected. The Stroop color–word conflict test is a mental stress test involving sensory rejection and has been used as a model of the defense reaction in humans (34). The Japanese words for "red," "blue," "green," and "yellow" are shown on paper in random order. The word is written in one of these four colors, but the name of the color and the color of the word are not necessarily the same. The subjects are instructed to recognize the color of a given word. The contradiction between the color of the word and the name of the color resulted in sensory rejection during cognitive processing of the color of the word.

Nine female subjects were used for the experiment. To monitor their psychological state, electron encephalograms were recorded during the examinations and especially contingent negative variation was evaluated as a signal of psychological stress (35). Contingent negative variation was larger in the stressed group than in the control subjects.

The barrier recovery rates of the subjects who took the Stroop color–word conflict test were lower than the rates in the control subjects, who did not take the test (33).

These results suggest that not only sustained stress, but also even a short period of mental stress can affect skin barrier homeostasis.

Long Period of Stress (36)

Chronic stress also affects human metabolism. In another model closely linked to daily life, Elias et al. demonstrated an impressive effect of long-term stress on skin barrier homeostasis. The skin barrier recovery rates were measured in 27 medical students immediately after winter vacation, six weeks after during their final examinations, and six weeks after during their spring vacation. Their psychological state was assessed using the perceived stress scale (PSS) and then by the profile of mood states (POMS). The PSS is a 14-item scale that assesses global perceptions of psychological stress, and measures the extent to which the subject appraises situations in her or his life as unpredictable, uncontrollable, and/or overloading. In contrast, the POMS consists of six individual subscales: Tension–Anxiety, Depression–Dejection, Anger–Hostility, Vigor–Activity, Fatigue–Inertia, and Confusion–Bewilderment. The total score of the POMS, referred to as total mood disturbance, represents a summation of the six subscale scores.

During the examination (high stress) period, the barrier recovery rates after tape stripping were slower than rates both after winter vacation and during the spring vacation (Fig. 8). Both the psychological tests showed the highest score of stress during the examination (Fig. 9). These studies provide a link between sustained psychological stress and skin barrier homeostasis.

Several type of dermatitis, such as atopic dermatitis, contact dermatitis, and psoriasis, are anecdotally provoked by enhanced psychological stress. Moreover, these disorders are also often triggered, sustained, or exacerbated by external physical insults to the epidermis. These insults, in turn, are known to lead to enhanced synthesis and release of cytokines from the epidermis. Moreover, epidermal hyperplasia, Langerhans cell activity, and inflammation develop rapidly following these insults. Thus, psychological stress could change the threshold for induction of cytokine release after physical insults, or it could simply prolong the recovery from such an insult.

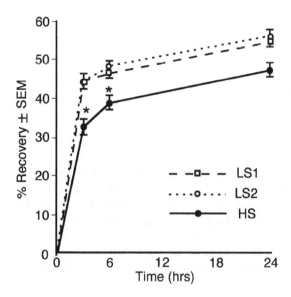

Figure 8 The mean percentage of permeability barrier recovery at three, six, and 24 hrs during the indicated psychological stress period. LS1 indicates low stress 1 (shortly after returning from winter vacation); HS, high stress (during final examination week); and LS2, low stress 2 (shortly after returning home from spring vacation).

Recently several models of stress and barrier recovery were reported. Altemus et al. (37) demonstrated that sleep deprivation and interview-induced stress also delayed the skin barrier recovery. Muizzuddin et al. (38) evaluated effects of marital dissolution–induced stress on the barrier function. They could not observe any

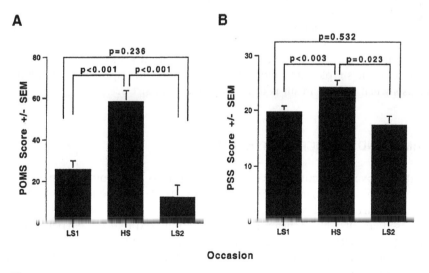

Figure 9 (A) Total mood disturbance on the profile of mood states (POMS). (B) Mean Perceived Stress Scale (PSS) scores for students during the indicated psychological stress period. The P values refer to the results of the post hoc tests. LS1 indicates low stress 1 (shortly after returning from winter vacation); HS, high stress (during final examination week); and LS2, low stress 2 (shortly after returning home from spring vacation).

correlation between the degree of stress and barrier recovery rate. Subjects with high stress showed slower barrier recovery than the subjects with low stress.

EFFECT OF ODORANT INHALATION ON BARRIER HOMEOSTASIS (39)

As described above, psychological stress–induced delay of the barrier repair was blocked by application of sedative drugs. On the other hand, olfactory stimulation can prolong the sleep time induced by pentobarbital administration in mice, and in some cases can itself act as a tranquilizer. Terpinyl acetate, phenythyl alcohol, dimethoxymethylbenzene (DMMB), and valerian oil each have a sedative effect, while lemon oil, jasmine oil, and phytol shorten the sleeping time (40–43). From these results, we hypothesized that inhalation of certain odorants could mitigate the psychological stress–induced deterioration of the skin barrier homeostasis.

Experiments were based on the new cage environment–induced stress described in the section on new environment-induced stress above. Five hairless mice were kept together in the same cage for 10 days. Then, each mouse was moved individually to a new cage with the same size, material, structure, and location in which it had been kept previously. One day before and after the change of cages, a plastic dish with a metal net, which included one odorant each, was placed in the cage. The mice in the control group were handled similarly, but returned to the cage in which they had been kept. A sham plastic dish covered with a metal net without odorant was placed in the cage of the control animals, which were not exposed to odorants. When we placed an odorant with a sedative effect in the animal's cage before and after moving the animals, the delay of the barrier recovery was significantly reversed. In contrast, an odorant that did not have a sedative effect did not reverse the delay in barrier repair induced by a change in environment (Fig. 10). We next evaluated the effects of the odorant in humans. The stress model based on the experiment was the Stroop color–word conflict test. A sedative odorant, DMMB was inhaled during the stress test. As shown in Figure 11, sedative odorant inhalation blocked the delay of the barrier repair induced by a short period of mental stress.

There are various methods to mitigate psychological stress. Yet, odorant inhalation is one of the simplest and most effective methods to improve the skin barrier homeostasis when the organism is under psychological stress.

EPIDERMIS AND ENDOCRINE SYSTEM

As described above, glucocorticoids play a crucial role as mediators between psychological condition and epidermal barrier homeostasis. Testosterone also affects the skin barrier homeostasis. Kao et al. (44) demonstrated that application of testosterone decreased lamellar body formation and secretion, and that the barrier recovery was delayed. Application of androgen receptor antagonist, flutamide, accelerated the barrier recovery in normal male mice. Previously, circadian alteration of the human barrier repair rate was reported (45). The alterations in barrier repair were independent of changes in the endogenous cortisol. Moreover, a previous report suggested that corticotropin-releasing factor might affect epidermal homeostasis (46). Potentially, a variety of endocrinological factors affect skin barrier homeostasis under various psychological conditions.

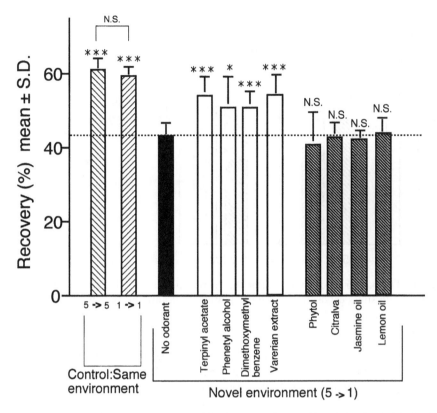

Figure 10 Inhalation of odorants, which have a sedative effect (*open bars*), blocked the delay of skin barrier recovery induced by a change of cages in hairless mice. Three hours after tape stripping, percentage recovery was evaluated. The dotted line shows the barrier recovery of the animals after a change of cages without any odorant inhalation. Respectively, 5→5 and 1→1 show the barrier recovery of animals which were kept continuously five per cage and one per cage respectively. In the new environment (5→1) animals were first kept five together per cage and then in a new cage separately one per cage. n = 5; *P < 0.05, ***P < 0.005. NS, not significant.

EPIDERMIS AND NEUROTRANSMITTERS

Not only endocrine factors, but also neural factors might influence the epidermal barrier homeostasis. Substance P influenced the ion distribution in the epidermis (46). Topical application of adrenergic β2-receptor agonists delayed the barrier repair, while antagonists of the receptor accelerated the barrier recovery (47). These results suggest that peripheral nerves or autonomic system is involved in the epidermal barrier homeostasis.

Ectoderm-derived central nerve cells and epidermal keratinocytes have similar components. Existence of receptors, such as cholinergic (48), purinergic (49), glutamate (50), GABA (51), and dopaminergic receptors (52), which were originally found in nerve cells, was reported in epidermal keratinocytes. Interestingly, most of them are involved in the skin barrier homeostasis. Topical application of nicotine, agonist of cholinergic receptor, delayed the barrier recovery and the delay was blocked by the receptor-specific antagonist (48). Agonist of purinergic receptor, ATP (49) and agonist

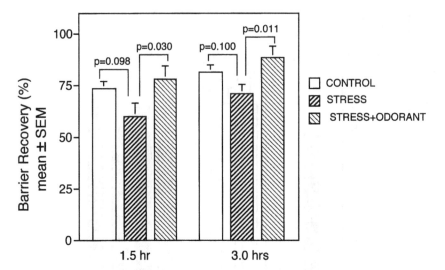

Figure 11 The barrier recovery rate after the barrier disruption. The barrier recovery rate was delayed with stress exposure and the delay was significantly blocked by the odorant.

of glutamate, NMDA (50) also delayed the barrier recovery. On the other hand, application of GABA accelerated barrier repair (51). Ion dynamics through these receptors play a crucial role in the barrier homeostasis. Further work is needed in this area.

CONCLUSION

In today's world, people often confront psychologically stressful situations. Drastic alteration of working and living conditions by modern technology, unstable economy, and friction between people of different backgrounds, potentially cause psychological stress.

The studies described in this chapter suggest that one mechanism by which stress could exacerbate skin disorders is to perturb permeability barrier homeostasis. Additionally, these studies suggest that the stress-induced stimulation of glucocorticoids by pathways that remain to be elucidated plays an important role in these alterations in permeability barrier homeostasis. Reduction of psychological stress by a sedative drug or odorant might be effective for barrier homeostasis under the stress (Fig. 12).

A number of common dermatologic disorders, including atopic dermatitis, psoriasis, and dyshindrotic eczema, are exacerbated by psychological stress. Alteration in permeability barrier function frequently occurs in these disorders, and by stimulating cytokine production and inducing epidermal hyperplasia, barrier function may trigger or sustain these cutaneous abnormalities. Stress reduction has been shown to accelerate barrier repair after the barrier disruption. It therefore may be possible to improve or ameliorate certain disorders by specifically blocking the pathways by which stress produces defects in permeability barrier homeostasis. This strategy could result in novel therapeutic approaches to treat cutaneous disorders.

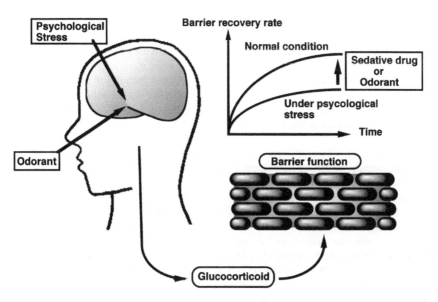

Figure 12 Scheme of the process between psychological stress and skin barrier function. Psychological stress increases glucocorticoid levels in serum and delays skin barrier recovery. Reduction of the stress by sedative drug or odorant reduces the delay of barrier recovery by the stress.

ACKNOWLEDGMENT

Most of our studies on stress presented in this chapter were carried out with helpful suggestions by Drs. Kenneth R. Feingold and Peter M. Elias. Some of the figures in this chapter were kindly provided by Dr. Peter M. Elias.

REFERENCES

1. Grice KA. Transepidermal water loss in pathologic skin. In: Jarrett A, ed. The Physiology and Pathophysiology of the Skin. London: Academic Press, 1980:2147–2155.
2. Wood LC, Jackson SM, Elias PM, Feingold KR. Cutaneous barrier perturbation stimulates cytokine production in the epidermis of mice. J Clin Invest 1992; 90:482–487.
3. Proksch E, Feingold KR, Man MQ, Elias PM. Barrier function regulates epidermal DNA synthesis. J Clin Invest 1991; 87:1668–1673.
4. Denda M, Wood LC, Emami S, Calhoun C, Brown BE, Elias PM, Feingold KR. The epidermal hyperplasia associated with repeated barrier disruption by acetone treatment or tape stripping cannot be attributed to increased water loss. Arch Dermatol Res 1996; 288:230–238.
5. Denda M, Sato J, Tsuchiya T, Elias PM, Feingold KR. Low humidity stimulates epidermal DNA synthesis and amplifies the hyperproliferative response to barrier disruption: implication for seasonal exacerbations of inflammatory dermatoses. J Invest Dermatol 1998; 111:873–878.
6. Glaser R, Kiecolt-Glaser JK, Speicher C. Stress, loneliness, and changes in herpesvirus latency. J Behav Med 1985; 8:249–260.
7. Glaser R, Rice J, Sheridan J. Stress-related immune suppression: health implications. Brain Behav Immun 1987; 1:7–20.

8. Glaser R, Kiecolt-Glaser JK, Malarkey WB, Sheridan JF. The influence of psychological stress on immune response to vaccines. Ann NY Acad Sci 1998; 840:649–655.

9. Palmblad KE. Stress-related modulation of immunity: a review of human studies. Cancer Detect Prev 1987; 1:57–64.

10. O'leary A. Stress, emotion, and human immune function. Psychol Bull 1990; 108:363–382.

11. Bonneau RH, Sheridan JF, Feng NG, Glaser R. Stress-induced suppression of herpes simplex virus (HSV)-specific cytotoxic T lymphocyte and natural killer cell activity and enhancement of acute pathogenesis following local HSV infection. Brain Behav Immun 1991; 5:170–194.

12. Kiecolt-Glaser JK, Glaser R, Gravenstein S, Malarkey WB, Sheridan J. Chronic stress alters the immune response to influenza virus vaccine in older adults. Proc Natl Acad Sci USA 1996; 93:3043–3047.

13. Sheridan JF, Dobbs C, Jung J. Stress-induced neuroendocrine modulation of viral pathogens and immunity. Ann NY Acad Sci 1998; 840:803–808.

14. Shavit Y, Terman GW, Martin FC, Lewis JW, Liebeskind JC, Gala RP. Stress, opioid peptides, the immune system, and cancer. J Immunol 1985; 135:827–834.

15. Spiegel D, Bloom JR, Kraemer HC, Gottheil E. Effect of psychological treatment on survival of patients with metastatic breast cancer. Lancet 1989; 2:888–891.

16. Spiegel D, Sephton SE, Terr AL, Stites DP. Effects of psychological treatment in prolonging cancer may be mediated by neuroimmune pathways. Ann NY Acad Sci 1998; 840:674–683.

17. Fawzy KI, Fawzy NW, Hyun A. Malignant melanoma: effects of an early structured psychiatric intervention, coping, and affective state on recurrence and survival 6 years later. Arch Gen Psychiatry 1993; 50:681–689.

18. Seville RH. Psoriasis and stress. Br J Dermatol 1977; 97:297–302.

19. Fava GA, Perini GI, Santonastaso P, Fornasa CV. Life events and psychological distress in dermatologic disorders: psoriasis, chronic urticaria and fungal infections. Br J Med Psychol 1980; 53:277–282.

20. Savin JA. Cotterill psychocutaneous disorders. In: Champion RH, Burton JL, Ebling FJG, eds. Textbook of Dermatology. Oxford: Blackwell Scientific Publications, 1992.

21. Gaston L, Lassonde M, Bernier-Buzzabga J, Hodgins S, Crombez JC. Psoriasis and stress: a perspective study. J Am Acad Dermatol 1987; 17:82–87.

22. Albadie MS, Kent GG, Gawkrodger DJ. The relationship between stress and the onset and excerbation of psoriasis and other skin conditions. Br J Dermatol 1994; 130:199–203.

23. Kodama A, Horikawa T, Suzuki T, Ajiki W, Takashima T, Harada S, Ichihashi M. Effect of stress on atopic dermatitis: investigation in patients after the great Hanshin earthquake. J Allergy Clin Immunol 1999; 104:173–176.

24. Denda M, Tsuchiya T, Hosoi J, Koyama J. Immobilization-induced and crowded environment-induced stress delay barrier recovery in murine skin. Br J Dermatol 1998; 138:780–785.

25. Pare WP, Glavin GB. Restraint stress in biomedical research: a review. Neurosci Biobehav Rev 1986; 10:339–370.

26. Tsuchiya T, Horii I. Immobilization induced stress decreases lipogenesis in sebaceous glands as well as plasma testosterone levels in male Syrian hamsters. Psychoneuroendocrinology 1996; 20:211–230.

27. Tsuchiya T, Horii I. Epidermal cell proliferative activity assessed by proliferating cell nuclear antigen (PCNA) decrease following immobilization-induced stress in male Syrian hamsters. Psychoneuroendocrinology 1996; 21:111–117.

28. Iwata N, Mikuni N. EEG change in the conscious rat during immobility induced by psychological stress. Psychopharmacology 1980; 71:117–122.

29. Takeuchi K, Okabe S, Takagi K. A new model of stress ulcer in the rat with pylous ligation and its pathogenesis. Dig Dis 1976; 21:782–788.

30. Lin AH, Castle CK, Melchiol GW, Marotti KR. The effect of population density on development of experimental atherosclerosis in female mice. Atherosclerosis 1995; 115:85 88.

31. Denda M, Tsuchiya T, Elias PM, Feingold KR. Stress alters cutaneous permeability barrier homeostasis. Am J Physiol 2000; 278:R367–R372.

32. Kao JS, Fluhr JW, Man MQ, Fowler AJ, Hachem JP, Crumrine D, Ahn SK, Brown BE, Elias PM, Feingold KR. Short-term glucocorticoid treatment compromises both permeability barrier homeostasis and stratum corneum integrity: inhibition of epidermal lipid synthesis accounts for functional abnormalities. J Invest Dermatol 2003; 120:456–464.

33. Denda M, Tanida M, Shoji K, Tsuchiya T. Inhalation of a sedative odorant prevents the delay in cutaneous barrier repair induced by psychological stress. Auton Nerv Syst 2000; 37:419–424.

34. Hoshikawa Y, Yamamoto Y. Effects of Stroop color–word conflict test on the autonomic nervous system responses. Am J Physiol 1997; 272:H1113–H1121.

35. Grey WW, Cooper R, Aldridge VJ, McCallum WC, Winter AL. Contingent negative variation: an electric sign of sensorimotor association and expectancy in the human brain. Nature 1964; 203:380–384.

36. Garg A, Chren M, Sands LP, Matsui MS, Marenus KD, Feingold KR, Elias PM. Psychological stress perturbs epidermal barrier homeostasis. Arch Dermatol 2001; 137: 53–59.

37. Altemus M, Rao B, Dhabhar FS, Ding W, Granstein RD. Stress-induced changes in skin barrier function in healthy women. J Invest Dermatol 2001; 117:309–317.

38. Muizzuddin N, Matsui MS, Marenus KD, Maes DH. Impact of stress of marital dissolution on skin barrier recovery: tape stripping and measurement of trans-epidermal water loss (TEWL). Skin Res Technol 2003; 9:34–38.

39. Denda M, Tsuchiya T, Shoji K, Tanida M. Odorant inhalation affects skin barrier homeostasis in mice and humans. Br J Dermatol 2000; 142:1007–1010.

40. Tsuchiya T, Tanida M, Uenoyama S, Ozawa T. Effects of olfactory stimulation on the sleep time induced by pentobarbital administration in mice. Brain Res Bull 1991; 26:397–401.

41. Tsuchiya T, Tanida M, Uenoyama S. Effects of olfactory stimulation with jasmine and its component chemicals on the duration of pentobarbital-induced sleep in mice. Life Sci 1992; 50:1097–1102.

42. Joichi A, Yomogida K, Nakamura S. The scent of roses: tea-scented modern roses and ancient Chinese roses. Proceedings of the 20th International Federation of the Societies of Cosmetic Chemists (Cannes) [Abstr]. September 1998:83.

43. Warren CB, Munteanu MA, Schwartz GE. Method of causing in the reduction of physiological and/or subjective reactivity to stress in humans being subjected to stress conditions. US Patent No. 4671959, 9 June 1987.

44. Kao JS, Garg A, Man MQ, Crumurine D, Ghadially R, Feingold KR, Elias PM. Testosterone perturbs epidermal permeability homeostasis. J Invest Dermatol 2001; 116: 443–451.

45. Denda M, Tsuchiya T. Barrier recovery rate varies time-dependently in human skin. Br J Dermatol 2000; 142:881–884.

46. Denda M, Ashida Y, Inoue K, Kumazawa N. Skin surface electric potential induced by ion-flux through epidermal cell layers. Biochem Biophys Res Commun 2001; 284:112–117.

47. Denda M, Fuziwara S, Inoue K. Beta-2-adrenergic receptor antagonist accelerates skin barrier recovery and reduces epidermal hyperplasia induced by barrier disruption. J Invest Dermatol 2003; 121:142–148.

48. Denda M, Fuziwara S, Inoue K. Influx of calcium and chloride ions into epidermal keratinocytes regulates exocytosis of epidermal lamellar bodies and skin permeability barrier homeostasis. J Invest Dermatol 2003; 121:362–367.

49. Denda M, Inoue K, Fuziwara S, Denda S. P2X purinergic receptor antagonist accelerates skin barrier repair and prevents epidermal hyperplasia induced by skin barrier disruption. J Invest Dermatol 2002; 119:1034–1040.

50. Fuziwara S, Inoue K, Denda M. NMDA-type glutamate receptor is associated with cutaneous barrier homeostasis. J Invest Dermatol 2003; 120:1023–1029.

51. Denda M, Inoue K, Inomata S, Denda S. GABA (A) receptor agonists accelerate cutaneous barrier recovery and prevent epidermal hyperplasia induced by barrier disruption. J Invest Dermatol 2002; 119:1041–1047.

52. Fuziwara S, Suzuki A, Inoue K, Denda M. Dopamine D2-like receptor agonists accelerate barrier repair and inhibit the epidermal hyperplasia indiced by barrier disruption. J Inverst Dermatol 2005 in press.

32

The Stratum Corneum of the Epidermis in Atopic Dermatitis

Jens-Michael Jensen and Ehrhardt Proksch
*Department of Dermatology, University Hospitals of Schleswig-Holstein,
Campus Kiel, Kiel, Germany*

Peter M. Elias
*Dermatology Service, VA Medical Center, and Department of Dermatology,
University of California, San Francisco, U.S.A.*

Atopic dermatitis (AD) is an inflammatory disease clinically characterized by marked pruritus, which typically assumes a chronic, relapsing course. AD affects 10% to 20% of the current U.S. population (1). In Asian populations, the incidence of AD exceeds 50% (2). Although AD is primarily a childhood disease, 60% to 70% of adults with AD suffer from more localized disease manifestations, such as hand eczema. The past three decades have witnessed a marked rise in the prevalence of atopic diseases in industrialized countries, and urban centers in less developed regions. This has led to an intense search for etiological factors that may explain such a pattern. A precise understanding of the genetic background and the disease pathophysiology is crucial to the development of effective treatment strategies for AD. An impaired stratum corneum (SC) and barrier function may be important for the pathophysiology of AD.

NORMAL STRATUM CORNEUM: COMPOSITION AND FUNCTION

The SC, the outermost layer of a keratinizing epithelium, protects terrestrial mammals from water loss and noxious physical, chemical, and microbial insults. This barrier between the body and the environment is constantly maintained by reproduction of inner living epidermal keratinocytes, which undergo a process of terminal differentiation and then migrate to the surface as SC cells. These cells provide the mechanical protection, and, together with their intercellular lipid surroundings, confer water-impermeability. A part of the barrier function is provided by the cornified cell envelope (CE), a protein/lipid polymer structure which is formed just below the cytoplasmic membrane and subsequently resides on the exterior of the cornified cells. It consists of a protein and a lipid envelope. The protein envelope is believed to contribute to the biomechanical properties of the CE as a result of the cross-linking of specialized CE structural proteins by both disulfide bonds and $N(\varepsilon)$-(γ-glutamyl)lysine isopeptide bonds formed by transglutaminases. Some of the structural proteins involved include involucrin, loricrin, small proline rich proteins, keratin intermediate filaments, elafin, cystatin A, and desmosomal proteins. The lipid envelope is located on the exterior of, and is covalently attached by ester bonds to, the protein envelope and consists of a monomolecular layer of ω-hydroxyceramides. The monomolecular ω-hydroxyceramide layer interdigitates with the intercellular lipid lamellae, perhaps in a Velcro-like fashion. A number of diseases which display defective epidermal barrier function, in particular the ichthyoses, are the result of genetic defects in either the synthesis of CE proteins, the transglutaminase 1 cross-linking enzyme, or the defective metabolism of skin lipids (3). The lipid composition is also crucially involved in stratum corneum structure and function as described in detail elsewhere.

ATOPIC DERMATITIS: GENETICS

A genetically impaired epidermal barrier has been proposed to be the primary cause of the rapid increase in the prevalence of AD and respiratory atopy. The subsequently increased exposure to irritants and allergens postnatally in predisposed individuals would lead, in a subset of these, to a specific TH2 cell activation favoring the development of IgE responses to atopens (4). Also, ichthyosis vulgaris, an autosomal dominant disorder causing defective epidermal filaggrin expression, is present in approximately 4% of AD cases. Due to the myriad of overlapping phenotypes, identification of a specific phenotype associated with AD is not yet possible. Predisposing genes may be present on the X-chromosome, as the incidence of AD in offspring of atopic mothers is significant. Mild asthma and AD is frequently related to X-linked hypohydrotic ectodermal dysplasia (5,6). Wiskott–Aldrich's syndrome, another syndrome linked to the X-chromosome, involves immunological deficiencies, low platelet counts, and co-morbid eczema. Although Wiskott–Aldrich patients have a relatively competent immune function, their immune system selectively attacks certain antigens, suggesting deficiencies in antigen presentation and processing (7,8). Eczema in Wiskott–Aldrich patients is clinically similar to AD and, as in AD, frequently evolves into eczema herpeticum manifesting in varicelliform eruptions.

A genetic propensity to AD can lead to decreased serine protease inhibitor (SPI) activity, as occurs in Netherton's syndrome, leading to increased serine-protease activity. Netherton's syndrome is a disease which is characterized by a profound permeability barrier abnormality and an AD-like dermatosis (9–13). Netherton's syndrome is caused by mutations in the SPINK 5 gene, which encodes the serine protease inhibitor pro-protein lympho-epithelial Kazal-type inhibitor 1 (LEKTI 1). LEKTI 1 is a marker of epithelial differentiation, strongly expressed in the granular and uppermost spinous layers of the epidermis, and in differentiated layers of stratified epithelia (14). In contrast to other SPI activities, such as those of elafin, PAI 2, and SLPI, this SPI is not found in the cornified envelope, and it is thought to be the major initiator of SCTE. In two recent studies, several independent panels of families with atopic diathesis (with and without AD) were found to have a single nucleotide polymorphism (SNP) in the SPINK 5 gene (11,15). Whether the SNPs for SPINK 5 in AD result in a loss of function and mutations in LEKTI 1, and therefore an increased sp (scte), is not known. SPI has also been shown to alleviate severe AD and induce barrier recovery after experimental barrier disruption (16,17). Western blotting revealed the degradation of desmoglein 1, a corneodesmosome structural protein, after rapid activation of serine proteases, which was followed by serine-protease–mediated degradation of corneodesmosomes (18).

Climate, ethnic background, and migration patterns may also contribute to the manifestation of atopic symptoms. It is suggested that the barrier function–driven cytokine cascade is always active regardless of the disease state, as atopic patients display an abnormal barrier function in uninvolved as well as involved skin (19–21). In examining AD manifestation in Asian populations, Denda et al. (22) demonstrated a connection between asymptomatic and subclinical disease states and residence in humid, tropical climates. With migration to different climate zones, previously asymptomatic patients were shown to suddenly develop AD symptoms. Mar et al. (2) contrasted genetic differences and environmental influences in the clinical expression of AD, reporting that many individuals predisposed to AD due to their genetic backgrounds may never accommodate to occupational or topical irritants due to favorable environmental conditions.

ATOPIC DERMATITIS: FUNCTION

Barrier Integrity and TEWL

In addition to inflammation and immunological abnormalities, AD is characterized by impaired SC differentiation and barrier function, resulting in scaling, roughness, and xerosis of the skin. A defective skin permeability barrier function is an accepted element of AD. Atopic patients display abnormal barrier function, and a 2-to 5-fold increase in basal TEWL, in both lesional and non-lesional skin (23,24). Severe barrier abnormalities may result from scratching, which removes parts of the stratum corneum (25). In contrast, TEWL levels and stratum corneum water content became normal in patients free from AD symptoms for more than five years (26). Abnormality in skin barrier function is often regarded as a consequence of inflammation (27). However, even in the asymptomatic skin of atopics, disturbance of epidermal barrier function promotes penetration. A lifestyle modification such as excessive use of detergents and shampoos removes skin lipids, irritates the skin, and impairs barrier function (28). Finally, psychological stress has been shown to increase skin irritability and abnormal barrier function (29–32). Disturbances in barrier function enable aeroallergens to penetrate the skin more easily, perpetuating the cycle of eczematous lesions (25,33).

Hydration

Dry skin surface and reduced water-holding capacity are hallmarks of AD (34,35). Even unaffected skin of atopic patients is universally recognized as dry and scaly. Changes in epidermal lipids and disruptions in epidermal differentiation have been shown to produce dry skin, while SC lipids are essential in regulating bound-water modulation (36–38). Atopic xerotic skin demonstrates higher TEWL and significantly lower surface hydration levels than healthy skin (39), which correlates with the lower content of molecules with water-retaining capacity in the superficial SC; e.g., the accelerated degradation of filaggrin into pyrolidone carboxyl acid and other disseminated amino acid humectants may contribute to dry skin conditions (40).

Reduced stratum corneum hydration in AD has been described in numerous publications (41–44). We found that hydration was significantly reduced in non-lesional (–24.5%) as well as lesional (–39.1%) epidermis of AD compared to controls (24). Recently, it has been proposed that residual detergents in cotton clothes may be a causative factor of deterioration of dry skin in winter in AD (45). An important goal in topical application of emollients is to increase stratum corneum hydration (46,47). Besides lipid-based water-containing emulsions, water-binding compounds like glycerol or urea are included to enhance hydration (48,49).

pH

Like other inflammatory dermatoses, AD shows an increase in surface pH (50). A higher pH leads to increased activity of serine protease, and SC chymotryptic and tryptic enzymes which regulate the SC integrity and cohesion (51,52). These proteases are also able to activate cytokines, which leads to premature corneo-desmosome lysis and degradation of constituent proteins, such as desmoglein 1 and corneodesmosine. SC neutralization not only leads to the activation of primary cytokines like interleukin 1-α but also involves inflammatory responses (53). Hachem et al. (18) demonstrated that SC neutralization alone provokes stratum corneum functional abnormalities, including abnormal permeability barrier homeostasis and decreased stratum corneum integrity and cohesion (18).

BASIS FOR BARRIER ABNORMALITIES

A well-maintained SC is critical for a functional skin barrier. The architecture of the SC, containing the lipid-depleted corneocytes and highly lipid-enriched extracellular bilayers, enables it to function as a border between the dry environment and the water-enriched organism. Abnormalities in the skin barrier result in an enhanced TEWL in one direction, and increased penetration of harmful substances from the environment into the skin in the other. This triggers the immune system, stimulating a cascade of cytokines and other mediators for repairing the physical barrier as well as influencing the innate and adaptive immune systems (54,55). Nevertheless, anti-microbial resistance is reduced in AD (56). Psychological stress, an inevitable factor of AD, results in further disturbance of the skin barrier (31,57). Even in "uninvolved" skin, AD patients display abnormal skin barrier function, which can persist for years after the disease has become dormant (24,58–60). It is possible that subclinical disease persists in sites with low-grade skin barrier abnormalities, mostly accompanied by xerotic skin conditions. The extent of the permeability barrier defect in AD largely correlates with the severity of the disease (34,61).

Lipids

The skin's primary permeability layer, the SC, composed of extracellular lipids and corneocytes, is formed during epidermal differentiation (62–66). In AD, a global reduction of SC lipid content has been identified as being potentially responsible for permeability barrier abnormalities. Older studies have shown that skin surface lipids, which are partially derived from sebaceous glands (depending on the method by which surface lipids are obtained) and different from the keratinocyte-derived barrier lipids, are significantly and consistently lower in AD patients than in normal controls, or in patients with ichthyosis vulgaris, suggesting a decrease in total SC lipids (67,68). The overall decrease in skin surface lipids in AD, as determined by the Sebumeter® (Courage & Khazaka, Cologne, Germany), has recently been confirmed (43). Mustakallio et al. (69) further characterized and quantified epidermal lipids in AD with thin-layer chromatography. Full-thickness epidermal sheets were obtained by the suction blister method during the winter months from the volar aspect of non-lichenified forearm skin of 12 patients with Besnier's prurigo (chronic, lichenified AD). As compared with epidermis from normal controls of the same age, AD epidermis displayed a decrease in total lipids, phospholipids, and sterol esters, as well as a relative increase in free fatty acids and free sterols. It is likely, based upon more recent work (see below), that the observed decrease in phospholipids reflects a decrease in sphingolipid content, specifically sphingomyelin. As sphingomyelin is a ubiquitous molecule essential for cell membrane function, a direct quantitative analysis of sphingomyelin content changes is rather difficult. The phospholipid and fatty acid content of lesional versus non-lesional epidermis was determined by Schäfer and Kragballe (70), who found increased activity of phospholipase A_2 and an incomplete transformation of phospholipids into other lipid classes in AD.

The three main classes of lipids form the lamellar membrane bilayers, which mediate the permeability barrier (62,71). Several studies have shown that SC cholesterol, ceramides, and free fatty acid content are all decreased in AD, but the most pronounced deficiency is in ceramides (38,72,73). In dry, non-eczematous skin of AD, Fartasch et al. (74) has described a disturbed extrusion of lamellar bodies, which could be responsible for the global decrease in SC lipids. Ceramides normally account for about 50% of SC lipids (by weight); cholesterol and free fatty acids represent together the other 50%, with less than 5% derived from other lipids (75).

The functions and requirements of specific SC ceramide types for skin barrier function in general, and for AD specifically, are not yet fully understood. Nine ceramide subclasses have been identified in human SC (76–79). Reduced ceramide 1 in the SC of clinically dry skin of AD without signs of eczema was described by Yamamoto et al. (80). Significantly lower levels of ceramide 1 and 3, and higher levels of cholesterol were found in lesional AD skin versus control subjects (73). The decrease in ceramide 3 significantly correlated with the degree of barrier impairment. A reduced amount of total ceramides and ceramide 1 was also found in the SC of atopic dry skin by Matsumoto et al. (81). Although the content of ceramide 2, 3, 4 plus 5, and 6 was also reduced, the differences were not of statistical significance.

In addition to free ceramides, covalently bound ceramides are also important for epidermal barrier homeostasis. The phospholipid-enriched plasma membrane is replaced by a ceramide-containing membrane bilayer during the process of cornification. This bilayer then attaches covalently to involucrin, envoplakin, and periplakin moieties on the extracellular surface of the cornified envelope by ω-hydroxyester bonds (75,82). The amount of covalently bound ceramides correlates with TEWL (as marker for skin permeability barrier function) levels (83). The levels of covalently bound ceramides have recently been determined in AD (84). While in healthy SC, ~50% of protein-bound lipids are ω-hydroxyceramides, in non-lesional and lesional AD, this proportion significantly declines to ~25% and ~15%, respectively. Furthermore, Macheleidt found that the amount of free extractable very long chain fatty acids with more than 24 carbon atoms was reduced in non-lesional SC and even more significantly reduced in lesional skin. In agreement with these results, metabolic labeling studies with [^{14}C]-serine in cultured epidermis revealed decreased biosynthesis of glucosylceramides and free ceramides in lesional skin of AD compared to in normal controls. In particular, the synthesis of ceramides containing very long chain N-acyl ω-hydroxy-fatty acids esterified with linoleic acid and 6-hydroxysphingosine as sphingoid base (ceramide 1, 4, and possibly 9) was reduced along with that of ceramides consisting of a non-hydroxy N-acyl fatty acid and phytosphingosine (ceramide 2 and 3). Based on this evidence, a defective corneocyte-bound lipid envelope, due to the increased in situ degradation of bound ceramides, could contribute to the abnormalities in hydration and barrier function in AD.

Alternatively, Bleck et al. (85) found two mono-hydroxylated and mono-unsaturated ceramide sub-fractions of different chain-length, containing C_{16} or C_{18} or C_{22}, C_{24}, C_{26} α-hydroxy fatty acids in whole SC of non-lesional skin in AD, using matrix-assisted laser desorption ionization time-of-flight (MALDI-TOF) mass spectrometry. In contrast, only a single peak occurred in the SC ceramides from senile xerosis, psoriasis, and seborrheic dermatitis. The authors suggested that an increase of a short chain Cer(AS) sub-fraction in non-lesional skin in AD may be a disease marker (85). It is worth noting that the relative amounts of all other SC lipid classes in AD, including squalene, cholesterol esters, triglycerides, free fatty acids, cholesterol, cholesterol sulfate, and phospholipids, did not differ significantly from controls in this study (80).

In contrast to data on ceramide metabolism, little is known about the activity of cholesterol and fatty acid–generating enzymes in AD. Epidermal ceramides derive from de novo synthesis by serine palmitoyl transferase as the rate-limiting enzyme, or by the hydrolysis of both glucosylceramides (β-glucocerebrosidase) and sphingomyelin (acid sphingomyelinase) (86–89). These precursors are degraded by ceramidase and a recently described enzyme called sphingomyelin deacylase (90). Due to the invasive nature of such studies and the sample size needed for such experiments, rates of ceramide synthesis and activity of serine palmitoyl transferase in the epidermis of AD have not yet been determined. In contrast, it has proven easier to examine hydrolytic enzymes, because their levels peak in the SC. Jin et al. (91) examined β-glucocerebrosidase and ceramidase activities in the SC of AD and age-related dry skin. As they did not find differences in either β-glucocerebrosidase or ceramidase activities in uninvolved SC of AD, the decrease of ceramides in AD could not be attributed to increased ceramide degradation. Likewise, Redoules et al. (92) confirmed the presence of unchanged β-glucocerebrosidase activity in the SC from non-eczematous dry skin of AD. Of the five enzymatic activities examined by these authors, AD displayed significantly reduced trypsin activity, increased acid phosphatase activity, and no changes in either secreted phospholipase A_2 or chymotryptic protease activity.

The epidermis contains two sphingomyelinase isoenzymes: acid sphingomyelinase, localized in epidermal lamellar bodies, which generates ceramides for the extracellular lipid bilayers of the SC; and neutral sphingomyelinase, important for cell signaling during permeability barrier repair (93). Kusuda et al. (94) measured the localization and amount of acid sphingomyelinase in lesional skin of AD. The authors generated a polyclonal antibody and found immunostaining extending from the upper spinous cell layers to the upper SC. Moreover, total amounts of enzyme protein measured by quantitative immunoblot analysis slightly increased in lesional versus non-lesional SC from AD patients.

Although these results suggest that acid sphingomyelinase activity is normal in AD, direct assays of enzyme activity were not performed. We recently determined epidermal sphingomyelinase activities in lesional and non-lesional skin of AD patients. In comparison to healthy controls, we found a decrease in epidermal acid sphingomyelinase activity in lesional and non-lesional skin of AD patients, which correlates with both reduced SC ceramide content and disturbed barrier function. In particular, ceramide 2, the quantitatively most important ceramide, and ceramide 5 are generated from sphingomyelin (89). Also, neutral sphingomyelinase activity was reduced in non-lesional skin and further reduced in lesional skin. For example, impaired expression of cornified envelope proteins and keratins, which are also important for skin barrier function, are impaired in AD (see below). Together, these results suggest that sphingomyelinase generates ceramides not only for structural function in the SC lipid bilayers, but also for lipid signaling in epidermal differentiation (24,60,95).

Decreased ceramide content in AD has been further explained by Ohnishi et al. (96). After collecting bacteria from the skin surfaces of eczematous and normal-appearing skin of AD, erythematous skin lesions of psoriasis, and normal control skin for selective bacterial culture, these authors assayed ceramidase and sphingomyelinase activities and found that more ceramidase was secreted from the bacterial flora of both lesional and non-lesional skin of AD than from either lesional psoriasis skin or skin from normal subjects. Sphingomyelinase secretion levels, in contrast, were similar in bacteria obtained from AD, psoriasis, and controls. Our recent study, showing reduced sphingomyelinase activity in AD (24), supports the view that bacterial sphingomyelinase does not substantially influence overall epidermal activity of this enzyme. However, bacteria-derived ceramidase could contribute to the SC ceramide deficiency in AD.

A current explanation for reduced ceramides in AD is that given by Imokawa (97), who found that the AD epidermis contains a novel enzyme, glucosylceramide/ sphingomyelin deacylase, which cleaves the N-acyl linkage of both sphingomyelins and glucosylceramides. They found that this enzyme is elevated in the SC of both uninvolved and involved skin in AD. Sphingomyelin deacylase reduces the ceramide amount by releasing free fatty acids and sphingosyl-phosphorylcholine (69,90,98,99). However, our recent experiments have shown much lesser activity of sphingomyelin deacylase than acid sphingomyelinase in human epidermis (24), which suggests a different and still unknown basis for sphingomyelin deacylase in atopic dermatitis pathophysiology.

Substantial indirect evidence points to the importance for permeability barrier function of the most non-polar species, ceramides 1 and 4, which contain linoleic acid ω-esterified to an unusually long-chain, N-acyl fatty acid (C ≥ 30; acylceramide) (77). The Ω-hydroxyceramides in the ceramide family are generated by a cytochrome P_{450}-dependent process (100). In essential fatty acid deficiency that results in a profound barrier abnormality, oleate substitutes for linoleate as the predominant ω-esterified species ceramide 1 and 4 (75,101–103). Only when acylceramides are added to model lipid mixtures of cholesterol, free fatty acids, and non–ω-esterified ceramides, do membrane structures form, which resemble those present in SC extracellular domains (104).

It has recently been postulated that linoleic acid and other unsaturated free fatty acids are potent, naturally occurring activators of peroxisome proliferator–activated receptor-α. Peroxisome proliferator–activated receptor-α ligands promote epidermal differentiation in vivo, and topical applications of peroxisome proliferator–activated receptor-α activators have been shown to restore tissue homeostasis in hyperplastic models resembling AD (105,106). As essential fatty acids are potential peroxisome proliferator–activated receptor-α activators, previous studies on the use of essential fatty acids in the treatment of AD should be re-examined. Research from the 1930s to the 1950s established that a deficit of n-6 essential fatty acids leads to an inflammatory skin condition. An essential fatty acid deficient diet was shown to induce extremely scaly, red skin and an up to 10-fold increase in TEWL rates in mice (101,107). The progressive increase in TEWL levels correlated with structural membrane alterations (108), explained by the replacement of linoleate by oleate in both epidermal ceramides and glucosylceramides (109). The signs of essential fatty acid deficiency in animals can be reversed by either systemic or topi-cal administration of n-6 essential fatty acids such as linoleic acid, γ-linolenic acid, or columbic acid (107). Although there is evidence for low blood essential fatty acid concentrations in AD, there is no deficiency of linoleic acid (110). Whereas linoleic acid concentrations tend to be elevated in blood, skin, and adipose tissue of patients with AD, levels of downstream metabolites of linoleic acid are substan-tially reduced (110). These observations suggested that conversion of linoleic acid into γ-linolenic acid might be impaired in AD (111). Although several studies have assessed the efficacy of systemic or topical n-6 essential fatty acids in AD, the results have not been conclusive. In most studies, administration of γ-linolenic acid appeared to reduce the clinical severity (112). However, the largest placebo-controlled trials of either n-6 or n-3 fatty acid supplementation in AD found no consistent benefit (113). Henz et al. (114) performed a double blind, multicenter analysis of the efficacy of borage oil (>23% γ-linolenic acid) in 160 patients with AD. Although overall response did not attain statistical significance, the authors described a subgroup of AD patients whose clinical symptoms significantly improved with borage oil treatment in comparison to placebo. The mechanisms of action of γ-linolenic acid are only partly understood. γ-Linolenic acid could influence epidermal barrier function, modulate eicosanoid metabolism, or modulate cell signal-ing (115). Although reduced content of linoleic acid in ceramide 1 has been reported in AD (80), it is not yet known whether topically or systemically applied n-6 fatty acids normalize linoleic or γ-linolenic acid content of ceramide 1. However, preliminary data from Michelsen (personal communication) showed that oral treatment with n-6 fatty acids did not significantly change ceramide content or composition.

Corneocytes

AD patients showed a thinner horny layer as well as a reduced mean corneocyte area in different types of clinically asymptomatic skin (116). Although the number of SC cell layers in atopic xerosis was substantially larger than that in controls, its turnover time was noticeably shorter (117). Superficial corneocytes in the skin of atopic xero-sis patients, as in skin with increased epidermal differentiation, are substantially smaller than in control samples (117). Various impairments in SC function are expressed in the atopic dry skin of AD patients, likely due to increased epidermal proliferation caused by persistent, low-level inflammatory reactions in the skin (118).

Proliferation and Differentiation

Atopic dermatitis is characterized by impaired SC differentiation, resulting in scal-ing, roughness, and xerosis of the skin. Protein synthesis, epidermal differentiation, and proliferation are highly important for the formation of the SC permeability barrier (66,82). A several-fold increase in epidermal proliferation in AD after in vitro incorporation with tritiated thymidine has been described (119). The results were confirmed by our recent study using the Ki-67 proliferation associated anti-body (24). Increased proliferation may be an attempt to compensate for cell loss, normalize barrier function, or remove invading antigens. Epidermal DNA synthesis increases during permeability barrier repair after experimental skin injury (120). In forced desquamation tests, atopic patients released more corneocyte clumps from the epidermis than did normal controls (117). These results suggest that, in addition to the known changes in lipid content, changes in epidermal differentiation occur in AD. As a result of both acute and chronic barrier disruption, hyperproliferation-associated keratins K6 and K10 are induced, along with inflammation-associated K17 in AD epidermis (24). Changes in the expression of differentiation-associated keratins are also related to barrier disruption (66,121).

Formation of the cornified envelope occurs through deposit and cross-linking of involucrin and envoplakin on the intracellular surface of the plasma membrane in the upper spinous and granular cell layers of the epidermis, which is then followed by the subjacent addition of elafin, small prolin-rich proteins, and loricrin. We very recently found that changes in keratins occurred in non-lesional and lesional AD skin (24). Extended expression of basal keratin K5 was already noted in non-lesional skin and was more pronounced in lesional skin of AD. The expression of the suprabasal/differentiation related K10 was reduced in lesional AD only. Staining for K10 was concentrated in the granular and upper spinous layers, but reduced in the lower spinous layers of the epidermis. In K10 deficient mice, a defect in permeability barrier function has been found (121). Reduced K10 was also noted in dry skin in our previous studies: Engelke et al. (122) showed decreased levels of keratins K1 and K10 and increased levels of basal keratins K-5 and K-14 in clinically dry skin. In dry skin, premature expression of involucrin, a cornified cell envelope precursor protein, has been observed without changes in loricrin expression. Therefore, reduced K10 could be related to both the dry skin condition and the disturbed barrier function in AD.

Differentiation of proteins	Healthy skin	Non-lesional skin	Lesional skin
Keratin 1 and 10	✓	✓	↓
Keratin 5 and 14	✓	↑	↑↑
Keratin 6	×	×	✓
Keratin 16	×	✓	↑
Keratin 17	×	×	✓
Involucrin	✓	↓	↓↓
Loricrin	✓	↑	↑↑
Filaggrin	✓	↓	↓↓
Proliferation	✓	↑	↑↑

Abbreviations: Strongly enhanced expression ↑↑; enhanced expression ↑; present ✓; not present ×; decreased expression ↓; strongly decreased expression ↓↓.

Decreased staining for involucrin and filaggrin has previously been described in non-lesional skin of AD and decreased filaggrin has been confirmed by the ELISA method (123). In our studies, total staining density of involucrin and filaggrin were reduced, thereby suggesting reduced protein content in diseased skin. In accordance, significantly reduced involucrin protein content was found by Western blot analysis in lesional skin, and even more pronouncedly in non-lesional skin of AD (24). As filaggrin expression is linked to SC hydration and filaggrin content is reduced in atopic skin, it has been suggested that the frequently seen skin dryness in atopic patients may derive from these filaggrin changes (40). Since involucrin serves as a substrate for the covalent attachment of ceramides to the cornified envelope (82,124) reduced involucrin content may also cause the reduced amount of ω-hydroxyceramides in AD by failing to provide sufficient involucrin as a substrate for the attachment of ceramides (84).

In contrast to involucrin and filaggrin, loricrin expression increased significantly in non-lesional and lesional epidermis of AD, as shown by Western blot analysis (24). Immunohistochemistry also revealed increased staining for loricrin in the upper epidermis of AD samples. Though the genes for filaggrin, involucrin, and loricrin are localized on the same gene, 1q21, known as the epidermal differentiation complex, the loricrin gene does not share all the regulatory elements of the filaggrin and involucrin genes (125). The reason for the increase in loricrin expression in AD is unclear. Hohl (126) described overexpression of loricrin and involucrin in orthokeratotic acanthotic conditions, such as lichen planus. However, in other forms of dermatitis, he found reduced loricrin expression. The altered expression of involucrin, filaggrin, and loricrin is in agreement with recently published work on genome screening for AD, where a genetic linkage to AD on chromosome 1q21 was found (127).

Signaling Abnormalities

Inside the keratinocytes, the most numerous of cell types in the epidermis, TNF activates two types of sphingomyelinases, the endosomal acid sphingomyelinase and a cell membrane–associated neutral sphingomyelinase (128)—assuming that cytokines such as TNF are also working at the high pH of AD. The mode of action of ceramides released as a result of TNF-stimulation appears to be determined by the subcellular site of production. We detected high levels of acid and neutral sphingomyelinase and ceramides after barrier disruption, as well as a significant delay in barrier repair after imipramine-induced inhibition of acid sphingomyelinase (88). Sphingomyelinase-produced ceramides not only are structurally important, but have also been recognized as an important second messenger in intracellular signaling of various cytokines and growth factors, depending on the cell type (93). For apoptosis Caspase-9 and -3 activation was shown to be partly dependent on acid sphingomyelinase and cathepsin D expression. Heinrich et al. (129) linked acid sphingomyelinase and the acid aspartate protease cathepsin D as novel endosomal intermediates to the mitochondrial TNF pathway.

Ceramide metabolism is even more complex. Prosaposin, a large precursor protein, is proteolytically cleaved, forming a group of sphingolipid activator proteins, which stimulate enzymatic hydrolysis of sphingolipids, including glucosylceramides and sphingomyelin. Prosaposin has been shown to be essential for normal epidermal barrier formation and function (130). ELISA studies of atopic epidermis using a polyclonal antibody to saposin D showed decreased levels of prosaposin. The authors suggested that the suppression of prosaposin synthesis might be related to the abnormal SC formation in atopic skin through lower activation of β-glucosylcerebrosidase or sphingomyelinase (131).

CLINICAL MANIFESTATIONS RESULTING FROM IMPAIRED BARRIER FUNCTION

As AD presents with such a broad symptomatology, different views on its pathogenesis exist. Ogawa and Yoshiike (25) argued that allergies and abnormalities in immunological function provide only incomplete explanations for the occurrence of AD and that barrier dysfunction may be centrally involved in disease manifestation. Most observers consider barrier dysfunction to be the result of underlying inflammation, although a minority argue that barrier dysfunction may be the primary initiator in the expression of atopic symptoms (25). Scratching injuries in both asymptomatic and affected skin of AD patients result in increased allergen penetration and subsequent eczematous dermatitis (132). Because we are unable to identify a clear single initiator for atopic reactions, we would argue that an interrelation exists between allergies, biochemical defects in barrier function, and immunological abnormalities, explaining the manifestation of AD.

Contact Allergies

AD patients showed an increased sensitivity to chemical irritants and increased epidermal thickness (133). Moreover, positive patch test reactions to aeroallergens, grass pollen, birch pollen, cat dander, and house dust mite were observed only in AD patients (33). After patch testing, patients developed positive skin reactions and showed a 2- to 4-fold increase in TEWL in the patch test area. As a consequence of alterations in barrier function, aeroallergens can penetrate the skin more easily, thereby perpetuating eczematous dermatitis (33). Several studies have shown a 2- to 5-fold increase in basal TEWL over clinically uninvolved skin in AD (23). The extent of the barrier abnormality appears to correlate with the state of dermatitis (i.e., acute, sub-acute, and chronic dermatitis) (134), as well as the degree of inflammation in lesional skin (44,135–137). Conversely, basal TEWL levels and SC water content eventually normalize in completely healed patients (free from symptoms of AD for more than five years) (26). However, stress-induced changes in TEWL levels were not examined and this could be different in patients with a history of AD. Together, these studies suggest that skin barrier function in AD undergoes fluctuations according to the phase of the disease. It has been suggested that the presence of active eczema provokes impaired barrier function in uninvolved skin, even at sites far from active lesions (137).

Barrier dysfunction in the mucous membranes in the atopy syndrome predisposes patients to the development of bronchial asthma, rhinitis, and type-1 allergic responses by enabling the penetration of allergens, haptens, and contact-sensitizing agents into the affected sites. While immunological tolerance develops normally, repeated contact with allergens can cause hypersensitivity, thereby initiating inflammatory allergic responses. Nishijima et al. (138) suggested that the interaction between immunologically induced inflammation and the resulting disruptions to barrier function are an essential dynamic in the manifestation of generalized atopic conditions. This hypothesis is supported by the increased frequency of positive patch tests to household antigens in AD patients, in turn due to enhanced percutaneous absorption of macromolecules (139–142). Attributable to barrier function deficiency in mucous membranes, higher levels of protein antigen immune complex in IgA, IgG, and IgE are found in the serum of AD patients than in control subjects after challenging with milk (143), although increased intestinal permeability and maldigestion have been implicated in this process (8,144–146).

Lifestyle, working conditions, and physical environment influence the incidence of skin irritability and barrier dysfunction (29–32). Increased attention to personal hygiene and sanitation is a generalized trend, leading to potentially excessive use of soaps and detergents whose residues may cause adverse skin reactions (28).

Increased exposure to airborne allergens such as dust mites and pollens due to air conditioning, central heating, and inadequate ventilation in working or living environments may also induce sensitization reactions, particularly in children with immunological inexperience and in individuals predisposed due to abnormalities in barrier function (144,147). Premature changes in infants' diets to include animal proteins and the penetration of those allergens through the intestinal barrier may induce hypersensitivity and type-1 allergic reactions (143).

Infections, Innate Immunity, and Lipids

Patterns of microbial colonization of the skin surface are severely altered in AD patients. Pathogenic microbes (bacterial, fungal, and viral) increase and the spectrum of pathogens is broader in AD compared to in normal skin. In addition to its physical and chemical functions, the SC contains antimicrobial agents that form a biological barrier as part of the innate immune system. Ongoing studies of the innate immune system suggest a function of the SC in the production or distribution of antimicrobial peptides and lipids. Defensins, RNase 7, and the cathelicidin-derived linear peptide LL-37 are potent agents against microbial infections of the skin (148–150). Clinical cases show that deficiencies in these peptides cause severe symptoms, as seen in Kostmann's disease and also in AD. Certain SC lipids, including free fatty acids, sphingosine, and polar lipids, such as glycosphingolipids, are also described as having antimicrobial functions (151–154). It is noteworthy that the increased deacylase activity in AD results in decreased sphingosin, which could, in part, account for increased infection. Although microbial infections are well known in AD, the innate immunity pathways and their interactions are to date insufficiently identified.

THERAPEUTIC IMPLICATIONS

Treatment strategies in AD often address immunogenic abnormalities and barrier function. Treatment with cyclosporin, corticosteroids, tacrolimus, and UV light therapy has been shown to reduce cell inflammation as well as to improve barrier function. Application of creams and ointments containing lipids and lipid-like substances, hydrocarbons, free fatty acids, cholesterol esters, and triglycerides artificially repairs barrier function and increases SC hydration. Hydrocarbons, most commonly petrolatum, have been shown to advance permeability barrier repair after artificial disruption through intercalation into the extracellular lamellar membranes of the SC (134). As AD is often accompanied by reduced lipid composition, topical application of lipids and hydrocarbons may partially correct permeability barrier in AD.

Experiments conducted by Aalto–Korte (155) showed a correlation between TEWL and systemic absorption of topical hydrocortisone in AD. Topical treatments with hydrocortisone ointments have been shown to produce rapid improvement in the barrier function in atopic skin. However, the role of the emollient base in this improvement has not yet been distinguished from the role of the hydrocortisone. However, improved barrier function in AD has been described after treatment with moisturizers only (39,46).

It has been proposed that lipids from emollients containing ceramides, cholesterol, and free fatty acids are able to permeate the disturbed SC and enter the nucleated cell layers. Keratinocytes then absorb the emollient mixture for release into nascent lamellar bilayers in SC interstices (156). In a recent study of stubborn-to-recalcitrant childhood AD, phase 1 application of a ceramide-dominant barrier moisturizer significantly reduced AD severity scoring, normalized TEWL, and improved SC integrity (157). In measurements at three and six weeks, involved skin showed a reduction in TEWL; uninvolved skin showed nearly normal TEWL levels at six weeks. Improvement in skin hydration takes place more slowly during the treatment process. Regeneration and rehydration of lamellar membrane bilayers through treatment with ceramide-containing mixtures can be measured in tape-stripped SC through electron microscopy. Berardesca et al. (158) measured the efficacy of ceramide 3 and patented nanoparticle cream in AD, finding improvement in erythema, pruritus, and fissure building in contrast to healthy controls. Improvements in skin dryness and desquamation were not evident during ceramide-nanoparticle treatment. Further research is necessary to determine the significance of ceramides in AD treatment and the treatment phase in which their application brings the most therapeutic benefit.

In addition to immunological changes, we conclude that changes in the SC as a result of impaired lipid synthesis and epidermal differentiation accompanied by disturbed skin barrier function are crucial in the pathogenesis of AD. Several well-accepted treatment regimens, especially topically applied lipid-based creams and ointments, aim to restore skin barrier function and normalize epidermal differentiation in the SC structure, while other treatment modalities including corticosteroids also target the immune system.

REFERENCES

1. Shultz LF, Hanifin JM. Epidemiology of atopic dermatitis. Immunol Allergy Clin North Am 2002; 22:1–24.
2. Mar A, Tam M, Jolley D, Marks R. The cumulative incidence of atopic dermatitis in the first 12 months among Chinese, Vietnamese, and Caucasian infants born in Melbourne, Australia. J Am Acad Dermatol 1999; 40(4):597–602.
3. Nemes Z, Steinert PM. Bricks and mortar of the epidermal barrier. Exp Mol Med 1999; 31:5–19.
4. Taieb A. Hypothesis: from epidermal barrier dysfunction to atopic disorders. Contact Dermatitis 1999; 41(4):177–180.
5. Vanselow NA, Yamate M, Adams MS, Callies Q. The increased prevalence of allergic disease in anhidrotic congenital ectodermal dysplasia. J Allergy 1970; 45(5):302–309.
6. Tupker RA, Pinnagoda J, Coenraads PJ, Nater JP. Susceptibility to irritants: role of barrier function, skin dryness and history of atopic dermatitis. Br J Dermatol 1990; 123(2):199–205.
7. Spitz JL. Genodermatosis. Baltimore: Williams and Wilkins, 1996:214–215.
8. Ochs HD. The Wiskott–Aldrich syndrome. Clin Rev Allergy Immunol 2001; 20(1): 61–86.
9. Schurer NY, Elias PM. The biochemistry and function of stratum corneum lipids. Adv Lipid Res 1991; 24:27–56.
10. Chavanas S, Bodemer C, Rochat A, Hamel-Teillac D, Ali M, Irvine AD, Bonafe JL, Wilkinson J, Taieb A, Barrandon Y, Harper JI, de Prost Y, Hovnanian A. Mutations in SPINK5, encoding a serine protease inhibitor, cause Netherton syndrome. Nat Genet 2000; 25(2):141–142.
11. Walley AJ, Chavanas S, Moffatt MF, Esnouf RM, Ubhi B, Lawrence R, Wong K, Abecasis GR, Jones EY, Harper JI, Hovnanian A, Cookson WO. Gene polymorphism in Netherton and common atopic disease. Nat Genet 2001; 29(2):175–178.

12. Sprecher E, Chavanas S, DiGiovanna JJ, Amin S, Nielsen K, Prendiville JS, Silverman R, Esterly NB, Spraker MK, Guelig E, de Luna ML, Williams ML, Buehler B, Siegfried EC, Van Maldergem L, Pfendner E, Bale SJ, Uitto J, Hovnanian A, Richard G. The spectrum of pathogenic mutations in SPINK5 in 19 families with Netherton syndrome: implications for mutation detection and first case of prenatal diagnosis. J Invest Dermatol 2001; 117(2):179–187.

13. Komatsu N, Takata M, Otsuki N, Ohka R, Amano O, Takehara K, Saijoh K. Elevated stratum corneum hydrolytic activity in Netherton syndrome suggests an inhibitory regulation of desquamation by SPINK5-derived peptides. J Invest Dermatol 2002; 118(3):436–443.

14. Bitoun E, Micheloni A, Lamant L, Bonnart C, Tartaglia-Polcini A, Cobbold C, Al Saati T, Mariotti F, Mazereeuw-Hautier J, Boralevi F, Hohl D, Harper J, Bodemer C, D'Alessio M, Hovnanian A. LEKTI proteolytic processing in human primary keratinocytes, tissue distribution and defective expression in Netherton syndrome. Hum Mol Genet 2003; 12(19):2417–2430.

15. Kato A, Fukai K, Oiso N, Hosomi N, Murakami T, Ishii M. Association of SPINK5 gene polymorphisms with atopic dermatitis in the Japanese population. Br J Dermatol 2003; 148:665–669.

16. Wachter AM, Lezdey J. Treatment of atopic dermatitis with alpha 1-proteinase inhibitor. Ann Allergy 1992; 69(5):407–414.

17. Denda M, Kitamura K, Elias PM, Feingold KR. Trans-4-(Aminomethyl)cyclohexane carboxylic acid (T-AMCHA), an anti-fibrinolytic agent, accelerates barrier recovery and prevents the epidermal hyperplasia induced by epidermal injury in hairless mice and humans. J Invest Dermatol 1997; 109(1):84–90.

18. Hachem JP, Crumrine D, Fluhr J, Brown BE, Feingold KR, Elias PM. pH directly regulates epidermal permeability barrier homeostasis, and stratum corneum integrity/ cohesion. J Invest Dermatol 2003; 121(2):345–353.

19. Wood LC, Jackson SM, Elias PM, Grunfeld C, Feingold KR. Cutaneous barrier perturbation stimulates cytokine production in the epidermis of mice. J Clin Invest 1992; 90(2):482–487.

20. Wood LC, Elias PM, Calhoun C, Tsai JC, Grunfeld C, Feingold KR. Barrier disruption stimulates interleukin-1 alpha expression and release from a pre-formed pool in murine epidermis. J Invest Dermatol 1996; 106(3):397–403.

21. Gfesser M, Rakoski J, Ring J. The disturbance of epidermal barrier function in atopy patch test reactions in atopic eczema. Br J Dermatol 1996; 135(4):560–565.

22. Denda M, Sato J, Masuda Y, Tsuchiya T, Koyama J, Kuramoto M, Elias PM, Feingold KR. Exposure to a dry environment enhances epidermal permeability barrier function. J Invest Dermatol 1998; 111(5):858–863.

23. Yoshiike T, Aikawa Y, Sindhvananda J, Suto H, Nishimura K, Kawamoto T, Ogawa H. Skin barrier defect in atopic dermatitis: increased permeability of the stratum corneum using dimethyl sulfoxide and theophylline. J Dermatol Sci 1993; 5(2):92–96.

24. Jensen JM, Folster-Holst R, Baranowsky A, Schunck M, Winoto-Morbach S, Neumann C, Schutze S, Proksch E. Impaired sphingomyelinase activity and epidermal differentiation in atopic dermatitis. J Invest Dermatol 2004. In press.

25. Ogawa H, Yoshiike T. A speculative view of atopic dermatitis: barrier dysfunction in pathogenesis. J Dermatol Sci 1993; 5(3):197–204.

26. Matsumoto M, Sugiura H, Uehara M. Skin barrier function in patients with completely healed atopic dermatitis. J Dermatol Sci 2000; 23(3):178–182.

27. Bos et al. 1994.

28. McNally NJ, Phillips DR, Williams HC. The problem of atopic eczema: aetiological clues from the environment and lifestyles. Soc Sci Med 1998; 46(6):729–741.

29. Elias PM, Wood LC, Feingold KR. Relationship of the epidermal barrier to irritant contact dermatitis. In: Beltrani V, ed. Immunology and Allergy Clinics of North America. Vol. 17. Philadelphia: Saunders, 1997:417–430.

30. Elias PM, Wood LC, Feingold KR. Epidermal pathogenesis of inflammatory dermatoses. Am J Contact Dermat 1999; 10(3):119–126.
31. Garg A, Chren MM, Sands LP, Matsui MS, Marenus KD, Feingold KR, Elias PM. Psychological stress perturbs epidermal permeability barrier homeostasis: implications for the pathogenesis of stress-associated skin disorders. Arch Dermatol 2001; 137(1): 53–59.
32. Altemus M, Rao B, Dhabhar FS, Ding W, Granstein RD. Stress-induced changes in skin barrier function in healthy women. J Invest Dermatol 2001; 117(2):309–317.
33. Darsow U, Ring J. Atopic patch test. Atopic eczema and allergy. Hautarzt 2003; 54(10): 930–936.
34. Werner Y, Lindberg M. Transepidermal water loss in dry and clinically normal skin in patients with atopic dermatitis. Acta Derm Venereol 1985; 65(2):102–105.
35. Imokawa G. Skin moisturizers: development and clinical use of ceramides. In: Loden M, ed. Dry skin and moisturizers. Boca Raton, FL: CRC Press, 1999:269–299.
36. Imokawa G, Hattori M. A possible function of structural lipids in the water-holding properties of the stratum corneum. J Invest Dermatol 1985; 84(4):282–284.
37. Imokawa G, Akasaki S, Hattori M, Yoshizuka N. Selective recovery of deranged water-holding properties by stratum corneum lipids. J Invest Dermatol 1986; 87(6):758–761.
38. Imokawa G, Abe A, Jin K, Higaki Y, Kawashima M, Hidano A. Decreased level of ceramides in stratum corneum of atopic dermatitis: an etiologic factor in atopic dry skin? J Invest Dermatol 1991; 96(4):523–526.
39. Tabata N, O'Goshi K, Zhen YX, Kligman AM, Tagami H. Biophysical assessment of persistent effects of moisturizers after their daily applications: evaluation of corneotherapy. Dermatology 2000; 200(4):308–313.
40. Scott IR, Harding CR. Filaggrin breakdown to water binding compounds during development of the rat stratum corneum is controlled by the water activity of the environment. Dev Biol 1986; 115(1):84–92.
41. Eberlein-Konig B, Schafer T, Huss-Marp J, Darsow U, Mohrenschlager M, Herbert O, Abeck D, Kramer U, Behrendt H, Ring J. Skin surface pH, stratum corneum hydration, trans-epidermal water loss and skin roughness related to atopic eczema and skin dryness in a population of primary school children. Acta Derm Venereol 2000; 80:188–191.
42. Choi SJ, Song MG, Sung WT, Lee DY, Lee JH, Lee ES, Yang JM. Comparison of transepidermal water loss, capacitance and pH values in the skin between intrinsic and extrinsic atopic dermatitis patients. J Korean Med Sci 2003; 18(1):93–96.
43. Sator PG, Schmidt JB, Honigsmann H. Comparison of epidermal hydration and skin surface lipids in healthy individuals and in patients with atopic dermatitis. J Am Acad Dermatol 2003; 48(3):352–358.
44. Sugarman JL, Fluhr JW, Fowler AJ, Bruckner T, Diepgen TL, Williams ML. The objective severity assessment of atopic dermatitis score: an objective measure using permeability barrier function and stratum corneum hydration with computer-assisted estimates for extent of disease. Arch Dermatol 2003; 139(11):1417–1422.
45. Kiriyama T, Sugiura H, Uehara M. Residual washing detergent in cotton clothes: a factor of winter deterioration of dry skin in atopic dermatitis. J Dermatol 2003; 30:708–712.
46. Loden M, Andersson AC, Lindberg M. Improvement in skin barrier function in patients with atopic dermatitis after treatment with a moisturizing cream (Canoderm). Br J Dermatol 1999; 140(2):264–267.
47. Peris K, Valeri P, Altobelli E, Fargnoli MC, Carrozzo AM, Chimenti S. Efficacy evaluation of an oil-in-water emulsion (Dermoflan) in atopic dermatitis. Acta Derm Venereol 2002; 82(6):465–466.
48. Loden M, Andersson AC, Anderson C, Bergbrant IM, Frodin T, Ohman H, Sandstrom MH, Sarnhult T, Voog E, Stenberg B, Pawlik E, Preisler-Haggqvist A, Svensson A, Lindberg M. A double-blind study comparing the effect of glycerin and urea on dry, eczematous skin in atopic patients. Acta Derm Venereol 2002; 82(1):45–47.

49. Loden M. Role of topical emollients and moisturizers in the treatment of dry skin barrier disorders. Am J Clin Dermatol 2003; 4(11):771–788.

50. Rippke F, Schreiner V, Schwanitz HJ. The acidic milieu of the horny layer: new findings on the physiology and pathophysiology of skin pH. Am J Clin Dermatol 2002; 3(4): 261–272.

51. Brattsand M, Egelrud T. Purification, molecular cloning, and expression of a human stratum corneum trypsin-like serine protease with possible function in desquamation. J Biol Chem 1999; 274(42):30033–30040.

52. Ekholm IE, Brattsand M, Egelrud T. Stratum corneum tryptic enzyme in normal epidermis: a missing link in the desquamation process? J Invest Dermatol 2000; 114(1): 56–63.

53. Lundqvist EN, Egelrud T. Biologically active, alternatively processed interleukin-1 beta in psoriatic scales. Eur J Immunol 1997; 27(9):2165–2171.

54. Hamid Q, Boguniewicz M, Leung DY. Differential in situ cytokine gene expression in acute versus chronic atopic dermatitis. J Clin Invest 1994; 94(2):870–876.

55. Engler RJ, Kenner J, Leung DY. Smallpox vaccination: risk considerations for patients with atopic dermatitis. J Allergy Clin Immunol 2002; 110(3):357–365.

56. Nomura I, Goleva E, Howell MD, Hamid QA, Ong PY, Hall CF, Darst MA, Gao B, Boguniewicz M, Travers JB, Leung DY. Cytokine milieu of atopic dermatitis, as compared to psoriasis, skin prevents induction of innate immune response genes. J Immunol 2003; 171(6):3262–3269.

57. Denda M, Tsuchiya T, Elias PM, Feingold KR. Stress alters cutaneous permeability barrier homeostasis. Am J Physiol Regul Integr Comp Physiol 2000; 278(2):R367–R372.

58. Toole JW, Hofstader SL, Ramsay CA. Darier's disease and Kaposi's varicelliform eruption. J Am Acad Dermatol 1979; 1(4):321–324.

59. Werner Y. The water content of the stratum corneum in patients with atopic dermatitis. Measurement with the Corneometer CM 420. Acta Derm Venereol 1986; 66(4):281–284.

60. Proksch E, Jensen JM, Elias PM. Skin lipids and epidermal differentiation in atopic dermatitis. Clin Dermatol 2003; 21(2):134–144.

61. Sugarman JH, Fleischer AB Jr, Feldman SR. Off-label prescribing in the treatment of dermatologic disease. J Am Acad Dermatol 2002; 47(2):217–223.

62. Elias PM, Menon GK. Structural and lipid biochemical correlates of the epidermal permeability barrier. Adv Lipid Res 1991; 24:1–26.

63. Lee SH, Elias PM, Proksch E, Menon GK, Mao-Quiang M, Feingold KR. Calcium and potassium are important regulators of barrier homeostasis in murine epidermis. J Clin Invest 1992; 89(2):530–538.

64. Mauro T, Bench G, Sidderas-Haddad E, Feingold K, Elias P, Cullander C. Acute barrier perturbation abolishes the Ca^{2+} and K^+ gradients in murine epidermis: quantitative measurement using PIXE. J Invest Dermatol 1998; 111(6):1198–201.

65. Mauro T, Holleran WM, Grayson S, Gao WN, Man MQ, Kriehuber E, Behne M, Feingold KR, Elias PM. Barrier recovery is impeded at neutral pH, independent of ionic effects: implications for extracellular lipid processing. Arch Dermatol Res 1998; 290(4):215–222. Erratum in: Arch Dermatol Res 1998; 290(7):405.

66. Ekanayake-Mudiyanselage S, Aschauer H, Schmook FP, Jensen JM, Meingassner JG, Proksch E. Expression of epidermal keratins and the cornified envelope protein involucrin is influenced by permeability barrier disruption. J Invest Dermatol 1998; 111(3):517–523.

67. Jakobza D, Reichmann G, Langnick W, Langnick A, Schulze P. Surface skin lipids in atopic dermatitis (author's transl). Dermatol Monatsschr 1981; 167(1):26–29.

68. Barth JH, Ridden J, Philpott MP, Greenall MJ, Kealey T. Lipogenesis by isolated human apocrine sweat glands: testosterone has no effect during long-term organ maintenance. J Invest Dermatol 1989; 92(3):333–336.

69. Mustakallio KK, Kiistala U, Piha HJ, Nieminen E. Epidermal lipids in Besnier's prurigo (atopic eczema). Ann Med Exp Biol Fenn 1967; 45(3):323–325.

70. Schafer L, Kragballe K. Abnormalities in epidermal lipid metabolism in patients with atopic dermatitis. J Invest Dermatol 1991; 96(1):10–15.

71. Schurer NY, Plewig G, Elias PM. Stratum corneum lipid function. Dermatologica 1991; 183(2):77–94.

72. Melnik B, Hollmann J, Hofmann U, Yuh MS, Plewig G. Lipid composition of outer stratum corneum and nails in atopic and control subjects. Arch Dermatol Res 1990; 282(8):549–551.

73. Di Nardo A, Wertz P, Giannetti A, Seidenari S. Ceramide and cholesterol composition of the skin of patients with atopic dermatitis. Acta Derm Venereol 1998; 78(1): 27–30.

74. Fartasch M, Bassukas ID, Diepgen TL. Disturbed extruding mechanism of lamellar bodies in dry non-eczematous skin of atopics. Br J Dermatol 1992; 127(3):221–227.

75. Madison KC. Barrier function of the skin: "la raison d'etre" of the epidermis. J Invest Dermatol 2003; 121(2):231–241.

76. Long SA, Wertz PW, Strauss JS, Downing DT. Human stratum corneum polar lipids and desquamation. Arch Dermatol Res 1985; 277(4):284–287.

77. Robson KJ, Stewart ME, Michelsen S, Lazo ND, Downing DT. 6-Hydroxy-4-sphingenine in human epidermal ceramides. J Lipid Res 1994; 35(11):2060–2068.

78. Stewart ME, Downing DT. A new 6-hydroxy-4-sphingenine-containing ceramide in human skin. J Lipid Res 1999; 40(8):1434–1439.

79. Ponec M, Weerheim A, Lankhorst P, Wertz P. New acylceramide in native and reconstructed epidermis. J Invest Dermatol 2003; 120(4):581–588.

80. Yamamoto A, Serizawa S, Ito M, Sato Y. Stratum corneum lipid abnormalities in atopic dermatitis. Arch Dermatol Res 1991; 283(4):219–223.

81. Matsumoto Y, Hamashima H, Masuda K, Shiojima K, Sasatsu M, Arai T. The antibacterial activity of plaunotol against Staphylococcus aureus isolated from the skin of patients with atopic dermatitis. Microbios 1998; 96(385):149–155.

82. Marekov LN, Steinert PM. Ceramides are bound to structural proteins of the human foreskin epidermal cornified cell envelope. J Biol Chem 1998; 273(28):17763–17770.

83. Meguro S, Arai Y, Masukawa Y, Uie K, Tokimitsu I. Relationship between covalently bound ceramides and transepidermal water loss (TEWL). Arch Dermatol Res 2000; 292(9):463–468.

84. Macheleidt O, Kaiser HW, Sandhoff K. Deficiency of epidermal protein-bound omega-hydroxyceramides in atopic dermatitis. J Invest Dermatol 2002; 119(1):166–173.

85. Bleck O, Abeck D, Ring J, Hoppe U, Vietzke JP, Wolber R, Brandt O, Schreiner V. Two ceramide subfractions detectable in Cer(AS) position by HPTLC in skin surface lipids of non-lesional skin of atopic eczema. J Invest Dermatol 1999; 113(6):894–900.

86. Holleran WM, Takagi Y, Menon GK, Legler G, Feingold KR, Elias PM. Processing of epidermal glucosylceramides is required for optimal mammalian cutaneous permeability barrier function. J Clin Invest 1993; 91(4):1656–1664.

87. Holleran WM, Ginns EI, Menon GK, Grundmann JU, Fartasch M, McKinney CE, Elias PM, Sidransky E. Consequences of beta-glucocerebrosidase deficiency in epidermis. Ultrastructure and permeability barrier alterations in Gaucher disease. J Clin Invest 1994; 93(4):1756–1764.

88. Jensen JM, Schutze S, Forl M, Kronke M, Proksch E. Roles for tumor necrosis factor receptor p55 and sphingomyelinase in repairing the cutaneous permeability barrier. J Clin Invest 1999; 104(12):1761–1770.

89. Uchida Y, Hara M, Nishio H, Sidransky E, Inoue S, Otsuka F, Suzuki A, Elias PM, Holleran WM, Hamanaka S. Epidermal sphingomyelins are precursors for selected stratum corneum ceramides. J Lipid Res 2000; 41(12):2071–2082.

90. Hara J, Higuchi K, Okamoto R, Kawashima M, Imokawa G. High-expression of sphingomyelin deacylase is an important determinant of ceramide deficiency leading to barrier disruption in atopic dermatitis. J Invest Dermatol 2000; 115(3):406–413.

91. Jin K, Higaki Y, Takagi Y, Higuchi K, Yada Y, Kawashima M, Imokawa G. Analysis of beta-glucocerebrosidase and ceramidase activities in atopic and aged dry skin. Acta Derm Venereol 1994; 74(5):337–340.

92. Redoules D, Tarroux R, Perie J. Epidermal enzymes: their role in homeostasis and their relationships with dermatoses. Skin Pharmacol Appl Skin Physiol 1998; 11(4–5): 183–192.

93. Kreder D, Krut O, Adam-Klages S, Wiegmann K, Scherer G, Plitz T, Jensen JM, Proksch E, Steinmann J, Pfeffer K, Kronke M. Impaired neutral sphingomyelinase activation and cutaneous barrier repair in FAN-deficient mice. EMBO J 1999; 18(9): 2472–2479.

94. Kusuda S, Cui CY, Takahashi M, Tezuka T. Localization of sphingomyelinase in lesional skin of atopic dermatitis patients. J Invest Dermatol 1998; 111(5):733–738.

95. Schmuth M, Man MQ, Weber F, Gao W, Feingold KR, Fritsch P, Elias PM, Holleran WM. Permeability barrier disorder in Niemann-Pick disease: sphingomyelin-ceramide processing required for normal barrier homeostasis. J Invest Dermatol 2000; 115(3):459–466.

96. Ohnishi Y, Okino N, Ito M, Imayama S. Ceramidase activity in bacterial skin flora as a possible cause of ceramide deficiency in atopic dermatitis. Clin Diagn Lab Immunol 1999; 6(1):101–104.

97. Murata Y, Ogata J, Higaki Y, Kawashima M, Yada Y, Higuchi K, Tsuchiya T, Kawainami S, Imokawa G. Abnormal expression of sphingomyelin acylase in atopic dermatitis: an etiologic factor for ceramide deficiency? J Invest Dermatol 1996; 106(6): 1242–1249.

98. Higuchi K, Hara J, Okamoto R, Kawashima M, Imokawa G. The skin of atopic dermatitis patients contains a novel enzyme, glucosylceramide sphingomyelin deacylase, which cleaves the N-acyl linkage of sphingomyelin and glucosylceramide. Biochem J 2000; 350(Pt 3):747–756.

99. Imokawa G. Lipid abnormalities in atopic dermatitis. J Am Acad Dermatol 2001; 45(suppl 1):S29–S32.

100. Behne M, Uchida Y, Seki T, de Montellano PO, Elias PM, Holleran WM. Omega-hydroxyceramides are required for corneocyte lipid envelope (CLE) formation and normal epidermal permeability barrier function. J Invest Dermatol 2000; 114(1):185–192.

101. Elias PM, Brown BE. The mammalian cutaneous permeability barrier: defective barrier function is essential fatty acid deficiency correlates with abnormal intercellular lipid deposition. Lab Invest 1978; 39(6):574–583.

102. Wertz PW, Cho ES, Downing DT. Effect of essential fatty acid deficiency on the epidermal sphingolipids of the rat. Biochim Biophys Acta 1983; 753(3):350–355.

103. Wertz PW, Swartzendruber DC, Abraham W, Madison KC, Downing DT. Essential fatty acids and epidermal integrity. Arch Dermatol 1987; 123(10):1381–1384.

104. Bouwstra JA, Gooris GS, Dubbelaar FE, Weerheim AM, Ponec M. pH, cholesterol sulfate, and fatty acids affect the stratum corneum lipid organization. J Investig Dermatol Symp Proc 1998; 3(2):69–74.

105. Komuves LG, Hanley K, Lefebvre AM, Man MQ, Ng DC, Bikle DD, Williams ML, Elias PM, Auwerx J, Feingold KR. Stimulation of PPARalpha promotes epidermal keratinocyte differentiation in vivo. J Invest Dermatol 2000; 115(3):353–360.

106. Komuves LG, Hanley K, Man MQ, Elias PM, Williams ML, Feingold KR. Keratinocyte differentiation in hyperproliferative epidermis: topical application of PPARalpha activators restores tissue homeostasis. J Invest Dermatol 2000; 115(3):361–367.

107. Proksch E, Feingold KR, Elias PM. Epidermal HMG CoA reductase activity in essential fatty acid deficiency: barrier requirements rather than eicosanoid generation regulate cholesterol synthesis. J Invest Dermatol 1992; 99(2):216–220.

108. Hou SY, Rehfeld SJ, Plachy WZ. X-ray diffraction and electron paramagnetic resonance spectroscopy of mammalian stratum corneum lipid domains. Adv Lipid Res 1991; 24:141–71.

109. Melton JL, Wertz PW, Swartzendruber DC, Downing DT. Effects of essential fatty acid deficiency on epidermal O-acylsphingolipids and transepidermal water loss in young pigs. Biochim Biophys Acta 1987; 921(2):191–197.
110. Horrobin DF. Essential fatty acid metabolism and its modification in atopic eczema. Am J Clin Nutr 2000; 71(suppl 1):367S–372S.
111. Melnik BC, Plewig G. Is the origin of atopy linked to deficient conversion of omega-6-fatty acids to prostaglandin E1? J Am Acad Dermatol 1989; 21(3 Pt 1):557–563.
112. Morse PF, Horrobin DF, Manku MS, Stewart JC, Allen R, Littlewood S, Wright S, Burton J, Gould DJ, Holt PJ, et al. Meta-analysis of placebo-controlled studies of the efficacy of Epogam in the treatment of atopic eczema. Relationship between plasma essential fatty acid changes and clinical response. Br J Dermatol 1989; 121(1):75–90.
113. Berth-Jones J, Graham-Brown RA. Placebo-controlled trial of essential fatty acid supplementation in atopic dermatitis. Lancet 1993; 341(8860):1557–1560. Erratum in: Lancet 1993; 342(8870):564.
114. Henz BM, Jablonska S, van de Kerkhof PC, Stingl G, Blaszczyk M, Vandervalk PG, Veenhuizen R, Muggli R, Raederstorff D. Double-blind, multicentre analysis of the efficacy of borage oil in patients with atopic eczema. Br J Dermatol 1999; 140(4):685–688.
115. Manku MS, Horrobin DF, Morse N, Kyte V, Jenkins K, Wright S, Burton JL. Reduced levels of prostaglandin precursors in the blood of atopic patients: defective delta-6-desaturase function as a biochemical basis for atopy. Prostaglandins Leukot Med 1982; 9(6):615–628.
116. Al-Jaberi H, Marks R. Studies of the clinically uninvolved skin in patients with dermatitis. Br J Dermatol 1984; 111(4):437–443.
117. Watanabe M, Tagami H, Horii I, Takahashi M, Kligman AM. Functional analyses of the superficial stratum corneum in atopic xerosis. Arch Dermatol 1991; 127(11): 1689–1692.
118. Fartasch M, Williams ML, Elias PM. Altered lamellar body secretion and stratum corneum membrane structure in Netherton syndrome: differentiation from other infantile erythrodermas and pathogenic implications. Arch Dermatol 1999; 135(7):823–832.
119. Van Neste D, Lachapelle JM, Desmons F. Atopic dermatitis: a histologic and radio-autographic study (after 3H-thymidine labelling) of epidermal and dermal lesions. Ann Dermatol Venereol 1979; 106(4):327–335.
120. Proksch E, Feingold KR, Man MQ, Elias PM. Barrier function regulates epidermal DNA synthesis. J Clin Invest 1991; 87(5):1668–1673.
121. Jensen JM, Schutze S, Neumann C, Proksch E. Impaired cutaneous permeability barrier function, skin hydration, and sphingomyelinase activity in keratin 10 deficient mice. J Invest Dermatol 2000; 115(4):708–713.
122. Engelke M, Jensen JM, Ekanayake-Mudiyanselage S, Proksch E. Effects of xerosis and ageing on epidermal proliferation and differentiation. Br J Dermatol 1997; 137(2): 219–225.
123. Seguchi T, Cui CY, Kusuda S, Takahashi M, Aisu K, Tezuka T. Decreased expression of filaggrin in atopic skin. Arch Dermatol Res 1996; 288(8):442–446.
124. Wertz PW, Madison KC, Downing DT. Covalently bound lipids of human stratum corneum. J Invest Dermatol 1989; 92(1):109–111.
125. Yoneda K, McBride OW, Korge BP, Kim IG, Steinert PM. The cornified cell envelope: loricrin and transglutaminases. J Dermatol 1992; 19(11):761–764.
126. Hohl D. Expression patterns of loricrin in dermatological disorders. Am J Dermatopathol 1993; 15(1):20–27.
127. Cookson WO, Ubhi B, Lawrence R, Abecasis GR, Walley AJ, Cox HE, Coleman R, Leaves NI, Trembath RC, Moffatt MF, Harper JI. Genetic linkage of childhood atopic dermatitis to psoriasis susceptibility loci. Nat Genet 2001; 27(4):372–373.
128. Wiegmann K, Schutze S, Machleidt T, Witte D, Kronke M. Functional dichotomy of neutral and acidic sphingomyelinases in tumor necrosis factor signaling. Cell 1994; 78(6):1005–1015.

129. Heinrich M, Neumeyer J, Jakob M, Hallas C, Tchikov V, Winoto-Morbach S, Wickel M, Schneider-Brachert W, Trauzold A, Hethke A, Schutze S. Cathepsin D links TNF-induced acid sphingomyelinase to Bid-mediated caspase-9 and -3 activation. Cell Death Differ 2004. In press.

130. Doering T, Holleran WM, Potratz A, Vielhaber G, Elias PM, Suzuki K, Sandhoff K. Sphingolipid activator proteins are required for epidermal permeability barrier formation. J Biol Chem 1999; 274(16):11038–11045.

131. Cui CY, Kusuda S, Seguchi T, Takahashi M, Aisu K, Tezuka T. Decreased level of prosaposin in atopic skin. J Invest Dermatol 1997; 109(3):319–323.

132. Gondo A, Saeki N, Tokuda Y. Challenge reactions in atopic dermatitis after percutaneous entry of mite antigen. Br J Dermatol 1986; 115(4):485–493.

133. Nassif A, Chan SC, Storrs FJ, Hanifin JM. Abnormal skin irritancy in atopic dermatitis and in atopy without dermatitis. Arch Dermatol 1994; 130:1402–1407.

134. Ghadially R, Halkier-Sorensen L, Elias PM. Effects of petrolatum on stratum corneum structure and function. J Am Acad Dermatol 1992; 26(3 Pt 2):387–396.

135. Shahidullah M, Raffle EJ, Rimmer AR, Frain-Bell W. Transepidermal water loss in patients with dermatitis. Br J Dermatol 1969; 81(10):722–730.

136. Agner T. Non-invasive measuring methods for the investigation of irritant patch test reactions. A study of patients with hand eczema, atopic dermatitis and controls. Acta Derm Venereol Suppl (Stockh) 1992; 173:1–26.

137. Seidenari S, Giusti G. Objective assessment of the skin of children affected by atopic dermatitis: a study of pH, capacitance and TEWL in eczematous and clinically uninvolved skin. Acta Derm Venereol 1995; 75(6):429–433.

138. Nishijima T, Tokura Y, Imokawa G, Seo N, Furukawa F, Takigawa M. Altered permeability and disordered cutaneous immunoregulatory function in mice with acute barrier disruption. J Invest Dermatol 1997; 109(2):175–182.

139. Mitchell EB, Crow J, Chapman MD, Jouhal SS, Pope FM, Platts-Mills TA. Basophils in allergen-induced patch test sites in atopic dermatitis. Lancet 1982; 1(8264):127–130.

140. Adinoff AD, Tellez P, Clark RA. Atopic dermatitis and aeroallergen contact sensitivity. J Allergy Clin Immunol 1988; 81(4):736–742.

141. Conti A, Di Nardo A, Seidenari S. No alteration of biophysical parameters in the skin of subjects with respiratory atopy. Dermatology 1996; 192(4):317–320.

142. Conti A, Seidenari S. No increased skin reactivity in subjects with allergic rhinitis during the active phase of the disease. Acta Derm Venereol 2000; 80(3):192–195.

143. Paganelli R, Atherton DJ, Levinsky RJ. Differences between normal and milk allergic subjects in their immune responses after milk ingestion. Arch Dis Child 1983; 58(3):201–206.

144. Ukabam SO, Mann RJ, Cooper BT. Small intestinal permeability to sugars in patients with atopic eczema. Br J Dermatol 1984; 110(6):649–652.

145. Pike MG, Heddle RJ, Boulton P, Turner MW, Atherton DJ. Increased intestinal permeability in atopic eczema. J Invest Dermatol 1986; 86(2):101–104.

146. Barba A, Schena D, Andreaus MC, Faccini G, Pasini F, Brocco G, Cavallini G, Scuro LA, Chieregato GC. Intestinal permeability in patients with atopic eczema. Br J Dermatol 1989; 120(1):71–75.

147. Arlian LG, Neal JS, Morgan MS, Vyszenski-Moher DL, Rapp CM, Alexander AK. Reducing relative humidity is a practical way to control dust mites and their allergens in homes in temperate climates. J Allergy Clin Immunol 2001; 107(1):99–104.

148. Harder J, Schroder JM. RNase 7, a novel innate immune defense antimicrobial protein of healthy human skin. J Biol Chem 2002; 277(48):46779–46784.

149. Ong PY, Ohtake T, Brandt C, Strickland I, Boguniewicz M, Ganz T, Gallo RL, Leung DY. Endogenous antimicrobial peptides and skin infections in atopic dermatitis. N Engl J Med 2002; 347(15):1151–1160.

150. Boman HG. Antibacterial peptides: basic facts and emerging concepts. J Intern Med 2003; 254(3):197–215.

151. Miller SJ, Aly R, Shinefeld HR, Elias PM. In vitro and in vivo antistaphylococcal activity of human stratum corneum lipids. Arch Dermatol 1988; 124(2):209–215.
152. Fluhr JW, Kao J, Jain M, Ahn SK, Feingold KR, Elias PM. Generation of free fatty acids from phospholipids regulates stratum corneum acidification and integrity. J Invest Dermatol 2001; 117(1):44–51.
153. Arikawa J, Ishibashi M, Kawashima M, Takagi Y, Ichikawa Y, Imokawa G. Decreased levels of sphingosine, a natural antimicrobial agent, may be associated with vulnerability of the stratum corneum from patients with atopic dermatitis to colonization by Staphylococcus aureus. J Invest Dermatol 2002; 119(2):433–439.
154. Schmuth M. Dropping lipids for epidermal defense. J Invest Dermatol 2003; 121(2):xi.
155. Aalto-Korte K. Improvement of skin barrier function during treatment of atopic dermatitis. J Am Acad Dermatol 1995; 33(6):969–972.
156. Mao-Qiang M, Brown BE, Wu-Pong S, Feingold KR, Elias PM. Exogenous nonphysiologic vs physiologic lipids. Divergent mechanisms for correction of permeability barrier dysfunction. Arch Dermatol 1995; 131(7):809–816.
157. Chamlin SL, Frieden IJ, Fowler A, Williams M, Kao J, Sheu M, Elias PM. Ceramide-dominant, barrier-repair lipids improve childhood atopic dermatitis. Arch Dermatol 2001; 137(8):1110–1112.
158. Berardesca E, Barbareschi M, Veraldi S, Pimpinelli N. Evaluation of efficacy of a skin lipid mixture in patients with irritant contact dermatitis, allergic contact dermatitis or atopic dermatitis: a multicenter study. Contact Dermatitis 2001; 45(5):280–285.
159. Elias PM, Feingold KR. Does the tail wag the dog? Role of the barrier in the pathogenesis of inflammatory dermatoses and therapeutic implications. Arch Dermatol 2001; 137(8):1079–1081.
160. Man MQ M, Feingold KR, Thornfeldt CR, Elias PM. Optimization of physiological lipid mixtures for barrier repair. J Invest Dermatol 1996; 106(5):1096–1101.

Epilogue: Fixing the Barrier—Theory and Rational Deployment

Peter M. Elias

Dermatology Service, VA Medical Center, and Department of Dermatology, University of California, San Francisco, California, U.S.A.

INTRODUCTION

As described elsewhere in this volume, the stratum corneum (SC) has many functions, but none is as important as its ability to serve as a protective barrier that prevents excess loss of fluids and electrolytes. Likewise, it is generally accepted that the permeability barrier is mediated by the organization of the extracellular lipids of the SC into a series of parallel membrane structures (1–3). Moreover, these membrane bilayers mediate not only permeability barrier function, but also additional, key protective function of the epidermis. Finally, it is the total lipid weight (= no. of extracellular bilayers); the hydrophobic characteristics of the constituent lipids; the presence of these lipids in an approximately equimolar ratio; and other features of these lipids that account for the ability of these membranes to mediate these barrier functions (Table 1). The extracellular lipids in the SC derive primarily from the secreted contents of epidermal lamellar bodies (LB), which are enriched in cholesterol, glucosylceramide, phospholipids, as well as their respective hydrolytic enzymes. These lipid processing enzymes catalyze the extracellular degradation of sphingomyelin and glucosylceramides to ceramides (Cer), as well as phospholipids to free fatty acids (FFA), respectively, that along with cholesterol (Chol), form the lamellar membranes required for permeability barrier function (1,2). Thus, the SC lamellar membrane comprises unique biological membranes, because they lack phospholipids.

DYNAMICS OF BARRIER RECOVERY

The skin barrier is often assaulted in daily life by hot water, detergents, solvents, mechanical trauma, and occupation-related chemicals. If not frequently and repeatedly and/or insufficiently repaired, these insults threaten the organism with desiccation due to accelerated transepidermal water loss. To avoid this outcome, the underlying epidermis mounts a coordinated metabolic response (Chap. 21), which ranges from increased lipid synthesis to accelerated lipid secretion, aimed at rapidly restoring

Table 1 How Lipids Mediate Barrier Function

Intercellular localization
Amount of lipid (lipid wt.%)
Elongated, tortuous, intercellular pathway (increases length of diffusion pathway)
Organization into lamellar membrane unit structures
Hydrophobic composition (absence of polar lipids and very long chain, saturated fatty acids)
Correct molar ratio (approximately 1:1:1 of three key lipids)
Unique molecular structures (e.g., acylceramides)

normal function. This response is elicited by any type of barrier insult (e.g., organic solvents, detergents, tape stripping) that depletes the SC of its complement of lipids (2,4). Although the total time required for barrier recovery varies according to age, there is an initial, rapid recovery phase that leads to 50–60% recovery in young humans in about 12 hours, with full recovery requiring about three days (Fig. 1). But in aged humans (>75 years), complete recovery from comparable insults is prolonged to about one week (5). Restoration of barrier function is accompanied by re-accumulation of lipids, visible with Nile red fluorescence, and by the reappearance of membrane structures within the SC interstices, as early as two hours after acute disruption (6,7). Since artificial restoration of the barrier with vapor-impermeable membranes inhibits barrier recovery as well as all of the metabolic process linked to it (7), the entire metabolic response represents a response that is aimed specifically at restoring normal permeability barrier homeostasis (2,4).

CLINICAL APPLICATIONS OF THE CUTANEOUS STRESS TEST

The kinetics of barrier recovery after acute perturbations (called the "Cutaneous Stress Test") can discern abnormal function or underlying pathology, even when basal parameters are normal (Chap. 2), analogous to the cardiac treadmill exam. Indeed, the cutaneous stress test reveals deficient barrier function both in aged (5)

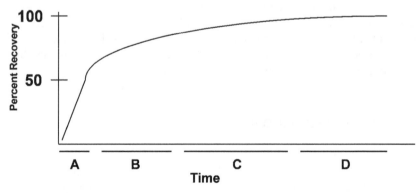

Figure 1 The cutaneous stress test and its applications.

and in neonatal (8) skin, despite deceptively normal function in both age groups under basal conditions. Further, it amplifies differences between other "normal" groups e.g., in testosterone-replete versus deficient individuals (9); in skin exposed to humid versus dry environments (10); and in individuals with type 5–6 versus 1–2 pigmentation (11). Finally, individuals subjected to increased psychologic stress reveal a defect in barrier recovery (12–14), explaining the propensity for stress and these other factors to exacerbate inflammatory dermatoses, such as psoriasis and atopic dermatitis, which already display barrier abnormalities. We have proposed that these factors further amplify the cytokine cascade that characterizes these disorders (15–17).

INDIVIDUAL LIPID REQUIREMENTS FOR THE BARRIER

The formation of LB by the epidermis requires a coordinated synthesis of the major lipid components of LB, i.e., cholesterol, glucosylceramides, and phospholipids (2,4). Although the epidermis is a very active site of lipid synthesis even under basal conditions (18), permeability barrier disruption stimulates a further, marked increase in the synthesis of all three key lipids [i.e., Chol, Cer, and FFA (6,19)], which provides the pool of lipids what is required for the formation of new LB. Yet, synthesis of these lipids is not only regulated by barrier requirements, but also required for normal function. For example, using specific inhibitors of key lipid synthetic enzymes, we demonstrated an individual requirement for Chol, FFA, Cer, and glucosylCer synthesis for barrier formation (reviewed in Refs. 4, 20). In fact, blockade of these enzymes always produces a similar result: decreased LB, as well as a paucity of extracellular lamellar membranes. Thus, each of the three key lipids is required individually for barrier function.

THE THREE KEY SC LIPIDS ARE REQUIRED IN AN EQUIMOLAR DISTRIBUTION

Although the above-described studies clearly demonstrate the individual requirement for Chol, FFA, and Cer for the permeability barrier, when applied topically, these lipids must be supplied in approximately equimolar proportions for normal barrier recovery to occur (21). In contrast, topical applications of any one or two of the three key lipids to acutely perturbed skin actually delays barrier recovery (21). Both incomplete and complete mixtures of the three key lipids rapidly traverse the SC, internalize within the granular cell layer, targeting the trans-Golgi network, where LBs are formed (22) (Fig. 2). Exogenous and endogenous lipids mix within nascent LB, producing normal or abnormal LB contents and derived lamellar membrane structures, depending on the molar distribution of the applied lipids. Barrier recovery can be further accelerated by increasing the proportion of any one of the three key lipids to a 3:1:1 ratio (23). Thus, physiologic mixtures of topical lipids influence barrier function, not by occluding the SC, as do non-physiologic lipids (see below), but rather by contributing to the lipid pool within the SC interstices.

NON-PHYSIOLOGIC LIPIDS—MECHANISM OF ACTION

In contrast to physiologic lipids, classic non-physiologic lipids, such as petrolatum, do not enter the lipid-secretory pathway of the granular cell. They do, however, fully

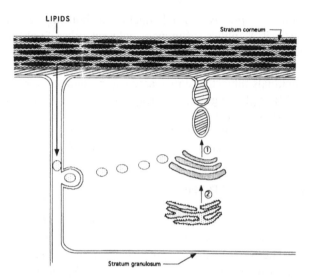

Figure 2 Physiologic lipids traverse the stratum corneum and traffic to trans-Golgi apparatus (1), where they blend with newly-synthesized (2) lipid.

penetrate the extracellular domains of the SC, where they form a hydrophobic, non-lamellar phase (24). These lipids, which include not only petrolatum, but also bees-wax, lanolin, and other hydrocarbons, form the equivalent of a vapor-permeable membrane, and as such, they reduce water loss immediately, while physiologic lipids display a lag time that reflects the time necessary for SC transport, endocytosis,

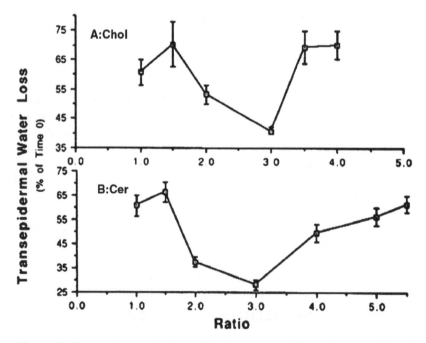

Figure 3 Progressive acceleration of barrier recovery (2 hrs after acute disruption) as molar ratios are increased to 3:1:1.

Table 2 Barrier Recovery after Various Topical Treatments

Treatment	% of Recovery			
	45 minutes	2 hours	4 hours	8 hours
Acetone + air exposure or vehicle	15	25	35	55
Acetone + physiologic lipids	10	55	75	90
Acetone + petrolatum	50	50	50	40
Acetone + physiologic lipids + petrolatum[a]	55	70	90	95

[a]Optimal molar ratio: 3:1:1 (Cer: free sterol: FFA).

secretion, and lamellar membrane formation (Table 2—compare petrolatum to physiologic lipids). Non-physiologic lipids have the further advantage that they do not discriminate among types of abnormalities—the same degree of correction is achieved in all cases. Finally, it should be noted that the non-physiologic lipids, though they are not components of the lamellar membranes, display a host of other, potentially-beneficial properties, e.g., anti-inflammatory, hydration, waterproofing, thermal insulation, etc.

POTENTIAL OF BARRIER REPAIR THERAPY

The contrasting features of non-physiologic and physiologic lipids dictate the clinical settings where each is uniquely useful. While non-physiologic lipids, like petrolatum, function like vapor-permeable membranes at the surface of the SC (22,24), physiologic lipids supplement the epidermis' own biosynthetic mechanism. As noted above, many skin diseases are associated with barrier abnormalities and other pathophysiologic insults, such as psychological stress or aging, can further aggravate these processes. Logically then, bolstering epidermal barrier status should decrease susceptibility to the large group of skin diseases that are triggered, sustained, or exacerbated by external perturbations, most notably, atopic dermatitis, contact dermatitis, and psoriasis (15) (Fig. 4). In fact, all these diseases are characterized by a barrier abnormality, whose extent parallels clinical severity (25–27).

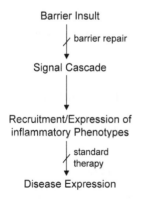

Figure 4 Disease pathogenesis and barrier repair: Alternate approaches to therapy.

Table 3 Logical Barrier Repair Strategies—Clinical Indications

Repair strategy	Clinical indication
Dressings	
Vapor permeable	Healing wounds
Vapor impermeable	Keloids
Non-physiologic lipids (NPL)	
Petrolatum or lanolin	Radiatin dermatitis or severe sunburn
	Premature infants (aged <34 weeks)
Physiologic lipids (PL): optimal molar ratio	
Chol-dominant	Aging or photoaging
Cer-dominant	Atopic dermatitis
FFA dominant	Neonatal skin, including psoriasis, diaper dermatitis (with added NPL)
Chol-, Cer-, or FFA-dominant	Irritant contact dermatitis (with added NPL)
	Glucocorticoid-treated (vehicle)
	Psychological stress

The recent emergence of "barrier repair" therapy represents a set of pathophysiologically based strategies that should decrease the susceptibility to these disorders. These repair approaches can be classified into three subcategories (17) (Table 3): (i) optimized mixtures of the three physiologic lipids (Cer, Chol, and FFA) in appropriate molar ratios that correct underlying biochemical abnormalities in the targeted disease; (ii) one or more non-physiologic lipids (e.g., petrolatum, lanolin), which restore function transiently without correcting specific abnormalities; (iii) dressings, either vapor-permeable, which allow metabolic (repair) processes to continue in the underlying epidermis, or vapor-impermeable, which shut down metabolic responses in the underlying epidermis.

But caveat emptor—the term "barrier repair" is frequently applied loosely and inappropriately by marketers to emollients, often based upon formulations of petrolatum or lanolin derivatives alone or emollients containing the physiologic lipids in incorrect proportions. These formulations can do more harm than good. As noted above, incomplete mixtures of physiologic lipids can impede rather than facilitate normalization of barrier function, and even optimized mixtures may not be beneficial, if the dominant lipid does not reflect the underlying biochemical abnormality

Table 4 Effects of Physiologic Lipid Mixtures on Barrier Recovery in Young versus Aged Human Skin

Physiologic lipids[a]	Young	Aged
Single lipid	Delays	Accelerates (cholesterol only)
Triple lipids (equimolar)	No change	Accelerates
Triple lipids (optimized)		
Fatty acid-dominant	Accelerates	Delays
Cer-dominant	Accelerates	Not studied
Chol-dominant	Accelerates	Accelerates

[a]Physiologic lipids = FFA, Chol, and Cer.

(Table 4). Moreover, occlusive, non-physiologic moisturizers can down-regulate repair mechanisms, i.e., they can send an important message suggesting incorrectly that barrier function is normal, though the underlying abnormality has not been addressed.

Nevertheless, all of these strategies have their appropriate use and clinical indications. In fact, we can now choose an appropriate barrier strategy, for a specific clinical indication, based upon knowledge of disease pathogenesis (17,28) (Table 3). For example, atopic dermatitis (AD) is characterized by a global decrease in SC lipids with a steep reduction in ceramides (26,29) attributable to increased sphingomyelin/glucosylceramide deacylase activity in affected epidermis (30). Hence, the logic and recent apparent success of a ceramide-dominant mixture of the three physiologic lipids as ancillary therapy in AD (31). In contrast, aged and photoaged epidermis exhibits a global reduction in SC lipids (5), with a further decrease in cholesterol synthesis (32). Hence, the success of a cholesterol-dominant mixture of physiological lipids in this setting (33). So critical is choice of proper formulation that substitution of an FFA-dominant mixture for the cholesterol-dominant version drastically delays barrier recovery in aged skin (Table 4).

Yet, there are several clinical situations where physiologic lipids might not be effective, if deployed alone, due to an impaired LB secretory system. These examples include: radiation dermatitis [both UV-B and x-irradiation (34,35)], very premature infants (i.e., < 33 weeks), and perhaps the initial stages of wound heading (17). In such situations, non-physiologic lipids or vapor-permeable dressing alone, with or without added physiologic lipids, would become the most logical choice (17).

REFERENCES

1. Elias PM, Menon GK. Structural and lipid biochemical correlates of the epidermal permeability barrier. Adv Lipid Res 1991; 24:1–26.
2. Elias PM, Feingold KR. Lipids and the epidermal water barrier: metabolism, regulation, and pathophysiology. Semin Dermatol 1992; 11:176–182.
3. Elias PM, Feingold KR. Skin as an organ of protection. In: Freedberg I, et al., eds. Fitzpatrick's Dermatology in General Medicine. Philadelphia: McGraw-Hill, 2003:164–174.
4. Feingold KR. The regulation and role of epidermal lipid synthesis. Adv Lipid Res 1991; 24:57–82.
5. Ghadially R, Brown BE, Sequeira-Martin SM, Feingold KR, Elias PM. The aged epidermal permeability barrier. Structural, functional, and lipid biochemical abnormalities in humans and a senescent murine model. J Clin Invest 1995; 95:2281–2290.
6. Grubauer G, Feingold KR, Elias PM. Relationship of epidermal lipogenesis to cutaneous barrier function. J Lipid Res 1987; 28:746–752.
7. Grubauer G, Elias PM, Feingold KR. Transepidermal water loss: the signal for recovery of barrier structure and function. J Lipid Res 1989; 30:323–333.
8. Fluhr J, Behne M, Brown BE, Moskowitz DG, Selden C, Mauro T, Elias PM, Feingold K Stratum corneum acidification in neonatal skin: I. secretory phospholipase A2 and the NHE1 antiporter acidify neonatal rat stratum corneum. J Invest Dermatol 2004; 122:320–329.
9. Kao JS, Garg A, Mao Qiang M, Crumrine D, Ghadially R, Feingold KR, Elias PM. Testosterone perturbs epidermal permeability barrier homeostasis. J Invest Dermatol 2001; 116:443–451.
10. Denda M, Sato J, Masuda Y, Tsuchiya T, Koyama J, Kuramoto M, Elias PM, Feingold KR. Exposure to a dry environment enhances epidermal permeability barrier function. J Invest Dermatol 1998; 111:858–863.

11. Reed JT, Ghadially R, Elias PM. Skin type, but neither race nor gender, influence epidermal permeability barrier function. Arch Dermatol 1995; 131:1134–1138.

12. Denda M, Tsuchiya T, Elias PM, Feingold KR. Stress alters cutaneous permeability barrier homeostasis. Am J Physiol Regul Integr Comp Physiol 2000; 278:R367–R372.

13. Altemus M, Rao B, Dhabhar FS, Ding W, Granstein RD. Stress-induced changes in skin barrier function in healthy women. J Invest Dermatol 2001; 117:309–317.

14. Garg A, Chren MM, Sands LP, Matsui MS, Marenus KD, Feingold KR, Elias PM. Psychological stress perturbs epidermal permeability barrier homeostasis: implications for the pathogenesis of stress-associated skin disorders. Arch Dermatol 2001; 137:53–59.

15. Elias PM, Wood LC, Feingold KR. Epidermal pathogenesis of inflammatory dermatoses. Am J Contact Dermat 1999; 10:119–126.

16. Elias PM, Feingold KR. Coordinate regulation of epidermal differentiation and barrier homeostasis. Skin Pharmacol Appl Skin Physiol 2001a; 14(suppl):28–34.

17. Elias PM, Feingold KR. Does the tail wag the dog? Role of the barrier in the pathogenesis of inflammatory dermatoses and therapeutic implications. Arch Dermatol 2001b; 137:1079–1081.

18. Feingold KR, Brown BE, Lear SR, Moser AH, Elias PM. Localization of de novo sterologenesis in mammalian skin. J Invest Dermatol 1983; 81:365–369.

19. Menon GK, Grayson S, Elias PM. Ionic calcium reservoirs in mammalian epidermis: ultrastructural localization by ion-capture cytochemistry. J Invest Dermatol 1985; 84:508–512.

20. Feingold KR, Man MQ, Proksch E, Menon GK, Brown BE, Elias PM. The lovastatin-treated rodent: a new model of barrier disruption and epidermal hyperplasia. J Invest Dermatol 1991; 96:201–209.

21. Man MQ, Feingold KR, Elias PM. Exogenous lipids influence permeability barrier recovery in acetone-treated murine skin. Arch Dermatol 1993; 129:728–738.

22. Mao-Qiang M, Brown BE, Wu-Pong S, Feingold KR, Elias PM. Exogenous nonphysiologic vs physiologic lipids. Divergent mechanisms for correction of permeability barrier dysfunction. Arch Dermatol 1995; 131:809–816.

23. Man MM, Feingold KR, Thornfeldt CR, Elias PM. Optimization of physiological lipid mixtures for barrier repair. J Invest Dermatol 1996; 106:1096–1101.

24. Ghadially R, Halkier-Sorensen L, Elias PM. Effects of petrolatum on stratum corneum structure and function. J Am Acad Dermatol 1992; 26:387–396.

25. Ghadially R, Reed JT, Elias PM. Stratum corneum structure and function correlates with phenotype in psoriasis. J Invest Dermatol 1996b; 107:558–564.

26. Proksch E, Jensen JM, Elias PM. Skin lipids and epidermal differentiation in atopic dermatitis. Clin Dermatol 2003; 21:134–144.

27. Sugarman JL, Fluhr JW, Fowler AJ, Bruckner T, Diepgen TL, Williams ML. The objective severity assessment of atopic dermatitis score: an objective measure using peermeability barrier function and stratum corneum hydration with computer-assisted estimates for extent of disease. Arch Dermatol 2003; 139:1417–1422.

28. Williams ML, Elias PM. Enlightened therapy of the disorders of cornification. Clin Dermatol 2003; 21:269–273.

29. Imokawa G, Abe A, Jin K, Higaki Y, Kawashima M, Hidano A. Decreased level of ceramides in stratum corneum of atopic dermatitis: an etiologic factor in atopic dry skin?. J Invest Dermatol 1991; 96:523–526.

30. Hara J, Higuchi K, Okamoto R, Kawashima M, Imokawa G. High-expression of sphingomyelin deacylase is an important determinant of ceramide deficiency leading to barrier disruption in atopic dermatitis. J Invest Dermatol 2000; 115:406–413.

31. Chamlin SL, Kao J, Frieden IJ, Sheu MY, Fowler AJ, Fluhr JW, Williams ML, Elias PM. Ceramide-dominant barrier repair lipids alleviate childhood atopic dermatitis: changes in barrier function provide a sensitive indicator of disease activity. J Am Acad Dermatol 2002; 47:198–208.

32. Ghadially R, Brown BE, Hanley K, Reed JT, Feingold KR, Elias PM. Decreased epidermal lipid synthesis accounts for altered barrier function in aged mice. J Invest Dermatol 1996a; 106:1064–1069.

33. Zettersten EM, Ghadially R, Feingold KR, Crumrine D, Elias PM. Optimal ratios of topical stratum corneum lipids improve barrier recovery in chronologically aged skin. J Am Acad Dermatol 1997; 37:403–408.

34. Holleran WM, Uchida Y, Halkier-Sorensen L, Haratake A, Hara M, Epstein JH, Elias PM. Structural and biochemical basis for the UVB-induced alterations in epidermal barrier function. Photodermatol Photoimmunol Photomed 1997; 13:117–128.

35. Schmuth M, Sztankay A, Weinlich G, Linder DM, Wimmer MA, Fritsch PO, Fritsch E. Permeability barrier function of skin exposed to ionizing radiation. Arch Dermatol 2001; 137:1019–1023.

Index

α-Defensin, 366, 369
α-MSH, 370
α-Tocopherol. *See also* Vitamin E.
β-Catenin, 172
β-Defensin, 5–6, 264, 300, 366, 367, 541
β-GlcCer'ase. *See* Beta-glucocerebrosidase.
β-Glucocerebrosidase, 262, 266, 348, 364 574
γ-Linolenic acid, action of, 576
ω-Glucosyl hydroxyceramide, 346
ω-Hydroxyceramides, 36, 262, 346, 578,

Acetyl CoA carboxylase, 38–39, 348, 350, 471, 542
Acidic sphingomyelinase, 348, 364, 540
Acral keratotic plaques, 342
Activated oxygen species, 380
 effects of, 380
Activator protein 1. *See* AP1.
Acylgalactosylceramides, 50
Acylglucosylceramide, 49–50
AD. *See* Atopic dermatitis.
Adherens junction, 172–173, 200, 279
Adipose differentiation-related protein (ADRP), 326
 role of, 326
Adrenomedullin, 371
Aged epidermis
 additional alterations, 541
 calcium gradient, 542
 clinical implications, 546
 functional changes, 538
  in pH levels, 540
  in women, 539
Aged skin
 cytokine effects, 538–539
 role of growth factors, 537
Aging, 392–393
 process of, 392, 544
Akt1, 326

Allergic contact dermatitis, 519
 analysis of, 455
 antioxidant, 526
 photoprotective effects of, 526
 vitamin C, 526
 vitamin E, 526
AM. *See* Adrenomedullin.
AMP. *See* Antimicrobial peptide.
Amphiregulin (AR), 353, 537
Animal model experiments, 554
Antimicrobial activity, 364, 366, 368
 in neuropeptides,
Antimicrobial barriers, 5, 7
Antimicrobial peptide, 365, 369
Antioxidant barrier systems, 379–395
 function of, 379
Antioxidant repair enzymes, 384
 methionine sulfoxide reductase, 384
 mode of action, 384
Antioxidant response element (ARE), 149
Antioxidant systems, 379, 381, 384
 defense systems against, 380
 oxidative stress, 379–380
  definition of,
  source of, 379
Antioxidants, 380–381
 nonenzymic, 381
  GSH and uric acid, 381
  L-ascorbic acid, 381
AP1, 123
Atopic dermatitis (AD), 352, 456, 522, 569–581
 barrier integrity and transepidermal water loss, 571–572
 effect of climate on, 571
 genetic factor causing, 572
 hydration, 571
 pH, 572
 response to allergens, 570
 therapeutic implications, 580

Atopic disposition
cause for, 523
ATP-binding cassette (ABC) transporter, 478
Autoimmune bullous dermatoses, 458
Autosomal dominant ichthyosis vulgaris, 458

B-glucocerebrosidase (GLC), 226
Bacillus, 364
Barrier abnormalities, 572
and lipids, 572
basis for, 572
metabolic basis, 542
Barrier disruption
causes, 519
Barrier dysfunction, 579
and allergens, 579
other causes, 579–580
Barrier function, 1
localization, 2
need for, 2
Barrier homeostasis, 337–361, 362, 364
odorant inhalation effects, 562
Barrier impairment, causes and effects, 573
Barrier perturbations, result, 535, 537
Barrier recovery, 346, 351–354, 591–597
Barrier repair, 352
role of melavonic acid, 542, 543
strategies, 545
Basement membrane zone, 98
Benign and malignant keratoses, 458
Benzoyl peroxide, 387
effect of, 388
Beta-chloroalanine, 350
Beta-glucocerebrosidase, 348
BHT. *See* butylated hydroxytoluene.
Biosensor concept, 2, 29–30
Biosynthesis of cholesterol, 37
BPO. *See* benzoyl peroxide.
Bullous dermatoses, 458
Butylated hydroxytoluene, 390
mechanism of, 390

C-fibers, 370
C1Orf10, 129
Ca^{++}
role in cohesion, 515
Calcitonin receptor-like receptor, 371
Calcium, 366–367
Calcium (Ca) signaling, 352
Calcium efflux, 367
Calcium gradient, 367, 372
Candida albicans, 369

[Calcium gradient]
extra-cellular, 367
regulation of, 297
Calcium response element, 435, 437
Calcium switch, 433
cytochalasin, 433
desmoplakin, 433
Calcium-sensing receptor (CaSR)
1, 25 dihydroxyvitamin D$_3$ interactions,
427
intercellular regulation of, 432
keratinocytes regulation, 432
mRNA levels, 433–434, 436
regulation of differentiation, 432
role in the epidermis, 431
role of receptor, 433
Calpain, 118
Catalase, 384, 393
structure of, 384
Cath peptide expression, 369
in psoriasis, 369
Cathelin
synthesis, 369
Cathepsin G, 371
Cathepsins
role of, 182–183
within intercorneocyte spaces, 183
Caveolin-1, 262
CCR6 receptor, 367
CD. *See* Corneodesmosomes.
CE. *See* Cornified envelope.
Cell envelope (CE), 569
Ceramide, 365, 447, 471, 484
See also pseudoceramides.
and abnormalities in hydration
and barrier function, 574
and glucosylceramide/ sphingomyelin
deacylase, 575
covalently bound, 573
definition of, 44, 55
function of, 43–48
in the stratum corneum
generation of, 48
localization of, 47
origin of, 49
molecular heterogeneity of, 45
production, stimulation of, 56
role in epidermal barrier function, 48
signaling, 574
subclasses in, 573
Ceramide synthesis, 348, 350
Chanarin Dorfman syndrome
clinical characteristics of, 485
molecular defect of, 485

[Chanarin Dorfman syndrome]
morphological and functional
consequences of, 485
Chemokines, 363, 369
CHH syndromes
clinical characteristics of, 482
morphological and functional
consequences of, 485
Chloroform-methanol extraction, 345
Cholesterol, 344, 348, 350, 352, 365, 373
Cholesterol ester transport protein (CETP),
329
Cholesterol sulfate, 35
cycle, 512
differentiation regulation, 513
effects on skin, 511
in stratum corneum, 511
processing of, 244
Cholesterol synthetic pathway, 348, 471
farnesyl diphosphate synthase, and, 471
HMG CoA synthase, 471
squalene synthase, 471
Chromofungin, 371
Chromophore, 379–380
reaction of, 379–380
type I photoreactions, 379
type II reaction, 380
Chymotryptic and tryptic serine proteases,
(SCCE and SCTE) in neutral pH, 227
Ciglitazone, 328–329
Cingulin, 196
Claudin 6, 201
Claudin 14, 196
Claudin 16 paracellin, 196
CLE. *See* Covalently bound lipid envelope.
CLE. *See* Corneocyte lipid envelope.
Clofibrate, 322
Clostridium difficile, 196
Clostridium perfringens, 196
CODA, 22
Colloidal lanthanum, 459
Concanavalin A, 153
Confocal microscopy, 369
Connexons, 171–172
Corneocyte, 337, 338, 471–472, 487, 576
maturation factor of, 414
parameters of, 418
properties, 417
water binding capacity
Corneocyte compartment, 472
Corneocyte cytosol, 341, 342
Corneocyte lipid envelope (CLE), 47, 239,
262, 345
comprised of, 471

[Corneocyte lipid envelope (CLE)]
functions of, 471
Corneocyte protein expression, 342
regulation of, 342
Corneocyte rigidity, 338
Corneocytes, 65–66, 262
Corneodesmolysis, 399, 413, 417
Corneodesmosin, 472
location, 172
role of, 181, 400
structure, 178
synthesis, 174
Corneodesmosomal Dsg1 and Dsc1, 177
Corneodesmosome protein desmoglein 1, 227
Corneodesmosomes 28, 98, 171–185, 225,
264–265, 391, 472,
components, 176
composition, 180
degradation, 181
hair follicle, in the, 176
proteolysis, 183–184
reasons for preferential loss, 176
role of, 181
specialized desmosomes of SC, 174
within intercorneocyte spaces, 183
Corneosome
degradation of, 525
Cornification, 261
Cornified cell envelope, 100
formation of, 100
Cornified envelope (CE), 97–106,
338, 469
catalyzed by, 473
composed of, 473
distinctive feature of, 473
formation, 100–105
proteins, 148
loricrin, 158
Cornified-lipid envelope, 97–106
Corticosteroids, 191
treatment of, 527
Covalently bound lipid envelope, 65
CRLR. *See* Calcitonin receptor-like
receptor.
Cryptosporidium, 368
Cutaneous stress test, 29, 346
Cystein protease activity, 391
Cysteine proteases
activity of, 368
Cytokine cascade, 29
Cytokines, 353–354
in lipid synthesis, 543
other effects of, 543
Cytoskeleton abnormality, 341

DAH, 524–526
Defensins, 366–367, 369
Dermatitis, influence of, 454
Desmocollins, 176, 472
Desmogleins, 172–173, 472
Desmoplakin, 173, 177, 341
Desmosomal cadherins, 472
Desmosome, 98, 100, 173
    desmoplakins, 173
    desmosomal plaques, 173–174
    structure, 173
    type of mechanical junction, 173
Desquamation, 264, 417
Detergents, 450
Differential irritation test, 524
    employed in, 525
DIT. *See* differential irritation test.
Domain structure, 146

E-cadherin hemidesmosomes, 172
Early fetal period, 280
EBS. *See* Epidermolysis bullosa simplex.
Eccrine gland, 364, 369
EFA. *See* Essential free fatty acid (EFA).
EDC. *See* Epidermal differentiation complex.
EFAD. *See* Essential fatty acid deficiency.
EFAD mice. *See* Essential fatty acid deficient
    mice.
EHK. *See* Epidermolytic hyperkeratosis.
Elafin, 182, 262
    product of LB, 262
Elastase, 368, 371
Electron microscopy, 366, 369
Embryonic fetal transition, 279
Embryonic period, 277
Endoplasmic reticulum, 349–351
Enkelytin, 370–371
Environmental factors
    impact of, 384
Enzymatic antioxidants, 383
        glutathione peroxidases, 384
        superoxide dismutases, 383–384
Enzymes, and antimicrobial activity,
        369–372
in profilaggrin modification, 118
Epidermal barrier function
    diseases related to, 53–55
    effect of ceramide application on, 53
    perturbation of, 369–372, 524–526
    pH, 526
    use of ceramides in, 54–55
Epidermal calcium gradient, 526
    implications of, 300

Epidermal cholesterol sulfate cycle, 512
Epidermal differentiation, 113, 131, 173, 431,
        410
Epidermal differentiation complex, 101
    role of 1, 25 dihydroxyvitamin D_3, 427
    role of calcium in, 111
    role of protein kinase C, 434
Epidermal lamallar bodies, enzymes in, 27
Epidermal lipids
    role, 332
    synthesis
Epidermal permeability barrier
    role of acidification, 225
Epidermal proliferation, in response to AD,
        576
Epidermal sphingolipids
    generation of, 48
Epidermis, 79
Epidermis, functional factors, 538
    abnormal cornification of, 475
    compoistion of, 431
        basal layer, 431
        granular layer, 431
        sinous layer, 431
    differentiation and cornification of, 469
    and neurotransmitters, 563
    and endocrine system, 562
    epidermal functions of, 472
Epidermolysis bullosa simplex, 147
Epidermolytic hyperkeratosis (EHK), 341, 460
    clinical characteristic of, 476
    molecular defect of, 474
    morphological and functional
        consequences of, 474
Epidermosides, 447
Epithelin tight functions in, 192–196
Erythrokeratodermia variabilis
    clinical characteristics of, 476
    morphological and functional
        consequences of, 476
Essential fatty acids (EFA), 75, 476
Essential fatty acid deficiency (EFAD), 485
    clinical characteristics of, 477
    morphological and functional
        consequences of, 478
Essential FFA, 343, 344
Estrogen, 460
Exocytosis, 266, 268, 344, 348
    of lamellar bodies, 344, 348
Extracellular compartment
    lamellar bodies (LBs), 470
Extracellular lipid lamellar structures,
    defects in, 477
Extracellular lipid matrix, 337

Extracellular lipid membranes, 480
Extracellular lipids, 226

F-actin filaments, 172
Fasting induced adipose factor (FIAF), 326
Fatty acid synthesis, 348, 349–350
Fatty aldehyde dehydrogenase (FALDH), 480
Fenofibrate, 322
FFA. *See* Free fatty acids.
Fibrils, 192
Filaggrin, 7, 450, 459, 469
  effect of AD on, 578
Filaggrin-2. *See Flg*-2.
Fiaggrin-histidine-urocanic acid (UCA)
    pathway, 28
  identification of, 122
  importance of, 123
  multiple functions of, 119
  structure, 115
Filagrin-derived histidine, 224
Histidase, 224
Flat electrode measurements, advantage of, 223
Flexural eczema, 522
Flg-2 repeats, 126
Fluorescence in situ hybridization (FISH), 477
Fluorscence life time imaging (FLIM), role of, 223
Free fatty acid (FFA), 66, 79, 224, 337, 364
  comprised of, 470
Furin, 119
Fused S100 gene family, 112

G-protein coupled receptor (GPCR), 300
Galactosylceramide, 56
  See also Pseudogalactosylceramide.
Gastricsin, 368
Gaucher's disease, 53, 262
  clinical characteristics of, 483
  molecular defect of, 483
  morphological and functional
      consequences of, 484
Gemfibrozil, 322
GlcCer'ase activity
  regulation of, 237
Glucosylceramide, 49–50, 39, 236
  signalling, 544
  synthase, 351
Glutathione, 382, 384
Glycerophospholipids, 365
  processing of, 242

Glycosphingolipids
Golgi apparatus, 349
Gram-positive bacteria, 371
Granulysin, 370
Growth factors, 353–354
  in aged skin, 544
GSH, 381

Hair follicles, inner root sheath, 185
  Henle's layer, 176
  Huxley's layer, 176
Hand dermatitis
  occur in, 519–520
Harlequin ichthyosis. *See* HI.
  clinical characteristics of, 482
  morphological and functional
      consequences of, 483
HBD. *See* Human β-defensins.
Health education, 527
Helicobacter pylori, 196
Hemidesmosomes, 172
Herpes virus, 458
HI, 123–124, 261, 269
High frequency conductometry
  technique for, 449
Histidase, 224
HMG CoA reductase, 348, 350
Homeostasis, 452–453
  keratins and, 141–159
Homeostatic repair response
  steps involved, 470, 475
Hornerin, 127
HUGO Gene Nomenclature Committee
    (HGNC), 142
Human β-defensins, 366, 368
Human epidermis, cell-cell junctions, 171
Human immunodeficiency virus 1, 371
Human skin equivalents, 78
  composition of, 66
  development of, 273
  function of, 78
  generation of
Human stratum corneum lipids, 33–39
  biosynthetic pathway of, 37
    ceramides and glucosylceramides in, 39
    cholesterol in, 37
    fatty acids, in, 38
  ceramides in, 34
  contaminants in, 36
  free long-chain bases in, 36
  history of, 33
  major components of, 33
  minor components of, 35

[Human stratum corneum lipids]
  sebaceous fatty acids in, 36
Hydration, effect on basser function, 11
  stratum corneum, 450
Hydrolytic enzymes, 262, 266
Hyperkeratosis, 474
Hyperplasia, 475, 477
Hypocholesteronemic drugs
  role of, 486
Hypothermia, 105

ICD. *See* Interdigital contact dermatitis.
Ichthyoses, 339, 341, 346
  effects of, 486
Ichthyosis keratinocytes, 341
Ichthyosis vulgaris
  clinical characteristics of, 492
  molecular defect of, 493
  morphological and functional
     consequences of, 493
IDS. *See* Interdigital space.
IF *See* Intermediate filament.
IFAP. *See* Intermediate filament-associated
  protein.
IL-1. *See* Interleukin-1.
IL-1α, characteristics, 537
IL-1ra, 537
IL-6. *See* Interleukin-6.
Imiquimod, 354
Immune response, 363, 373
  of skin, 373
Immune-mediated inflammatory dermatoses,
  456
Immunocytochemistry, 369
Immunogold staining, 366
Immunolocalization, 342
Inflammatory and keratinizing disorders, 265
  atopic dermatitis, 265
  ichthyoses, 265
Inflammatory dermatoses, stimuli, 450
Inflammatory pathway, 363
Intercellular junctions, 171–172
  communication junction, 171
  connexins, 171
  glycine loops, 180
  mechanical junctions, 171–172
Interdigital contact dermatitis, 524
  occurrence of, 525
  precursor of, 525
Interdigital dermatitis, 522
Interferon-γ (IFNγ), role of, 430, 371
Interfollicular epidermis, histo-architecture
  of, 98

Interleukin-1, 305
Interleukin-1α, 366, 371
Interleukin-1β, 366, 371
Interleukin-6, 309
Intermediate filament, 141
Intermediate filament-associated protein, 114
Involucrin, 323–324, 339, 447
  effect of AD on, 577
Irritant contact dermatitis
  analysis of, 455
Irritant dermatitis
  caused by, 450–452
Irritated skin
  effects of treatment, 522
IV. *See* Ichthyosis vulgaris.

KAPs. *See* Keratin-associated
    proteins.
Keratin, 338, 341
  complexity, 141
  fibers, 450
  filaments, 469, 480
  nomeclature, 142
  role of, 141–154
Keratin-associated proteins, 142
Keratinization disorders
  Darier's disease, 460
  erythrokeratoderma variablilis, 460
Keratinocyte. *See* PPAR delta.
Keratinocytes, differentiation of, 65, 225
Keratinocytes, life cycle of, 98
  autolysis of, 173
  calcium receptor, 433–434
  in cell cycle activation, 363–366
Keratinopathies, 151–152
Keratins, 338, 341
  assembly of, 158
  classification of functions of, 159
    hard principles, 159
    soft principles, 159
  domain structure of, 146
  expression of, 150, 577
  gene
    density of, 142, 146
    K3, 146
    Ka17, 158
    regulation of, 148
  IF, 147–148
  modifications of, 148
  mutations
    effect of, 147
  nomenclature of, 141, 142
  organization in cells, 141

[Keratins]
  signaling, 152–153
  structure of, 146
  types of, 474
Keratoderma, 339, 342
Keratohyalin, 339, 342, 431, 437.
Keratohyalin granules. See KHGs.
KHGs, 117
KID syndrome
  clinical characteristics of, 496
  molecular defect of, 496

L-ascorbic acid, 381
Lactic acid, 364
  eccrine gland derived, 364
Lamellae, lipid layers of, 75, 78
Lamellar body (LB), 66, 261–269, 337
  description of, 469–470
  enzymes in, 264
  formation by SG cells, 470
  functions of, 261–265
  lipids, processing of, 470
Lamellar body secretion, 344, 353
  cementsome, 262
  keratinosome, 262
  membrane coating granules, 262
  Odland bodies, 262
  functions of, 261
  regulation of, 265
  secretions of, 265
  pathophysiology of, 269
  structure of, 261, 263
Lamellar ichthyosis, 100, 459
Lamellar ichthyosis/congenital
      ichthyosiform erythroderma
      (LI/CIE)
  clinical characteristics of, 478, 494
  molecular defect of, 478, 494
  morphological and functional
      consequences of, 494
Langerhans cells (LC), 370
Late fetal period, 281
  keratinization, 281
  periderm disaggregation, 283
  skin barrier formation, 282
LB secretion,kinetics of, 265
LB. See Lamellar body.
Leukocyte motility, 369
Lichenoid dermatoses, 458
Ligands, 322
  liposensors, 322
  nature of, 322
Light microscopy, 366

Linoleic acid, 79, 471, 481
Lipid
  and barrier abnormalities, 572
  barrier function 400
  classes, 573–574
  coralentty bound, 36
  composition and organization, 66–75
  altered, 75–76
  in diseased skin, 75
  in humans 33–36
    in xerotic skin, 88
  Lipid layers
    leakage of, 78
    of lamellae, 75, 78
  Lipid peroxidation, 382, 384, 386
  Lipid phase behavior
    ceramide subclasses in, 82
    CHOL:pigCER molar ratio role in, 81
    cholesterol sulfate role in, 82
    difference in, 84
    dipalmitoylphosphatidylcholine mixtures
        role in, 81
    effect of pH on, 82
    human CER1 role in, 83
    role of CER, CHOL and FFA in, 81
  Lipid processing, 231–249
  Lipid synthesis, 27, 348–349, 354
    epidermal, 348–349
      transcriptional regulation of, 349
  Liposensors, 343
  Lips, TEWL in, 449
  Liver X receptor (LXR), 329, 343
    activation, 329
    anti-inflammatory effects of, 329
    deficiency, 329
    effects, 330
    epidermal consequences of, 322
    expression
      in human keratinocytes, 323, 328
    in vivo effects of, 328
    role in epidermal development, 329
    types of, 329
  Long periodicity phase, 85
  Loricrin, 101–103, 323–324, 339,
      474, 578
  Loricrin keratoderma
    clinical characteristics of, 487
    molecular defect of, 487
    morphological and functional
        consequences of, 487
  Loricrin, increase of, 431, 434–437
  LPP. See long periodicity phase.
  LXR. See Liver X receptor.
  Lyell-syndrome, 191

Lympho-epithelial Kazal-type inhibitor 1
    (LEKTI 1), 570

Macrofibrils, 469, 474
Maculae occludentes, 201
Mammalian epidermis, 111
Mammalian keratin clusters
    type I, 142
    type II, 145
Mast cells, 367–368, 370
Matriptase, 119
Melanin, 428
    role in D_3 production, 431
Metabolism adaptations, 268
    facilitate, 267
Mevalonate, 350
MIC. See Minimum Inhibitory
    concentration
Microbial growth, 363, 366
Micrococcus, 364–365
Mid fetal period, 280
Minimum inhibitory
    concentration, 364
Molecular models
    basis of, 74
    domain mosaic model, 87
    liposome models, 85
    sandwich model, 87
    single gel phase model, 87
    Swarzendruber's model, 87
    trilayer models of L, 87
Monocytes, 369, 371
Motta system, advantages of, 35
MSRA. See Methionine sulfoxide
    reductase.
Multiple sulfatase defeciency, 477–478
Myelocytes, 368
Myeloid cells, 368

Natural moisturizing factor. See NMF
    and corneocytes, 407
    and profilaggrin-filaggrin protein, 408
    composition, 407
NEFA. See Non-essential FFA.
Neonatal Gaucher's disease, 477
Netherton syndrome, 269, 570
    clinical characteristics of, 497
    molecular defect of, 497
    morphological and functional
        consequences of, 498
Neuropeptide, 370
Neuropeptide Y (NPY), 370

Neutrophils, 366, 368
NHE1, 225
NHE1-mediated acidification, 225
NHE1. See Sodium/hydrogen
    antiporter-1 (NHE1).
NHR. See Nuclear hormone
    receptors (NHR).
Niacin, 57
Niemann-Pick disease, 49, 53
    clinical characteristics of, 484
    molecular defect of, 484
    morphological and functional
        consequences of, 484
Nile red fluorescence, 346
NMF, 119
Non-epidermolytic palmo-plantar
    keratoderma (NSPPK), 342
Non-essential FFA (NEFA), 344, 471
Non-palmar-plantar lesions, 342
Non-physiologic lipids, 351–352
Nonbullous ichthyosisform erythroderma,
    459
Nonoxidative pathway, 366
NSPPK. See Non-epidermolytic
    palmo-plantar keratoderma.
Nuclear hormone, 319
Nuclear hormone receptors (NHR), 342
    class II
        regulatory role of PPAR and LXR, 319
        regulatory role of PPAR and
            LXR activation of, 325
    liposensors, 322, 325
    mechanism of action, 319
    effects by DNA-binding independent
        mechanisms, 322
Nuclear receptors
    class II constitutive androstane
        receptor (CAR), 319
    class II farnesol X receptor (FXR), 319
    class II liver X receptor (LXR), 319
    class II peroxisome proliferator-activated
        receptors (PPAR), 319–322
    class II pregnane X receptor (PXR), 319
    composition of, 319–320
        retinoic acid receptor (RAR), 319
        thyroid receptor(TR), 319
        vitamin D receptor (VDR), 319

Occludin, 193
    effect of, 522
Oddland bodies, 373
Omega-hydroxycermides, 471
Ontogenesis, 342

Organellogenesis, 348
Orphan receptors. *See* Nuclear receptors.
OSD
  influenced by, 522
  prevalence of, 522
  prevention of, 520
    primary prevention, 521
    secondary prevention, 520–521
Osmolytes, role of. *See also* Natural
    moisturizing factor.
Oxygen radicals, 380
  effects of, 380
Ozone, 384–386

Palmoplantar skin, 449–451
Paneth cells, 366
Parathyroid hormone, 430
  effects of, 430
  role in production of 1, 25(OH)$_2$D, 430
Pathogenesis, 475
Pathogenic bacteria, 364, 372
PCA. *See* Pyrrolidone carboxylic acid.
PEAP. *See* Proenkephalin A derived peptide.
Pepsin C. *See also* Gastricsin.
Percutaneous absorption, 198, 525
Percutaneous penetration, 25
Permeability barrier, 337–361, 1–3
Permeability barrier homeostasis, 364
  function, criterion, 2
  homeostasis, 350–352
  status alterations, 2–3
Permeabilization, 367
Peroxisome proliferator activator receptor
    (PPAR),
  types of isotopes, 322
Peroxisomes, 384
pH-sensitive enzymes, 226
  B-glucocerebrosidase, 226
  sphingomyelinase (ACM), 226
  trans-urocanic acid (tUCA), 224
pH-sensitive fluroscent dyes, 223–224
Phorbol, 325
Phorbol 12-myristate-13-acetate (TPA), 324
Phosphoinositide, 436
Phospholipase
  C-γ1, 434
  role of, 434
Phospholipids-derived NEFA, 471
Phosphorylation, 148
Photoaging, role of ROS, 545
Photo-protection, 389–392
Photoprotective barriers, 389
  melanin barrier, 389

[Photoprotective barriers]
  protein barrier, 389
Photosensitizers
  initiatation of, 379, 387
Physical insults, 451
Phytosphingosine, 471
Placental sulfatase deficiency syndrome, 477
Plakoglobin, 172
Plaque proteins ZO-1 and ZO-2, 195–196
Plasminogen activator inhibitor type 3
    (PAI-2), 472
Plastic wrap model, 25
PLE. *See* polymorphous light eruption.
PMN. *See* Polymorphonuclear leukocyte.
Polymorphonuclear leukocyte, 371
Polymorphous light eruption, 384
POMC peptides, 370
PP2A. *See* Protein phosphatase type 2A.
PPAR-alpha activators
  clofibrate and farnesol, 323
  role in epidermal development, 324
PPAR-alpha agonists
  activation of, 323
  consequences of, 322
  deficiency, 323
  expression of, 323
  in vivo effects of, 323
  location of, 321–322
  role in epidermal development, 324
PPAR-beta
  activation of, 327
  anti-inflammatory effects of, 327
PPAR-delta
  activation of, 326
  deficiency of, 325
  epidermal consequences
    in human keratinocyte, 325
  in vitro effects of, 326
  in vivo effects of, 325
  protein kinase B-alpha, 326
  role of, 326
PPAR-gamma agonists
  anti-inflammatory effects of, 329
  activation of, 327
  epidermal consequences of, 328
  expression of, 328
  in vitro effects of, 328
  in vivo effects of, 328
  key role of, 327
  role in epidermal development, 329
PPAR. *See* Peroxisome proliferator activator
    receptor.
Pre-D$_3$, 429
Premature aging diseases, 380

Primary cytokines, 30
Primary individual prevention, 521
Primary, secondary, and tertiary
  prevention
  strategies of, 521
Proenkephalin A, 370
Profilaggrin, 111–131, 323, 474
  comparison of, 116
  composition of, 120
  dephosphorylation of, 117
  evolutionary aspects of, 124
  expression, 124
  function of, 119–120
  immunoreactivity, 117
  localization of, 120
  N-terminal peptide, 120
    potential functions, 120
    structure, 120
  phosphorylation of, 117
  processing of, 117
  proteolytic processing of, 118
  regulation of, 122
  structural similarity of *Flg*-2 to, 127
  structure of, 115
  synthesis of, 123
Progeria, 380, 392
Pseudomonas aeruginosa, 367
Protein, 380
  targets for, 380
Protein carbonyls, 380
Protein kinase C
  effect of activation, 434–435
Protein oxidation gradient, 391
Protein phosphatase type 2A, 117
Proton-induced X-ray emission analysis
  (PIXE), 290
Pseudo-ainhum, 339
Pseudoceramides, 55
Pseudogalactosylceramide, 57
pseudosphingolipids, clinical trials, 54
Psoriasis, 185, 456
Pyrrolidone carboxylic acid, 120

RA. *See* Retinoic acid.
Reactive oxygen species, 379, 385–386
  formation of, 379
Recessive X-linked ichthyosis (RXLI), 511
  abnormal desquamation mechanisms, 514
  barrier perturbation mechanisms, 514
    types, 515
  causes of, 514
  clinical characteristics of, 477, 514
  molecular defect of, 477

[Recessive X-linked ichthyosis (RXLI)]
  morphological and functional
    consequences of, 478
Refsum disease
  clinical characteristics of, 480
  molecular defect of, 481
  morphological and functional
    consequences of, 481
Repetin, 128
Retinoic acid, 123
ROS. *See* reactive oxygen species.

S100 Ca^{2+}-binding proteins, 124
Saran® wrap analogy, 25–27
SC acidity
  antimicrobial activity, 226
  desquamation, 225, 227
  factors contributing, 224–225
  importance of, 225
  inflammation of, 226
SC barrier function, 451
SC chymotryptic enzyme (SCCE), 472
SC H+, 225
SC lipids, composition, 471, 535
SC tryptic enzyme (SCTE), 264, 472
SCAP. *See* SREBP cleavage-activating
  protein (SCAP).
Sebaceous gland, 365, 371
Sebum, constituents of, 69
Secondary individual prevention
  aim of, 527
Secondary or tertiary reaction products, 381
Secretory leukocyte protease inhibitor
  (SLPI), 367, 472
Secretory phopholipases (sPLA2), 348
  function of, 224–225
  location of, 224–225
Serine palmitoyl transferase (SPT), 348, 350,
  535
Serine palmityl transferase, 39
Serine protease inhibitors (SPI), 264, 472
SG-SC interface, 344, 348
SG. *See* Stratum granulosum.
SIP. *See* Secondary individual
  prevention.
Site 1 protease (S1P), 349
Site 2 protease (S2P), 350
Sjögren-Larsson syndrome
  clinical characteristics of, 479
  molecular defect of, 480
  morphological and functional
    consequences of, 480
SKALP, 5, 264, 572

Skin barrier
  Function, 69, 81, 103
  structure, 65–88
  tight junctions, 99
Skin equivalents, 78–80
Skin, human, development of, 273–284
Skin surface lipids, 386, 388
  derived from, 386
  photooxidation of, 384
Skin surface, reflections by, 69
Skin's permeability barrier, 191
  functions of, 191
  stratum corneum, 191
Skin, role of, 99
Skin, dry, causes of, 571–572
Skin-derived antileukocyte proteinase
        (SKALP) or elafin, 472
SLPI. See Secretory leukocyte protease
    inhibitor.
SLS-induced hardening phenomenon, 523
Small proline-rich proteins (SPRRs), 473
Sodium lauryl sulphate
  induces, 450
Sodium/hydrogen antiporter-1 (NHE1), 364
Solar elastosis, 393
Sphingolipids, 43–45
  clinical trials, 54
Sphingomyelin, 44–52, 345, 348
Sphingomyelin deacylase activity, 352
Sphingomyelinase, 364, 372
  acid, 574
  neutral, 574–575
Sphingosine, 365, 373, 471
SPLA2. See Secretory phospholipase A2.
Squalene, 386–388
Squalene wax, 365
Squamous cell carcinomas, 430
  1, 25 Dihydroxyvitamin D3, 429
  24, 25(OH)2D3, 430
  and VDR mRNA, 430
SREBP cleavage-activating
        protein, 349
SREBP. See Sterol regulatory element
    binding proteins.
Staphylococcus aureus, 364
Staphylococcus epidermidis, 364
Steroid sulfatase (SSase) activity, 511
  LB secretory system, 513
  impact of deficiency in, 511
Sterol regulatory element binding proteins,
        349, 350
  in cholesterol synthesis, 348, 350
Stevens-Johnson syndrome, 458
Stratified epithelia, 149–156

Stratum corneum (SC), 337, 344
Stratum corneum barrier, 337
Stratum corneum
  age factor, 417
  antimicrobial activity in, 226–227
  at birth, 364
  barrier function, 79, 364
  biological activity, 25, 27
  compartments of, 447
  components of, 450
  concepts of, 2, 26
  coordinated formation of, 332
  cytosol, 28
  defensive function of, 5–11
  defunction of, 1–3
  desquamation, 182
  dry skin, 411, 414, 418, 420–421
  electron diffraction, 72
  enzymes, 417
  extracellular lipids of, 343
  free fatty acids in, 35
  frozen sections, 25
  functions of, 28, 450
    water-holding capacity, 451
  hydration of, 399–421, 525
  lipid classes, 79, 81
  lipid organization in, 68
  lower, 175
  origin of ceramides
  pH, 28, 223
  photo-oxidation, 386
  protease activities, 472
  redox properties of, 390
  sebaceous lipids in, 36
  signaling mechanisms, 29
  structure of, 28, 458
  surface area of, 75
  synchrotron, 69
  transport of molecules, through, 37
Stratum granulosum, 174,
        197–198, 322, 337
Stratum granulosum-stratum corneum
        (SG-SC), 212
Streptococcus, 364–365
Stress, and barrier function, 553–565
  environment-induced, 555
  immobilization-induced, 554
  new environment-induced, 555
Structural adaptations, 267
  facilitate, 267
Substance P (SP), 370
Suprabasal bulla, 191
Symplekin, 195–197
Synopsis, 393

T lymphocytes, 369–370
Terminal cornification, involves, 469
Terminal differentiation, 117
Tertiary individual prevention (TIP), 529
Testosterone, 460
TEWL. *See* Transepithelial water loss.
TEWL, measurement of, 191, 451–452
TG1 deficiency, 341
Thin layer chromatography, 365
Thyroid, 460
Tight junctions
  role of, 191–202
  typical structures of, 198
TJ proteins
  in normal epidermis, 199
  in various diseases, 199–200
  localizations of, 196
  signal transduction functions, 196
TNF-α receptor-associated death domain
    (TRADD), 152–153, 156
TNF. *See* Tumor necrosis factor.
TOFA. *See* Topical 5- (tetradecyloxy)-
    2-furancarboxylic acid.
Topical 5-(tetradecyloxy)-2-furancarboxylic
    acid, 350
TRADD, 152–153
Trans-epidermal water loss (TEWL), 348,
    212, 283, 522
Trans-urocanic acid, 224
Transepidermal water loss. *See* TEWL.
Transepithelial water loss, 97, 475
Transforming growth factor-β1, 371
Transglutaminase, 78
Transglutaminase 1 (TG1), 473
  deficiency of, 339
Transglutaminases, 100
  formation of, 391
Traumatic injuries influence of, 452
Trichohyalin, 127
Troglitazone, 329
Trypsin activity, 574
TTP. *See* alpha-tocopherol-transfer
    protein.
Tumor necrosis factor (TNF), 324, 371
  role of, 371
Type 2 Gaucher's disease, 460

UCA. *See* Urocanic acid.
Ultraviolet irradiation, 385
  desquamation, 385
  erythema, 385
  hyperproliferation, 385
Uric acid, 381–383
Urocanic acid (UCA), 364
UV irradiation, epidermal impact, 545
UVA, effect of, 384, 386
UVB-irradiation, 523

VALA, 524
Vasostatin-I, 371
Vertebrate integument, adaptive features of,
    211
Vibrio cholerae, 196
Vitamin 1, 25 dihydroxyvitamin D_3
Vitamin C, 390
Vitamin D, 427–437
Vitamin E, 381–382, 386, 388, 390
Vitamin E esters, 390–391
  effect of, 390
  regulation of, 391
Vohwinkel disease, 339, 496
  clinical characteristics of, 496

Water, as a plasticizer in stratum corneum,
    401
Water retention capacity of sc, 405–409
Waterproofing facultative, 215–219
Wax esters, 365
Werner's syndrome, 380, 392
Western blot analysis, 366
Wiskott-Aldrich's syndrome, 570
Water content, in sc, 401–405

X ray irradiation, 451
X-Linked dominant ichthyosis, 459, 481
X-linked ichthyosis (RXLI), 182, 476–477
X-linked recessive ichthyosis, 476

Zonulae occludentes, 198